PSYCHIATRY UPDATE

The American Psychiatric Association Annual Review

VOL. III

Edited by Lester Grinspoon, M.D.

American
Psychiatric
Press, Inc.

Washington, D.C. 1984

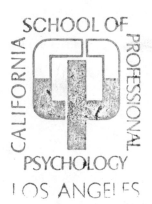

SCHOOL OF
CALIFORNIA
PROFESSIONAL
PSYCHOLOGY
LOS ANGELES

American Psychiatric Press, Inc.

1400 K STREET, N.W.
WASHINGTON, D.C. 20005

Psychiatry Update: Volume III
ISSN 0736-1866
ISBN 0-88048-015-7

Printed and bound in the United States of America.

To
Joshua and Peter
two young men
on whom the future can depend

PSYCHIATRY UPDATE: VOLUME I
The American Psychiatric Association Annual Review (1982)

Lester Grinspoon, M.D., Editor
The Psychiatric Aspects of Sexuality
Virginia A. Sadock, M.D., Preceptor
The Schizophrenic Disorders
Robert Cancro, M.D., Med.D.Sc., Preceptor
Depression in Childhood and Adolescence
Henry H. Work, M.D., Preceptor
Law and Psychiatry
Alan A. Stone, M.D., Preceptor
Borderline and Narcissistic Personality Disorders
Otto F. Kernberg, M.D., Preceptor

PSYCHIATRY UPDATE: VOLUME II
The American Psychiatric Association Annual Review (1983)

Lester Grinspoon, M.D., Editor
New Issues in Psychoanalysis
Arnold M. Cooper, M.D., Preceptor
Geriatric Psychiatry
Ewald W. Busse, M.D., Preceptor
Family Psychiatry
Henry Grunebaum, M.D., Preceptor
Bipolar Illness
Paula J. Clayton, M.D., Preceptor
Depressive Disorders
Gerald L. Klerman, M.D., Preceptor

CONTENTS

Page

Introduction to Psychiatry Update: Volume III   xiii
Lester Grinspoon, M.D., Editor

Part

I

Brief Psychotherapies

Introduction to Part One		7
	Toksoz Byram Karasu, M.D., Preceptor	
Chapter 1	Intensive Brief and Emergency Psychotherapy	11
	Leopold Bellak, M.D.	
Chapter 2	Short-Term Anxiety-Provoking Psychotherapy	24
	Peter E. Sifneos, M.D.	
Chapter 3	Time Limited Psychotherapy	35
	James Mann, M.D.	
Chapter 4	Cognitive Therapy	44
	A. John Rush, M.D.	
Chapter 5	Interpersonal Psychotherapy for Depression	56
	Gerald L. Klerman, M.D., Myrna M. Weissman, Ph.D., Bruce Rounsaville, M.D., Eve S. Chevron, M.S.	
Chapter 6	Multimodal Therapy	67
	Arnold A. Lazarus, Ph.D.	
References for Part One		77

Part

II

Children at Risk

Introduction to Part Two		87
	Irving Philips, M.D., Preceptor	
Chapter 7	Children Vulnerable to Major Mental Disorders: Risk and Protective Factors	91
	Norman Garmezy, Ph.D.	
Chapter 8	Children at Acute Risk: Psychic Trauma	104
	Lenore Cagen Terr, M.D.	

Chapter 9 Children with Mental Retardation 120
 Irving Philips, M.D.

Chapter 10 Parenting and Children at Risk 129
 Henry Grunebaum, M.D.

Chapter 11 Children of Divorce: The Dilemma
 of a Decade 144
 Judith S. Wallerstein, Ph.D.

References *for Part Two* 159

Part

III

Consultation-Liaison Psychiatry

Introduction *to Part Three* 177
 Zbigniew J. Lipowski, M.D.,
  Preceptor

Chapter 12 History, Definition, and Scope of
 Consultation-Liaison Psychiatry 179
 Zbigniew J. Lipowski, M.D.

Chapter 13 Prevalence of Psychiatric Morbidity
 in Medical Populations 187
 Stephanie Cavanaugh, M.D.,
 Robert M. Wettstein, M.D.

Chapter 14 Clinical Research at the Interface of
 Medicine and Psychiatry 215
 Harvey Moldofsky, M.D.

Chapter 15 Psychiatry and Geriatric Medicine 231
 Charles V. Ford, M.D.

Chapter 16 Psychiatry and Oncology 239
 Mary Jane Massie, M.D.,
 Jimmie C. Holland, M.D.

Chapter 17 Psychiatry and Surgery 256
 Michael R. Milano, M.D.,
 Donald S. Kornfeld, M.D.

References *for Part Three* 278

Part

IV

Alcohol Abuse and Dependence

Introduction *to Part Four* 299
 George E. Vaillant, M.D.,
  Preceptor

Chapter 18 The Diagnosis of Alcoholism
 After DSM-III 301
 Lee N. Robins, Ph.D.

Chapter 19 The Course of Alcoholism and
 Lessons for Treatment 311
 George E. Vaillant, M.D.

Chapter 20   Genetic and Biochemical Factors
              in the Etiology of Alcoholism   320
                 Marc A. Schuckit, M.D.

Chapter 21   Contributions of Learning Theory
              to the Diagnosis and Treatment
              of Alcoholism   328
                 Peter E. Nathan, Ph.D.

Chapter 22   Psychotherapy in the Treatment
              of Alcoholism   338
                 Sheila B. Blume, M.D.

Chapter 23   Pharmacotherapy in the
              Detoxification and Treatment
              of Alcoholism   346
                 Ernest P. Noble, Ph.D., M.D.

Chapter 24   Alcohol Policy: Preventive Options   359
                 Dean Gerstein, Ph.D.

References for Part Four   371

Part

V

The Anxiety Disorders

Introduction to Part Five   390
                 Donald F. Klein, M.D.,
                    Preceptor

Chapter 25   Diagnostic Issues in the
              DSM-III Classification of the
              Anxiety Disorders   392
                 Robert L. Spitzer, M.D.,
                 Janet B.W. Williams, D.S.W.

Chapter 26   The Role of Genetics in the
              Etiology of Panic Disorder   402
                 Raymond R. Crowe, M.D.

Chapter 27   Anxiety Disorders in Children   410
                 Rachel Gittelman, Ph.D.

Chapter 28   The Psychotherapy of Anxiety   418
                 Jerome D. Frank, M.D., Ph.D.

Chapter 29   Anxiety and Psychodynamic
              Theory   426
                 John C. Nemiah, M.D.

Chapter 30   The Relaxation Response and the
              Treatment of Anxiety   440
                 Herbert Benson, M.D.

Chapter 31   Exposure Treatment of
              Agoraphobia   448
                 Matig Mavissakalian, M.D.

Chapter 32   Mortality After Thirty to Forty
              Years: Panic Disorder Compared
              with Other Psychiatric Illnesses   460
                 William Coryell, M.D.

Chapter 33   The Biology of Anxiety   467
        Jack M. Gorman, M.D.

Chapter 34   The Biochemistry of Anxiety:
        From Pharmacotherapy
        to Pathophysiology   482
        Steven M. Paul, M.D.,
        Phil Skolnick, Ph.D.

Chapter 35   β-Adrenergic Blockers and
        Buspirone   490
        Jonathan O. Cole, M.D.

Chapter 36   The Efficacy of Antidepressants
        in Anxiety Disorders   503
        Michael R. Liebowitz, M.D.

Unresolved Questions   519
        Donald F. Klein, M.D.

References for Part Five   526

Index   541

Introduction

Psychiatry Update:
Volume III

Psychiatry Update:
Volume III

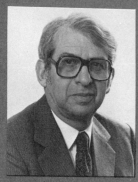

Lester Grinspoon, M.D.,
Editor

Associate Professor of Psychiatry
Harvard Medical School
Massachusetts Mental Health Center

Introduction

by Lester Grinspoon, M.D., Editor

With the publication of this volume, I complete my tenure as the Editor of *Psychiatry Update: The Annual Review of the American Psychiatric Association*. It has been my great pleasure to shepherd the *Annual Review* from an idea to three bound volumes.

This third volume of the *Annual Review* embodies the same spirit that animated the first two volumes: it presents a fresh and consolidated view of what we have learned and are still learning about several major topics in psychiatry. Like the first two volumes, Volume III addresses the need of mental health professionals for comprehensive and current knowledge in a complex and rapidly changing field. Again, the volume covers five major topics, each developed by a Preceptor and faculty members who are known for their contributions in the field. And again, the 1984 *Annual Review* is designed to mirror and magnify the Psychiatry Update program of the Annual Meeting of the American Psychiatric Association.

This year's topics should interest a wide range of mental health professionals: "Brief Psychotherapies," with Dr. Toksoz Byram Karasu as Preceptor; "Children at Risk," with Dr. Irving Philips as Preceptor; "Consultation-Liaison Psychiatry," with Dr. Zbigniew J. Lipowski as Preceptor; "Alcohol Abuse and Dependence," with Dr. George E. Vaillant as Preceptor; and "The Anxiety Disorders," with Dr. Donald F. Klein as Preceptor.

The choice of this year's topics follows a scheme I have used since the beginning of this series. Each volume covers two diagnostic categories in depth: Volume III covers the alcohol abuse and dependence and the anxiety disorders categories; Volume II, the interrelated categories of bipolar illness and depressive disorders; and Volume I, the schizophrenic disorders and the borderline and narcissistic personality disorders.

Two Parts in each volume review recent developments in the theory and practice of psychiatry: this volume reviews the brief psychotherapies and consultation-liaison psychiatry; the 1983 volume, new issues in psychoanalysis and developments in family psychiatry; and the 1982 volume, the psychiatric aspects of sexuality and the new interdisciplinary speciality of law and psychiatry.

Finally, each volume contains a Part devoted to a particular population of interest to mental health professionals: this year's volume includes the Part on children at risk; last year's, the Part on geriatric psychiatry; and the first year's, the Part on depression in childhood and adolescence.

As in the past, I have included in Volume III some Editor's notes that suggest where within the three volumes the reader may find further information on a given topic. Beginning with Volume II, we also developed a detailed cumulative index covering the subjects of both volumes. We have continued that practice with this year's volume, so that all three volumes are linked through the cumulative index that appears at the end of Volume III.

Producing an annual volume of this scope and depth in just one year has required the attention and cooperation of many people. In putting together their Parts, this year's Preceptors, like their predecessors, have in effect served as associate editors. Their faculty members have worked hard to prepare material that will be useful to the whole spectrum of mental health practitioners and researchers. This volume is therefore the fruition of much work on the part of the Preceptors and their faculties. Their only reward is the pleasure they take in sharing knowledge with their colleagues. All of us who learn from what they have written are indebted to them.

There are others to whom I should like to express gratitude for the help they have given in launching this idea and producing the first three volumes. Various members of the staff supported the idea wholeheartedly and contributed to the solution of the many problems that any new project of this magnitude is bound to encounter. The members of the Scientific Program Committee, and particularly the members of the Long-Range Planning Subcommittee, were most generous in sharing their thoughts and suggestions with me. The staff of the American Psychiatric Press played a key role, attending to the many details of copy editing, as well as to the numerous responsibilities involved in design and production.

I especially appreciate the contribution of Ms. Ruth Cross, who is responsible for the expertly conceived and executed cumulative index.

Nancy Palmer, my assistant, has served not only as an invaluable aid to me in the coordination of the scientific program, but also as an essential and highly effective liaison between the production of the book and the development of the program.

I am most indebted to my editorial assistant, Carolyn Mercer-McFadden. If this volume enjoys the same success as the first two volumes, much of the credit will again belong to her. Again, she has examined every sentence of the manuscript with exceptional intelligence and caring attention.

It is my pleasure to introduce *Psychiatry Update: Volume III*, the third of the Annual Review series from the American Psychiatric Association. I hope that under its new Editors, the *Annual Review* will continue to grow in reputation and readership.

November 1983
Boston, Massachusetts

I

Brief Psychotherapies

Brief Psychotherapies

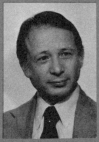

Toksoz Byram Karasu, M.D., Preceptor

Professor and Deputy Chairman
Department of Psychiatry
Albert Einstein College of Medicine/
    Montefiore Medical Center
Director
Department of Psychiatry
Bronx Municipal Hospital Center

Authors for Part I

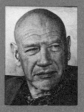

Leopold Bellak, M.D.
Clinical Professor of Psychiatry
Albert Einstein College
    of Medicine
Clinical Professor of Psychology
Postdoctoral Program
    in Psychotherapy
New York University

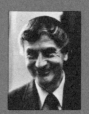

Peter E. Sifneos, M.D.
Associate Director
Psychiatry Service
Beth Israel Hospital
Professor of Psychiatry
Harvard Medical School

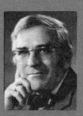

James Mann, M.D.
Professor Emeritus
School of Medicine
Boston University
Training and Supervising Psychoanalyst
Boston Psychoanalytic Institute

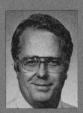

A. John Rush, M.D.

Betty Jo Hay Professor
 of Psychiatry
Department of Psychiatry
University of Texas Health
 Science Center at Dallas

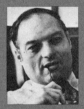

Gerald L. Klerman, M.D.

George Harrington Professor
 of Psychiatry
Harvard Medical School
Director of Research
Department of Psychiatry
Massachusetts General Hospital

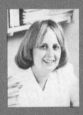

Myrna M. Weissman, Ph.D.

Professor of Psychiatry
 and Epidemiology
Director
Depression Research Unit
Department of Psychiatry
Yale University
 School of Medicine

Bruce Rounsaville, M.D.

Assistant Professor of Psychiatry
Department of Psychiatry
Yale University
 School of Medicine

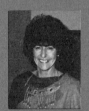

Eve S. Chevron, M.S.

Clinical Psychologist
Department of Psychiatry
Yale University
 School of Medicine

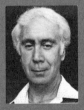

Arnold A. Lazarus, Ph.D.

Professor of Psychology
Graduate School of Applied
 and Professional Psychology
Rutgers, the State University

I

Brief Psycho-therapies

	Page
Introduction to Part One	7
Toksoz Byram Karasu, M.D.	
Chapter 1	11
Intensive Brief and Emergency Psychotherapy	
Leopold Bellak, M.D.	
Background	11
Basic Concepts and Tenets of BEP	12
The Sequence of the Sessions	14
The Therapeutic Process	17
Summary	22
Appendix 1. Specific Considerations in the Management of Selected Problems	22
Chapter 2	24
Short-Term Anxiety-Provoking Psychotherapy	
Peter E. Sifneos, M.D.	
Patient Selection Criteria	25
Evaluation Tasks	27
Technical Requirements of STAPP	29
Recent Developments	32
Conclusion	35
Chapter 3	35
Time Limited Psychotherapy	
James Mann, M.D.	
The Meaning and Significance of Time	35
The Bridge Between Time and the Central Issue	37
Time, the Central Issue, and Therapeutic Change	39
Clinical Technique in TLP	40
Indications and Limitations	43
Chapter 4	44
Cognitive Therapy	
A. John Rush, M.D.	
Theoretical Background	44
Therapeutic Technique in Cognitive Therapy	46
Indications	48
Applications	50
Conclusions	56

Chapter 5   56

Interpersonal Psychotherapy for Depression
  Gerald L. Klerman, M.D.,
  Myrna M. Weissman, Ph.D.,
  Bruce Rounsaville, M.D.,
  Eve S. Chevron, M.S.
Theoretical and Empirical Bases   56
Psychotherapeutic Goals   59
Phases in IPT   60
IPT Compared With Other Psychotherapies   63
IPT and Psychodynamic Theory   66

Chapter 6   67

Multimodal Therapy
  Arnold A. Lazarus, Ph.D.
Introduction   67
Multimodal Diagnosis and Assessment   68
Bridging and Tracking   75
Final Comment   76

References for Part One   77

Introduction
by Toksoz Byram Karasu, M.D.

A proliferating literature suggests that brief psychotherapy is a mode of treatment whose time has certainly come. The literature on brief psychotherapy describes widespread clinical applications, increasing research investigations, and a striking assortment of approaches. Viewed historically, these developments in large part reflect the capacity of brief psychotherapies to meet several contemporary needs simultaneously: the need for short-term techniques in light of socioeconomic considerations which make protracted (and costlier) treatments less viable; the need to serve larger numbers of patients who may not be characterologically amenable to long-term therapy or diagnostically suitable; the need for accountability and for systematic studies of psychotherapy outcomes within specific formats and circumscribed time frames; and the need for innovative treatment strategies that are tailor-made for individual patients based on our new knowledge of what is most efficacious with specific patient populations. Moreover, as the spectrum of patients in brief psychotherapy has expanded, we are learning that its goals need not be superficial nor its effects short-lived. As an added analytic attraction, the earlier fear of symptom substitution as an inevitable consequence of such treatment has essentially been quelled. Thus, short-term treatment may meet yet another need: the need to retain flexibly the enduring strengths of the Freudian legacy, by combining its psychodynamic assets with newer, more expedient techniques.

Although brief treatments have only recently emerged as primary, preferred modalities in their own right, they are far from new. Their appearance on the psychotherapeutic horizon can be traced from ancient (Egyptian and Greek) history to the major methods of the early twentieth century; even the original Freudian techniques were brief. When Franz Alexander challenged the validity of long-term treatment as an essential ingredient of reconstructive therapy and questioned the basic assumptions of classical psychoanalysis (Alexander and French, 1946), he (like Adler, Ferenczi, Stekel, and Rank before him) was repudiated in analytic circles. However, Alexander and French persevered in this area and provided much of the foundation for the development of subsequent systems of dynamic, short-term therapy. Thus, Malan (1963) evolved his "active interpretive" technique for use with carefully screened patients who could withstand the rigors of uncovering therapy. In 1965, Bellak and Small, departing from more limited conceptualizations of crisis intervention, developed their principles of brief, emergency psychotherapy in answer to both crisis and noncrisis needs. Later, following along the lines of Malan, Sifneos (1972) focused on the issue of locating more specific patient selection criteria (like above-average intelligence, a willingness to reveal and understand oneself, the ability to have an affective interaction with the interviewer), and he formulated another brief dynamic therapy, based especially on "anxiety-provoking" techniques. At about the same time, Mann (1973), directly concerned with man's temporal concepts in relation to treatment, developed his fixed-session, "time limited psychotherapy." And Davanloo (1978), directing himself to the needs of patients in outpatient clinics, developed additional evaluation criteria and psychoanalytically oriented strategies resembling those of Sifneos and Malan. Davanloo particularly emphasized the vital importance of having a therapeutic focus in short-term treatment while retaining the basic psychodynamic context.

Also spurred by compelling community need and increasing dissatisfaction with lengthy treatments during the 1960s and 1970s, others explored the application of more varied systems, but they, too, incorporated dynamic formulations, restructuring or conceptualizing them along short-term lines. Of a more eclectic nature are the contributions of Wolberg (1977) and Lazarus (1981), the former an outgrowth of the analytic tradition, the latter of the behavioral model. Both use broad selection criteria and techniques. Wolberg uses many supportive-educational techniques, with hypnosis as an adjunct to brief psychotherapy, and especially emphasizes the use of methods that are applicable after the therapy is over. Lazarus employs a behavioral array including anxiety-management training, imagery, modeling, biofeedback, and meditation, and he applies his "multimodal" techniques to specific marital and sexual disorders. Finally and most tailor-made for a particular diagnostic population, special attention to depressive disorders has resulted in the establishment of two short-term therapies of increasing popularity and interest. Very different in both theory and technique, the "cognitive therapy" of Beck, Rush, and associates (1979) addresses the patient's false, irrational beliefs, while Klerman and his associates' (1979) "interpersonal psychotherapy" aims at the social context and the interactions within which the illness occurs.

Short-term modalities now cover a rich and varied spectrum, as the six chapters in this Part demonstrate. Prominent contributions to the field are discussed here by their originators: intensive brief and emergency psychotherapy by Dr. Leopold Bellak; short-term anxiety-provoking psychotherapy by Dr. Peter E. Sifneos; time limited psychotherapy by Dr. James Mann; cognitive therapy by Dr. A. John Rush; interpersonal psychotherapy by Dr. Gerald L. Klerman, Dr. Myrna M. Weissman, Dr. Bruce Rounsaville, and Ms. Eve S. Chevron; and multimodal therapy by Dr. Arnold A. Lazarus.

Dr. Bellak's intensive brief and emergency psychotherapy (BEP) is rooted in community psychiatry, psychoanalytic theory, ego psychology, and emergency treatment. Basically a five-session therapy (but by no means fixed), BEP derives from the author's long experience that most patients at outpatient clinics break off treatment after five visits. On a conceptual level, Dr. Bellak transcends earlier notions of crisis intervention by departing from the more limiting belief that emergency psychotherapy can only return the patient to his or her previous level of functioning. He opts to reconstitute the patient at a higher level of integration, believing in the capacity of the individual, through attempts at adaptation and problem solving, to become stronger than before the traumatic situation. In addition, BEP is a systematic, focused, and highly conceptualized approach that uses dynamic therapy as a foundation from which to understand the patient. Through scrupulous elucidation of BEP in therapeutic management, Dr. Bellak demonstrates its application to an array of specific disorders from depression, physical illness, phobias, and catastrophic events to acting out, incipient psychotic states, and feelings of unreality and depression.

Dr. Peter E. Sifneos's short-term anxiety-provoking psychotherapy (STAPP) shares with Dr. Bellak's and others' a psychodynamic framework, but it is distinctive regarding patient evaluation and specific technique. It was Dr. Sifneos who recognized a first-priority need to formulate selection criteria that would delineate appropriate patients for short-term treatment. He made gradual revisions through careful clinical observation until he came up with a set of evaluation standards that he was able to apply to over 500 patients: a past meaningful relationship, a circumscribed chief complaint, good motivation, a capacity for insight and above-average intelligence, and flexibility. STAPP is also special in its aggressive approach to treatment. Videotapes and follow-up research have demonstrated that the systematic use of anxiety-provoking confrontations and clarifications are effective ways of urging patients to face their maladaptive defense mechanisms.

Also within the psychoanalytic tradition, Dr. James Mann's time limited psychotherapy (TLP) departs from the treatments of Drs. Malan and Sifneos in having broad selection criteria, a focus on separation and re-union as opposed to oedipal issues, and less reliance on insight as the curative agent. But most original, of course, is the development of a short-term treatment modality pivoted upon the crucial meaning of *time*. It is Dr. Mann's innovation to have acknowledged the unconscious experience of time in the past, present, and future life of the individual, and to have recognized the perils of a false sense of unlimited time in therapy (as in life itself). Directly translated into technical terms, Dr. Mann is therefore responsible for the incorporation into the therapeutic endeavor of two structural features that are unprecedented in the domain of brief psychotherapy: (1) the strict limit of a *set* number of 12 sessions and, perhaps more important for the patient, (2) the establishment of the *exact termination date* at the start of treatment. Moreover, Dr. Mann's TLP heightens the therapist's sensitivity to time throughout the patient's progress and the total treatment process by selecting and stating a crucial "central issue" from the start, around which treatment (and time) are pivoted.

In contrast to these brief therapies based upon psychoanalytic foundations, the cognitive therapy discussed by Dr. A. John Rush goes back to the Greek Stoic philosophers and the later phenomenological approach to psychology. Yet cognitive therapy shares with TLP its major goal of resolving or minimizing negative feelings about the self. Viewing psychopathology as the consequence of negative cognitions or assumptions, cognitive therapy uses symptoms as clues to the definition of specific cognitive schemata to which the patient is vulnerable. The initial phase of treatment, which aims at symptom reduction, teaches the patient to recognize these destructive thought patterns, while the second half of the therapy, which aims at prophylaxis, focuses on the modification of specific assumptions (which, as in psychoanalytic theory, are assumed to derive from early life experiences). As such, the cognitive approach has been especially effective for altering depressogenic ideation in affective disorders. But it is by no means limited to a diagnosis of depression. The method has now been used successfully for a wide variety of psychiatric disturbances, including generalized anxiety, phobias, obesity, alcoholism, drug dependency, and chronic pain. Adding to the method's applicability, its originators have described the technique in a manual (Beck et al., 1979).

Dr. Gerald L. Klerman, Dr. Myrna M. Weissman, Dr. Bruce Rounsaville, and Ms. Eve S. Chevron developed their interpersonal psychotherapy (IPT) primarily for treating depressive disorders. In contrast to cognitive theory, IPT reflects an understanding of depression from an interpersonal point of view. Although such a vantage point is not new to the thinking about depressive disorders, IPT does make the unique attempt to depart from those former treatments that necessarily opted for personality alteration and that had a long-term course. More specifically, IPT represents a significant advance over other modalities in the following ways: first, of course, it is short-term; second, it is oriented only toward interpersonal or social problems and symptom relief; and third, it is based upon controlled clinical trials (both as maintenance and acute treatment). Of special importance, as in cognitive therapy, the originators have helped to standardize the treatment in two ways, through a manual which systematically specifies IPT's techniques and their sequence (Klerman et al., 1979; 1984) and through specific training programs that are based on manual-specified procedures and are designed to increase consistency among therapists. The treatment itself expressly clarifies and renegotiates with the patient the interpersonal context associated with the symptom formation, and the evidence is growing that such an approach is not only therapeutic, but also preventive of future episodes.

Finally, in contrast to the therapies delineated above, Dr. Arnold A. Lazarus's multimodal therapy most represents both a theoretical and a technical eclecticism (albeit from a basically behavioral background). The multimodal assessment, BASIC ID, evolved directly from Dr. Lazarus's attempt to tap therapeutically the broad array of personality dimensions (behavior, affect, etc.) that constitute the individual and to use an assortment of techniques in their behalf. This means that Dr. Lazarus puts into practice what one would hope other therapists would do implicitly. He draws from a variety of sources, applies techniques with flexibility and versatility, and is sensitive to individual differences in patients' needs. In addition, just as he relinquishes partisan allegiance to a specific theory or technique, he replaces conventional diagnostic labels with "modality profiles," which systematically relate a particular personality dimension, or modality, with a specific problem and a specific proposed treatment. Therapeutic methods range from assertiveness training, biofeedback, self-hypnosis, and abdominal breathing exercises, to medication, family therapy, and support groups. Dr. Lazarus's approach thus brings together the advantages of systematic flexibility but remains cognizant of the limitations of unsystematic eclecticism.

All told, the short-term therapies discussed in this Part have each added something special to the field and have together contributed an array of impressive innovations. Selection criteria are available for better matching the patient with a suitable therapy, greater explicitness exists regarding the relationship between theory and clinical practice, well-defined protocols and standardized training programs have been designed, and the field is more capable of rigorous scientific research and of responding to the current pressures for proof of efficacy. Most critically, these therapies and their originators exemplify the courage to explore the old and the new in a search for more effective methods of treatment. Their contributions not only further our knowledge in this special field, but they also augur well for the future of short-term psychotherapy and the futures of its patients.

Chapter *1*

Intensive Brief and Emergency Psychotherapy
by Leopold Bellak, M.D.

BACKGROUND

From 1935 to 1938, I passed nearly daily, on my way to my training analysis with Ernst Kris, W. Stekel's "Institut für Aktive Analyse," which was the first specific attempt at a psychoanalytically based brief psychotherapy. Later on those mornings in Vienna (my session started at 7:00 A.M.), I walked another few blocks to the Anatomical Institute and then by the Physiological Institute, which stood across the street from the beginning of the Berggasse, where Freud resided at No. 19.

I do not know whether Stekel's attempts at brief therapy remained with me as a preconscious mental set. I do know that when I opened an office in New York in late 1946, I was glad to have the Veterans Administration send me patients. As a contract psychiatrist, I was at first authorized to see these veterans for only three visits, and after a little while for six visits. I found it especially frustrating to diagnose them only or merely write out dispositions; therefore, I soon attempted to give at least a minimum of help in those six sessions.

From 1948 to 1958, I was the psychiatrist for ALTRO Health and Rehabilitation services. For a long time the only psychiatrist for a large number of patients, I tried to provide some help for the multitude of tubercular, cardiac, and eventually psychotic patients included in the agency's program. It was then that the Director of Social Work there, Celia Benney, pointed out to me that I seemed to have developed a special technique of brief intervention. In fact, three decades ago I published my first paper on emergency psychotherapy (of depression) (Bellak, 1952). I left ALTRO to organize the Department of Psychiatry at the City Hospital at Elmhurst, New York, of which an outstanding part became my "Trouble-Shooting Clinic," by some accounts the first fully staffed, 24-hour walk-in clinic in the United States. It offered primarily brief and emergency psychotherapy, since it was at the time the only public clinic that offered dynamic psychotherapy in Queens with its population of 2 million (Bellak, 1960).

Thus, my method grew from the needs of veterans, of ALTRO, and of the Trouble-Shooting Clinic. With great limitations of available staff, my method had to offer something for every problem in every condition and for large numbers of patients in need, many of them severely ill. The method followed the principle of community psychiatry laid down by Leighton (1960), "Action on behalf of one must be within the framework of calculation for the many."

My method of brief psychotherapy thus differs from that of Sifneos (1972), who selects patients who are specifically capable of having their anxiety aroused and who have an oedipal level of development. I gather that this method is useful with only a small percentage of patients, especially of patients coming to a public clinic. My method also differs from that of Mann (1973), who focuses on separation anxiety. Such a theoretical constraint would not have been useful, for instance, for the chronic psychotic who turned up because people were sending electric shooting pains into her leg. I could also not have used Davanloo's (1978) technique of confrontation by videotaped material because videotape had, of course, not as yet been invented. Even today, most clinics can afford neither the technology nor the time. Furthermore, I do not believe that confrontation is useful for every patient.

My method has some similarities to Malan's (1963), who published his first book shortly before Small and I, unaware of his, published our own (Bellak and Small, 1965). We both had a psychoanalytic background, and eventually Malan came to share my willingness to take on virtually all comers (Malan, 1973). Malan's technique, however, was developed in the relative tranquility of the Tavistock Clinic. Thus, not only could Malan offer more time to his patients than I had available in my original settings, but he was also probably dealing with patients who were not as sick as mine.

My form of brief psychotherapy, then, is often closely related to emergency psychotherapy, and it is rooted in community psychiatry. Unlike some crisis intervention theorists, though, I believe that emergency psychotherapy may be able to help a patient reconstitute on a higher level of integration than before the emergency.

BASIC CONCEPTS AND TENETS OF BEP

The method of intensive brief and emergency psychotherapy (BEP) is delineated as follows. For a more detailed discussion of the basic propositions discussed in this chapter, see Bellak and Small (1978), Bellak and Faithorn (1981), and Bellak and Siegel (1983).

1. BEP focuses on the crucial features of the presenting disorder.
2. BEP attempts to understand the patients in terms of the psychoanalytic theory of dynamics and structure, and specifically to understand why the patient comes to see a therapist at a particular time.
3. BEP views the major contribution of psychoanalysis as the establishment of continuity between the present and the past, specifically between childhood and adulthood, between sleeping and waking thought, between pathology and health.
4. BEP attempts to understand the patient's presenting problem by establishing the continuity with his or her past, the precipitating situation, and various biological, familial, social, and other aspects.
5. In a broader sense, BEP sees all symptoms as attempts at problem solving, at coping with conflict and with deficit.
6. Like all psychotherapy, BEP is seen as a form of learning, unlearning, and relearning by various means (Bellak, 1977). Therefore, BEP

focuses on what has been poorly coped with, what has been poorly learned, and what needs to be unlearned and relearned in a most efficacious manner.

7. The essence of BEP lies not in the limited number of sessions, but in a systematic, focused, and highly conceptualized approach.
8. BEP generally uses five sessions because this is the number of times most patients in a clinic are willing to return.
9. Indications for BEP are very broad. BEP selects the problem for treatment, not the patient. In that sense, BEP is useful for primary, as well as secondary and tertiary, prevention of a wide range of problems. (Thus, some patients certainly fare better with BEP and some worse, as they do with all forms of therapy.)
10. BEP does not necessarily offer dynamic therapy only. BEP does insist that the therapist first understand the patient psychodynamically. Therapy itself may take any number of different forms.

BEP is not a band-aid; nor is it second-rate treatment. Anyone who enjoys short stories knows that it is often more difficult to write a good short story than a novel. The same holds true for the relationship between brief therapy and long-term therapy. At times, there may be a tendency to denigrate BEP by comparing it with what Freud practiced in his early, uninformed days. But the fact is that Freud had not at the time developed ego psychology. BEP, on the other hand, is a skilled technology which uses all that ego psychology has to offer.

BEP must be based on an extensive guided history, in which the history taking is guided by clearly formulated concepts and uses a suitable style of communication. With a patient complaining of depression, for example, the guided history would entail keeping in mind the various factors listed in Table 3, listening for them, and using them as a guide to further exploration. The idea is to have a frame of reference that does not, however, lead to rigid prejudgment. In a general sense, the principles are those of emergency medicine. When a medical technician approaches an unconscious patient, he or she knows to follow certain definite procedures and is quite clear about what the proper sequence is. It should be the same with brief psychotherapy, and especially with emergency psychotherapy.

Administratively, BEP could be considered the intake procedure of choice. Long-term therapy is indicated if the patient has failed to improve with brief therapy or if one has other special reasons for choosing a longer therapy. While BEP will certainly be effective with some problem area in virtually any patient, one may still, of course, wish to aim for a more extensive therapeutic change than is feasible with brief psychotherapy.

A final general feature of concern is that some of the factors that distinguish BEP from traditional treatment can incur resistance. The resistance frequently stems from the mistaken notion that BEP is a second-rate therapy. Another source of resistance may be characterological. Therapists are by and large probably less aggressive than lawyers or businessmen, and they have chosen their profession in part because passive-receptive listening attitudes come to them easily. Insofar as BEP demands some active intervention, it does not suit their personality style.

Finally, the extensive training therapists receive in long-term and psychoanalytic therapy also makes it difficult for them to engage in the active interventions that are especially called for in emergency therapy.

THE SEQUENCE OF THE SESSIONS

The Initial Session

BEP sessions are usually fifty minutes long and occur once a week, unless the patient has a need to return sooner or conditions are very acute. Table 1 lists the features of the initial session.

Table 1. Features of the Initial Session in BEP

1. Chief complaint	
2. History of chief complaint	
3. Secondary complaints	
4. Life history	
5. Family history	
6. Dynamic formulation	
7. Transference	
8. Therapeutic alliance	The Three Factors in the Therapeutic Relationship
9. Therapeutic contract	
10. Review and planning	

Note: Reproduced from Bellak L, Siegel H: Handbook of Intensive Brief and Emergency Psychotherapy, Larchmont, New York: C.P.S., Inc., Box 83, 1983, with permission of the publisher and the authors.

The initial interview is by far the most interesting, the one which demands the hardest work from both therapist and patient, and probably the most crucial. One can obtain an exhaustive history from the patient if the interview contains a reasonable and appropriate mixture of spontaneous talking by the patient and guidance by the therapist toward relevant areas of information. In eliciting the history, the therapist should look for common denominators between the onset of the patient's chief complaint and earlier situations in the patient's life. The best guide to taking a history is that the therapist should visualize the patient at different times in his or her life, especially in childhood, within his or her physical setting and particular subculture, and in relation to significant others. A sense of the prevailing home atmosphere should be gained, as well as information about parents and siblings. In every instance, the therapist must learn as much as possible about the ethnic and cultural aspects of the patient's life.

In the broad meaning of the term *transference relationship*, the patient comes to treatment programmed with certain apperceptive distortions derived from the past, which he or she ascribes to the as-yet-unknown therapist (e.g., by dreaming the preceding night of going to the dentist). A useful routine is to question the patient concerning any dream of the night before the appointment; this may give an idea of the preformed transference expectations.

In the course of the history taking, a significant interpersonal relationship is established that includes positive or negative countertransference features, more or less of a rescue fantasy on the therapist's part, with cognitive closure and possible critical feelings. For the patient, the intensive interest in his or her history is often a form of narcissistic gratification. It conveys the genuine interest of the interviewer and thus contributes to the establishment of a positive transference. In addition, more personal transference/countertransference relations form as soon as the patient and therapist meet in the waiting room.

Another part of the first session is to review at its end the salient features of the history and the complaint or problems which brought the patient into therapy. Here, the therapist points out some easily perceived common denominators between the history and the current problem, and their relationship to the therapist, as expressed by the patient. The patient should gain at least an intellectual understanding of what his or her problem might be, thus decreasing any feelings of helplessness and giving the patient the feeling that, whatever the problem, it can at least be understood and that the therapist can understand it. This further contributes to the development of an interpersonal relationship between the patient and the therapist. At the same time, the therapist is formulating a general notion about the dynamics and structure of the patient's personality and problem. While the therapist later attempts to follow up on these heuristic hunches, they should remain flexible as other data come in.

The careful history taking and review of salient features creates an atmosphere of compassionate empathy. In the author's experience, empathy can be entirely genuine if one conceives of life somewhat in terms of a Greek drama. All of us are more or less helpless victims of circumstances to which we adapt in various ways, and the therapist's job is to help the patient achieve a little better adaptation. The atmosphere should also have some feeling of hope, predicated upon the therapist's understanding of the patient's problems and mixed with realistic limitations as formulated in the therapeutic contract.

The therapeutic alliance can be introduced to the patient with a specific formula: "The rational and intelligent part of you needs to sit together with me to help understand the irrational and unconscious part of you that causes you problems." In the first or second session, the therapist may briefly explain the nature of the therapeutic process, as he or she sees it, to increase this alliance. A basic idea to convey is that we understand behavior if we understand that there is continuity between childhood and adulthood, between waking and sleeping thought, and between normal and pathological behavior. This can be illustrated with an example or two from the patient's account. Dreams, of course, are especially valuable for this purpose as one can show the relationship between the day residue, the dream, and the past history.

The therapeutic contract in brief psychotherapy is much more clear-cut and specifically stated than in longer forms of psychotherapy. The therapist expresses the hope that the patient will be able to deal with the problems in five sessions, each of them lasting approximately fifty minutes. Patients are always expected to communicate with the therapist about a month after the fifth session, by telephone, letter, or in person, to say how they are faring. Generally, the therapist will have reason to believe that the five sessions will be sufficient and successful, and should express this to the patient. The therapist should also convey that if the five sessions are not enough, he or she will see that the patient gets whatever further therapy is necessary.

Six Sessions: From Plan to Follow-Up

During the manifest and verbal part of the initial session, a silent, but equally important, process is simultaneously at work. While listening to the patient, the therapist is formulating hypotheses regarding the interaction of genetic, familial, social, and medical factors with experiential factors. The therapist should also be deciding on the best plan of treatment, such as dyadic treatment, conjoint sessions, family therapy, team approach, use of drugs, use of community resources, and so forth. If brief therapy is to play the primary therapeutic role, the therapist should select the areas and methods of intervention and their sequences. The range of possibilities can be seen in Tables 3 and 4 and in the Appendix.

During *the second session*, the therapist further explores the patient's dynamics and structure, aiming at better closure, and reexamines the basis for choosing the areas and methods of intervention. The therapist should ask how the patient felt during the intervening week and elicit any additional complaints. Making connections from session to session is important for the therapist and especially for the patient. This connection increases the synthetic-integrative functioning of the ego as well as the therapeutic alliance. In short, the therapeutic process serves to formulate progressively better-fitting hypotheses and to establish progressively more continuity for both patient and therapist.

In *the third session*, the therapist should make a special attempt to work through what has already been learned, allowing additions whenever possible. This may be an opportune time for a conjoint interview, if the therapist decides that would be the most useful way to gather further information and to effect changes between two people, such as spouses. On the other hand, the therapist may decide that a family session would be more useful at this time.

During the third session, the therapist should start referring to the impending separation. The therapist should specify that the patient will probably feel worse during the next visit, possibly because of a fear of separation and abandonment. If this session is dyadic, it should be used specifically to work through separation problems.

The fourth session is dedicated to understanding more about the patient's problem, adding insights, and intervening whenever necessary. Once again, discussion of termination and the patient's reactions is necessary.

The fifth and final session begins as usual, with establishing the patient's present emotional state and his or her feelings during the intervening week. The patient should then verbally review the entire treatment period, and the patient and therapist should work through any additional material, especially regarding termination of therapy or other plans.

Termination should be accomplished with the positive relationship intact. The therapist may request that the patient make contact by telephone, letter, or personally at least one month following therapy. To prevent further dependency, the therapist should indicate the problems that termination itself may produce. In addition, the therapist may suggest that if the patient tolerates the immediate discomfort, it will strengthen the therapeutic achievements.

During *the sixth session* (follow-up), the therapist should evaluate the therapeutic achievements and make dispositions accordingly. Once again, it is important to leave the patient with a positive transference and the feeling that the therapist or a substitute will be available. As Oberndorf (1953) stated, the positive transference is valuable for the long-term maintenance of therapeutic improvement.

In very disturbed patients, especially psychotics, an ordinary structural appraisal of the strength of the superego, the nature of the introjects, and so forth may not be enough. Under these circumstances, the recommended approach is a systematic, albeit informal, appraisal of the 12 ego functions that the author has found useful in previous research (Bellak et al., 1973). Such an appraisal may also guide other therapeutic decisions, such as how active a role the therapist may have to play, whether drugs are indicated, or whether significant others have to be drawn in.

THE THERAPEUTIC PROCESS

Features of the therapeutic process appear in Table 2. The first four features listed follow the basic steps of dynamic psychotherapy. Once the patient begins to communicate verbally, the therapist can formulate some common denominators between the patient's present behavior, past history, and the therapeutic relationship. When the timing is correct, as determined by several technical criteria, the therapist should inform the patient of these common denominators. The process of indicating the common denominators between the patient's behavioral and affective patterns in the past, present, and transference situations is generally known as *interpretation*. If the patient is able to recognize these common denominators, he or she is applying *insight*. The patient's verbal re-

Table 2. Features of the Therapeutic Process in BEP

1. Forming common denominators via communication between the patient and the therapist
2. Interpretation
3. Insight
4. Working through

   } Basic Steps of Dynamic Psychotherapy

5. Guiding and controlling the intensity of the therapeutic process
6. Facilitating communication (Appropriate style is essential.)
7. Explaining the therapeutic process in simplified terms at the end of the initial session
8. Facilitating learning (Appropriate intellectual, conceptual, and linguistic style is recommended.)
9. Using projective techniques
10. Educating the patient as part of the therapeutic process (e.g., having the patient sketch the diseased organ in emergency treatment of emotional reactions to physical illness)

Note: Reproduced from Bellak L, Siegel H: Handbook of Intensive Brief and Emergency Psychotherapy, Larchmont, New York: C.P.S., Inc., Box 83, 1983, with permission of the publisher and the authors.

sponse to the interpretation must have strong affective components and not merely signify an intellectual recognition. When the patient is able to apply acquired insights to life situations, he or she is considered to be *working through* the problems. This is basically a process of learning by conditioning. Ultimately, a different reaction to the situation will be automatic as a result of the newly learned mechanisms and insight.

Brief therapy gains much of its effectiveness from the nature and guidance of the therapeutic process, which includes facilitating communication and learning.

Facilitating Communication

For dynamic psychotherapy to take place, the patient must above all be able to communicate. In order to do this, the therapist usually introduces patients to the concept of self-reporting. The author sometimes tells patients a variant of Freud's story of two passengers in a train compartment. One man is sitting near the window, able to look out, and the other is sitting on the inside, unable to see the landscape. The passenger near the window has a perfect view, but is unfamiliar with the landscape. The passenger away from the window is unable to see any of the scenery, but is very familiar with the particular area through which they are passing. The two men make a contract: they agree that the man at the window will call out the scenery, and the man away from the window will then try to designate their location. The man at the window says, "I see a small village square with a monument to the left and an inn behind it." The man away from the window replies, "Aha, in that case I expect a little church to the right, and we must be in Petersburg." The man at the window says, "No, there isn't a church to the right, but there is a movie house." Whereupon the man away from the window says, "Ah, in that case we are in North Walden." This story demonstrates the necessity of collaboration between the patient and therapist if they are to arrive at the best hypotheses concerning the significance and nature of the patient's symptoms and thoughts.

The therapist should ask very specific questions to elicit information, such as the patient's thoughts following the last session and immediately prior to the present session. Emphasis should be placed on thoughts the patient has during semiautomatic activities such as shaving, driving, applying makeup, and cooking, since much can be learned from the thoughts during such activities. In addition, the therapist may ask the patient what he or she thinks about immediately before falling asleep, upon awakening, and when arising from bed. Dreams are also important and can be encouraged by inquiring about the patient's recall of some feeling, word, or picture.

It is a good idea to explain the therapeutic process in simplified terms at the conclusion of the first session. The author prefers to use the approach of apperceptive distortion (Bellak and Small, 1978). One explains that the patient's past experiences have been stored in the memory as images. When the patient confronts a contemporary scene or figure, a male foreman at work, for example, the patient is likely to view this figure through a collage of past apperceptions of superior male figures, of father, of uncles, of older brother, of teachers, as if through a kaleidoscope. Thus, neurotic or other pathological distortions result from an excessive influence of past apperceptions on contemporary cognition.

Psychotherapy's goal is to identify and understand the distortion of present cognition according to past experiences and thus produce a perceptual correction and structural change.

Facilitating Learning

Psychotherapy is a process of learning, unlearning, and relearning; the therapist's task is to facilitate this process by making it as concrete, vivid, and colorful as possible. Interpretations can be understood by using vivid examples to explain concepts.

Projective techniques can sometimes be useful as vehicles for communication as well as for interpretation. For example, showing the patient Rorschach blots or pictures from the Thematic Apperception Test may produce responses that indicate latent aggression. Projective techniques may thus be used to increase the patient's psychological mindedness and to change ego-syntonic to ego-alien behavior.

In the emergency treatment of emotional reactions to physical illness, asking the patient to sketch the diseased organ is often helpful. This enables the therapist to observe a concrete illustration of the patient's distortions of reality. It presents an opportunity for the therapist to inform the patient about the realities of the disorder, which are almost always easier to bear than the irrational notions and fantasies that he or she has imagined.

Managing Specific Clinical Conditions

Depression, acting out, suicidal danger, and management of acute psychosis are among the conditions which the clinician most frequently encounters. Only the first two can be discussed here. For the others and six additional major problems, Appendix 1 lists the main factors to be kept in mind. A more detailed discussion of all of these can be found elsewhere (Bellak and Siegel, 1983).

DEPRESSION More than 50 percent of all the people who come to outpatient clinics are said to complain of depression. As suggested elsewhere (Bellak, 1981), the author has never seen a depression which did not have a clearly related precipitating factor, be it a neurotic depression, an endogenous depression with a familial history, or a depressive phase in a bipolar affective condition.

The ten factors enumerated on Table 3 are relevant to all depressions, and they are rank ordered in terms of their importance. Insult to self-esteem very frequently plays the major role in depression. Since persons with affective disorders have developed complex mechanisms for regulating their self-esteem, understanding and working through the trauma to a depressed patient's self-esteem is often crucial in relieving the depression.

Depressed people often have a good deal of anger, primarily of an oral nature, a rage which may be directly related to the experience of someone lowering the patient's self-esteem. This aggression often conflicts with a very severe superego. Under the latter's influence, the aggression readily turns into intraaggression and self-denigration and, in extreme cases, a self-accusatory tendency.

Loss of a love object, of a job, or of anything emotionally significant often precipitates depressions. It was Edith Jacobson (1971) who pointed

Table 3.   Ten Specific Considerations in the Therapeutic Management of Depression

Dealing With:
1. Problems of self-esteem regulation
2. Severe superego
3. Intraaggression
4. Loss
5. Disappointment
6. Deception
7. Stimulus hunger (orality) and dependence on external nutrients
8. The dyadic unit or system
9. Denial
10. Disturbances in object relations

Note: Reproduced from Bellak L, Siegel H: Handbook of Intensive Brief and Emergency Psychotherapy, Larchmont, New York: C.P.S., Inc., Box 83, 1983, with permission of the publisher and the authors.

out the importance of a feeling of disappointment in depressed people and who connected this disappointment to a feeling of having been deceived.

Historically, orality has played an important role in the classical psychoanalytic conception of depression. The role of oral needs can sometimes be very concretely and plainly seen, for example in housewives. They may typically complain that they have been unable to go to the supermarket to buy food for the family. They may also not feel like eating at home, but have excellent appetites when taken out to a restaurant. The dynamics are clearly that they wish not to have to feed the family anymore nor even to feed themselves, but rather to be fed.

The depressed person alternates from a normal mood to a depression as part of an interaction with another significant person. For instance, one woman frequently suffered from depression because her husband made excessive demands on her, enraged her, and denigrated her. Her first response, lasting several weeks, would always be compliance. Then she would become depressed and unable to perform the household tasks or other chores her husband found for her. At that point, the husband would become very solicitous. Once helped out of her depression, she would become slightly elated and somewhat assertive and would engage in shopping sprees and a good deal of social activity. In due course, though, the husband would become severely critical of her. She would enter her compliance cycle again, only to become depressed once again. In such cases it rarely suffices to treat only the identified patient. The other person must be included in the treatment, and this may, sometimes but not necessarily, take the therapeutic situation out of the range of brief therapy. In other cases, the depressed patient is part of a more complex system with similar interactions, sometimes familial and sometimes in relation to work.

The outstanding defense mechanism in all affective disorders is denial. In fact, the main task in therapy must often be finding out just what the precipitating factor was, since the patient is not aware of it and is often actively denying it. It is probably this very lack of ability to see or look for subtle events at the onset of depression that has led some to believe that the so-called endogenous depressions have no clearly reactive factors in their onset.

Finally, depressed people have some disturbance in their object relations, which are usually markedly anaclitic and even considerably narcissistic, as Jacobson (1971) points out in great detail. While depressions are eminently suited for brief psychotherapy and the author has had unusual success with them, brief therapy cannot usually do much to change the nature of object relations. Regrettably, this is also often impossible even in long-term therapy.

ACTING OUT   Acting-out patients present a particular challenge to the clinician. Table 4 lists some of the strategies for dealing with patients who act out. Bargaining for a delay is one useful tactic. Consulting to a suicide prevention service, the author encountered some difficult situations referred from the hot line. Someone would call up the clinic and say, "Listen, I am sitting on the windowsill on the fifth floor and just want you to know that I am about to jump off." The best advice in such situations is to tell the person, "Look, I'm awfully sorry you feel that bad. I'm afraid I can't do anything about your jumping off, since, after all, it is your life. On the other hand, you can always jump tomorrow, when I can't do anything about it either. So, if you will come in and discuss it, you still have your options open." This tactic is intended to bring the patient in. Once one has successfully bargained for a delay, the chances are good that the patient who is prone to momentary impulses will rather easily give up, at least for the time being, the idea of self-harm. One must then hope that the treatment will be effective in decreasing the suicidal danger generally.

Impulsive people enjoy the feeling of omnipotence. They can do what they want to do when they want to do it. If one can make their acting out ego-alien, one is well on the road to changing their acting-out behavior. With these patients, a useful strategy is to point out how they are the helpless victims of their past, how they are programmed much like a computer without even knowing it. In other words, one makes of what feels to them ego-syntonic (acting out) something that is ego-alien (helplessness). This change interferes with a great deal of their pleasure in acting out (Bellak, 1965).

To decrease the future tendencies to act out, one must ensure that the patient understands the particular set of circumstances, such as lowering of self-esteem or a particular temptation, that leads to his or her

---

Table 4.   Ten Specific Considerations in the Therapeutic Management of Acting Out

1. Bargaining for a delay
2. Making the act ego-alien
3. Making a "cathartic" interpretation of the underlying drive
4. Increasing signal awareness and sensitizing the patient to cues
5. Predicting when a patient will act out
6. Strengthening the superego
7. Removing the patient from a provocative setting
8. Enlisting the help of others
9. Utilizing drugs
10. Utilizing brief hospitalization

Note: Reproduced from Bellak L., Siegel H: Handbook of Intensive Brief and Emergency Psychotherapy, Larchmont, New York: C.P.S., Inc., Box 83, 1983, with permission of the publisher and the authors.

acting out. This is called sensitizing the patient to cues and increasing the signal awareness. Such cues have the added advantage of enabling one to predict when a patient may act out. Shared with the patient, such predictions may help the patient to ward off any temptation and not have it come true. At times, preventing impulsive acts may require pointing out the harm they will do others, thus involving the superego.

When a patient again and again acts out because an occupational or other life situation is conducive and in fact seems likely to precipitate the acting-out behavior, one may take the unusual step of suggesting, or even insisting, that the patient change the situation.

SUMMARY

Intensive brief and emergency psychotherapy usually involves five sessions. It is a method applicable to the broadest scope of psychopathology. The understanding of the patient must be predicated upon psychoanalytic theory. The types of interventions may be of many different forms, as long as they are well conceptualized and understood analytically. A special style is necessary to make complex dynamic factors understandable to some patients. The very clear-cut conceptualizations discussed throughout this chapter are essential for an optimal resolution of psychopathology.

APPENDIX 1.
SPECIFIC CONSIDERATIONS IN THE MANAGEMENT OF SELECTED PROBLEMS

The Therapeutic Management of Panic
1. Establishment of the cause of the panic
2. Continuity between immediate panic, precipitating factors, and life history
3. Intellectual explanation as part of establishing continuity
4. Exogenous panic: the unconscious meaning of the external event
5. Conversion of exogenous panic to endogenous, making it ego-alien
6. Endogenous panic as part of an incipient psychosis
7. Need to be completely available to patient
8. Need to provide a structure
9. Interpretation of denial
10. Use of catharsis or mediate catharsis

The Therapeutic Management of Physical Illness or Surgery
Dealing with:
1. The patient's concept of the illness or impending surgery
2. The personal meaning and role of illness (secondary gains, etc.)
3. Educating the patient
4. Contact with the treating physician or surgeon
5. The meaning of anesthesia
6. Specific notions and fears of death
7. Specific types of illness and surgery
Special Problems:
8. Organs of sexual significance
9. Malignancies
10. Heart disease

The Therapeutic Management of Phobias

Dealing with:
1. Specific dynamics of different phobias
2. Specific phobias as part of a family and cultural context
3. Overdetermined pathogenesis for the phobia
4. The need to face the phobic situation and reporting back
5. The working through of insights in the actual phobic situation
6. Drugs for symptomatic relief of some phobias
7. Counterphobic symbols and defenses
8. Migratory phobias: looking for the common denominator
9. Panphobias
10. Somatic delusions

The Therapeutic Management of Incipient Psychotic States

1. Establishing contact
2. Establishing continuity
3. Reassuring by understanding and interpretation
4. Structuring the patient's life
5. Being available
6. Involving significant others
7. Splinting
8. The therapist as auxiliary ego
9. Utilizing drugs
10. Utilizing brief hospitalization

The Therapeutic Management of Feelings of Unreality of the Self and of the World

1. Dealing with coexistence of feelings of unreality of the self and of the world
2. Recognizing a continuum of pathology
3. Addressing states of heightened and changed awareness of the self or body
4. Addressing aggressive, sexual, exhibitionistic, and separation aspects
5. Dealing with disturbances of sense of self as intrasystemic ego disturbance
6. Understanding estrangement related to physical factors
7. Realizing drug-induced states of unreality (prescription and street drugs)
8. Explaining déjà vu and déjà reconnu phenomena
9. Utilizing psychotherapeutic interventions
10. Utilizing drug management

Enabling the Brief Intensive Ambulatory Psychotherapy of Psychotic Patients

1. A reasonably cooperative, nonassaultive patient
2. At least one stable relationship in the patient's life
3. Optimally, a family network
4. A close relationship with a nearby hospital
5. Availability of an auxiliary therapist
6. Awareness of community resources (YMCA, YWCA, OVR, etc.)

7. Hot lines and emergency centers
8. Access to an alarm system: Do not be a hero!
9. A suitable housing situation
10. Drug therapy in combination with psychotherapy

The Therapeutic Management of Suicide
1. Dealing with precipitating factor or situation (depression or panic)
2. Considering content, concreteness, and primitivity of fantasies and plans
3. Weighing previous attempts (or plans) and attending circumstances
4. Evaluating family history of suicidality and/or depression
5. In acute suicidal patients, abandoning therapeutic neutrality, etc.
6. Working with tunnel vision
7. Bargaining for a delay and using other tactics involved in dealing with acting out
8. Working with factors pertaining to depression or panic
9. Drawing significant others into the situation and using community resources
10. Utilizing drugs, hospitalization

The Therapeutic Management of Catastrophic Events
1. Catharsis
2. Specific meaning of the event
3. Exploration of "liability"
4. Chronic sequelae "recognition"
5. Superego aspects
6. Ego aspects
7. Specific responses to mugging
8. Specific responses to burglary
9. Specific responses to rape
10. Specific responses to accidents[1]

Chapter 2

Short-Term Anxiety-Provoking Psychotherapy
by Peter E. Sifneos, M.D.

This chapter begins by discussing the development and change in the patient selection criteria for short-term anxiety-provoking psychotherapy (STAPP), a psychodynamic therapy of brief duration. Current criteria for selecting appropriate patients and the technical requirements and results of STAPP are then reviewed in some detail.

[1]Appendix 1 is based on material from Bellak L, Siegel H: Handbook of Intensive Brief and Emergency Psychotherapy, Larchmont, New York: C.P.S. Inc., Box 83, 1983, with permission of the publisher and the authors.

PATIENT SELECTION CRITERIA

Initial Assumptions

An early priority in the development of STAPP was to formulate criteria for selecting appropriate candidates for short-term therapy. Initially, the requirements were that a patient show an ability to relate well to other people, demonstrate that love and affection had been received and reciprocated in the past, and express affect during the evaluation interview. In addition, the patient had to show flexibility and possess good motivation for psychotherapy. Finally, with regard to symptoms, the patient had to have a circumscribed chief complaint and be in a state of emotional crisis. Using these criteria, the author and his colleagues selected fifty patients between 1954 and 1958. All of them received short-term dynamic psychotherapy consisting of weekly sessions over a period of two to nine months (Sifneos, 1961).

Most of these patients were young people, ranging in age from 19 to 36, and most were students. It was at first thought that only younger patients would benefit from STAPP and that older patients would not be good candidates because they were more rigid. However, this assumption proved to be erroneous. When older patients were subsequently selected according to the same criteria used with the younger individuals, the author and his colleagues discovered, to their surprise and delight, that elderly patients were also able to use this treatment effectively. Elderly patients worked as hard as younger ones to overcome their emotional conflicts, and when they were seen in follow-up interviews they exhibited the same kinds of outcomes as their younger counterparts.

Of the 50 patients from the first study, 21 were seen in follow-up interviews six months to two years (1958 to 1960) after the termination of their treatment. The findings pointed to moderate symptomatic relief and improved self-esteem. The patients' original expectations of the results of their therapy had become more realistic, and they described their treatment as a "new learning experience." Finally, they demonstrated that they had been able to overcome the psychological crisis that they had been unable to resolve in the past.

Despite these encouraging results, the criteria for selection were clearly too rigid. Fifty patients over a four-year period was a small number indeed. The various criteria were examined closely to assess which ones should remain and which could be eliminated. As a result of this reevaluation, the emotional crisis criterion was eliminated. Most of the patients in a state of emotional crisis tended to be seen in the hospital's emergency unit, and only rarely did they make an appointment at the psychiatric clinic.

As a consequence of this change, more than 500 patients were treated and studied over the next four years (1960 to 1964). At the same time that the results of this investigation were presented at the International Congress of Psychotherapy in London in 1964, Malan was making similar observations from the Tavistock Clinic in London. Encouraged by the similarities of approaches, the author and his colleagues then decided to set up a controlled study of STAPP with appropriate candidates selected according to the five current selection criteria (Sifneos,

1972). (The results of this and a subsequent study are reviewed at the end of the chapter.)

Current Criteria

1. *The patient must have a specific circumscribed chief complaint.* A systematic effort should be made to help the patient select one symptom or psychological difficulty, such as a problem in interpersonal relations, and assign to it a top priority. Such a selection signifies that the patient is able to choose one from a variety of problems, and this ability to focus is seen as evidence of ego strength.

2. *The patient must be able to indicate that during childhood he or she had at least one meaningful relationship.* A person who, during early life, was able to have an "altruistic relationship" suggests a person who is capable of trust, who can reciprocate positive feelings, and who has learned somewhere along the way to interact in a give and take with other people. Such a patient is not expected to be seriously disturbed, and neurotic difficulties are likely to be limited.

3. *The patient must interact flexibly with the evaluator.* This third criterion is a test of the second one. If a patient has had a meaningful relationship in the past, he or she should presumably be able to interact with another in a first meeting and to express feelings freely.

4. *The patient must have the ability to recognize that his or her problems are psychological in origin and to demonstrate above-average intelligence.* These attributes reveal a psychological sophistication and a capacity for using in a meaningful way what is learned during treatment. This capacity for insight, if discovered at this time, eventually becomes a critical factor in the success of the therapy, and it will also be found at follow-up.

5. *The patient must show motivation for change.* Probably the most important of all the selection requirements is demonstration on the part of the patient that he or she possesses the motivation for psychological change. The word *change* is of particular significance. It should not be confused with a wish for symptom relief. If relief is all that the patient wants, this signifies passivity and an expectation that the therapist will perform some kind of miraculous cure. Such expectations are evidence of poor motivation and can lead to future disappointments and treatment failures. Because motivation for change was found to be correlated with a successful treatment outcome, the author and his colleagues have since formulated seven more specific criteria for its assessment. These are (1) the ability to recognize that problems are psychological in origin, (2) introspection and willingness to give a truthful account of difficulties, (3) curiosity and willingness to understand oneself, (4) realistic expectations of the outcome of the treatment, (5) willingness to explore and to experiment, (6) the capacity to make a tangible sacrifice even if this means a certain degree of discomfort, and finally (7) an ability to participate actively in the therapeutic process.

An additional advantage of such a specific assessment of the motivation for change is that it gives the therapist a basis for monitoring the progress of treatment. For example, a patient who during the evaluation meets all seven motivation criteria is viewed initially as having excellent motivation. But if the motivation score decreases to five (fair motivation) by the fourth session and three (unmotivated) by the eighth session, the outcome is potentially poor, unless the therapist can motivate the patient. Thus, the ongoing assessment of motivation for change can be a valuable prognostic criterion for the success of the therapy.

EVALUATION TASKS

In addition to assessing the patient according to the selection criteria, the evaluator has two other initial tasks before starting treatment. The first is to present the patient with a psychodynamic formulation of those conflicts which appear to underlie the patient's psychological problem. This formulation, derived from a systematic history taking, eventually becomes the focus around which the therapy revolves. It is therefore important that the patient agree to work in this circumscibed area of conflicts. Even if he or she might want help with other difficulties, the patient must, for the sake of brevity, forgo such help. Later, it is expected, the patient will be able to use what he or she has learned during the brief treatment of circumscribed conflicts to solve these additional problems. Second, the evaluator should specify in writing the changes that he or she expects the patient to achieve as a result of STAPP.

While the evaluation process does have discrete tasks, the evaluation process and the psychotherapy do not necessarily have a clear-cut demarcation. The patient's responses to interpretations during the evaluation interview already may have therapeutic impact. Occasionally, such interpretations are so effective that some patients, as Malan (1976) has also observed, do not require any further psychotherapy. They are able to disentangle their conflicts all by themselves subsequent only to this evaluation interview. With a few patients seen only for an evaluation interview, the author and his colleagues found several years later that they showed ample evidence of psychodynamic change and of overcoming their original problems.

Case Illustration

A 23-year-old female graduate student came to the clinic because she was anxious and depressed about her current relations with two of her boyfriends, Jim and Todd. She was very fond of Jim, to whom she was engaged; the only problem had to do with their sexual relations. She reported that as soon as she had become engaged to Jim and started to think about her future married life, sexual intercourse had become unsatisfactory to her. At the same time, having met Todd, a garage mechanic with a grade-school education, she was extremely attracted to him, made frequent love with him, and felt "very satisfied." She talked at length about her annoyance at her inability to resolve these problems by herself, emphasizing repeatedly that her sense of competence and independence were at stake.

During the history taking, she specified that she was clearly her father's favorite. She remembered, with much feeling, the weekly walks they took on Sundays after church while her mother and her younger sister returned home. She felt that her father enjoyed having this special time with her, and she proudly remarked that he had never asked either her mother or her sister to accompany him on these walks. She described her father as "an intellectual giant" who had been a judge and was currently a professor at a prestigious law school. She also emphasized that her father was particularly interested in education. He had told her on many occasions that the primary responsibility of society was "to educate its less fortunate, but nevertheless likable, members."

When the evaluator inquired more extensively about her fiancé, she said that he reminded her very much of her father. Then the following exchange with the evaluator took place.

Evaluator:	In what way does Jim remind you of your father?
Patient:	Well, they are both lawyers, but Jim is also very well educated and places the same kind of emphasis on it as my father does.
Evaluator:	What does your father look like?
Patient:	*(With feeling)* He is tall and thin, with dark hair. He is a very distinctive man.
Evaluator:	And what does Todd look like?
Patient:	Oh, no. He doesn't look like my father.
Evaluator:	Did you think I thought he did?
Patient:	Hm . . . maybe, yes. In any case, he does not. He, if anything, seems to be very different; short, with curly red hair and not very distinctive. He is a warm guy and eager to learn a great deal from me.
Evaluator:	Now, let's get back to Jim. What does he look like?
Patient:	Jim is also tall, not as tall as my father, and not as distinctive, but he is very bright. The queer thing, also, is that he has the same name as I do.
Evaluator:	Why is it queer?
Patient:	When I get married, I wouldn't have to change my name.
Evaluator:	You'd have the same name as your mother.
Patient:	Yes. I had thought of that.
Evaluator:	What would that make you in reference to your father?
Patient:	. . . It's interesting that I haven't thought of that.
Evaluator:	Why?
Patient:	. . . I don't know.
Evaluator:	It would . . .
Patient:	I'd be like a second wife to him! No! No!
Evaluator:	Precisely! This is the reason why you cannot enjoy sexual relations with Jim, who is very much like your father, while you enjoy sex with Todd, who is very different, who is not well educated, who is eager to learn, and who is also the kind of person your father likes.
Patient:	This is amazing! I have thought a great deal about my relationship with Jim, and all the problems about our sex relations; I have never wanted to think at all about my relationship with Todd. My mind is always blank when we have sex. I thought that it was so because it was so pleasurable, but . . .
Evaluator:	But it is because you wanted to avoid thinking of your father under similar circumstances.
Patient:	Oh, my God!

The evaluation interview proceeded along the same lines for a while, with the patient giving additional details about splitting her feelings for her father into two different directions as far as her two male boyfriends were concerned.

When she was called to commence her psychotherapy three weeks later, she mentioned that she did not feel the need for it, because during the intervening time she had decided to end her relationship with Todd and to set the date for her marriage with Jim. Furthermore, she added, her sexual relationship with her fiancé had greatly improved, and she felt that she had a better insight about her feelings for her father. When asked what did she attribute all these changes to, she exclaimed that her evaluation interview was clearly responsible for setting in motion a problem-solving process. She added, "I have been vaguely aware of all the issues which were discussed, but the whole thing jelled during that interview. From then on, I realized that I could solve my own riddle, and I am pleased that I did."

TECHNICAL REQUIREMENTS OF STAPP

STAPP uses many of the classic dynamic interventions, but also differs in some fundamental ways from the technical requirements of long-term psychotherapy and psychoanalysis. The technical requirements used in STAPP are briefly detailed below (Sifneos, 1979).

The *interviews* are *face-to-face*, are *held weekly*, and last *45 minutes*.

The *working alliance* established during the evaluation interview develops into a true *therapeutic alliance*. Here, both therapist and patient actively engage in working together to resolve the psychological conflicts in the area chosen as the focus of the treatment. This implies that the information the patient gives in terms of memories, fantasies, episodes from the past, associations, and so on, is brought into the session for the therapist to analyze. At the same time, by using his or her clinical expertness, the therapist presents the information back to the patient in a different way, e.g., challenging the patient's behavior patterns, emphasizing paradoxical contradictions, and interpreting defensive maneuvers. Thus, the patient and the therapist collaborate in disentangling the patient's emotional problem.

In the early phase of the treatment, the therapist systematically uses *confrontations and clarifications*. These techniques tend to be anxiety provoking at times because they serve the purpose of keeping the patient within the confines of the psychodynamic focus chosen during the evaluation interview. In a sense, the patient is in the dual position of having to work to resolve the problem, but at the same time having to resist this resolution because it gives rise to anxiety. It may appear paradoxical, therefore, that the therapist behaves in a way that will further increase the patient's unpleasant feelings, e.g., anxiety. But the therapist is confident of the patient's motivation, as a result of having systematically assessed it, and feels that the increased anxiety will stimulate the patient to look even more closely into the areas of conflict that he or she tends to avoid.

The *therapist's activity* is another special characteristic of this kind of brief dynamic psychotherapy. Active interpretations were described and used by Ferenczi (1952) during the early years of psychoanalysis. Certain distinctions should be made, however, between active therapeutic interventions offered as physical rewards to the patient and the verbal activity of the therapist in STAPP. The activity in STAPP is more associated with making interpretations that relate to the focal problem as well as with stopping the patient's efforts to escape by various defensive maneuvers. This verbal activity does share with Ferenczi's reinforcements and rewards to encourage the patient to pursue his or her efforts, and it therefore has characteristics in common with learning theory and behavior modification.

Staying within the therapeutic focus is a vital aspect of STAPP. The patient, feeling anxious, wants to avoid dealing with the problem despite strong motivation to inquire into it. The therapist, on the other hand, using anxiety-provoking confrontations and clarifications, tries to urge the patient to face the maladaptive defense mechanisms which give rise to the neurotic difficulties. At times, the therapist may interpret the conflicts relating to the focus even before dealing with the defense used to avoid it. This unorthodox maneuver intensifies the anxiety, but with a well-motivated patient produces rapid results.

The types of therapeutic foci that have been found to respond best to short-term dynamic interventions like STAPP include unresolved oedipal conflicts, grief reactions, and problems about separation and loss. Some investigators have claimed that broad-focused brief psychotherapy has been used successfully with sicker patients, such as individuals suffering from multiple phobias, chronic obsessive-compulsive symptoms, or borderline personalities, but no systematic research has been done to justify these claims.

The interpretation of transference feelings during the early stage of therapy is one of the most useful technical requirements of STAPP. Moreover, the early attention paid to the patient's transference feelings, which are predominantly positive at this stage, has changed certain preconceived ideas about the general handling of transference. In psychoanalytic psychotherapy, it was thought that the therapist did not have to worry about the patient's transference except when it appeared in the form of resistance. But patients with good ego strength, unless encouraged to do so, will take a long time to bring up such feelings. When the feelings are not brought up, it tends to create complications, and it can eventually lead to the development of a transference neurosis. The short-term therapist is unable to analyze a transference neurosis; unlike the analyst, he or she does not use free association and thus has no access to all the patient's fantasies and thoughts. Face-to-face, once-a-week psychotherapy limits the therapist's freedom of interpretation, except in the area of the therapeutic focus. Thus, the therapist must work fast, interpret transference reactions, and end the therapy before complications set in.

Early transference clarifications become an important aspect of another technical requirement basic to all forms of brief dynamic psychotherapy, namely, *parent-transference links.* Links between feelings the patient had in the past for parents or parent surrogates and similar feelings transferred to the therapist can be examined "live" during the sessions and may lead to "a corrective emotional experience" (Alexander and French, 1946). For example, the patient's expectation that the therapist will in some way react like a parent figure perpetuates the neurotic tendencies the patient has displaced on other people. If, on the other hand, the therapist can demonstrate that the emotions the patient experiences toward him or her have been transferred from the past and are identical to those the patient experienced toward a parent, then the patient has the opportunity not only to examine the feelings systematically, but also to alter attitudes about them. When this occurs, the maladaptive defense reactions that the patient has used may be changed, neurotic distortions may be altered, and solutions can be found to old unresolved problems.

Parent-transference links made often and early in the course of brief dynamic psychotherapy have been found to correlate meaningfully with a successful therapeutic outcome. A prerequisite for making such links, however, is not only based on the *early* utilization by the therapist of transference feelings, but also on good motivation for change on the part of the patient. This is yet another reason why motivation is so carefully evaluated.

Avoidance of pregenital characterological issues in STAPP is another of its distinct technical aspects. This entails avoiding discussions of subjects unrelated to the focus where the patient is more or less attempting to resist interpretation and to avoid anxiety. When the patient does bring up such material, particularly during or after a session where meaningful work has been done and much anxiety has been aroused, the therapist should point out that the patient's maneuvers are being used defensively to avoid anxiety and that they are not related to the therapeutic focus.

STAPP also uses *recapitulation* in order to bypass resistance. On occasion, as would be expected, the therapist's interpretations may cause the patient's resistance to become so strong that a clash with the therapist is unavoidable. One way to deal with such a situation is for the therapist not to persist with the confrontations or interpretations, but rather to try to bypass the resistance by recapitulating what had transpired up to the point when the resistance became manifest. When the therapist attempts this recapitulation, the material must be presented very systematically. For example, the patient's exact words should always be repeated verbatim. To be ready to do this effectively, the therapist should be taking notes throughout the treatment. Note taking offers a golden opportunity to review past sessions and to observe how the material discussed has been presented during the interviews. Admittedly, note taking is controversial. Some claim that it interferes with doctor-patient interactions and the spontaneity of communication. It has also been suggested that therapists sometimes use note taking as a mask for strong countertransference feelings toward the patient. Despite these potential hazards, the advantages of note taking clearly outweigh the disadvantages. When parent-transference links are being made, the notes enable the therapist to enumerate the times the patient has used the same words for transference feelings and feelings toward the parents. The impact of this is profound.

STAPP promotes *problem solving*. Problem solving is a way of helping the patient to develop insight. Material offered during previous sessions is systematically analyzed, synthesized, and presented back to the patient with a potential solution. This offers new learning possibilities and is instrumental in enhancing self-understanding and in the development of new and more adaptive attitudes. As a result, the patient's self-esteem is greatly improved.

STAPP requires *tangible evidence of change*. Specific evidence of progress in the therapy comes from the patient's own tangible examples of new attitudes and behavioral changes. These changes can be in the form of diminished symptoms or new ways of reacting to people with whom the patient had difficulties in the past. Other evidence might include the patient's demonstration of more adaptive defense mechanisms in contrast to the maladaptive and neurotic patterns of the past.

STAPP opts for *early termination*. Termination should be considered when the therapist sees enough tangible examples of change and feels that the patient is not fleeing into health. These are the indicators that focal conflicts have actually been resolved.

RECENT DEVELOPMENTS

Two major developments during the 1970s are worthy of note. The first is videotaping, and the second is follow-up research assessing the results of short-term dynamic psychotherapy.

Videotaping

Videotapes have been valuable research tools in STAPP because they depict changes in the patients selected for STAPP and show tangible evidence of improvement after treatment. In a sense, videotaped patients are under a "psychiatric microscope," as they help document our findings. Clinically, videotaping the entire length of the therapy offers innumerable advantages to the therapist who wants to scrutinize his or her interventions, and it helps demonstrate what actually takes place during the therapy. Videotapes are also useful as educational tools, not only in demonstrating to trainees how an experienced therapist goes about treating patients, but also in showing them how they are progressing. By scrutinizing tapes with their supervisor, trainees can review their mistakes and learn from them. Because of these educational advantages, videotapes have also been made of supervisory sessions. The comments and short-term predictions made during supervisory sessions can be tested for accuracy.

Follow-Up Studies

After the first ten years of experience with STAPP, the author and his colleagues undertook a controlled outcome study (1964 to 1968) (Sifneos, 1968). Patients were selected according to the five major criteria described above and were matched for age and sex. After being seen by two independent evaluators, the experimental patients entered STAPP immediately without waiting. Upon termination of treatment, these patients were again seen by the original evaluators. The matched controls were also seen by two independent evaluators and waited without receiving any therapy at all. Control patients were seen again a few months later in order to assess what had happened to them during the waiting period. Following this assessment, the control patients also entered STAPP, and after the end of their therapy, they also were seen by the original evaluators and compared with their experimental counterparts. Both groups were seen subsequently in follow-up interviews when possible.

Despite sophistication regarding the well-known difficulties inherent in psychotherapy research, the study encountered several problems. One was the potential bias of both evaluators and patients in favor of obtaining good results. Topics that were discussed during the first evaluation interview sometimes affected the second session, either positively or negatively, thus altering the score that the second evaluator gave to a patient. Another difficulty concerned the loss of the sample. Because many of the patients were students who eventually left the Boston area, it was difficult to see them in long-term follow-up. In the first study of

35 experimental and 36 control patients, only 14 experimental and 18 control patients were seen at the end of their therapy, and only 12 experimental and 9 control patients were seen in the follow-up interviews six months to four years after the end of their treatment. A related difficulty in evaluating outcome underlines the importance of being able to follow the treatment groups. Responses given during the immediate posttreatment follow-up may result from the termination itself, e.g., the patient's transference feelings over the loss of the therapist. These feelings can initially obscure improvements, but usually disappear in longer-term follow-up when enough time has elapsed. (Since this study, the author and his colleagues have initiated a similar study in Norway, where long-term follow-up interviews are much easier to organize than in the United States. Early results are encouraging, and preliminary reports have been presented at various international congresses [Sifneos, 1970; 1975b]).

The results of the follow-up study were nonetheless significant in that they showed that intrapsychic, psychodynamic, and interpersonal changes had occurred in the STAPP patients. This study used specific outcome criteria focusing on the assessment of changes in the patient's physical and/or psychological symptoms, self-esteem, learning, attitudes, and problem solving. As well as scrutinizing the patient's self-understanding and expectations of the treatment results, the outcome criteria emphasized assessments of interpersonal relations and the replacement of maladaptive defense mechanisms with more adaptive ones. Finally, a formulation was specified regarding potential resolutions of original conflicts underlying the focus chosen as the central issue.

Among the 21 experimental and control patients seen in the longer-term follow-up interviews, while only moderate symptomatic relief had taken place, impressive changes had occurred in patients' attitudes about their symptoms, and their symptoms clearly did not interfere as much with their overall functioning. More striking, however, was the finding that 80 to 90 percent of the patients had improved self-esteem, developed new attitudes, and increased self-understanding. New learning, better interpersonal relations, and improved problem solving were found in 70 to 80 percent. Finally and most significantly, 62 percent of patients were actually using their new learning, and 67 percent were using their new problem-solving skills, to solve emotional problems encountered long after the treatment had ended. With this finding, the patients showed that they had incorporated certain aspects of their therapy and were applying them effectively in their everyday lives. It was interesting to hear the patients describe how, when faced with a current psychological difficulty, they would recreate the therapeutic situation mentally in the form of "an internalized dialogue." One part would ask the questions and make the confrontations that the therapist had made during STAPP, while the other part would provide information and associations, thus reinforcing and facilitating the problem-solving process.

Of particular interest was the status of the control patients at the end of their waiting period and before STAPP. Less than half had any symptomatic improvement while waiting, as a result either of actions they took or of beneficial environmental changes. What was more striking was that no other characterological changes had taken place. There were, for example, no changes in the patients' underlying conflicts, and because of this, they were motivated to undertake psychotherapy. Furthermore, no patients showed evidence of improvement on any of the other outcome criteria that have been enumerated.

After these same control patients had completed their therapy, though, they compared favorably with their experimental counterparts on all three dimensions of the outcome criteria. They also mentioned that they were using what they had learned in order to solve new emotional problems.

During the 1970s, the author and his colleagues repeated this kind of control study at the Beth Israel Hospital's Department of Psychiatry clinic in Boston (Sifneos, 1975a; Sifneos et al. 1980). Only patients who had as their focus an unresolved oedipal problem were chosen, and all the therapists, both male and female, were supervised individually by the author and Dr. George Fishman to make sure that they were acquainted with and were correctly using all the technical requirements of STAPP. Patients again were seen by two independent evaluators, and they were accepted for study only when it was unanimously agreed that they fulfilled the criteria for STAPP and had an unresolved oedipal problem.

This study used nine outcome criteria similar to the ones used in the earlier study. The first eight criteria accounted for 50 percent of the total score and included specification of improvement or changes in (1) symptoms, (2) interpersonal relations, (3) self-esteem, (4) attitudes, (5) learning, (6) problem solving, (7) self-understanding, and (8) work performance. The ninth was referred to as SIP (Special Internal Predisposition), and it accounted for the other 50 percent of the total score. The SIP criterion involved a change in the basic predisposing factors that were specific to each patient and believed to be responsible for his or her unresolved oedipal problem. Finally, based on the patient's scores on the criteria, the evaluators rated the overall improvement of the patient as "recovered," "much better," "a little better," or "unchanged."

Out of the total of 29 patients (22 experimental and 7 control), 28 were seen in follow-up interviews. Of these, 18 patients (14 experimental and 4 control) were considered "recovered"; 6 patients (4 experimental and 2 control) were "much better"; 3 experimental patients were "a little better," and 1 experimental patient was "unchanged." When the 7 control patients were seen at the end of their waiting period, 3 were a little better, having had some symptomatic improvement without any other noticeable change, while 4 were unchanged. (One control patient seen after the end of the waiting period withdrew although unchanged, having decided to leave the Boston area.)

These findings, again involving small numbers, were similar to those from the earlier study. An important component of the later study, however, was that the patient group was homogeneous; they were all individuals with unresolved oedipal problems who also fulfilled the criteria for selection. It was thus concluded that STAPP was a treatment especially indicated for the needs of such patients.

Our failures, it should be noted, can in many ways be viewed as more instructive than our successes. Three of the experimental patients who were rated only "a little better" and one patient who was rated "unchanged" were individuals in whom we had inadequately evaluated "motivation for change." With these patients, when their anxiety diminished during therapy, their motivation seemed also to decrease; the outcome of their therapy was therefore not as satisfactory as might have been expected.

CONCLUSION
STAPP has opened the door to the systematic investigation of the outcome of psychotherapy, has introduced innovative techniques, and has emphasized the systematic selection of appropriate patients with circumscribed problems. In addition, STAPP has demonstrated its technique for everyone to see and has in this way provided a promising teaching experience for younger therapists. Finally, STAPP has considerably reduced the costs of psychotherapy, a problem which is becoming increasingly important during the 1980s.

Chapter 3 # Time Limited Psychotherapy
by James Mann, M.D.

THE MEANING AND SIGNIFICANCE OF TIME
Time and our concept of time are the means by which we integrate in our minds and in our feelings what was, what is, and what will be. In his first book (Mann, 1973), the author reviewed some of the fascinating aspects of time and time perception in their psychological meaning, particularly on the unconscious level. Hartocollis (1972) has studied and written extensively about the unconscious meaning of time and its contribution to superego and ego development and also about the important connection between time and affects. Memories, something from the past, cannot be separated from time, and as we recall memories, knowledge about ourselves increases little by little. Knowledge and memory are one and the same thing. As the patient reviews and picks up threads of his or her past, present, and future, the patient is at the same time expanding his or her awareness of what was, what is, and what will be. In every case, our interventions and our interviewing techniques serve to stimulate this kind of temporal review. Regardless of the patient's current problems, any kind of psychological treatment aims toward helping the patient confront the past so that he or she may gain confidence in mastering the present, and then feel freer in deciding upon the future.*

Time and the development of reality sense go hand in hand. The child's accomplishment in learning to tell time on the clock constitutes a significant addition to the child's sense of reality. Time now no longer has infinite duration, but clearly has various durations, all of which are limited. Time as having an end now has meaning, and with this meaning comes the awareness that there is a specific end to time known as death. We experience time both as duration and as intensity. These will vary

*Editor's note: Dr. Robert Michels, in his review of contemporary psychoanalytic thought regarding interpretation (*Psychiatry Update: Volume II*, Part I, pages 61–70), explores the concept of the past with a particular emphasis on its meaningful, but not causal, relationship to the patient's present.

in relation to each other in accord with our immediate state of mind. Furthermore, since we are considering time in its psychological meaning and not in its physical or philosophical frame, we may think of two major types of time: categorical time and existential time. The first is the time that we know by reference to clocks and calendars; the second is the time that is lived in, experienced.

When we offer a patient any kind of treatment, whether for physical ailments or for psychological ailments or both, we know that the patient has certain conscious and unconscious expectations. Consciously, the patient wishes for relief from physical or psychological pain and for a restoration of the previously experienced self. Unconsciously, the expectations are far more global. In all instances, there is the expectation of magical cure, of some kind of total fulfillment, an unconscious search for a change from what one is into what one always wished to be. In any case, our patients' conscious and unconscious hopes are that we will turn back time, that we will repair what was so that what is will be so altered as to make certain a different and better future.

The greater the ambiguity with respect to the duration of treatment, the more does child time predominate, that is, the idea that time is endless and has the constant possibility of fulfillment. Clinically, we recognize this child time in the regression that is a regular and expected occurrence in any kind of long-term psychotherapy or in psychoanalysis. The greater the specificity with respect to the duration of treatment, the more rapidly is child time confronted with real time and the work to be done. This leads to an important element in time limited psychotherapy (TLP): the patient knows in advance the end date of treatment.

Insofar as each present moment immediately becomes something of the past and each moment that lies ahead becomes an element of the future, it is quite impossible to think of any "now" that does not include past, present, and future. By the same token, this conglomerate now carries conscious and unconscious affects that are attached to all three dimensions of time. Thus, we see the patient speaking of painful events or situations of the past or present and holding the expectation that the future may bring the same pain, with sadness or with tears or with anger. We also see the patient relating what we recognize as painful recollections and expectations without any of these manifest affects. In this latter patient, we understand the need to repress or otherwise defend against the affects that are located in time. The classical example of this patient is the obsessional patient whose affects are totally isolated from thoughts; the work of therapy is to undo defenses so that what the patient thinks and feels are experienced as a unity. This very same obsessional patient may also be obsessed with time, punctilious about appointments, wedded to clocks and calendars, constantly aware of the pressure of time. The opposite is also seen, an obsessive need to be late, to ignore clocks and calendars, and to live as though time did not exist. In brief, we live within a framework of time that always includes painful recollections of the past and the present along with painful expectations of the future. The pain is avoided by a variety of psychological and physical defense mechanisms. When these begin to fail and the pain becomes intolerable, the patient seeks our help.

With the patient now before us, we come to the second major foundation of TLP, the selection of the central issue. As soon as possible, any psychotherapy that is to be brief must of necessity zero in on some particular issue that will be the work of the therapy. In the literature, this is referred to as establishing a focus. The author uses the term *central issue*, rather than focus, in order to distinguish it as something quite different in its construction, its meaning to the patient, its connection with time, and its function in the therapeutic process.

THE BRIDGE BETWEEN TIME AND THE CENTRAL ISSUE

In the usual course of events, patients come to us and elaborate, or we help them to elaborate, their reasons for seeking help. In general, they will enlighten us with a symptom or a series of symptoms and complaints. In some instances, the patient can only disclose a vague sense of unease or uncertainty.

The first step, then, is to evaluate the patient's status so that two decisions may be made, a tentative diagnostic decision regarding the severity of the patient's mental state and whether TLP would be suitable and a decision about what would be the central issue. In most instances, this can be accomplished in one to three interviews. Bypassing the question of suitability for TLP for the present, let us look to the selection of the central issue, that issue which will be the center of attention throughout the 12 sessions of treatment.

The Selection of the Central Issue

The evaluation searches for those recurrent events in the patient's life which may appear factually to be very different one from the other, but which may be understood psychodynamically to be symbolically very similar for the patient. That is to say, although these events appear different, the patient's response is invariably similar. Discerning this requires that the therapist listen in a particular way. Too often we pay close attention to the facts of the patient's history, but neglect to ask ourselves the question, In the light of what this person is telling me about some life event or circumstance, how must this person have felt about him- or herself while experiencing or living that event or circumstance? Answering this question, the therapist can recognize a present and chronically endured pain, with repetitive experiences that may differ in character, but that are similar in the way the patient experienced them. Out of these data, the therapist recognizes that for this patient there has always been *an affective statement to him- or herself about how he or she feels and has always felt about the self.* At times, this statement is preconscious: for fleeting moments in a given situation, the patient may be consciously aware of this chronic pain about the self, only to ward off immediately any further consideration of it by bringing into play characteristic adaptive modes that will obscure from him- or herself that painful self-statement. For example, the ever-smiling and gracious person may conceal an exquisitely poignant sensitivity to rejection as an unworthy person by continuing to smile and be gracious. The central issue is one that is linked with time sense and with the various affects that are attached to the particular patient's time line or history. As a result, the central issue in every case will be totally different from the complaints that bring the patient for help. The central issue is thus vastly different from the usual "focus," which generally directs attention to one or another of the patient's complaints as the work of the treatment.

A 45-year-old woman asked for help in managing her rebellious teenage daughter who was driving her to distraction, despite the patient's very genuine efforts to be understanding and helpful. The evaluation revealed a series of life events beginning when the patient was 3. Her parents and others imposed an enormous amount of unusual control over her, and this was subsequently reenacted in a variety of environmental situations. The feeling of being controlled, manipulated as though she were a puppet, with the feelings of helplessness that followed, were once more being experienced in a way that only a rebellious teenager could arouse.

The central issue for this patient was not therefore how she might contrive better management methods for her daughter, but rather how she might deal with her old feelings of being controlled and helpless.

The Formulation of the Central Issue

Elsewhere the author and Goldman (1982) have proposed a scheme of the varieties of feelings in order to indicate the limited range available and therefore identifiable in any person. In this scheme, any feeling about the self can be placed under one of five headings: (1) glad, (2) sad, (3) mad, (4) frightened, or (5) guilty. The importance of this scheme for the present discussion is that it makes easier the formulation of the central issue. The central issue is always formulated so as to include time, affects, and the image of the self, and the image of the self will always be found under one of the five headings.

The therapist's statement of the central issue does not include anything about the patient's conflict with any significant others. These conflicts will emerge soon enough with diminished defensiveness and with a greater sense of trust in the therapist. The patient must not only feel understood, but must also feel that the therapist is on his or her side. If the therapist states that the patient's problem lies in a conflict with some other, the patient will tend to respond with the same automatic defensiveness that has always marked his or her response to that particular issue. The central issue, on the other hand, is an empathic statement, in which the therapist discloses that he or she understands how much the patient has struggled to master pain. The patient feels understood as never before.

ILLUSTRATIVE CENTRAL ISSUES

1. You have had a very difficult time and have put in a lot of hard work to get where you are. . . . What troubles you and always has is the feeling that too much is always demanded of you . . . more than you feel you should give since you get so little in return. [A 34-year-old man complaining of depression and multiple hypochondriacal concerns about melanoma, leukemia, heart disease, and hypertension that interfere with his work.]

2. You are a talented woman and you've achieved a good deal of success. Nevertheless, you are troubled now and always have been troubled with the feeling that there is something about you that is bad and unworthy. [A 49-year-old woman complaining of both anxiety and depression, with particular emphasis on her fear of oncoming menopause.]

Each of these central issues carries specific messages. They begin with the therapist's recognition of the patient's genuine efforts, in part successful, to achieve certain goals. These are not messages of false assurance, since they accurately describe what the therapist has learned about the patient from the patient. The central issue then informs the patient that the therapist is aware of how the patient feels and has always felt about the self despite his or her best efforts. In each instance, the work of treatment will confine itself to learning together what happened that led the patient to feel in this particularly negative way about the self. It may be noted now that each of these central issues includes time, affects, and the image of the self.

TIME, THE CENTRAL ISSUE, AND THERAPEUTIC CHANGE

The particular importance of time in TLP is that the relatively short duration of treatment limits regression and subsequently short-circuits infantile expectation. The more indefinite the length of therapy, the more likely the development of an underlying, fixed maternal transference. The power of such a transference, with its promise of uninterrupted gratification, security, and even immortality, supports the patient's refusal to give up that for which he or she came to treatment in the first place. Prolonged therapeutic stalemates may occur, with the patient unconsciously fighting improvement in order to ward off the dreaded termination, which always reinvokes the reality principle. The anticipation of termination also means a confrontation with separation, an end to the timeless state, and the renewed awareness that time, in life, has its intensities, but even more so its distinct durations, including aging and death.

For a child to grow up and confront reality, to renounce infantile wishes and replace them with more aim-inhibited ones, and finally to accept mortality, it is necessary to strike a bargain with life. The bargain involves the promise of future gratification as the price for renouncing the old. In our patients, the road has been littered with broken promises and repeated, even unending, disappointments. Growing up the first time was sufficiently difficult; betrayal will not occur a second time. TLP aims at both a dynamic and a genetic experiential appreciation of the conflicts involved in the guiding fiction about the self within the context of powerful transference reactions, which in turn reflect intense childhood wishes toward primary figures.

A special attempt is made at the very beginning of TLP to link a profound notion about the self to factors of time (as duration) and time (as intensity) in the intense affect present. Even though we may not be able to detect whether the important etiologic traumas occurred at a specific age or ages, the patient will invariably state that he or she has always felt this way about the self. Powerful traumas, at least through adolescence, profoundly influence either unconscious guilt or narcissistic equilibriums or, most often, both. Negative influences on either of these then affect relationships back to the primary internal objects, the parents. Since the relationships hark back to childhood, when the earliest introjections occur, objective time is obliterated as far as affective experience is concerned. The felt myth about the self is experienced as always having been there. This adds to the patient's sense of hopelessness, for the patient cannot believe that something experienced so powerfully for so long can easily be removed. The result is a forever quality to the pain and the sense that resolution in the future is impossible. The therapeutic impact of the central issue embraces the always, the intensity of the pain, the way in which the patient has experienced it, and the efforts at adaptation. The therapeutic work proceeds at a rapid pace as a result of the therapeutic alliance and positive transference and the knowledge that time is limited.

Early in treatment, the patient subjectively experiences the duration of treatment as unrealistically long. When the midpoint comes and passes, time seems to be flying, as the patient perceives the relationship to the therapist rapidly coming to a close. Deep transference experiences profoundly affect one's relationship to one's internal objects. Without this occurrence, there would likely be no therapeutic progress. Repeated interpretations link the loss of the therapist with past losses, with past and present symptoms, and with misconceptions about the self and the resulting maladaptive behavior, which are in turn more permanently reduced. The patient becomes more confident of making it alone.

CLINICAL TECHNIQUE IN TLP

The Treatment Proposal
The evaluation is complete when the information is sufficient to enable the formulation of a central issue in the terms noted. The formulation is done in the therapist's time, and the central issue is presented exactly as planned at the next meeting. If the patient does not respond when the central issue is presented, the therapist asks for a reaction. In most cases, patients respond that they have been read correctly. Others may not be so certain, but are sufficiently touched to want to consider it further.

The full treatment proposal is then offered to the patient. The therapist tells the patient that treatment will consist of 12 meetings, with this one (at which the central issue is stated) being the first and the final one being on a date already determined by previous study of the calendar. Again, response from the patient is solicited if none is forthcoming. Since it is not possible here to review all the various responses patients may give, suffice it to say that the empathic pertinence of the central issue and the patient's optimism on hearing that he or she can be helped in such a short time results in almost zero refusals to continue. The therapist then goes on to propose that meetings will occur once each week for 45, 50, or 60 minutes (whichever is the therapist's usual procedure) and that the work will center on learning what happened in the patient's life that led the patient to feel this way about him- or herself. Then the therapist seeks the patient's approval for the full treatment proposal and asks the patient to begin the work.

With the 12 meetings once each week, and with the one or more evaluation sessions already held, the total period of contact between patient and therapist will extend over a period of about three or four months. The end date now known to the patient seems to be far into the future. More immediately, the patient is moved by the impact of the central issue and by the optimism generated through the treatment proposal, and a process is set in motion in which the guidelines for the therapist are very clear in the pursuit of a specific treatment goal. The exact beginning of treatment is evident, and equally clear are the midpoint and the precise end. Further, the therapist can expect that the patient will respond in reasonably predictable ways to the beginning phase of treatment, to the middle phase especially as the midpoint is reached, and to the approaching end or termination of treatment.

The Phases of Treatment

The description of the TLP treatment phases serves as a guide for the therapist in learning the sources of the patient's negative self-image, their repetition in the patient's current life, and their experience in the transference to the therapist. In all three phases of treatment, it is obligatory for the therapist to attend only to those expressions of thoughts, feelings, and behavior that relate directly or derivatively to the central issue. A word of caution: since no two patients are alike in the biological and the psychological schemata that have fashioned them as individuals, it should not be expected that the phases of treatment will always be similar.

The first phase of treatment is determined by the patient's response to the central issue and the time limit. Most often, the patient will present a spontaneous flow of associations and recollections that corroborate the precision of the stated central issue. A sense of optimism follows, as the abreaction that is taking place confers a sense of relief and trust. Barring the appearance of resistance, which must be met promptly, the therapist's interventions are only in the direction of stimulating further associations and recollections to be mentally recorded for later use.

The second phase of treatment is marked by the patient's awareness, sometimes conscious and sometimes totally repressed, that the midpoint of treatment is about to come or has already come. The patient usually responds with expressed discouragement, ambivalence, and loss of optimism, and often with the return of the initial complaints. This is the familiar situation in which the patient says, "I have told you all I know about myself, so where do we go from here?" Rather than responding with reassurance (or with sinking inner feelings), the therapist understands the patient's reaction to be a return of ambivalence experienced with earlier important figures as the patient begins to perceive dimly that separation and loss are in the offing. The patient's unconscious pathological need is to attempt a separation that will be similar to the one earlier experienced, and hence ambivalent, to conclude with the same negative feelings about the self as earlier and since repeatedly experienced. The therapist therefore neither reassures nor becomes discouraged. Rather, by encouraging the patient's ambivalence and disappointment in the process, the therapist learns still more about the pertinent circumstances and feelings that have given rise to the patient's dysfunction. The therapist is also very much aware that the patient is engaged in powerful transference reactions. For example, one may here see directly in the patient's behavior the manner in which the patient managed relationships to the important earlier persons as well as to people in his or her current life. The therapist may or may not offer transference interpretations, depending again upon the particular patient, the intensity of his or her reactions, and the therapist's judgment about the need to diminish the patient's reaction to manageable levels or to overcome major resistance.

The end phase of treatment is the most difficult for both patient and therapist. It is imperative that the last two or three meetings be devoted to exploring and dealing with the patient's reactions to the end of treatment. Invariably, patients are surprised that the end is near; the end date, known from the start, is usually denied and in some instances totally repressed. If, by the ninth or tenth session at the latest, the patient has made no mention of the end either directly or indirectly through associations, the therapist is obliged to raise this issue.

Transference and Countertransference

The major problem then becomes the patient's transference and the therapist's countertransference. In the opening phase of treatment, transference is usually very positive. The patient feels the therapist's confidence in him or her, the central issue has touched deeply, and trust in the therapist is very high. In the middle phase, the transference tends to become ambivalent, as skepticism about the result of treatment and symptomatic regression are likely to be present. In the end phase of treatment, the affective tenor changes once more. In all the sessions prior to the end phase, the affective tone has been maintained at a high level, and the patient's involvement has been constantly intense. In the end phase, that intensity becomes even greater, as the patient is confronted with an agreed-upon end date and cannot help yielding to a mixture of emotions, all of which are directly related to the central issue. The patient does not wish to end, to separate and tolerate still another loss. In all the patient's previous encounters with separations, he or she has been impelled unconsciously to respond not only ambivalently, but also with repetitively experienced damaged feelings about the self. The patient struggles with the therapist in the accustomed manner, but with a major difference. That difference consists in all that the patient has learned about him- or herself up to that point and in all that the therapist now knows about the patient's image of the self with its mélange of feelings. Most important, the therapist knows that the patient's transference makes the patient feel toward the therapist precisely as he or she had felt toward the important earlier person(s) and that the patient expects to be disposed of in the very terms of the central issue. With the earlier example of the patient in whom the central issue was too much having been demanded of him, more than he felt he should give since he has gotten so little in return, that patient will in the end phase experience this same feeling toward the therapist. He has worked hard, he has given of himself to the therapist, and now he must be left.

The patient is caught up in a mixture of feelings, including a minimal trace of being glad and maximal expressions of being mad, sad, frightened, and guilty. The therapist is enforcing a separation that repeats for the patient the situation which the patient left originally and then repeatedly left with damaged feelings about the self. This time, however, there is the opportunity to correct the reaction and the response to separation and loss. The therapist speaks directly to the transference reactions of the patient: how the patient has come to regard the therapist as he or she regarded father (or mother or some other significant earlier person), the kinds of feelings that person aroused, how as a child the patient had little recourse but to conclude that there was something lacking about him or her, how this negative feeling about the self gave rise to coping efforts which continue into present relationships, and how these efforts continually fail to spare the patient from pervasive, chronic pain. These interpretations are reinforced by rich illustrations from the patient's accounts in the preceding sessions. They are illustrations from the patient's life which point up how the misconception about the self arose, was always maintained, and is now experienced with the therapist.

The therapist makes every effort to help the patient recognize the mixture of feelings regarding the therapist. As might be expected, anger is likely to be the most difficult for the patient to expose. In this connection, it may not be until the 10th or 11th session that the patient reports some kind of regressive acting-out response. The time limit and the particular kind of central issue used in TLP are remarkably effective in almost eliminating acting out. If acting out does occur in TLP, it occurs at this point and is an expression of unspoken anger toward the therapist.

The time limit and the central issue combine to bring about a telescoping of psychodynamic events that results not only in a proliferation of data, but also in a constant heightened affective state within the treatment. Both the patient and the therapist come to the end phase highly involved with each other. It is not just the patient who must confront separation and loss with its attendant psychological consequences. All human beings suffer the scars of the multiple separations and losses we must all endure, and none of us manages these events totally successfully. The patient's reactions to the termination of treatment reverberate within the therapist. Each therapist cannot help being subject to the vicissitudes of his or her own separation experiences. Again, the time limit, the awareness that treatment will indeed end on the known date, forecloses stalling on the part of the therapist. Still, the therapist may seek ways of delaying the end. Perhaps, if so much has been done for the patient, would not a little more be even more helpful? Perhaps the patient is right about not being ready to stop treatment. Or perhaps, in the 11th session, the patient may complain of the return of an old symptom or even of a new one. Might it not be better to continue? More properly, the therapist recognizes that both patient and therapist are resistant to enduring the separation and that both have their own particular reasons.

Another important countertransference element lies in the central issue itself. It is probably a truism that each person carries within some question about some aspect of the integrity of the self. The particular central issue presented to a patient may touch upon a similar issue in the therapist. Both the time limit and this particular central issue may serve as major countertransference difficulties for the therapist.

INDICATIONS AND LIMITATIONS

A close study of TLP in practice would soon reveal that the same kind of central issue seems appropriate for an inordinate number of patients. The question then arises whether we are fitting patients to a procrustean couch. The fact is that the same kind of central issue will indeed be applicable to a large number of patients. The reason for this lies in our understanding that only a limited number of feelings are available to all human beings. Since every self-image is conceptualized in terms of words which denote a feeling about the self, it follows that similar central issues will apply. The central issue should also be understood as the gateway to the unique manner in which each patient has come to feel about him- or herself. Nonetheless, although many other feelings will emerge which may seem to deviate sharply from the central issue, in the course of treatment a great variety of feelings about the self will be subsumed under the dominant one of the central issue.

In regard to the selection of cases, space limitation here allows only for some specific contraindications and several generalizations about suitability. Conditions such as schizophrenia, manic-depressive states, psychotic depressions, severe borderline states, and severe narcissistic disorders should not be treated in any short form of psychotherapy. Borderline states and narcissistic disorders possessing a number of effective neurotic defenses are suitable cases. In addition, two major generalizations regarding suitability are applicable. First, the patient's history should reveal a capacity for engaging quickly and disengaging quickly without suffering unduly, which may be determined by his or her history of managing successive losses. Second, regardless of the degree of disruption in the early environment, the patient should, for reasons unknown, have nevertheless managed to achieve a satisfactory state of stability as manifested in current work and relationships. TLP is thus a suitable therapeutic method for a wide variety of patients in whom one makes a positive assessment of ego strength despite known developmental difficulties. In any case, the process of TLP is such that the therapist will always know enough by the third or fourth treatment session either to warrant continuing on to the prescribed end, or to recognize a serious diagnostic error has been made and that the mode of treatment must be changed accordingly.

Chapter 4

Cognitive Therapy†
by A. John Rush, M.D.

THEORETICAL BACKGROUND
Cognitive therapy derives from the so-called phenomenological approach to psychology (Spiegelberg, 1971; 1972). The phenomenological emphasis assigns a central role to one's view of oneself and of the world as determinants of behavior, an idea initially proposed by the Greek Stoic philosophers. Alfred Adler emphasized the idea that each person lives in a personal conceptualization of the objective world (Ansbacher and Ansbacher, 1956). The profusion of stimuli that bombard us are immediately organized, conceptualized, and given meaning based upon our individual and very personal prior experiences. Adler termed this constructed representation of objective reality the "phenomenal field." The

†The author wishes to express his appreciation to Ms. Marie Marks and Ms. Judy Bement for secretarial assistance and to Dr. Kenneth Z. Altshuler, Professor and Chairman of the Department of Psychiatry, for his administrative support.

phenomenal field as a construct is used to explain why different people respond differently to the same event or series of events. For example, one person might see moving to a new city as an adventure, while another might see the same move as a loss. Thus, it is not things in themselves, but rather the views that we take of things, that upset or please us.

The phenomenological emphasis apparently arose in part from a dissatisfaction with the concept of unconscious motivation for explaining and predicting various behaviors. Generally speaking, unconscious motivation is inferred from a behavior or a series of behaviors by examining the end products of the behavior(s). The clinician assumes that these end products are expressions of the individual's unconscious wishes and desires. Thus, even if the person denies actually desiring the end products of a behavioral sequence, the testimony may be discounted.

If the consequence(s) of a behavior constitute the *sole* basis for inferring unconscious motivations, diagnostic errors may result. For instance, one may erroneously infer an unconscious desire from a behavioral consequence that the individual actually neither desired nor foresaw. Motivational inferences that rely exclusively upon the consequences of a behavior assume (1) that a person can make anything happen that he or she wants, (2) that nothing happens that a person does not want, and (3) that a person can consciously or unconsciously foresee all the consequences of any particular behavioral sequence before undertaking it. Obviously, these assumptions are rarely applicable to everyday situations.

On the other hand, the cognitive perspective assumes that a person chooses those options that are in his or her own best interest, based upon a particular, albeit idiosyncratic, view of things. Not only are these views rarely objective, but they are often highly biased in a stereotyped fashion. Thus, self-defeating behaviors do not come from a desire to lose, for example, but from the person's inability to either conceive of, or to act upon and carry out, more constructive alternative plans of action.

Initially, the cognitive therapist clarifies how the patient views things (that is, how the patient conceptualizes and gives meaning to particular events). What are the bases for these views? Are they accurate? To what behaviors and feelings do these views lead? For instance, a depressed patient often fails to undertake specific measures that might relieve the depression. In the cognitive view, this is not because the patient wants to suffer (one of several possible unconscious motivational assumptions). Rather, it is because the patient does not conceive of undertaking particular steps to reduce the depression, does not believe that any action will result in relief, or does not believe that he or she could successfully undertake these steps or actions. If a patient is convinced that corrective actions are unavailable or doomed to failure, this conviction logically leads to a decision not to try.

The cognitive explanatory system allows for direct empirical testing of many of the presumed determinants of behavior. If a patient's view of events leads to particular responses, and if this view is available to consciousness, then the relationship between this view and the observed behaviors can be evaluated. Indeed, the cognitive theory is supported by a variety of empirical data. (For a detailed review, see Beck and Rush, 1978.)

THERAPEUTIC TECHNIQUE IN COGNITIVE THERAPY

Cognitive therapy is a generic term which refers to a variety of psychotherapeutic techniques developed and applied within the perspective of cognitive theory. The techniques are designed to accomplish the following specific objectives. (1) Patients learn to become aware of the views that they take of various events, particularly of upsetting events. (The therapist leads the patient to recognize and examine his or her "phenomenal field.") (2) Patients learn to assess, reality test, and correct these views, to make a better match between objective reality and the particular meanings they attribute to specific events. Thus, stereotyped perceptions are identified and corrected. (3) Patients learn to identify specific schemata or silent assumptions by inferring general rules from what they say and think in various situations. These schemata are not conscious thoughts or behaviors; rather, they are the premises by which a person weighs, encodes, and gives meaning to specific events. (4) Patients practice various cognitive and behavioral responses to anticipated and unusual stresses. (5) Patients generate new assumptions and apply them to actual and anticipated circumstances.

The therapist acts as a guide. The data of therapy consist of cognitions or thoughts, as well as behaviors and feelings, that the patient records or reports. The therapist uses both the experiences within the therapeutic relationship and the data provided by the patient about ongoing interpersonal relationships to teach the patient to recognize and correct stereotyped, biased thinking and self-defeating behavioral patterns.

The relationship between cognitions, schemata, and logical errors, the three critical elements in cognitive theory, deserves further comment. *Cognitions* are thoughts or images that are available to consciousness. They are the immediate, nearly automatic ideas to which each person is subject when confronted with any situation. Their content reflects the meaning the person gives to any situation. Cognitions are not what a person thinks *about* a situation; rather, they are what a person thinks *in* a situation. These cognitions are closely tied to and are said to account for both the feelings raised and the behaviors displayed in the situation.

The relationship between *schemata* and cognitions may be illustrated by the cognititve theory of depression (see Table 1). Depressed persons have negatively biased views of themselves, their world, and their future (Beck, 1976; Beck and Rush, 1978; Rush and Beck, 1978a; 1978b). Much empirical data support this contention (Beck and Rush, 1978; Rush and Giles, 1982). Schemata are silent assumptions or beliefs derived from early experience that direct the person to attend to certain events, to ignore others, and to value and encode these events in particular ways. Thus, schemata account for cognitions. A careful, logical analysis of a series of cognitions enables the inference of the schema, which is typically an if-then statement. This statement is not thought by the patient, but is a rule that guides the patient's thinking. For example, "If I am not loved and valued by others, then my life has no meaning" might constitute such a rule. Depressed persons endorse a variety of such illogical notions. When an event occurs that would lead most people to transient dysphoria (for example, breaking up with a loved one or experiencing the death of a spouse), the person who bases his or her happiness and self-worth largely upon attention from this other person will develop a depressive syndrome that exceeds normal dysphoria. A schema

Table 1.   Cognitions and Schemata in Beck's Cognitive Theory of Depression

Cognitions	Consist of thoughts and images
	Reflect unrealistically negative views of self, world, and future
	Are based on schemata
	Are reinforced by current interpretations of events
	Explain symptoms of depressive syndrome
	Covary with severity of depression
	Show logical errors that are negatively distorted
Schemata	Consist of unspoken, inflexible assumptions or beliefs
	Result from past (early) experience
	Form the basis for screening, discriminating, weighing, and encoding stimuli
	Form the basis for categorizing and evaluating experiences, making judgments, and distorting actual experience
	Determine the content of cognitions formed in situations and the affective response to them
	Increase vulnerability to relapse

Source: Reprinted with permission from Rush AJ: Cognitive therapy of depression: Rationale, techniques, and efficacy. Psychiatr Clin North Am 6:105–127, 1983.

is activated and begins to influence how the person thinks about analogous events (for example, a friend forgetting to call at a specific time). Notions such as "I am generally unlovable" or "My life has no meaning" begin to enter consciousness. The depressed person construes otherwise neutral events as further evidence that these negative notions are true. For example, being ignored by a salesperson in a department store may stimulate such thoughts as "No one cares about me" or "I'll never get what I want." Schemata thus direct the content of cognitions and with depressed persons account for vulnerability to recurrence of depressive episodes.

Logical errors become evident when one examines the logical relationship between cognitions and the associated events. Consider the above case. When the friend forgets to call, the event is a nonevent; nothing at all actually happens. Furthermore, the patient's thought, "My life has no meaning," is unrelated to the nonevent. This arbitrary inference is a conclusion drawn on insufficient evidence. The thought, "I'll never get what I want," is an overgeneralization from the current frustrating circumstance in the store. Other logical errors include personalization (a neutral event given personal meaning), magnification, and selective attention (ignoring the positive aspects of a situation, and so on). These logical errors are the consequences, not the causes, of negatively biased thinking (Rush and Beck, 1978a; 1978b).

The Therapeutic Relationship

The therapeutic relationship must be carefully attended to in cognitive therapy (Beck et al., 1979; Rush, 1980; 1982a; 1982b). In fact, cognitive therapy (at least when limited to twenty sessions) is contraindicated with patients who have difficulty forming a working alliance within a short period of time (such as borderline patients). The therapist must be both empathic and objective. Empathically, the therapist must be able to think as the patient does, to understand both the cognitive and the emotional responses and to see the world as the patient does. At the same time, the therapist must remain objective and logical about the events reported and the patient's thinking.

Similarly, great tact is required in helping patients to become objective about their views. Depressed patients, for example, are notorious for overpersonalizing their interactions with others. When the therapist identifies and points out negatively biased thinking, many patients may feel as if they are being attacked. As one patient put it, "When I came here, I thought I had just a depression. Now you tell me I can't think straight either."

In developing a collaborative alliance, the therapist spends a great deal of time introducing the patient to the rationale for treatment. With depressed patients, the pamphlet, *Coping with Depression* (Beck and Greenberg, 1974), is a useful part of this introduction. In addition, patients are strongly encouraged to point out when they feel criticized or attacked during a session. Each session begins with a review of the patient's responses to the previous session, and each session is reviewed before the patient is dismissed.

Negative transference is dealt with through a cognitive framework (Beck, 1976; Beck et al., 1979; Rush, 1980). The patient's views of the therapist, the therapy, or specific transactions that were associated with increased dysphoria are elicited, evaluated collaboratively, and considered objectively. One patient, who was particularly sensitive to the therapist's behavior, reported thinking, "He doesn't want to see me," while she waited for ten minutes one day when the therapist was late. On another occasion, when the therapist was early, she thought, "I must be especially ill." On most occasions, when the therapist was punctual, she thought, "He's just running a factory and not taking a personal interest in me." When this pattern was elicited and examined, the patient readily saw that she came out the loser regardless of the therapist's behavior. Careful attention to the therapeutic relationship is essential to ensure compliance with homework, to reduce premature termination, and also to reveal negative cognitions and dysfunctional attitudes.

INDICATIONS
Cognitive therapy has been applied to a variety of psychopathological conditions, including major nonpsychotic, unipolar depressions, generalized anxiety disorders, phobic disorders, obesity, alcoholism, drug dependency, and chronic pain. Specific techniques will differ according to the condition and the phase of therapy. Cognitive theory (Beck, 1976) predicts the kinds of thinking patterns encountered with each disorder. For example, anxious patients frequently perceive danger in situations that are not dangerous, while depressed patients often see evidence for personal defects in situations in which no objective reasons for self-depreciation exist. Paranoid patients may misconstrue situations in terms of being gypped or attacked. Cognitive theory also suggests that specific beliefs are more commonly found in certain disorders. For example, the need for love, approval, or success is likely to underlie the negatively biased thinking in depression.

Most empirical data have documented the efficacy of this approach in depression. Outcome studies suggest that the depressed patients most suitable for this approach suffer from mild to moderate unipolar, nonpsychotic depressions and that they have the capacity to establish a working alliance in a short period of time. These patients appear most likely to obtain significant symptom reduction in ten weeks of treatment. Chronic depressions are not more responsive and may be less responsive than the acute disorders (Rush et al., 1978). Depressions with melancholic features (American Psychiatric Association, 1980) have not been systematically evaluated. At this point, such patients should receive pharmacotherapy or electroconvulsive therapy as a primary treatment.

Patients with endogenous features according to the Research Diagnostic Criteria (Spitzer et al., 1978) may or may not respond to cognitive therapy (Blackburn et al., 1981; Kovacs et al., 1981). While the answer to this controversial question awaits further research, the clinician is well advised not to use cognitive therapy as the sole therapeutic modality for symptom reduction with such patients. On the other hand, cognitive therapy may conceivably help some of these patients reach a better level of interepisode recovery, even if antidepressant medications are essential for initially obtaining symptom reduction. For example, consider a man who has endured three episodes of major depression with substantial, but not total, interepisode recovery. He may have obtained almost total symptomatic remission with amitriptyline. This patient has still spent a good deal of time in the recent past in a depressed state. This experience is likely to have affected his view of himself, his sense of competence, and his view of his future. Pharmacotherapy may not be as effective as cognitive psychotherapy in modifying such views, at least in the short run (Rush et al., 1982). He might profit from a short course (five to ten weeks) of cognitive therapy to help him to become more objective about both himself and his illness. Cognitive therapy may thus be indicated with patients who require antidepressants for symptom reduction, prophylaxis, or both, and who also need to modify specific self-defeating views or notions that either preceded or arose in conjunction with the depressive episodes.

While Beck and co-workers caution that many depressed patients may require medication or may not respond to cognitive therapy (Beck et al., 1979), specific contraindications to this treatment are yet to be identified. Clinical experience does suggest that patients with impaired reasoning abilities or memory function (e.g., organic brain syndromes), borderline personality structures, and schizoaffective disorder will not respond to brief cognitive therapy (Beck et al., 1979; Rush, 1980; 1982a). Whether antisocial personalities with major depression or other forms of secondary depressions will respond to cognitive therapy is yet to be empirically established.

Clinical experience also suggests that major depressions which accompany medical disorders may respond rapidly to cognitive therapy, except when the depression is biologically caused by the medical disorder (i.e., Organic Affective Disorder in DSM-III). Especially likely to benefit are patients who have no history of preexisting psychopathology. For example, patients with their first myocardial infarction, with some forms of cancer, or with physical injuries that require substantial psychological readjustment (e.g., blindness, loss of limb) can profit from this approach in as short a time as five weeks. Patients with more chronic, disabling, and progressive medical illnesses may profit to some degree, but will respond more slowly.

APPLICATIONS

The specific techniques of cognitive therapy for depression have been detailed elsewhere (Beck et al., 1979). The following case examples illustrate the application of some of these techniques to commonly encountered clinical situations. The first case illustrates a straightforward depression treated with medication and cognitive therapy.

Cognitive Therapy and Antidepressant Medication

Mr. L., a 52-year-old married father of two and a retired naval officer, referred himself, stating, "Maybe I am a manic-depressive and need lithium." He complained of guilt, difficulty concentrating, suicidal ideation, early morning and sleep-onset insomnia, anorexia, a 15-pound weight loss, social withdrawal, decreased libido, intermittent impotency, lack of interest in formerly enjoyable activities, and mild psychomotor retardation. Although he had no history of alcohol addiction, he had been given to excessive drinking since the onset of the depression.

His depression had been triggered three years previously when he discovered his wife's extramarital affair with a fellow officer. His wife terminated the affair when Mr. L. found out. A year later, he resigned from the service as a consequence of his depression.

Mr. L. believed he had forced his wife to stay with him by his discovery, although there was no evidence, even after several interviews with her, that this was a valid belief. She stated she chose to stay with him because she loved him. She saw the affair as a symptom of difficulties in the relationship. He spent most of his waking moments thinking about the affair, which he interpreted in terms of personal failure and inadequacy.

Mr. L. had had two other episodes of depressive syndrome in the past. Each episode lasted one year, each remitted without formal treatment, and each was associated with the failure to get promoted on time. He construed each of these events as evidence of his incompetence.

There was also suggestive evidence of hypomanic episodes, with increased activity, euphoria, energy and feelings of creativity, but these episodes failed to meet criteria for hypomania. The patient presented evidence by history and mental status of obsessive-compulsive personality. He showed significant concern over issues of respect, control, and time.

Treatment for this patient consisted of simultaneous pharmacotherapy and cognitive therapy. The cognitive therapy consisted of hourly sessions once weekly for a total of 16 sessions. Pharmacotherapy consisted of amitriptyline maintained at 100 to 150 mg/day until the 16th week of treatment, when it was discontinued. The therapy sessions initially included only the patient, but subsequently included his spouse as well. The patient's response to this treatment, measured by the Beck Depression Inventory (BDI), is shown below.

Week No.:	Initial	2	5	6	8	10	12	16	24
BDI Score:	19	10	7	4	5	1	0	2	7

Pharmacotherapy was intended to provide rapid symptomatic relief, since the patient appeared suicidal and hopeless at the beginning of treatment. Without rapid symptomatic relief, hospitalization appeared imminent. Another rationale for pharmacotherapy was to create a milieu in which psychological treatment might be better accepted by the patient; he expected, indeed nearly insisted on, drug treatment.

Cognitive therapy was designed to help this patient (1) identify and record his negative automatic thinking; (2) identify stimuli which triggered those negative thoughts; (3) provide methods to control these thoughts; (4) provide methods for the patient to refute and correct these thoughts; and (5) identify and correct the silent assumptions or themes which ran throughout and supported his negative thinking.

Step 1. Recording Cognitions. The patient recorded his thoughts and associated environmental events in his notebook. He reported a profusion of negative automatic thoughts or cognitions. These cognitions were repetitious, upsetting, distorted, and generally reflected a very negative view of himself. The content consisted of such statements as "I am a failure in my occupation . . . My wife has shown me I'm a failure in marriage . . . I can't get a job in civilian life . . . No one respects me . . . I've never succeeded at anything . . . Why bother to apply for a job, they'll never hire someone as old as I am . . . I can't even play tennis anymore."

Step 2. Recording Environmental Stimuli. By recording the environmental events associated with his negative thinking, the patient identified stimuli for this thinking. Exacerbating stimuli included playing tennis, having dinner with his wife, and looking at old Navy pictures. Drinking alcohol or walking in the woods alone decreased the frequency of this recurrent stream of self-critical thinking.

Step 3. Monitoring and Controlling Cognitions. The patient used a wrist counter to monitor the frequency of these thoughts and the stimuli associated with them. On the average, these thoughts occurred about sixty times per hour during most of the day. The patient then used a stopwatch and counter to record and graph the exact number of negative thoughts per minute for four days for every waking minute. With this technique, he gained some control over these thoughts, reducing them to as few as three to seven per hour. In addition, he began to look at his thinking more objectively (i.e., he began to regard these thoughts as upsetting, yet repetitious, psychological events, rather than as accurate reflections of reality).

Step 4. Correcting, Validating, and Refuting Cognitions. After he learned to control and to become more objective about his negative thoughts, he was able to begin to correct, validate, or refute each thought. When asked for evidence that these thoughts were true, he repeated the previous experiences of delayed promotion, failure to make admiral, and his current difficulty with sexual performance. He felt that his wife was too ashamed of her affair to seek a divorce and that this explained why she would go on living with him while she still loved her former lover. Furthermore, this lover had been of a higher rank than the patient, and the patient saw this as evidence that he was not good enough for his wife. He saw his wife as a bright, attractive, talented, artistic, and much admired and respected woman. In comparison, he saw himself as an occupational, marital, sexual, and social failure. He attributed his many military honors to "the system," while he attributed occupational failures to himself. In reviewing these thoughts, he learned to identify and correct the cognitive distortions of overgeneralization, arbitrary inference, and magnification.

Step 5. Identifying and Correcting Themes. He learned to identify specific themes which were inferred from the negative automatic thoughts he recorded. He learned to evaluate these themes with logic and, at times, with experimental testing. Examples of these themes are "Unless I do everything perfectly, I'm a failure . . . If I am not rewarded and respected, I'm a failure . . . If I make a mistake, it means I'm defective . . . Because my wife had an affair, she no longer loves or respects me . . . I can't enjoy anything if I'm not the best."

Initially, the patient enumerated a plethora of specific events from his past, each of which he construed as supporting these themes. Often his evidence went back 5 to 25 years prior to treatment. By reviewing the evidence point by point and suggesting alternative interpretations of the events reported, the patient developed enough doubt in his thinking that he would consider running an experiment to test the assumption or theme under consideration. For example, he was directed to lose intentionally at several sets of tennis with a mediocre player and at the same time to identify what else he might be enjoying while playing. He reported enjoying the exercise, conversation, weather, and other players at the club, and he thereby disentangled the issues of achievement and enjoyment.

He learned to see his wife's affair more as a reflection of her view of herself and the marriage, rather than as conclusive proof of some permanent defect in himself. By learning how he had inadvertently blocked communication (at least from his wife's viewpoint), he could take corrective action to discuss and solve problems, rather than concluding that he was a total failure by overgeneralizing from a few complaints from his wife.

At six-month follow-up the patient's BDI score was 6. He was taking no medication. He was employed full-time, still married, and not drinking excessively. He and his wife both reported a dramatic improvement in marital satisfaction.

This case illustrates the use of combined pharmacotherapy and cognitive therapy. The combination treatment may have certain advantages. Pharmacotherapy may provide rapid symptomatic relief (e.g., for insomnia), and it may also match the patient's expectations in such a way that the cognitive and behavioral change techniques can be applied. In this case, the cognitive therapy may have sufficiently corrected the patient's chronic negative distortion of past and present events to provide prophylaxis against future depressions.

This case further illustrates the value of involving a spouse in cognitive therapy. Often the spouse can provide information to correct cognitive distortions (Rush et al., 1975). Furthermore, as the spouse becomes aware of the patient's negative thinking, he or she can resort to verbal and nonverbal behaviors that will consistently disconfirm the patient's negative automatic thinking. These points are illustrated further in the discussion and case example which follow.

Couples Cognitive Therapy

There are both practical and theoretical reasons for involving the partner or significant other in cognitive therapy with selected depressed patients. Half the patients requesting psychotherapy do so because of marital difficulties (Sager et al., 1968). In addition, spouses are often concerned about their role in helping the patient. Neglecting the spouse may mean missing an opportunity to engage an ally or to disarm an inadvertent enemy of treatment.*

Theoretically, improved efficacy of treatment may result if the spouse actively supports therapy. For example, in behavioral treatment of obese outpatients, a significantly greater weight loss resulted when treatment was delivered in a couples format than when the spouse was uncooperative or refused to participate in treatment (Brownell et al., 1977). Behavioral techniques for the treatment of sexual dysfunctions have also been adapted to a dyadic format to improve efficacy (Masters and Johnson, 1970; Kaplan, 1974). In addition, the depression and the marriage may be closely related. Berman and Lief (1975) have detailed the nature of marital relationships and the various stages of development. In theory, depression can be conceptualized to result from a failure to resolve these developmental stages or to correct a maladaptive relationship. Thus the treatment of depression would logically involve the marital system. The relationship may also serve to maintain idiosyncratic beliefs and distorted cognitions that in turn maintain the depression. The importance of social systems in preserving selected beliefs has been emphasized both by social anthropologists (Spradley, 1972) and by psychotherapy researchers (Khatami and Rush, 1978; Bergner, 1977).

Interaction between the members of a couple has important effects on the beliefs and perceptions of each spouse. The spouse of the depressed patient cannot be considered neutral. He or she becomes frustrated, confused, overly solicitous, or angry, or withdraws emotionally. These attitudes and behaviors may readily serve to reinforce the depressed patient's negative view of self and the world. Thus the spouse's behavior can reinforce and maintain the very cognitive distortions alleged to contribute to a depression. An essential objective of engaging the nondepressed spouse in treatment consists of reversing this potentially negative environmental input. In assessment, the spouse may provide information about specific events preceding the depressive reaction. During treatment, the spouse may assist in collecting behavioral data or in providing positive reinforcement for compliance with homework assignments. Often the spouse can serve as a more objective reporter of events or provide more realistic perceptions and conceptualizations of specific situations. In some cases, the spouse can articulate idiosyncratic beliefs or silent assumptions upon which the patient bases behavior. For example, the spouse may readily identify the patient's insistence on achievement as a necessary condition for feeling happy or satisfied.

Finally, by directly observing the couple, the therapist can discern patterns of interaction that are aggravating the depression. For example, the therapist can identify the depressed person's tendency to present his or her viewpoint apologetically or to fail to participate in decision making affecting the couple. The therapist may then elicit distorted cognitions that support this type of behavior (e.g., "I don't want to hurt his/her feelings" or "My opinion is less important"). When these thoughts

*Editor's note: In Part III of *Psychiatry Update: Volume II,* Dr. Ellen Berman discusses several conceptual models and techniques of marital therapy (pages 215–228). Couples' sexual problems and various treatment approaches are among the topics of Part I of *Psychiatry 1982 (Psychiatry Update: Volume I),* "The Psychiatric Aspects of Sexuality."

are brought to the attention of both spouses, the nondepressed member can frequently offer alternative perceptions of these behaviors and provide information to correct the distorted cognitions. The following case illustrates how cognitive techniques can be used in a couples format.

Mrs. X., a 33-year-old married mother of four, was referred with a severe depressive syndrome of 4½ months' duration. She had had three previous episodes of depression, each lasting approximately 4 months. Her mother had died of leukemia when the patient was 12. She described her father as "strict and cold." She saw her stepmother as loving but very critical and demanding.

At evaluation, Mrs. X. complained that she was a burden to her family, that she wanted to be "close" to her husband and children, but that she was unable to express her love. She reported fearing visits from her parents and in-laws because she was "in terrible shape." She was extremely nonassertive and had a very poor repertoire of parenting skills. She feared that she would lose control and hurt her children. The children habitually expressed their love for their mother in response to her questions. She discounted these expressions of affection, while feeling extremely guilty about having struck her eldest child in anger.

Mrs. X.'s husband was an easygoing, successful professional who rarely expressed feelings and was generally oversolicitious. Nine years previously the couple had separated for several months, believing that they were incompatible. The results of cognitive treatment are shown below as measured by the patient's BDI scores.

Week No.:	Initial	1	4	7	10	13	16	24	30
BDI Score:	41	22	26	17	24	22	3	18	7

Step 1. Recording Cognitions. The patient recorded her depressive cognitions for several weeks. She learned that she continually read rejection into her family's behavior (e.g., in one day, she recorded 27 instances of thinking, "No one really cares for me"). She believed that she was "worthless," which served to explain why no one could care about her. The evidence for these beliefs included her inability to demonstrate affection, her withdrawal from and criticism of her husband, and her continual requests for love.

Step 2. Identifying Cognitions and Behaviors Within the Couples System. To facilitate cognitive correction, treatment sessions were tape-recorded. The patient and her husband reviewed these tapes between sessions.

The couple's communication was virtually unidirectional as in her husband stating, "I've told you before that the problem's in your head." The therapist decided to train the couple to recognize their own cognitions. Thus, their communication pattern and their cognitive distortions became the initial targets for treatment. Table 2 illustrates one sequence of interaction between the spouses.

Step 3. Correcting Cognitive Distortions. Therapy sessions focused on the patient's automatic thought, "No one cares." A meeting was held to clarify family roles and expectations. Her husband's notion that she simply had to work her way out of her depression ("Just do things, and you'll be happy") was identified and challenged. He recognized the paradox between his previously unstated expectations of her and his fear of "putting too much pressure on her," and he agreed to work on his verbal and nonverbal communications. In fact, as the patient recognized that her husband did not want just a "housecleaner," she began

Table 2. Illustration of an Interaction in a Couple

Situation	Wife's responses		Husband's responses	
	Affect	Cognition	Affect	Cognition
She wants to go shopping. He agrees, but starts to work on another project.	Anger	First, he promises to go shopping and then he lets me down. He doesn't really care.	Happiness	I'm glad she is feeling good today. I'll finish up this job and then we'll handle the shopping.
She withdraws to bedroom. He continues working.	Sadness	Nobody cares about what I want. I don't really deserve to go because he has more important things to do. I shouldn't make requests of him. I'm too selfish.	Anxiety	She's going into one of her moods again. I wonder, what upset her? I'd better leave her alone or she'll lose her temper.
She sits upstairs. Having finished the other job, he makes coffee for the couple.	Guilt	I don't deserve to be his wife. I'm just a burden on him. It would be better if I were dead.	Anxiety	I'd better make the dinner tonight to take off some pressure.
He makes dinner.	Sadness	He doesn't even need me to cook anymore. The kids didn't even notice I wasn't around. I'm totally useless to my family.	Anger	Well, if she's going to pout all night, I'm going out for a beer.

to reconsider some of her own ideas. She realized that her behavior was geared toward "cleaning house to get approval."

Each member of the couple began to ask, "What do I want? What does my spouse want? How can we achieve our goal?" Communication generally improved as the spouses learned about each other's thinking styles. The patient became more confident and less dependent by learning to verbalize her needs directly. Her husband appreciated these clear messages and willingly recognized that she did not have to follow his prescriptions for coping with depressed feelings.

This case illustrates how both spouses can be engaged in correcting cognitive distortions. As each partner learned to identify maladaptive interactions and associated cognitive distortions, each could see how cognitive distortions and problematic behaviors developed. Therapy allowed both spouses to recognize and correct individual contributions to marital misperceptions and dissatisfactions.

CONCLUSIONS

Cognitive theory and the therapeutic techniques associated with it represent a significant paradigm shift in viewing and intervening with selected psychiatric disorders. The indications and contraindications for these methods in various conditions are currently under study. Whether this treatment is differentially effective compared with other short-term treatments, and in which conditions, if any, it offers specific advantages remain to be clarified. Since the cognitive approach does aim specifically at symptom reduction and prophylaxis, its efficacy can be empirically evaluated. Further, the theory itself allows therapists to create techniques that are especially tailored for the individual patient. Thus, the therapeutic techniques subsumed by the term cognitive therapy are not limited to those published in a particular treatment manual (e.g., Beck et al., 1979). Rather, these published techniques should provide clinicians with a sense of the approaches that are logically derived from the theory. Therapy always involves judgment and creativity. The therapist must always choose the cognitive, attitudinal, or symptom targets to be addressed with each patient and select or create the methods to address these target problems with that patient. In the author's opinion, we have seen only the very beginnings of the therapeutic opportunities offered by this theoretical leap.

Chapter 5

Interpersonal Psychotherapy for Depression †

by Gerald L. Klerman, M.D., Myrna M. Weissman, Ph.D., Bruce Rounsaville, M.D., Eve S. Chevron, M.S.

THEORETICAL AND EMPIRICAL BASES

Interpersonal psychotherapy (IPT) is a psychological treatment especially designed and evaluated for depressed patients. It is a short-term,

†Supported by grants from the National Institute of Mental Health, Alcohol, Drug Abuse and Mental Health Administration, United States Public Health Service, Department of Health and Human Services, and by the George Harrington Program in Clinical and Epidemiologic Psychiatry.

time-limited psychotherapy which focuses on the patient's current interpersonal relations. While genetic, biochemical, developmental, and personality factors have a role in the vulnerability to depression, clinical depression occurs in an interpersonal context.* The authors are convinced, based on clinical experience and research evidence, that psychotherapeutic intervention directed at this interpersonal context will facilitate the patient's recovery from the acute episode and may possibly have preventive effects against relapse and recurrence.

Theoretical Basis

The theoretical basis for IPT derives from the interpersonal school of psychiatry, a distinctly American contribution to psychiatry and mental health. The earliest theoretical source was Adolf Meyer, whose psychobiological approach to understanding psychiatric disorders placed great emphasis on the patient's experiences (Meyer, 1957). In contrast to Kraepelin's concept of disease entities, derived from continental European psychiatry, Meyer applied Darwin's concept of adaptation to understanding psychiatric illness. Meyer saw psychiatric illnesses as part of the patient's attempt to adapt to the environment, usually the psychosocial environment, and considered that a patient's particular response to environmental changes reflected early developmental experiences, especially experiences in the family and social groups.

Among Meyer's associates, Harry Stack Sullivan stands out for his articulation of the theory of interpersonal relations. His writings linked clinical psychiatry to anthropology, sociology, and social psychology (Sullivan, 1953a; 1953b). Sullivan asserted that psychiatry is the scientific study of people and interpersonal processes, as distinct from the exclusive study of mind, society, or brain. In its emphasis on interpersonal and social factors in the understanding and treatment of the depressive disorders, IPT has drawn from the work of many other clinicians, especially the work of Fromm-Reichmann (1960) and Cohen et al. (1954) and more recently that of Arieti and Bemporad (1978). Becker (1974) and Chodoff (1970) are also among those who have emphasized the social roots of depression and the need to attend to the interpersonal aspects of the disorder, and Frank (1973) has stressed the general importance in psychotherapy of focusing on current interpersonal situations.

Empirical Basis

The empirical basis for the interpersonal approach to depression derives from several areas of research, including ethological and experimental work with animals, developmental research with children, and clinical and epidemiologic studies of adults.

Attachment theory has emphasized that the most intense human emotions are associated with the formation, disruption, and renewal of affectional attachment bonds. Based on findings of the animal ethologists, Bowlby studied mother-child relationships, and he demonstrated that attachment bonds were important in human functioning and that their disruption made individuals vulnerable to depression or despair (Bowlby, 1969). The individual learns to form these bonds largely through

*Editor's note: Part V of *Psychiatry Update: Volume II* presents a review and update on the epidemiology, etiology, and treatment of the depressive disorders. Dr. Klerman served as the Preceptor for that Part.

experience within the family, especially, but not exclusively, during early childhood. Bowlby's work has since been extended by Rutter (1972), who showed that relationships other than those between the mother and child have an impact on the formation of attachment bonds. The related work of Henderson and his colleagues (1978a; 1978b; 1978c) has shown that a deficiency of social bonds in an individual's current environment is associated with neurotic distress. Based on these observations, Bowlby (1977) has more recently proposed a rationale for interpersonal psychotherapy. Psychotherapy should assist the patient in examining current interpersonal relationships and how these relationships are based on experiences with attachment figures in childhood, adolescence, and adulthood.

Focusing on one aspect of attachment bonds, Brown et al. (1977) examined confiding relationships in connection with the development of depression. In a community survey of women living in the Camberwell section of London, they found that the presence of an intimate, confiding relationship with a man, usually the spouse, was an important protection against developing a depression in the face of life stress.

A considerable body of research has demonstrated a relationship between "stress," usually studied as recent life events, and the onset of psychiatric illness, particularly depression. The studies of the Yale group are most relevant to understanding stressful life events and depression (Klerman, 1979; Paykel et al., 1969). Exits of persons from the social field occurred more frequently with depressed patients than with normal subjects in the six months prior to the onset of depression. This group also found that marital friction was the most common stress reported by depressed patients prior to the onset of depression. Several studies relate to the emotional consequences of marital disputes, separation, and divorce, linking marital disruption with a wide variety of emotional disorders, including depression (Bloom et al., 1978). Ilfeld (1977) made similar observations in a survey of about 3,000 adults in Chicago. Depressive symptoms were closely related to stress, particularly to stress in marriage and, less frequently, to the stresses of parenting. In another study, chronic problems within intact marriages were as likely to produce distress and depressive symptoms as was the total disruption of the marriage by divorce or separation (Pearlin and Lieberman, 1977).

Impaired interpersonal relations can thus predispose to or precipitate mental disorders; at the same time, mental disorders have been found to produce interpersonal deficits.* The impairment in close interpersonal relations of depressed women has been studied in considerable detail (Weissman and Paykel, 1974). Depressed women are considerably impaired in most aspects of their role functioning, as workers, wives, mothers, family members, and friends. This role impairment is greatest with close family members, particularly spouses and children, with whom considerable hostility, disaffection, and poor communication were evident. With recovery from symptoms, most, but not all, of the social impairments are diminished. Marital relationships often remain chronically unhappy and easily disrupted.

*Editor's note: In Part V of Psychiatry Update: Volume II, Dr. Robert M.A. Hirschfeld and Ms. Christine K. Cross present four causal models for understanding the relationship between depressive disorders and psychosocial factors, and they review the findings related to each model (pages 382–405).

There has been debate about whether the marital difficulties associated with depression are antecedents or consequences of the disorder (Briscoe and Smith, 1973). Studying the interactions of depressed patients and normal subjects, Coyne (1976) has demonstrated that depressed patients characteristically elicit unhelpful responses from others.

Empirical findings add to the theoretical rationale for an interpersonal approach to understanding depression and for a psychotherapeutic approach based on interpersonal concepts. The research has documented both the importance of close and satisfactory attachments in the prevention of depression and the role of disrupted attachments in the development of depression.

PSYCHOTHERAPEUTIC GOALS

IPT assumes that the episode of clinical depression has three component processes. (1) *Symptom formation,* the development of depressive affect and other symptoms, stems from psychobiological and/or psychological mechanisms. (2) *Social and interpersonal relations,* which are based on learning from childhood experiences, concurrent social reinforcement, and/or personal mastery and competence, are disrupted, usually by an event. (3) *Personality problems* form part of the person's predisposition to depressive symptom episodes, particularly enduring traits such as inhibited expression of anger, guilt, poor psychological communication with significant others, and/or difficulty with self-esteem. IPT intervenes in the first two of these three processes, symptom formation and social and interpersonal relations. Because of IPT's relatively brief duration and low level of psychotherapeutic intensity, IPT is not expected to have a marked impact upon enduring aspects of personality structure, although personality functioning is assessed. While some longer-term psychotherapies have been designed to achieve personality change using the interpersonal approach (Arieti and Bemporad, 1978), these treatments have not been assessed in controlled trials.

IPT facilitates recovery from acute depression by relieving depressive symptoms and by helping the patient become more effective in dealing with those current interpersonal problems that are associated with the onset of symptoms. Symptom relief begins with helping the patient understand that the vague and uncomfortable symptoms are part of a known syndrome, which is well described, understood, and relatively common, and which responds to a variety of treatments and has a good prognosis. Psychopharmacologic approaches may be used in conjunction with IPT to alleviate symptoms more rapidly. Improvement in interpersonal relations begins with exploring which of four problem areas commonly associated with the onset of depression—grief, role disputes, role transition, or interpersonal deficits—is related to this particular patient's depression. IPT then focuses on the particular interpersonal problem as it relates to the onset of depression.

In the authors' experience, the psychotherapy of depressed patients has paid insufficient attention to techniques for reducing symptoms, for facilitating the patient's current social adjustment, and for improving interpersonal relations. With IPT, personality reconstruction is not attempted in the symptomatic state; instead, the technique emphasizes reassurance, clarification of emotional states, improvement of interpersonal communication, testing of perceptions, and performance in interpersonal settings. These techniques are conventionally grouped under the rubric of "supportive psychotherapy." In the authors' view, however, the term supportive psychotherapy is a misnomer. Most of what is called supportive psychotherapy attempts to assist the patient to modify interpersonal relations, to change perceptions and cognitions, and to reward behavioral contingencies.

PHASES IN IPT

As shown in Table 1, the conduct of IPT is best discussed in terms of three phases. The three phases include (1) an early phase devoted to assessment and the negotiation of the therapeutic contract, (2) a middle phase, which has the longest duration and which entails psychotherapeutic work on one or another of the four problem areas, and (3) the termination phase.

Table 1.   Phases and Tasks in the Conduct of IPT

Phases	Tasks
EARLY	Treatment of depressive symptoms
	Review of symptoms
	Confirmation of diagnosis
	Communication of diagnosis to patient
	Evaluation of medication need
	Education of patient about depression (epidemiology, symptoms, clinical causes, treatments, prognosis)
	Legitimation of patient's "sick role"
	Assessment of interpersonal relations
	Inventory of current relationships
	Choice of interpersonal problem area
	Therapeutic contract
	Statement of goals, diagnosis, problem area
	Medication plan
	Agreement
MIDDLE	Treatment focusing on problem area
	Grief reaction
	Interpersonal disputes
	Role transition
	Interpersonal deficits
TERMINATION	

The Early Phase

The tasks of the early phase are to deal with the depression, to assess the interpersonal problems, and to negotiate a mutually agreeable therapeutic contract.

The first task, *dealing with the depression,* has a high priority during the early phase. To accomplish this, six more specific tasks are recommended.

First, the symptoms should be reviewed systematically, going through the DSM-III inclusion and exclusion criteria. A structured interview such as the SADS, DIS, or SKID is often helpful. The time course of a current episode should be reconstructed, with attention to the current sequence of symptoms, their intensity, and their characteristics. Assessment should also inquire into any current life event that may relate to the onset of the episode. A family history should be taken, with a systematic inquiry into the medical and psychiatric status of all first-degree relatives, particularly parents, siblings, and offspring.

Second, the diagnostic possibilities should be assessed using standard operational criteria, particularly DSM-III. Differential diagnosis from anxiety conditions and alcoholism should receive particular attention. Within the DSM-III category of Affective Disorders, an attempt should be made to assign the patient to one of the subcategories such as Bipolar Disorder, Major Depression, or Dysthymic Disorder. Within Major Depression, attention should be given to the presence or absence of delusions and melancholic symptoms.

Third, if the patient does meet the criteria for a DSM-III diagnosis, the patient should hear the diagnosis confirmed with a statement such as, "We have reviewed your symptoms, and it appears that you meet the criteria for [diagnosis] and that you should receive treatment for this."

Fourth, as the symptoms and diagnosis are considered, the possible value of medication should be assessed. With IPT, in contrast to many other forms of psychotherapy, the authors do not believe that medication is theoretically or clinically contraindicated. Medication is indicated when the patient's symptoms are of sufficient intensity and when the syndrome shows features of the melancholic pattern or delusional symptoms. The authors have found that melancholic and delusional patients do not respond to psychotherapy alone, but will respond to the combination of medication and IPT.

Fifth, during one of the early interviews, the patient should receive explicit information about the nature of depression as a clinical condition and should learn something about its symptom pattern, frequency, and clinical course and about the alternative treatments and essentially good prognosis for depression. Many patients will have read about depression in the lay literature or in such books as *Moodswing* (Fieve, 1975) or *Unfinished Business* (Scarf, 1980).

Sixth, and finally, this whole process legitimizes the patient in the sick role. The authors place IPT, unlike other psychotherapies, in the general medical model and believe that an important part of the therapeutic improvement comes from the patient being legitimized in the sick role. Efforts should be made, nonetheless, to minimize dependency. If the patient is in the labor force, treatment should encourage the patient to keep working. The patient should also maintain a reasonable schedule of social and family activities. The tendency to withdraw socially and to avoid activity should be countered by explicit suggestion.

The second major task of the early phase is *assessment of the interpersonal problem area*, with a systematic inventory of the significant persons in the patient's current and past life. This assessment especially emphasizes the current relationships, their stability, and their possible disruption. On the basis of this, one can often make a judgment about which of the four problem areas is associated with the patient's depression and which requires further therapeutic work.

The formation of *the therapeutic contract* with the statement of goals constitutes the third and final main task of the first phase. When the other two tasks are completed, the patient should receive an explicit statement reiterating the diagnosis of the depressive symptoms and identifying the interpersonal problem area. If the patient agrees on both of these matters, a treatment plan should be proposed, including a medication plan where appropriate, and focusing on the interpersonal problem. The proposal to the patient might say, "There is good evidence that episodes of depression like yours are often related to interpersonal problems, and your problem seems to be [statement of interpersonal problem]. If you agree, we will work on these issues over the next few months."

The Middle Phase: Problem Areas and Treatment Tasks

Previous research indicates general and specific techniques for dealing with each of the four interpersonal problem areas in IPT—abnormal grief reaction, interpersonal role disputes, role transition, and interpersonal deficits.

Many depressions involve an *abnormal grief reaction*. This is not identical with normal bereavement, which is usually self-limiting and has approximately six to nine months' duration of symptoms, with a shorter period of social disability. Most people experiencing grief adapt without professional assistance. However, about 15 percent of patients have symptoms that persist beyond six to nine months, and others have anniversary reactions.

The tasks in treating abnormal grief reactions are to facilitate the mourning process which has been suppressed, delayed, or prolonged, to assist the patient with establishing new relationships, and to offer an attachment which may serve as a partial and temporary substitute for the lost relationship with the significant other. Along with these tasks, IPT with grief reactions entails reconstruction of the relationship with the dead person, with special attention to the patient's expression of positive and negative affects, unfulfilled expectations, and any guilt or self-remorse.

In clinical practice, *interpersonal role disputes* are among the interpersonal difficulties most commonly associated with depression, particularly for women. Role disputes develop when the patient and at least one significant other have nonreciprocal expectations about their role interactions and relationships. Specifically, they take the form of marital disputes, disputes between parent and child, disputes between work colleagues, or disputes within the extended family or friendship network.

The first treatment task with interpersonal role disputes is to help the patient identify the existence of a dispute and the issues involved. Since such disputes are very often masked, simply identifying the existence of a dispute and relating it to the onset and perpetuation of the depression can be of considerable assistance to a depressed patient (Spiegel, 1957). The task then is to guide and encourage the patient in examining and choosing alternative courses of action, which will include renegotiating the relationship and modifying any maladaptive communication patterns and expectations. The most important task is to facilitate the renegotiation of role expectations between the patient and the significant other. Often, as with a marital dispute, this will be accomplished best by bringing the other person into the session. When disputes require negotiations that cannot take place in the therapeutic session, as with disputes involving occupations and friends, IPT will entail the ongoing monitoring of the interactions.

Role transitions occur normally with the life changes that require a person to move from one social role to another. The developmental life cycle often includes such changes as graduating from high school or college, leaving home for college, entering the military, entering the labor force, being promoted or demoted, losing a job, having a child, changing residency, and retiring. Most people adapt to these role transitions with minimal difficulty. Some develop depressive symptoms, however, which under DSM-III may be considered an Adjustment Disorder with Depressed Mood or a Major Depressive Episode. Those who fail to cope adequately with transitions and develop symptoms often experience the role transition as a loss, and accordingly some psychodynamic theorists have interpreted these transitions as being akin to grief and bereavement. For work with IPT, however, the authors believe that grief reactions and role transitions should be distinguished.

IPT with the patient whose depression is related to a role transition includes the task of enabling the patient to regard the new role in a positive, less restricted manner and to view it as opportunity for growth. Other tasks are to restore self-esteem by encouraging the patient's sense of mastery and to explore the positive and negative aspects of the previous role. Disruptions of previous interpersonal relations with work colleagues, friends, and family are also explored, and the patient is helped to initiate new relationships and to examine the repertoire of social skills that may be involved in the new role.

Interpersonal deficits constitute the fourth and final area of IPT's focus. People often lack the skills for initiating or sustaining interpersonal relations. Some have the skills to initiate relationships, but cannot sustain them, particularly the close attachments that require commitment, intimacy, and expectations of fidelity and loyalty. Others have trouble initiating relationships because they lack the repertoire of skills and are shy, isolated, and lonely. In the authors' experience, depressed patients whose symptoms are associated with social isolation tend to have more severe disturbances, and IPT has been less successful with these patients. Long-term treatment is often necessary, to work on their underlying personality problems and to help them develop new social skills.

In IPT with patients who have interpersonal deficits, one can expect to accomplish the preliminary task of helping the patient identify past positive relationships and experiences which may serve as a model. Patients may also be guided to consider opportunities for forming new relationships. Beyond this, the techniques and therapeutic maneuvers for helping such patients cannot be detailed in this brief discussion. A manual has been available in unpublished form for some time (Klerman et al., 1979) and has recently been elaborated in a published volume (Klerman et al., 1984).

IPT COMPARED WITH OTHER PSYCHOTHERAPIES

The authors agree with Jerome Frank (1973) that the procedures and techniques in many of the different psychotherapies have much in common.* Many of the therapies emphasize helping the patient to develop a sense of mastery, combating social isolation, restoring the patient's feeling of group belonging, and helping the patient to rediscover meaning in life. The psychotherapies differ, however, on whether the patient's problems lie in the far past, the immediate past, or the present.

IPT focuses primarily on the patient's present, and it differs from other psychotherapies in its limited duration and its attention to current depressive symptoms and the current depression-related interpersonal context. Given this frame of reference, IPT includes a systematic review of the patient's current relations with significant others. IPT also differs in that it was developed for the treatment of a single group of disorders—the depressive disorders. Table 2 summarizes the similarities and differences in the approaches of IPT and other psychotherapies.

Table 2. Comparison of IPT with Other Psychotherapies

	IPT	*Other Psychotherapies*
ASSESSMENT QUESTIONS	What has contributed to this patient's depression right now?	Why did the patient become what he or she is, and/or where is the patient going?
	What are the current stresses?	What was the patient's childhood like?
	Who are the key persons involved in the current stress? What are the patient's current disputes and disappointments?	What is the patient's character?
	What are the patient's assets?	What are the patient's defenses?
TREATMENT QUESTIONS	How can I help the patient clarify his or her wishes and have more satisfying relationships with others?	How can I understand the patient's fantasy life and help the patient get insight into the origins of his or her behavior?
	How can I help the patient ventilate and unburden himself or herself of painful emotions (i.e., guilt, shame, resentment)?	How can I find out why this patient feels guilty, shameful, or resentful?
	How can I correct misinformation and suggest alternatives?	How can I help the patient discover false or incorrect ideas on his or her own?
OUTCOME QUESTION	Is the patient learning how to cope with the problem?	Is the patient cured?

*Editors note: In Part V of this volume, Frank reviews a number of the common features of the various psychotherapies.

IPT is *time limited and not long-term.* Considerable research has demonstrated the value for most patients' current problems and for most symptom states of short-term, time-limited psychotherapies (usually once a week for less than 9 to 12 months). While long-term treatment may still be required for changing personality dysfunctions, particularly maladaptive interpersonal and cognitive patterns, and for ameliorating or replacing dysfunctional social skills, evidence for the efficacy of long-term psychotherapy is limited. Long-term treatment also has the inherent potential disadvantages of promoting dependency and reinforcing avoidance behavior. Psychotherapies that are short-term or time limited aim to minimize these adverse effects.

IPT is *focused and not open-ended.* In common with other brief psychotherapies, IPT focuses on one or two problem areas in the patient's current interpersonal functioning, and these are agreed upon by the patient and the psychotherapist after several evaluation sessions. The content of sessions is therefore focused and not open-ended.

IPT deals with *current and not past interpersonal relationships.* The IPT therapist focuses the sessions on the patient's immediate social context, as it was just before and as it has been since the onset of the current depressive episode. Past depressive episodes, early family relationships, and previous significant relationships and friendship patterns are, however, assessed in order to understand overall patterns in the patient's interpersonal relationships.

IPT is concerned with *interpersonal, not intrapsychic* phenomena. In exploring current interpersonal problems with the patient, the psychotherapist may observe the operation of intrapsychic defense mechanisms such as projection, denial, isolation, undoing, or repression. In IPT, however, the psychotherapist does not work on helping the patient see the current situation as a manifestation of internal conflict. Rather, the therapist explores the patient's behavior in terms of interpersonal relations. The example of how dreams are handled is analogous. Although the therapist does not usually ask the patient to recall dreams, patients may spontaneously report them. When this occurs, the psychotherapist may work on the dream by relating its manifest content and associated affects to relevant current interpersonal problems.

IPT is concerned with *interpersonal relationships, not cognitive-behavioral phenomena* per se. IPT attempts to change how the patient thinks, feels, and acts in problematic interpersonal relationships. Specific negative cognitions or behaviors such as lack of assertiveness and lack of social skills are not in themselves a treatment focus in IPT. They are considered only in relationship to significant persons in the patient's life and for the ways that they impinge upon these interpersonal relationships.

In common with cognitive-behavioral therapy, IPT is concerned with the patient's distorted thinking about him or herself and others and with the relevant options for change. The IPT therapist may work with the patient about his or her distorted thinking by calling attention to discrepancies between what the patient is saying and doing or between the patient's standards and those of society in general. Unlike cognitive-behavioral therapies, however, IPT does not attempt systematically to uncover such distorted thoughts, give homework, or prescribe methods of developing alternative thought patterns. Rather, the IPT psychothera-

pist calls the patient's attention to distorted thinking in relation to significant others as the evidence arises during the psychotherapy. The IPT
psychotherapist will often visit with the patient to explore the effect of
his or her maladaptive thinking on interpersonal relationships.

In IPT, *personality is recognized but is not the focus.* The patient's personality is very frequently the major focus in psychotherapy. IPT does not
expect to make an impact on personality. It recognizes, but does not
focus on, the patient's personality characteristics. Moreover, IPT does
not make the assumption that persons who become depressed have
unique personality traits. This assumption is still questionable and requires further testing; so far, research on this question has not yielded
any conclusive answers.

IPT AND PSYCHODYNAMIC THEORY

The authors' goal in developing IPT was not to create a new psychotherapy, but to make explicit and operational a systematic approach to
depression and to base that approach on accepted theory and empirical
evidence. Much of IPT resembles what many, perhaps most, psychoanalytic and dynamic psychotherapists do. This reflects the extent to
which the interpersonal approach has permeated American psychotherapeutic practice, a trend whose historical roots are probably twofold. In the first place, most of the founding psychotherapists and practitioners of the interpersonal approach, including Sullivan, Fromm-
Reichmann, Cohen, and Stanton, were initially trained in Freudian psychoanalysis. While they disagreed with some aspects of psychoanalytic
theory and practice, the role of early childhood experience and the existence of unconscious mental processes were not the sources of this
disagreement. Their disagreement arose over the existence of libido, the
dual instinct theory (eros and death instincts), and the relative importance of biological, instinctive forces, compared with social and cultural
influences, on personal development and current functioning. A second
historical force was the expansion of psychotherapy following World War
II, which coincided with widespread national concerns about social
change, racial and sexual equality, personal well-being, and the enhancement of personal potential and individual happiness. Such cultural values are highly compatible with scientific and professional pur-
suits that focus on interpersonal relations and personal development
throughout the life cycle.

For purposes of theoretical clarity and research design, the authors
have nonetheless often found it useful to highlight the differences between the interpersonal and the psychodynamic approaches to human
behavior and mental illness. The essential focus of a pure psychodynamic approach is on unconscious mental processes and the role of intrapsychic memories, wishes, fantasies, and conflicts in determining behavior and psychopathology. The essential focus of a pure interpersonal
approach is on social roles and interpersonal interactions in the individual's past and current life experiences. Both the interpersonal and the
psychodynamic approaches are concerned with the person's life span
and the important role of early experiences and persistent personality
patterns at all developmental stages and in all areas of personal functioning. However, in understanding personal functioning, the psychodynamic psychotherapist is concerned with object relations, while the

interpersonal psychotherapist is concerned with interpersonal relations. Put another way, the psychodynamic psychotherapist listens for the patient's intrapsychic wishes and conflicts, while the interpersonal psychotherapist listens for the patient's role expectations and disputes.

A comprehensive theory would ideally incorporate both these approaches, along with biological, behavioral, and other views. Given the current state of knowledge, however, the authors believe it timely and valuable to focus clearly on one approach, to explore its validity, and to examine its utility through systematic research, especially through controlled trials of efficacy and other outcomes.

Chapter 6

Multimodal Therapy †

by Arnold A. Lazarus, Ph.D.

INTRODUCTION

Multimodal therapy is the outgrowth of more than twenty years of clinical research into systematic, short-term, and yet comprehensive psychotherapeutic strategies. A fundamental premise of the multimodal approach is that patients are troubled by at least several specific problems that may require a wide range of specific treatments. Another basic assumption is that the durability of results is a function of the effort expended by patient and therapist across seven dimensions of personality: behavior, affect, sensation, imagery, cognition, interpersonal relationships, and biological factors.

Since the publication of Brentano's *Psychologie vom empirischen Standpunkte* in 1874, the subject matter of general psychology (the scientific study of human behavior) has been concerned with sensation, imagery, perception, cognition, emotion, and interpersonal relationships. Most of our experiences consist of moving, feeling, sensing, imagining, thinking, and relating to one another. In the final analysis, though, we are biochemical, neurophysiological entities. Human life and conduct thus are products of ongoing *b*ehaviors, *a*ffective processes, *s*ensations, *im*ages, *c*ognitions, and *i*nterpersonal relationships, springing from a *b*iological matrix. (BASIC IB is the acronym directly corresponding to this sequence, but for convenience and euphony the letter D [for drugs] stands for the biological modality. This also generates the more compelling acronym BASIC ID [ID as in identity].) "If we examine psychotherapeutic processes in the light of each of these basic modalities," the author has written elsewhere, "seemingly disparate systems are brought into clearer focus, and the necessary and sufficient conditions for long-lasting therapeutic change might readily be discerned" (Lazarus, 1983, 406).

Multimodal therapy is pluralistic and personalistic. It emphasizes that human disquietude is multileveled and multilayered and that few, if any, problems have a single cause or a unitary "cure." A sensitivity to individual differences and exceptions to general rules and principles obviates the need to apply preconceived treatments to patients with simi-

† The first draft of this chapter profited enormously from incisive criticisms and cogent suggestions provided by Allen Fay, M.D.

lar "diagnoses." Rather, the multimodal clinician searches for appropriate interventions for each patient. Clinical effectiveness is predicated on the therapist's flexibility, versatility, and *technical* eclecticism.

The *theoretical* eclectic may subscribe to theories or disciplines that are epistemologically incompatible. The limitations of orthodoxy have become apparent, and many clinicians embrace multidimensional and multifaceted assessment and treatment procedures. Yet those who endeavor to unite the morass of competing systems, models, vocabularies, and personal idiosyncrasies into a unified whole tend to end up with an agglomerate of incompatible and contradictory notions (Lazarus, 1981; Messer and Winokur, 1980). The *technical* eclectic uses many techniques drawn from different sources without adhering to the theories or systems that spawned them. One need not believe in gestalt principles to use gestalt techniques; one may employ behavioral methods without subscribing to the tenets of social learning theory.

While a recent survey (Smith, 1982) indicated that the majority of therapists are eclectic and multimodal in outlook, in the author's view, only a few are *multimodal therapists*. The distinction is important. Multimodal therapy has a well-defined history, a systematic theoretical base, a coherent framework, and a wide range of specific techniques (Lazarus, 1976; 1981; 1983). The principles of multimodal therapy are expressed in terms that can be tested, and its procedures are consonant with current scientific findings. Multimodal therapists constantly adjust to the patient in terms of that mode of interaction most likely to achieve the desired aims of the therapy. The essential and distinguishing features of multimodal therapy are its comprehensive scope and its systematic methodology. Whereas some therapies are multifaceted and espouse "multimodalism" in principle, multimodal therapy alone uses the exhaustive BASIC ID schema. "The aim of Multimodal Therapy (MMT) is to come up with the best methods for each client rather than force all clients to fit the same therapy. . . . Three depressed clients might be given very different treatments depending on their therapists' assessments and the methods they prefer. . . . The only goal is helping clients make desired changes as rapidly as possible" (Zilbergeld, 1982, 86).

MULTIMODAL DIAGNOSIS AND ASSESSMENT

The multimodal approach to diagnosis and treatment is similar to "the problem-oriented record approach." The emphasis upon problem specification in psychiatry was underscored by Hayes-Roth et al. (1972). This approach to record keeping and treatment had been introduced to medicine somewhat earlier and is best illustrated by Weed's (1968) work.

The Modality Profile

The cliché "diagnosis must precede treatment" points to the obvious fact that when the real problems have been identified, effective remedies (if they exist) can be administered. Conventional diagnostic labels and nosological categories are less valuable for treatment planning than the construction of modality profiles (i.e., a chart that lists problems and proposed treatments across the BASIC ID). For illustrative purposes, Table 1 shows the modality profile of a 32-year-old woman diagnosed as suffering from Alcohol Dependence (DSM-III 303.9x).

Table 1. Illustrative Modality Profile

Modality	Problem	Proposed Treatment
Behavior	Excessive drinking	Aversive imagery
	Avoids confronting most people	Assertiveness training
	Negative self-statements	Positive self-talk assignments
	Always drinks excessively when alone at home at night	Develop social outlets
	Screams at her children	Instruction in parenting skills
Affect	Holds back anger (except with her children)	Assertiveness training Anger expression exercises
	Anxiety reactions	Self-hypnosis and/or positive imagery
	Depression	Increase range of positive reinforcement
Sensation	Butterflies in stomach	Abdominal breathing exercises
	Tension headaches	Relaxation or biofeedback
Imagery	Vivid pictures of parents fighting	Desensitization
	Being locked in bedroom as a child	Images of escape and/or release of anger
Cognition	Irrational self-talk about low self-worth	Cognitive disputation
	Numerous regrets	Reduction of categorical imperatives (shoulds, oughts, musts, etc.)
Interpersonal relationships	Ambivalent responses to husband and children	Possible family therapy and specific training in use of positive reinforcement Support group to control alcohol abuse (AA)
	Secretive and suspicious	Self-disclosure training
Drugs	Reliance on alcohol to alleviate depression, anxiety, tension	Possible use of disulfiram and antidepressant medication

The following paragraphs describe the typical anamnestic procedures that enable a therapist to construct modality profiles. (The present chapter addresses adult outpatients. For the multimodal therapy approach to children, see Keat [1979], and for its use with inpatients see Brunell and Young [1982].) The initial interview, as in most psychotherapeutic approaches, is devoted to eliciting and evaluating presenting complaints, establishing rapport, and formulating the optimal treatment. The multimodal therapist remains alert to dysfunctions across the entire BASIC ID. Immediate antecedent events and the presymptomatic environment are carefully evaluated. In examining the postsymptomatic environment, a key question is, "Who or what appears to be maintaining the problems?"

At the end of the initial interview, patients are usually given the 12-page Multimodal Life History Questionnaire (Lazarus, 1981), which they complete at home and then bring to their next session. The questionnaire, in addition to reviewing the patient's early development, family interactions, educational, sexual, occupational, and marital experiences, specifically assesses the most salient aspects of the BASIC ID. Ambiguous or incomplete answers are usually discussed with the patient during the second session.

With notes from the first two meetings and the patient's responses on the Life History Questionnaire, the construction of the modality profile is relatively straightforward. Generally patients are asked to do their own modality profiles; it is often particularly valuable for therapist and patient to perform this exercise independently, and then compare notes. Before being asked to draw up their profiles, patients are provided with a brief explanation of each term in the BASIC ID (see Table 2).

Patients are not assumed to be capable of identifying or articulating all problem areas throughout the BASIC ID. Obviously, different people display different degrees of awareness and disclosure, so that many thoughts, beliefs, wishes, feelings, impulses, and actions may not be immediately ascertained from the initial profile. During the course of multimodal therapy, nonconscious processes and defensive reactions are addressed whenever indicated (Lazarus, 1981). Indeed, part of the purpose of the therapy is to discover certain hitherto unrecognized factors that fit into one or more categories of the BASIC ID (one form of "insight"). Assessment and therapy are both reciprocal and continuous. The technique of second-order BASIC ID assessment often uncovers material that has been inaccessible to other avenues of inquiry.

Second-Order BASIC ID Assessment

The initial BASIC ID or modality profile provides a macroscopic overview of personality. A complete diagnosis calls for an accurate and thorough assessment of each modality and the interactions among and between the seven modalities. A second-order BASIC ID consists of subjecting any item on the initial modality profile to a more detailed inquiry in terms of behavior, affect, sensation, imagery, cognition, interpersonal factors, and drugs or biological considerations. This recursive application of the BASIC ID to itself is usually conducted when problematic items result in treatment impasses.

For example, a patient being treated for generalized anxiety listed four areas of discomfort in his sensation modality: tension headaches, tightness in chest, sweaty palms, and pain in the jaws (temporomandibular joint syndrome, or TMJ). He showed improvement in the first three complaints as his general anxiety level decreased, and as he grew proficient at relaxation and diaphragmatic breathing exercises. His TMJ problem, however, persisted despite the use of special biofeedback procedures to alleviate the pain. He kept careful notes of specific times of day, places and situations, and thoughts and activities that preceded and followed those occasions when his jaws felt especially tight or painful.

Table 2. Patients' Instructions for Constructing a Modality Profile

Behavior
This refers mainly to overt behaviors: to acts, habits, gestures, responses, and reactions that are observable and measurable. Make a list of those acts, habits, etc., that you want to increase and those you would like to decrease. What would you like to start doing? What would you like to stop doing?

Affect
This refers to emotions, moods, and strong feelings. What emotions do you experience most often? Write down your unwanted emotions (e.g., anxiety, guilt, anger, depression, etc.). Note under Behavior what you tend to *do* when you feel a certain way.

Sensation
Touching, tasting, smelling, seeing, and hearing are our five basic senses. Make a list of any negative sensations (tension, dizziness, pain, blushing, sweating, butterflies in stomach, etc.) that apply to you. If any of these sensations cause you to act or feel in certain ways, make sure you note them under Behavior or Affect.

Imagery
Write down any recurring dreams and any vivid memories that may be bothersome. Include any negative features about the way you see yourself, your "self-image." Make a list of "mental pictures," past, present, or future, that may be troubling you. If any "auditory images," tunes or sounds that you keep hearing, constitute a problem, jot them down. If your images arouse any significant actions, feelings, or sensations, make sure these items are added to Behavior, Affect, and Sensation.

Cognition
What types of attitudes, values, opinions, and ideas get in the way of your happiness? Make a list of negative things you often say to yourself (e.g., "I am a failure," or "I am stupid," or "Others dislike me," or "I am no good"). Write down some of your most irrational ideas. Be sure to note how these ideas and thoughts influence your Behavior, Affect, Sensation, and Imagery.

Interpersonal Relationships
Write down any interactions with other people (relatives, friends, lovers, employers, acquaintances, etc.) that bother you. Any concerns you have about the way other people treat you should appear here. Check through the items under Behavior, Affect, Sensation, Imagery, and Cognition, and try to determine how they influence, and are influenced by, your interpersonal relationships. (Note that there is some overlap between the modalities, but don't hesitate to list the same problem more than once, e.g., under Behavior and Interpersonal Relationships.)

Drugs
Make a list of all drugs, whether prescribed by a doctor or not, that you are taking. Include any health problems, medical concerns, and illnesses that you have now or have had in the past.

No discernible pattern could be traced. A second-order BASIC ID was conducted.

Therapist: What do you *do* when your jaws become extremely painful?
Patient: Well, it depends. When it's not too bad, I get by with extra-strength Excedrin and perhaps 2 mg of Valium, but sometimes I take some pills my doctor gave me. They contain codeine. I rarely use the codeine pills more than once a week, but sometimes I take Excedrin two or three times a day.

Therapist:	Do you do anything else?
Patient:	Sometimes it helps if I catnap.
Therapist:	How would you describe your mood or feelings when your jaws ache so badly?
Patient:	I get damn despondent!
Therapist:	Depressed?
Patient:	Yes, and angry. I feel, why me? But mainly I feel sort of discouraged.
Therapist:	You have told me exactly how and where you get the pains. Have you observed any other sensations that accompany the tightness in the jaws and the pain—"like hot spikes being driven in," that's what you said.
Patient:	That's right. The shooting pains go right into my ears.
Therapist:	Any other sensations?
Patient:	Yes, nausea. That's probably more from the pills than anything else.
Therapist:	Okay, now try to imagine that your jaws are feeling very tight and painful. *(Five-second pause)* What picture comes to mind?
Patient:	I don't know why, but my grandfather came to mind.
Therapist:	Your grandfather. Maternal or paternal? Was there something distinctive about him?
Patient:	Yes, my dad's dad. He was very British. *(Affecting an accent)* Stiff upper lip and all that sort of thing!
Therapist:	Stiff upper lip. How about a tight lower jaw?
Patient:	*(Laughs)* Actually my dad's expression was, "Grit your teeth, men!" I haven't thought about that in years. He used to coach our track team when I was in sixth grade. I remember him saying, "Grit your teeth and put in that extra effort!"
Therapist:	Well, here's the obvious question. I wonder if there's some connection between being a man, gritting your teeth, putting in that extra effort, and your aching jaws?
Patient:	Well, as I mentioned when I first came to see you, I'm always sizing myself up, seeing where I rank on the pecking order.
Therapist:	And where would you rate in your grandfather's eyes and in your father's estimation?
Patient:	Well, my grandfather died more than ten years ago . . .
Therapist:	But if he were alive today, what would he think of you?
Patient:	Gee. That's hard. *(Pause)* I guess he wouldn't think too much of me. The truth is I've never been much of an athlete. I guess I make up for it by earning more money in a year than my dad and his dad both made in ten years.
Therapist:	I think we have to cool your head before we can loosen your jaw.
Patient:	What does that mean?
Therapist:	I don't want to read too much into it, but it is my guess that your fiercely overcompetitive strivings are tied into proving your manliness or adequacy. You are less anxious than you were three months ago, and this is reflected by the fact that your tension headaches are less frequent and your chest pains and sweaty palms are no longer a problem. But the tension in your jaws still bothers you. This is the last frontier, and you may need to achieve a relaxed frame of mind before your jaw muscles will let up.
Patient:	And how do we do that?
Therapist:	Well, for now, I want to put the sensory mode on hold, al-

though I want to be sure that you will continue doing your relaxation and breathing exercises. I want to take a closer look at some of your assumptions, and also at the images that tie into your thought processes.

The second-order BASIC ID for this patient's TMJ syndrome would read as follows:

B   Takes medication
    Catnaps

A   Despondent
    Angry
    Discouraged

S   Shooting pains into ears
    Nausea

I   Paternal grandfather (stiff upper lip)

C   Grit your teeth, men (from father)

I   Fiercely overcompetitive

D   Analgesic and antianxiety drugs, self-prescribed and physician prescribed

When selecting techniques, a multimodal axiom is: "Begin with the most obvious and logical procedures." It is important to eschew simplistic panaceas, but it is also important to avoid the penchant for making straightforward problems needlessly complicated. Thus, in the foregoing case, the best established methods of anxiety reduction were administered first, i.e., relaxation training, biofeedback, self-monitoring. But when an impasse was reached, a second-order BASIC ID underscored fundamental identifications and an adversarial interpersonal stance that called for correction. While the initial modality profile had reflected overcompetitive strivings, it had not revealed the patient's concerns about his manhood and his attempts to meet real or imagined standards set by his father and grandfather. Accordingly, the treatment focused on the "scripts" that he had abstracted from his male models. With guidance from the therapist, the patient enacted several imaginary dialogues with his father and grandfather in which he persuaded them (and thus convinced himself) that their standards of manliness were irrational and obsolete. Subsequently, a second course of biofeedback successfully mitigated his TMJ discomfort.

The Structural Profile

Whereas modality profiles list specific problems in each dimension of the BASIC ID, structural profiles provide a quantitative self-rating of the patient's proclivities in each of the seven modalities (see Table 3). In everyday terms, some people are primarily doers, whereas others are thinkers, or feelers, or people-oriented relaters, and so forth. By using a ten-point scale for each modality, patients may be asked to rate the

Table 3. Structural Profile

Here are seven rating scales that pertain to various tendencies that people have. Using a scale of 0 to 10, please rate yourself in the seven areas. (A 10 is high; it characterizes you, or you rely on it greatly. A 0 means that it does not describe you, or you rarely rely on it.)

1. *Behavior*
How active are you? How much of a "doer" are you? Do you like to keep busy?
Rating: 0 1 2 3 4 5 6 7 8 9 10

2. *Affect*
How emotional are you? How deeply do you feel things? Are you inclined to impassioned or soul-stirring reactions?
Rating: 0 1 2 3 4 5 6 7 8 9 10

3. *Sensation*
How much do you focus on the pleasures and pains derived from your senses? How "tuned-in" are you to your bodily sensations—to sex, food, music, art, etc.?
Rating: 0 1 2 3 4 5 6 7 8 9 10

4. *Imagery*
Do you have a vivid imagination? Do you engage in fantasy and daydreaming a great deal? Do you "think in pictures"?
Rating: 0 1 2 3 4 5 6 7 8 9 10

5. *Cognition*
How much of a "thinker" are you? Do you like to analyze things, make plans, reason things through?
Rating: 0 1 2 3 4 5 6 7 8 9 10

6. *Interpersonal Relationships*
How much of a "social being" are you? How important are other people to you? Do you gravitate to people? Do you desire intimacy with others?
Rating: 0 1 2 3 4 5 6 7 8 9 10

7. *Drugs/Biology*
Are you healthy and health conscious? Do you take good care of your body and physical health? Do you avoid overeating, ingestion of unnecessary drugs, excessive amounts of alcohol, and exposure to other substances that may be harmful?
Rating: 0 1 2 3 4 5 6 7 8 9 10

extent to which they perceive themselves as doing, feeling, sensing, imagining, thinking, and relating. They are also asked to rate the extent to which they observe and practice "health habits" such as regular exercise, good nutrition, abstinence from cigarettes. A high D score on the structural profile indicates a healthy and health-minded individual.

Simple bar diagrams or graphs may be constructed from the profile. Structural profiles are especially useful in marriage therapy. Spouses may be asked to draw up their own profiles, their estimate of how their mate might perceive them, and a profile of how they see their spouse. This frequently provides a springboard for a fruitful discussion of specific areas of incompatibility and precise measures for remedying particular discrepancies (see Lazarus, 1981). Moreover, when therapist and patient explore the meanings and relevance behind each rating, important insights are often gained. In addition to global self-ratings, structural profiles may be obtained for specific areas of functioning (akin to second-order modality profiles). For example, in the realm of sexuality, the degree of activity, emotionality, sensuality, and imagery or fantasy may be rated on separate scales, together with questions about how highly valued sexual participation is (cognition), its specific interpersonal importance, and the patient's biological adequacy.

BRIDGING AND TRACKING

Bridging refers to a procedure in which the therapist deliberately responds to the patient in his or her dominant modality before branching off into other dimensions that seem likely to be more productive. Bridging thus contrasts with the tactic of challenging or confronting patients whose style is to avoid the expression of feelings and to present an intellectual facade. Labeling these patients resistant or exhorting them to produce "gut feelings" (as some gestalt therapists do) is seldom as fruitful as bridging, and often has disturbing, if not painful, consequences (Lazarus and Fay, 1982). Here is a brief example:

> *Therapist:* I want to know how you felt when your mother compared you to Sue.
>
> *Patient:* I think she was only trying to be impartial. Let me tell you how her mind works. . . .

Instead of truncating the patient's intellectualizations and emphasizing that the therapist was interested in her feelings, not in her post hoc rationalizations, the therapist allowed the patient to complete her explanation. This took about five minutes. The therapist then continued to address her preferred modality (cognition) for a while.

> *Therapist:* So your mother sometimes bends over backwards to be fair. I guess that she thinks that Sue is particularly vulnerable. She sees you as the stronger of the two, so you sometimes get dumped on.
>
> *Patient:* Well, it's not that I get dumped on exactly.
>
> *Therapist:* Of course, your mother's reasoning is that to be fair-minded, she must not take sides, but she does sometimes make comparisons.
>
> *Patient:* (*Laughs*) And sometimes I don't come out smelling like a rose.
>
> *Therapist:* You're laughing, but do you really find it amusing?
>
> *Patient:* Well, I understand her.
>
> *Therapist:* Nevertheless . . . Are you in touch with any feelings or sensations right now?
>
> *Patient:* (*Rubbing her neck*) I've got a slight headache.
>
> *Therapist:* Let's focus on the headache. What can you tell me about it?
>
> *Patient:* Nothing much. It's just throbbing a bit.
>
> *Therapist:* Where is it throbbing?
>
> *Patient:* (*Touches her temples and runs her fingers down the back of her neck*) Sort of here and here.
>
> *Therapist:* Can you get in touch with any feelings, any emotions?
>
> *Patient:* (*Pause*) I don't know. (*She covers her eyes, puts her head down, and begins to cry. She takes a handkerchief from her pocketbook and dries her tears.*) It makes me sad. I understand it, but it still upsets me.
>
> *Therapist:* Let's talk about the sadness.

The bridging maneuver commenced when the therapist switched from the cognitive emphasis and inquired, "Are you in touch with any feelings or sensations right now?" This elicited a sensory response from the patient, "I've got a slight headache." The therapist then focused on the sensory modality which rapidly elicited affective reactions. Thus, a five-minute "detour" avoided unnecessary confrontations, permitted the patient to be "heard," and brought forth the feeling states that the therapist was initially interested in pursuing.

Similarly, in treating a man who was highly visual and who created vivid images that preceded and accompanied virtually every encounter, it was necessary first to discuss his mental pictures before bridging to his thoughts and feelings. Referring to a person as visual or as a sensory reactor or a cognitive reactor, does not mean that the person will always respond in that given modality. Clinically, however, the author has noted that people tend to favor one or two modalities (which often correlates with their quantitative ratings on a structural profile). By joining the patient in his or her preferred modality, it is usually simple to guide him or her into other areas of discourse.

Tracking refers scrutinizing carefully the "firing order" of the different modalities. For example, some patients tend to generate negative emotions by dwelling first on catastrophic ideas (cognitions), immediately followed by unpleasant mental pictures (images), that lead to tension and heart palpitations (sensations), culminating in avoidance or withdrawal (behavior). The foregoing pattern of cognitions to images to sensations to behavior may call for different treatment strategies than, say, a pattern going from sensations to cognitions to images to behavior. In practice, it is usually more productive to administer techniques in the same sequence as the patient's own "firing order." Thus, relaxation and biofeedback would be favored as initial treatments for a patient with sensations in the first order (i.e., predominantly sensory techniques to meet the patient's sensory trigger). The patient whose pattern goes from cognitions to images to sensations to behavior would be expected to respond less well to sensory techniques until some improvement was evident in cognitive and imagery areas. Some experimental support for these observations has recently been presented (Öst et al., 1981; 1982).

FINAL COMMENT

This has been a brief overview of multimodal therapy. Halleck (1982), commenting on the multimodal orientation, stated that "it should cause us to ponder the limits of our current practices and convince us that the goal of rational multidimensional practice is achievable" (24). The author hopes that the BASIC ID framework will appeal to those who are interested in multidimensional and multifaceted interventions, but who are also cognizant of the limitations of unsystematic eclecticism. Above all, the multimodal approach permits the clinician to identify idiosyncratic variables and thereby avoids molding patients to preconceived treatments.

References for Part I

References for the Introduction

Alexander F, French TM: Psychoanalytic Therapy. New York, Ronald Press, 1946

Beck AT, Rush AJ, Shaw BF, Emery G: Cognitive Therapy of Depression. New York, Guilford Press, 1979

Bellak L, Small L (eds): Emergency Psychotherapy and Brief Psychotherapy, 1st ed. New York, Grune & Stratton, 1965

Davanloo H (ed): Short-Term Dynamic Psychotherapy. New York, Spectrum Publications, 1978

Klerman GL, Rounsaville BJ, Chevron ES, Neu C, Weissman MM: Manual for Short-Term Interpersonal Psychotherapy (IPT) of Depression. Unpublished manuscript, fourth draft, June 1979

Klerman GL, Weissman MM, Rounsaville BJ, Chevron ES: Interpersonal Psychotherapy of Depression. New York, Basic Books, 1984

Lazarus AA: The Practice of Multimodal Therapy. New York, McGraw-Hill, 1981

Malan DH: A Study of Brief Psychotherapy. London, Tavistock Publications, 1963

Mann J: Time-Limited Psychotherapy. Cambridge MA, Harvard University Press, 1973

Sifneos PE: Short-Term Psychotherapy and Emotional Crisis. Cambridge MA, Harvard University Press, 1972

Wolberg LR: The Technique of Psychotherapy, 3rd ed. New York, Grune & Stratton, 1977

References for Chapter 1

Intensive Brief and Emergency Psychotherapy

Bellak L: The emergency psychotherapy of depression, in Specialized Techniques in Psychotherapy. Edited by Bychowski G, Despert JL. New York, Basic Books, 1952

Bellak L: A general hospital as a focus of community psychiatry. JAMA 174:2214–2217, 1960

Bellak L: The concept of acting out: Theoretical considerations in Acting Out—Theoretical and Clinical Aspects. Edited by Abt L, Weissman S. New York, Grune & Stratton, 1965

Bellak L: Once over: What is psychotherapy? J Nerv Ment Dis 165:295–299, 1977

Bellak L: Brief psychoanalytic psychotherapy of non-psychotic depression. Amer J Psychother 35:160–172, 1981

Bellak L, Faithorn EP: Crisis and Special Problems in Psychoanalysis and Psychotherapy. New York, Brunner/Mazel, 1981

Bellak L, Siegel H: Handbook of Intensive Brief and Emergency Psychotherapy. Larchmont NY, C.P.S. Inc, 1983

Bellak L, Small L (eds): Emergency Psychotherapy and Brief Psychotherapy, 1st ed. New York, Grune & Stratton, 1965

Bellak L, Small L (eds): Emergency Psychotherapy and Brief Psychotherapy, 2nd ed. New York, Grune & Stratton, 1978

Bellak L, Hurvich M, Gediman H: Ego Functions in Schizophrenics, Neurotics, and Normals. New York, John Wiley & Sons, 1973

Davanloo H: Basic Principles and Techniques in Short-Term Dynamic Psychotherapy. New York, Spectrum Publications, 1978

Jacobson E: Depression: Comparative Studies of Normal, Neurotic and Psychotic Conditions. New York, International Universities Press, 1971

Leighton AH: An Introduction to Social Psychiatry. Springfield IL, Charles C Thomas, 1960

Malan DH: A Study of Brief Psychotherapy. Springfield IL, Charles C Thomas, 1963

Malan DH: Therapeutic factors in analytically oriented brief psychotherapy, in Support, Innovation, and Autonomy. Edited by Gosling R. London, Tavistock Publications, 1973

Mann J: Time Limited Psychotherapy. Cambridge MA, Harvard University Press, 1973

Oberndorf CP: A History of Psychoanalysis in America. New York, Grune & Stratton, 1953

Sifneos PE: Short-Term Psychotherapy and Emotional Crisis. Cambridge MA, Harvard University Press, 1972

References for Chapter 2

Short-Term Anxiety-Provoking Psychotherapy

Alexander F, French T: Psychoanalytic Psychotherapy. New York, Ronald Press, 1946

Ferenczi S: Further Contributions to the Theory and Technique of Psycho-Analysis. 1926. New York, Basic Books, 1952

Malan DH: The Frontier of Brief Psychotherapy. New York, Plenum Press, 1976

Sifneos PE: Dynamic psychotherapy in a psychiatric clinic, in Current Psychiatric Therapies. New York, Grune & Stratton, 1961

Sifneos PE: Learning to solve emotional problems—A controlled study of short-term psychotherapy, in The Role of Learning in Psychotherapy. Edited by Porter R. London, J&A Churchill Ltd. (Ciba Foundation Publication), 1968

Sifneos PE: Psychodynamics and psychotherapy: The cornerstones for the education of the psychiatrist. Nordisk Psykiatrisk Tiddskrift, Bind 24 (Hoefle 2): 116–129, 1970

Sifneos PE: Criteria for psychotherapeutic outcome. Psychother Psychosom 26:49–59, 1975a

Sifneos PE: A research study of short-term anxiety-provoking psychotherapy. Proceedings of the 9th International Congress of Psychotherapy. New York/Basel, S Karger AG, 1975b

Sifneos PE: Short-Term Psychotherapy and Emotional Crisis. Cambridge MA, Harvard University Press, 1972

Sifneos PE: Short-Term Dynamic Psychotherapy Evaluation and Technique. New York, Plenum Press, 1979

Sifneos PE, Apfel R, Bassuk E, Fishman G, Gill A: Ongoing outcome research in short-term dynamic psychotherapy. Psychother Psychosom 4:233–242, 1980

References for Chapter 3

Time Limited Psychotherapy

Hartocollis P: Time as a dimension of affects. J Am Psychoanal Assoc 20:92–108, 1972

Mann J: Time Limited Psychotherapy. Cambridge MA, Harvard University Press, 1973

Mann J, Goldman R: A Casebook in Time Limited Psychotherapy. New York, McGraw-Hill, 1982

References for Chapter 4

Cognitive Therapy

American Psychiatric Association: Diagnostic and Statistical Manual of Mental Disorders, 3rd ed. Washington DC, American Psychiatric Association, 1980

Ansbacher HL, Ansbacher RR (eds): The Individual Psychology of Alfred Adler: A Systematic Presentation in Selection from his Writings. New York, Basic Books, 1956

Beck AT: Cognitive Therapy and the Emotional Disorders. New York, International Universities Press, 1976

Beck AT, Greenberg RL: Coping with Depression. Philadelphia, University of Pennsylvania, Center for Cognitive Therapy, 1974

Beck AT, Rush AJ: Cognitive approaches to depression and suicide, in Cognitive Defects in the Development of Mental Illness. Edited by Serban G. New York, Brunner/Mazel, 1978

Beck AT, Rush AJ, Shaw BF, Emery G: Cognitive Therapy of Depression. New York, Guilford Press, 1979

Bergner RM: The marital system of the hysterical individual. Fam Process, 16:85–95, 1977

Berman EM, Lief HI: Marital therapy from a psychiatric perspective: An overview. Am J Psychiatry 132:583–592, 1975

Blackburn I, Bishop S, Glen AIM, Whalley LJ, Christie JE: The efficacy of cognitive therapy in depression: A treatment trial using cognitive therapy and pharmacotherapy, each alone and in combination. Br J Psychiatry 139:181–189, 1981

Brownell K, Heckerman CL, Westlake RJ: The effect of couples training and spouse cooperativeness in the behavioral treatment of obesity. Paper presented at the annual meeting of the Association for the Advancement of Behavior Therapy, Atlanta, December 1977

Kaplan HS: The New Sex Therapy. New York, Brunner/Mazel, 1974

Khatami M, Rush AJ: A pilot study of the treatment of outpatients with chronic pain: Symptom control, stimulus control, and social system intervention. Pain 5:163–172, 1978

Khatami M, Rush AJ: One year follow-up of multimodal treatment of chronic pain. Pain 14:45–52, 1982

Kovacs M, Rush AJ, Beck AT, Hollon SD: Depressed outpatients treated with cognitive therapy or pharmacotherapy. A one-year follow-up. Arch Gen Psychiatry 38:33–39, 1981

Masters WH, Johnson VE: Human Sexual Inadequacy. Boston, Little Brown & Co, 1970

Rush AJ: Psychotherapy of the affective psychoses. Am J Psychoanal 40:99–123, 1980

Rush AJ: Cognitive therapy for depression, in Affective and Schizophrenic Disorders: New Approaches to Diagnosis. Edited by Zales MR. New York, Brunner/Mazel, 1982a

Rush AJ (ed): Short-Term Psychotherapies for Depression. New York, Guilford Press, 1982b

Rush AJ, Beck AT: Cognitive therapy of depression and suicide. Am J Psychother 32:201–219, 1978a

Rush AJ, Beck AT: Adults with affective disorders, in Behavioral Therapy in the Psychiatric Setting. Edited by Hersen M, Bellack AS. Baltimore, Williams & Wilkins Co, 1978b

Rush AJ, Giles DE: Cognitive therapy: Theory and research, in Short-Term Psychotherapies in Depression. Edited by Rush AJ. New York, Guilford Press, 1982

Rush AJ, Khatami M, Beck AT: Cognitive and behavioral therapy in chronic depression. Behav Ther 6:398–404, 1975

Rush AJ, Holon SD, Beck AT, Kovacs M: Depression: Must pharmacotherapy fail for cognitive therapy to succeed? Cognitive Therapy and Research 2:199–206, 1978

Rush AJ, Beck AT, Kovacs M, Weissenburger J, Hollon SD: Differential effects of cognitive therapy and pharmacotherapy on hopelessness and self concept. Am J Psychiatry 139:862–866, 1982

Sager CJ, Gundlach R, Kremer M: The married intriguement. Arch Gen Psychiatry 19:205–217, 1968

Spiegelberg H: The Phenomenological Movement, vols 1 and 2. The Hague, Nijhoff, 1971

Spiegelberg H: Phenomenology in Psychology and Psychiatry. Evanston IL, Northwestern University Press, 1972

Spitzer RL, Endicott J, Robins E: Research diagnostic criteria: Rationale and reliability. Arch Gen Psychiatry 3:773–782, 1978

Spradley JP (ed): Culture and Cognition: Rules, Maps and Plans. San Francisco, Chandler, 1972

References for Chapter 5

Interpersonal Psychotherapy for Depression

Arieti S, Bemporad J: Severe and Mild Depression. The Psychotherapeutic Approach. New York, Basic Books, 1978

Becker J: Depression: Theory and Research. New York, John Wiley & Sons, 1974

Bloom BL, Asher SJ, White SW: Marital disruption as a stressor: A review and analysis. Psychol Bull 85:867–894, 1978

Bowlby J: Attachment and Loss, vol 1: Attachment. New York, Basic Books, 1969

Bowlby J: The making and breaking of affectional bonds: II. Some principles of psychotherapy. Br J Psychiatry 130:421–431, 1977

Briscoe CW, Smith JB: Depression and marital turmoil. Arch Gen Psychiatry 28:811–817, 1973

Brown GW, Harris T, Copeland JR: Depression and loss. Br J Psychiatry 130:1–18, 1977

Chodoff P: The core problem in depression, in Science and Psychoanalysis. Edited by Masserman J. New York, Grune & Stratton, 1970

Cohen MB, Blake G, Cohen R, Fromm-Reichmann F, Weigert E: An intensive study of twelve cases of manic-depressive psychosis. Psychiatry 17:103–137, 1954

Coyne JC: Depression and the response of others. J Abnorm Psychol 85:186–193, 1976

Fieve RR: Moodswing. New York, Bantam Books, 1975

Frank J: Persuasion and Healing: A Comparative Study of Psychotherapy. Baltimore, Johns Hopkins University Press, 1973

Fromm-Reichmann F: Principles of Intensive Psychotherapy. Chicago, Phoenix Books, 1960

Henderson S, Duncan-Jones P, McAuley H, Ritchie K: The patient's primary group. Br J Psychiatry 132:74–86, 1978a

Henderson S, Duncan-Jones P, Byrne DG, Scott R, Adcock S: Social bonds, adversity, and neurosis. Presented at World Psychiatric Association, Comm on Epidemiology and Community Psychiatry, St. Louis, Oct 18–20, 1978b

Henderson S, Byrne DG, Duncan-Jones P, Adcock S, Scott R, Steele GP: Social bonds in the epidemiology of neurosis. Br J Psychiatry 132:463–466, 1978c

Ilfeld FW: Current social stressors and symptoms of depression. Am J Psychiatry 134:161–166, 1977

Klerman GL: Stress, adaptation and affective disorders, in Stress and Mental Disorder. Edited by Barrett JE, Rose RM, Klerman GL. New York, Raven Press, 1979

Klerman GL, Rounsaville BJ, Chevron ES, Neu C, Weissman MM: Manual for Short-Term Interpersonal Psychotherapy (IPT) of Depression. Unpublished manuscript, fourth draft, June 1979

Klerman GL, Weissman MM, Rounsaville BJ, Chevron ES: Interpersonal Psychotherapy of Depression. New York, Basic Books, 1984

Meyer A: Psychobiology: A Science of Man. Springfield IL, Charles C Thomas, 1957

Paykel ES, Myers JK, Dienelt MN, Klerman GL, Lindenthal JJ, Pepper MP: Life events and depression: A controlled study. Arch Gen Psychiatry 21:753–760, 1969

Pearlin LI, Lieberman MA: Social sources of emotional distress, in Research in Community and Mental Health. Edited by Simmons R. Greenwich CT, JAI Press, 1977

Rutter M: Maternal Deprivation Reassessed. London, Penguin Books, 1972

Scarf M: Unfinished Business: Pressure Points in the Lives of Women. New York, Doubleday & Co, 1980

Spiegel JP: The resolution of role conflict within families. Psychiatry 20:1–16, 1957

Sullivan HS: Conceptions of Modern Psychiatry. New York, WW Norton & Co, 1953a

Sullivan HS: The Interpersonal Theory of Psychiatry. New York, WW Norton & Co, 1953b

Weissman MM, Paykel ES: The Depressed Woman: A Study of Social Relationships. Chicago, University of Chicago Press, 1974

References for Chapter 6

Multimodal Therapy

Brunell LF, Young WT: Multimodal Handbook for a Mental Hospital. New York, Springer, 1982

Halleck SL: The search for competent eclecticism. Contemp Psychiatry 1:22–24, 1982

Hayes-Roth F, Longabaugh R, Ryback R: The problem-oriented medical record and psychiatry. Br J Psychiatry 121:27–34, 1972

Keat DB: Multimodal Therapy with Children. New York, Pergamon Press, 1979

Lazarus AA: Multimodal behavior therapy: Treating the BASIC ID. J Nerv Ment Dis 156:404–411, 1973

Lazarus AA: Multimodal Behavior Therapy. New York, Springer, 1976

Lazarus AA: The Practice of Multimodal Therapy. New York, McGraw-Hill, 1981

Lazarus AA: Multimodal therapy, in Current Psychotherapies, 3rd ed. Edited by Corsini RJ. Itasca IL, Peacock, 1983

Lazarus AA, Fay A: Resistance or rationalization? A cognitive-behavioral perspective, in Resistance: Psychodynamic and Behavioral Approaches. Edited by Wachtel PL. New York, Plenum, 1982

Messer SB, Winokur M: Some limits to the integration of psychoanalytic and behavior therapy. Am Psychol 35:818–827, 1980

Öst LG, Jerrelmalm A, Johansson J: Individual response patterns and the effects of different behavioral methods in the treatment of social phobia. Behav Res Ther 19:1–16, 1981

Öst LG, Johansson J, Jerrelmalm A: Individual response patterns and the effects of different behavioral methods in the treatment of claustrophobia. Behav Res Ther 20:445–460, 1982

Smith D: Trends in counseling and psychotherapy. Am Psychol 37:802–809, 1982

Weed LL: Medical records that guide and teach. N Engl J Med 278:593–600, 1968

Zilbergeld B: Bespoke therapy. Psychol Today 16:85–86, 1982

II
Children at Risk

Part II
Children at Risk

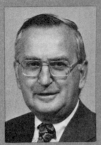

Irving Philips, M.D.,
Preceptor

Director and Professor
Child and Adolescent Psychiatry
University of California
  at San Francisco

Authors for Part II

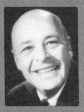

Norman Garmezy, Ph.D.
Professor of Psychology
University of Minnesota

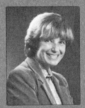

Lenore Cagen Terr, M.D.
Associate Clinical Professor
  of Psychiatry
University of California
  at San Francisco

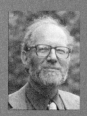

Henry Grunebaum, M.D.

Clinical Professor
  of Psychiatry
Harvard Medical School
Director, Group and Family
  Psychotherapy Training
Cambridge Hospital

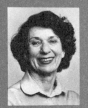

Judith S. Wallerstein, Ph.D.

Executive Director
Center for the Family
  in Transition

	Page
Introduction to Part Two	87
Irving Philips, M.D.	
Chapter 7	*91*
Children Vulnerable to Major Mental	
Disorders: Risk and Protective Factors	
Norman Garmezy, Ph.D.	
Introduction	91
Risk Concepts in the History	
of Psychiatry	93
Research on the Risk for	
Specific Disorders	95
Methodological Issues in	
Risk Research	101
The Search for Protective Factors	102
Chapter 8	*104*
Children at Acute Risk:	
Psychic Trauma	
Lenore Cagen Terr, M.D.	
Review of the Literature	104
Recent Research	111
Interventions	117
Summary	120
Chapter 9	*120*
Children with Mental Retardation	
Irving Philips, M.D.	
Introduction	· 120
Epidemiology of Emotional Disorder	123
Intervention and Prevention	125
Chapter 10	*129*
Parenting and Children at Risk	
Henry Grunebaum, M.D.	
Introduction	129
Children with Mentally Ill Parents	130
Children with Parents Under Stress	135
Issues in Preventive Intervention	136
Interventions and their Outcomes	138
Epilogue	143

Chapter 11   *144*
Children of Divorce:
   The Dilemma of a Decade
   Judith S. Wallerstein, Ph.D.
Incidence and Social Impacts
   of Divorce   144
The Nature of Divorce   147
Children's Reactions to Divorce   150
Disputed Custody and Visitation   154
Future Directions   157

References for Part Two   *159*

Introduction
by Irving Philips, M.D.

Children at risk as a research endeavor is both old and new. There have always been efforts to help developing children avoid injury and achieve their maximum potentials. A relatively new effort is the systematic research that aims to determine risk factors in relation to vulnerability and outcome as well as protective factors and competencies in the face of similar stressors. Reflecting these old and new endeavors are two sometimes overlapping definitions of *children at risk.* In the first place, children at risk can simply mean children who, because of particular physical, psychosocial, or socioeconomic conditions, are at risk of future difficulty or danger. Associated with the newer research endeavors, children at risk can also mean the children of a parent (or parents) with major mental disorder. The chapters in this Part reflect the currency of both definitions and both the older and newer research concerns.

Research on children at risk has evolved rapidly during the past several decades. Garmezy's 1974 article, "Children at Risk: The Search for the Antecedents of Schizophrenia," is a classic in the field and has stimulated the work of many. In that article, Garmezy cited communications with the pioneering researcher, Barbara Fish. In the 1950s, Fish and Alpert had in a limited sample affirmed the predictive power of deviant neurological development as an indicator of vulnerability to schizophrenia, but their study was criticized as requiring a larger sample. However, as Fish privately communicated to Garmezy, "plans for a larger scale study with appropriate controls failed to receive support in 1958 because these risk studies were then viewed as too 'farfetched' " (Garmezy, 1974, 19). More recently, the chapter, "A Taxonomy of Psychosocial Risks in Infancy," contained 48 pages of single-spaced references to approximately 1,100 published research reports in the field (Swain et al., 1980b). From an idea too farfetched to be productive, this area of research has grown to encompass a broad spectrum that ranges from studies of biopsychosocial stressors on infants to studies of untoward, unexpected, and unplanned stressors on the developing child.

A conceptual framework for addressing the major features of psychosocial risk today must be comprehensive. Such a scheme, duplicated in Figure 1, has been offered by Swain et al. (1980a). Based on this model, many developmental outcomes are possible. Again, Swain et al. (1980a) have offered a useful enumeration. Outcomes for the infant or young child include the following.

1. "Normal" child
2. Developmental disabilities and mental retardation
3. Emotional and psychophysiological disorders
4. Hyperactivity and conduct disorders
5. Depression
6. Physical growth problems (obesity, failure to thrive)
7. Abuse
8. Psychosis (including early infantile autism)
9. "Invulnerable" child

For parents and families, Swain et al. list five possible outcomes.

1. "Normal" parents and families
2. Parental reactive disorders
3. Marital discord
4. Disturbed family relations
5. "Invulnerable" parents and families[1]

Broad as are these lists and the model presented in Figure 1, they do not consider the untoward and unexpected tragedies of life often referred to in insurance terminology as acts of God: hurricanes, fires, tornadoes, and floods; kidnappings of the innocent; the witnessing of murder and bloodshed. Nor do they incorporate the sudden emergence in a parent of major affective disorder or psychosis or the growing problems of divorce, neglect, or desertion. But even these additions would not exhaust the list. The field has grown considerably, even since 1980.

Many aspects of vulnerability are being studied today: the genetic, the psychogenetic, and the sociogenetic and the interactions of each of these with each other. As Werner and Smith noted in their impressive study on the children of Kauai, "to venture a guess at (or predict) the probabilities of developmental outcomes we had to consider both the child's constitutional makeup and the quality of his or her caretaking environment" (1982, 7). This model thus reinforces the earlier transactional model of Sameroff and Chandler (1975), which focuses on the organism's ability, over time and development, to organize the world adaptively in the face of the quality of the caregiving environment. Werner and Smith (1982) have particularly emphasized the protective factors in a child's experience that can lead to invincibility even though the child encounters the same biopsychosocial stressors that make for risk in others. Protective factors have often been overlooked in the search for stressors that result in vulnerability and subsequent pathology. Although this Part does not consider protective factors in depth, it does emphasize the intervention programs for those who are vulnerable and who are not so fortunately resilient as their more favored peers.

Dr. Norman Garmezy, a pioneer in the search for both risk and protective factors, has prepared a chapter that delves into the current knowledge about children at risk for the major mental disorders of antisocial personality disorder, affective disorder, and schizophrenia. He especially emphasizes studies of the vulnerability of children who have a schizophrenic parent. He precedes his discussion of this research with an exploration of the roots of the risk concept in the history of psychiatry and concludes it with a synopsis of the methodological difficulties in studying risk factors. Finally, he touches on the emerging knowledge of protective factors.

Dr. Lenore Cagen Terr presents current data and a number of historical observations on the effects on children of psychic trauma pursuant to wars, disasters, and other unexpected events. As she points out in her review of the psychic trauma concept, its history of definition and redefinition has led to some quiet periods and some confusion in this

[1]Permission to reproduce lists granted by the publisher. Material originally appeared in Swain DB, Hawkins RC II, Walker LO, Penticuff JH (editors): Preface, in Exceptional Infant, Vol. 4. New York, Brunner/Mazel, 1980, ix, Figure 2.

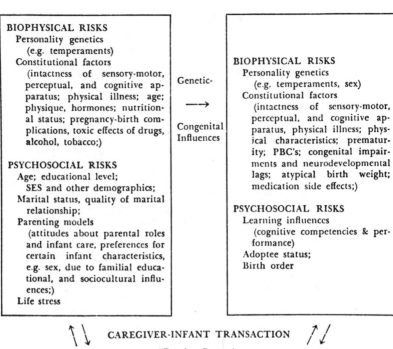

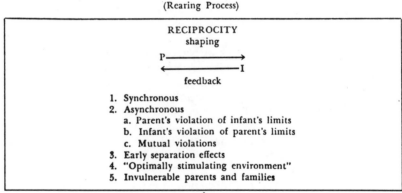

Figure 1. Psychosocial risks in pregnancy and early infancy

Source: Swain DB, Hawkins RC II, Walker LO, Penticuff JH (editors): Preface, in Exceptional Infant, Vol 4. New York, Brunner / Mazel, 1980, viii, Figure 1. Permission to reprint granted by the publisher.

area of risk research. Nonetheless, as she illustrates, recent research has been fruitful, and some critical new areas for study are beginning to draw attention. At the end of her chapter, Dr. Terr offers some guidelines for group, family, and individual interventions toward minimizing the long-range psychological harm that children may suffer posttraumatically.

The Preceptor chose to write a chapter on a group all too frequently avoided and often misunderstood by mental health professionals—children with mental retardation. As the data in the chapter indicate, these children are at high risk for developing a wide range of mental disorders, along with the developmental difficulties which they have by definition. With a minority of these children, the mental retardation is severe, and a protected life outside the family may be necessary. For most, the trend is community living, where possible with the natural family. Child psychiatrists and mental health professionals have many roles to play, from helping the family adjust to having a retarded child, to helping the retarded individual directly with his or her emotional difficulties. The chapter concludes with a review of the wide variety of primary, secondary, and tertiary prevention measures addressed to this multietiologic condition.

Dr. Henry Grunebaum focuses primarily on the processes of parenting and child rearing and examines the possibilities for intervention, both with children who have a mentally ill parent and with children whose parent or parents are experiencing stress without identified psychopathology. With the specific attention to parental behavior of mentally ill adults, Dr. Grunebaum's first topic thus complements some of Garmezy's review. From here the chapter explores the stresses on mothers and families which may lead to a child's emotional or behavioral difficulties. Finally, the chapter includes a detailed review of programmatic interventions which have been attempted with the two populations of interest.

In the last chapter of the Part, Dr. Judith S. Wallerstein reviews the research and the research agenda pertaining to a particularly large group of children at risk for emotional difficulty—the children of divorce. As well as examining current knowledge concerning the process of divorce, the changes in parent-child relationships, and short- and long-range effects on children's psychological development, she reviews some startling statistics on divorce and its social impacts. As Dr. Wallerstein emphasizes, psychosocial knowledge in this area is not keeping pace with the rapidly changing field of family law. Consequently, the long-term effects of such popular interventions as mediation and joint custody are undocumented. Not surprisingly in light of her perspective, she ends her chapter with an outline of research and intervention priorities.

There will never be enough psychiatrists or mental health workers to care adequately for those children at risk who become impaired. Interventions must therefore be directed toward primary, secondary, and tertiary prevention. The major benefit of risk research is in its preventive potential, or the neutralization of stressors by intervention. Interventions may support protective factors through enrichment, or they may ameliorate stressors either to reduce impairment or disability or to prevent the emergence of disorder. We know that children respond to adequate and sustained intervention. Although too few psychiatrists or mental health workers are involved in either research or prevention, many opportunities for prevention do exist. Given a clear delineation of where best to intervene, the practitioner, of whatever discipline, may become more attentive to research findings and apply them to individual situations. Through the chapters in this Part and their discussions of biopsychosocial stressors and associated interventions, the Preceptor hopes that some of this delineation has occurred. "It is essential to translate research findings into methodology that will improve not only practice but also the plight of individuals who are in need . . . and vulnerable, so that prevention will become an integral consideration of all treatment programs" (Philips, 1983, 394).

Chapter 7

Children Vulnerable to Major Mental Disorders: Risk and Protective Factors[†]
by Norman Garmezy, Ph.D.

INTRODUCTION

The concept of *risk* has a universal meaning. From its seventeenth century origins in the world of commerce and insurance to its contemporary use in medicine, risk has implied hazard, danger (often of unknown origin), and loss. In contrast, the concept of *protective factors* is of recent origin and has but a modest recognition within the scientific community. There is a research literature associated with risk, although it often travels under other names; in comparison, research on the protective factors that may modify risk shows evidence of benign neglect, despite recognition of its potential significance.

Epidemiology is the core science concerned with both risk and protective factors. That is evident in the three fundamental questions Gruenberg (1981) has cited as epidemiology's province. (1) Who gets sick? Who does not? (2) Why? (What are the risk factors?) (3) What can be done to reduce the incidence of sickness? To question (2) we can add, What are the protective factors? Obviously, protective factors can restrict the incidence of illness and thus have direct relevance for both question (1) and question (3). These research issues are the heart of the current movement to investigate risk and protective factors in the major mental disorders. Research is emphasizing the predisposing factors in disorder (i.e., the assessment of risk and vulnerability indices) and the search for protective factors (i.e., the assessment of indicators that reflect resistance to disorder). The ultimate goal is to integrate knowledge drawn from both areas into a sound strategy for identifying vulnerable

[†]Preparation of this chapter was facilitated by a grant from the William T. Grant Foundation, by Grant No. MH 33222 from the National Institute of Mental Health, and by National Institute of Mental Health Research Career Award No. MH 14914.

The chapter includes materials originally published by the author in:

Garmezy N: Children at risk: The search for the antecedents to schizophrenia. Part II. Ongoing research programs, issues and intervention. Schizophr Bull 9:55–125, 1974

Garmezy N: The experimental study of children vulnerable to psychopathology, in Child Personality and Psychopathology, vol. 2. Edited by Davids A. New York, John Wiley & Sons, 1975

Garmezy N: On some risks in research. Editorial. Psychol Med 7:1–6, 1977

Garmezy N: The current status of research with children at risk for schizophrenia and other forms of psychopathology, in Risk Factor Research in the Major Mental Disorders. Edited by Regier DA, Allen G. Washington DC, US Government Printing Office. DHHS Publication No. (ADM) 81–1068, 1981

Garmezy N: Stress-resistant children: The search for protective factors, in Proceedings of the 10th International Congress of the International Association for Child and Adolescent Psychiatry and Allied Professions. Edited by Rutter M, Hersov L. Elmsford NY, Pergamon Press, 1983 individuals and for initiating preventive interventions to contain the emergence of disorder in such persons.

Risk and vulnerability have often been used as synonyms. Holzman (1982) has urged that a distinction be made between them. He has suggested that *vulnerability* be used to describe a "perceivable, palpable, or measurable variation in structure or function that represents a predisposition to a specific disease process" (Holzman, 1982, 19). Vulnerability is identifiable prior to the onset of disease and heightens the individual's susceptibility to it, provided that certain as yet unknown environmental conditions are present. Such traits are necessary but not sufficient conditions for the development of disease. In contrast, *risk* factors are neither necessary nor sufficient, but they express statistical probabilities that some groups of people will become affected by a particular disorder. Whether that probability eventuates in disorder will be a function of whether the underlying structural predisposition is present in the individual's makeup.

The relative neglect of epidemiology in psychiatry in the United States compared with Great Britain and western Europe is now being transformed into a growing awareness of its power to generate clues about risk, vulnerability, and protective factors. The National Institute of Mental Health (NIMH) is newly committed to measuring the scope of America's mental health problem through the Epidemiologic Catchment Area (ECA) Program and grants to several major university departments. The program aims to assess the scope of the nation's problem and its use of psychiatric services, to identify individual and environmental characteristics which place people at greater risk for developing mental disorders, and ultimately to advance the knowledge of multiple causation and to put forth suitable strategies for intervention. Darrel Regier, Director of the NIMH Division of Biometry and Epidemiology, has elaborated on four more specific objectives for the program. A first objective is to identify risk factors beyond those usually studied (demographic factors and life events) to locate biological as well as social, environmental, and psychological variables that have a higher specificity for the major mental disorders. Next, the Institute seeks to assess the potential utility of each factor in a program of trials similar to that of the Heart Institute. The final two objectives, according to Regier, are "to develop criteria for deciding when a potential risk factor should be subjected to a large-scale epidemiologic trial . . . [and] . . . to promote a close alliance between neurobiology and general psychiatry, sociology and psychology in research on the etiology of mental disorders" (Regier, 1981, 6–7).

Several observations about this laudable research movement are relevant to the subject of this chapter. First is the program's current restriction to studies of the adult population. This emphasis will, of necessity, devolve on contemporary demographic status and potential dispositional (biological and behavioral) variables. Possible developmental antecedents, if they are studied, may well be contaminated by the frequently noted errors that stem from adults' retrospective recall of childhood behaviors and significant early life events. A developmental and longitudinal orientation should have a place in these catchment area programs, and the identification of children presumed to be at risk for behavioral pathology should become an integral part of the catchment research programs that are now being mounted.

Second, the programmatic emphasis is on etiology, always a driving force in medical research. A risk factor can, however, be nonetiologic but still predictive in its ability to potentiate a vulnerability to disorder. The issue of causation in the mental disorders is critical, but a handsome correlate need not carry the basic properties of an etiologic agent to have status as a valuable risk factor.

Third, the emphasis on risk should be matched by equivalent emphasis on protective elements, just as Gruenberg's (1981) triad of research questions gives equal importance to those who get sick (risk) and to those who do not (resistance). To develop a meaningful program of prevention requires knowledge in both domains, data on risk factors that lead to the development of illness and data on protective factors. Protective factors can be detected in individuals who, although exposed to risk factors, do not manifest psychopathology and remain functionally competent and adaptive. These individuals can be viewed as the resilient or stress-resistant individuals within a population deemed to be at risk.

RISK CONCEPTS IN THE HISTORY OF PSYCHIATRY

The early beginnings of psychiatry's interest in risk are evident in the work of the field's most luminous figures. Four examples, among many that could be offered, should suffice.

Freud's search for the sexual trauma, real or fantasied, to account for symptoms in hysteria, constituted a milestone not only for dynamic psychiatry, but for risk research as well.* The power of such a trauma as a risk factor had been known to other distinguished figures such as Charcot and Kraepelin.

Kraepelin's own awareness of the concept of risk is revealed in his scholarly treatise, *Dementia Praecox and Paraphrenia* (Kraepelin, 1919). For the first 250 pages of that volume, Kraepelin offered a masterly description of the phenomenology of dementia praecox. Then, in a brief concluding section devoted to coping with the disease, he presented his view of possible risk factors.

> In children of such characteristics as we so very frequently find in the previous history of *dementia praecox* one might think of an attempt at prophylaxis especially if the malady had been already observed in the parents or brothers or sisters. Whether it is possible in such circumstances to ward off the outbreak of the threatening disease, we do not know. But in any case it would be advisable to promote to the utmost of one's power general bodily development and to avoid one-sided training in brain work, as it may well be assumed that a vigorous body grown up under natural conditions will be in a better position to overcome the danger than a child exposed to the influences of effeminacy, of poverty, and of exact routine, and especially of city education. Childhood spent in the country with plenty of open air, bodily exercise, escalation beginning late without ambitious aims, simple food, would be the principal points to keep in view (Kraepelin, 1919, 253).

Kraepelin's statement incorporates the view of a genetic diathesis and a set of potentiating stressors, a formulation common today. His suggested interventions, although stylistically different, can be readily

*Editor's note: In Part V, Nemiah presents a review and examination of Freud's theories on hysteria and anxiety.

translated into the present idiom of dispositional and environmental risk: gender confusion and gender identity, social isolation, overideational obsessiveness, rigid compulsivity, disadvantaged social class status, and the disabling effects of limited educational opportunities and experiences.

Adolf Meyer (1919) also perceived stressful events as risk factors, and he formalized their significance in the "life chart," an instrument that graphically depicted possible temporal relationships between stressful antecedent events and maladaptive consequences. Meyer's method was the forerunner of the current life events schedules (e.g., Holmes and Rahe, 1967; Coddington, 1972a; 1972b; Dohrenwend and Dohrenwend, 1974). These schedules catalogue stressors presumed to be potentially destabilizing in the lives of normal and vulnerable children. Their moderate correlations with a broad band of physical and mental disturbances provide a window into the relationship between event and disease, but the processes underlying these modest relationships require (and typically have not received) explication from researchers using the method.

Add to this distinguished group Manfred Bleuler and his recent contribution, *The Schizophrenic Disorders: Long-Term Patient and Family Studies* (Bleuler, 1978). This extraordinary volume summarizes the results of Bleuler's longitudinal 22-year study of 208 schizophrenic probands. The book is replete with data related to potential risk factors evident in the backgrounds of the patient cohort. An important bonus is the volume's lengthy chapter on the adaptation of the probands' offspring, the stress they have endured, and their adaptive methods for coping with their disadvantaged status. Bleuler's contribution is also noteworthy in that it anticipated the focus of many recent research programs on the development of children born to parents diagnosed schizophrenic (Watt et al., 1984). Another noteworthy feature is Bleuler's citation of the many adaptational successes of the probands' offspring. "The majority of them are healthy and socially competent, even though many . . . have lived through miserable childhoods, and even though there are reasons to suspect adverse hereditary traits . . . One is even left with the impression that pain and suffering has a steeling—a hardening—effect on the personalities of some children, making them capable of mastering their lives with all its obstacles, in defiance of all their disadvantages" (Bleuler, 1978, 409). Such observations speak to the importance of searching vigorously for the strengths that are contributed by protective factors in the lives of patients and family members.

The historical continuity evident in the foregoing examples is also evident in the expanding research on risk factors in the major mental disorders. The material that follows focuses on developmental studies of children deemed to be at risk. Space limitations force the author to ignore explorations into risk factors beyond the precursor periods of childhood and adolescence. One can study risk at various points in the life span of the mental patient. For example, the many studies of prognostic indicators also provide important data on risk and protective factors.

One specific example is provided by the investigations of the adaptation of patients discharged back to the community. Who relapses? Who recovers? These questions parallel those posed by Gruenberg, indicating that investigations addressed to these issues also lie in the domain of risk research. A distinguished group of British investigators have combined clinical sensitivity with rigorous methodology to develop a carefully designed, reliable clinical interview with family members (parents/spouse) of patients who have returned to the community (Birley and Brown, 1970; Brown et al., 1972; Leff, 1976; Vaughn and Leff, 1976a; 1976b; Vaughn et al., 1982). Their findings indicate a pronounced relationship between florid schizophrenic symptomatology in the course of a year-long follow-up period and a home atmosphere marked by intense "expressed emotion" (EE). This index of emotional interaction is made up of three ratings: hostility, marked emotional involvement, and the number of critical comments made by relatives when talking about the patient and his or her illness.*

Family settings marked by high EE constituted a risk factor for the patient, one indexed by a heightened probability of return to the hospital. Low-EE settings apparently served as a protective factor, as measured by greater retention rates in the community of patients residing with such families. The studies reveal other protective factors as well. EE can be dampened by training the ex-patient and family members in needed social skills. Drug maintenance and reduced contact with family members apparently are additional protective factors. Still another is the availability of support systems in the community, a protective factor that has been repeatedly validated in a literature focused on adaptation of patients following their discharge from a mental hospital.

Of particular interest here is the demonstrated utility of EE in investigations with nonschizophrenic adolescents referred to a University clinic. At the UCLA risk research program, Goldstein, Rodnick, and their colleagues have shown that EE has predictive status as a risk variable with disturbed adolescents. Family interactions in the laboratory were coded for EE, and they predicted the psychiatric status of adolescents five years after they were first seen for diagnosis and treatment. The offspring of consistently negative (high EE) parent pairs were frequently diagnosed as schizophrenia spectrum disorder cases; in contrast, the offspring of benign parent (low EE) pairs had favorable outcomes (Lewis et al., 1981; Rodnick et al., 1982).

The diversity of risk studies that cross developmental stages is more than equaled by the diversity of contexts in which risk studies are conducted. In the three sections that follow, aspects of current research on three of the severe major mental disorders are briefly described. The first section deals with one of the most refractory, antisocial personality disorder, and subsequent sections explore the research on risk for the affective disorders and schizophrenia.

RESEARCH ON THE RISK FOR SPECIFIC DISORDERS

Antisocial Personality Disorder

Investigators have for a long time been trying to develop predictors from childhood behavior of a later diagnosis of antisocial or sociopathic per-

*Editor's note: These studies are reviewed by Dr. Robert Paul Liberman in Part II of *Psychiatry 1982 (Psychiatry Update: Volume I)*, pages 103–106, and family therapies are discussed in Part III of Volume II by Dr. William R. McFarlane, Dr. C. Christian Beels, and Mr. Stephen Rosenheck, pages 242–249.

sonality. Lee Robins's classic study, *Deviant Children Grown Up*, contains a telling paragraph enumerating 15 such predictors for boys.

> If one wishes to choose the most likely candidate for a later diagnosis of sociopathic personality from among children appearing in a child guidance clinic, the best choices appear to be (1) the boy [Note: Sex is a risk factor, with the incidence of male delinquents five times in excess of females] referred for theft or aggression who has shown (2) a diversity of antisocial behavior in many episodes, (3) at least one of which could be grounds for a Juvenile Court appearance and whose antisocial behavior involves him with (4) strangers and organizations as well as with (5) teachers and parents. With these characteristics more than half of the boys appearing at the clinic were later diagnosed sociopathic personality. Such boys had a history of (6) truancy, (7) theft, (8) staying out late, and (9) refusing to obey parents. They (10) lied gratuitously, and (11) showed little guilt over their behavior. They generally were irresponsible about (12) being where they were supposed to be or (13) taking care of money. They were (14) interested in sexual activities and had (15) experimented with homosexual relationships (Robins, 1966, 157, numbers added).

These risk indicators are based on childhood behavioral antecedents to a formal adult diagnosis of antisocial personality disorder. How reliable are these indicators? The research findings may vary somewhat, but a strong consistency has been demonstrated for a number of these factors in studies conducted in Great Britain (Bennett, 1960; West, 1967; West and Farrington, 1973), in the United States (Glueck and Glueck, 1968; Guze, 1976; Conger and Miller, 1966), and in Norway (Olweus, 1978). These citations are merely illustrative, and the list can be readily and extensively expanded.

Other risk factors are revealed by studies of family structure, home atmosphere, parental personality, and neighborhood setting, and they also show marked reliability (McCord and McCord, 1959; Hersov et al., 1978; Patterson, 1982). Robins (1978) analyzed data from four longitudinal studies to compare the power of three classes of factors for predicting adult antisocial specific behaviors: the number of antisocial behaviors exhibited in childhood, specific behaviors, and family variables. The most powerful proved to be the first group, which included a history of childhood arrests, truancy, alcohol use, fighting, sexual activity, school dropout, bad friends, incarceration, and early drug use.

Finally, there have been an increasing number of reports on genetic risk factors which interact with environmental factors in antisocial disorder (Hutchings and Mednick, 1974; Reid, 1978; Cloninger, et al., 1978).

The stability, breadth, and multiplicity of risk factors that characterize antisocial children and their families thus enhance predictions of the continuity of such behavior into adulthood (Rutter, 1972). In this respect, antisocial personality disorder is without peer among the psychopathologies.

Affective Disorders

The study of children at risk for affective disorders is a comparative newcomer, and it adds appreciably to the potential research significance of the area. Several reasons can be suggested for the emergence of this research interest. In the first place, research and clinical activity in the adult affective disorders has increased significantly. Identified with this upswing are a greater rigor of classification, a larger role for epidemiology as the high prevalence rate is observed across social classes, and the discovery of successful drug and behavioral interventions for alleviating the distressing symptomatology of depression. With the growth of research attention to the adult affective disorders, interest inevitably began to turn to severe forms of the disorder and the ramifications for children (e.g., Beardslee et al., 1983; Kashani et al., 1981; McKnew et al., 1979).

Recently, Hirschfeld and Cross (1981) evaluated psychosocial and psychological risk variables that accompany adult depression (see also Hirschfeld and Cross, 1982; 1983). In the same 1981 publication, Prange and Loosen offered a comparable review of somatic risk factors. But none of these reviews referred specifically to risk factors for affective disorder in children.

An overarching vulnerability factor in the affective disorders appears to be genetic. Twin studies, family pedigree data, and adoption studies of offspring born to affectively disordered parents all strongly implicate a genetic factor in bipolar and (to a lesser extent) unipolar affective disease. (For reviews see Slater and Cowie, 1971; Rosenthal, 1970; Gershon, 1983; Nurnberger and Gershon, 1982; Cadoret and Winokur, 1975; Winokur et al., 1969).

The genetic data are robust. From the standpoint of risk research with children, the genetic findings of Gershon et al. (1982) related to the offspring of affectively disordered parents are particularly significant. They showed that if one parent was ill, the age-corrected risk to 614 adult children of patients with major affective illness was 27 percent. For 300 children, each with one bipolar parent and one well parent, the risk was 29.5 percent. If two parents were ill, the risk of major affective disorder rose to 74 percent in 28 offspring. Zerbin-Rudin estimated the morbidity risk of affective disorder in the offspring of manic-depressive index patients at 14.8 percent (cited in Slater and Cowie, 1971). Rosenthal (1970) cited studies of the same diagnosis that revealed a range of risk from 6 percent to 24.1 percent, with a median rate of 11.2 percent. It is thus evident that adult offspring of parents with affective illness have increased rates of morbidity relative to control cases.

Most psychopathologists would endorse Gershon's summary statement that the evidence favoring genetic factors is "persuasive and generally accepted" (Gershon, 1983, 435). Whether or not young children of such parents show precursor signs of disordered mood or more severe depressive symptomatology is only now beginning to be investigated. Particularly relevant to this issue are Gershon's suggestions for programmatic research to isolate characteristics that could serve as etiologic (genetic) markers and the four criteria he offered for determining their power as predisposing vulnerability indicators. The characteristic should (1) be associated with an increased likelihood of the presence of the specific psychiatric illness; (2) be heritable and not exert a secondary effect on the disorder; (3) be observable or capable of being evoked in the well state, thus permitting it to be measured in well relatives; and (4) be related to illness within the pedigree, i.e., transmission of the illness and presence of the marker should be invariant. These criteria for marker status are noteworthy for the precision they demand; to date, risk research has lacked such exactitude.

A number of research programs on children at risk for affective disorders are now underway in the departments of psychiatry at Columbia, Harvard, Yale, Pittsburgh, Washington University, and UCLA and within the NIMH Intramural Research Program. Their range of approaches to the study of risk for depression is commendable. Most of the programs strongly emphasize careful diagnostic assessments of the children. The vexing issue about whether childhood depression exists seems to have been resolved in the affirmative, but the history of its denial has reinforced the need for careful clinical evaluations of children using structured-interview and questionnaire procedures. Diagnostic appraisals of the children of depressed parents and of depressed children in comparison with other clinical groups of children, manifestly disturbed or at risk, may also help to resolve the concept of "masked" depression, with its assumption that hyperactivity, somatization, anxiety, and antisocial behavior may serve to cloak affective disorder in children. Another emphasis in a number of these programs is on the acquisition of epidemiologic, biological, and genetic data, an orientation that has not been central in many of the programs of research with children at risk for schizophrenia.

Early reports from these various programs also demonstrate their breadth of procedures and contexts. In some programs, for example, measurements include extensive batteries of tests to evaluate children's intelligence, sensorimotor integration, memory, achievement, self-concept, and personality characteristics. In-depth interviews are conducted with parents and children, and family psychiatric histories and pedigrees are sought. Stressful events that have impinged on parents and child are being ascertained. Measures of the children's functional competence are joined with assessments of their adaptational difficulties. In one project, mother-child interactions are videotaped in a laboratory set up as a homelike apartment; researchers can observe the recovering patient's activities with her children in the context of routine household activities and the initiation of perturbing events. Other variables being studied include peer interaction and measures of affective arousal, expression, and control. One program has been examining the psychobiological correlates of prepubertal major depressive disorder, including such variables as cortisol secretion, sleep alteration, growth hormone in response to insulin-induced hypoglycemia, and so forth (Puig-Antich and Gittelman, 1982).*

Some projects are using multiple comparison groups. For example, one program is comparing the performance of school-aged children of parents with affective disorder with the performance of those whose parents manifest secondary depression, schizoaffective disorder, and chronic medical illness, as well as with matched community controls. Such multiple comparison groups are essential to determining the specificity of risk variables. Finally, longitudinal studies and follow-up evaluations are considered necessary in order to observe the effects of symptomatic changes that may occur in parents and children over time. Work over the next few years should yield data that will begin to shed light on the competencies and the adaptational successes and failures of children at risk for affective disorders and related states.

*Editor's note: Psychiatry 1982 (Psychiatry Update: Volume I) includes a chapter in Part III by Dr. Joaquim Puig-Antich reviewing the findings to date from these studies (pages 288–296).

Schizophrenia

Nearly half a century has passed since Bender (1937) wrote a monograph on the behavior problems of children of psychotic and criminal parents. Two decades later, Fish (1957) produced the initial account of her longitudinal study of biological deviations in infants who were presumed to be vulnerable to schizophrenia because of the disordered status of their mothers. The recently published volume, *Children at Risk for Schizophrenia: A Longitudinal Perspective* (Watt et al., 1984), reviews the current status of 15 ongoing research programs. In addition to this complete appraisal of studies currently underway in various nations, a series of earlier reviews make it unnecessary here to offer a broad-gauged overview of the research (Garmezy and Streitman, 1974; Garmezy, 1974; 1981; Wynne et al., 1978; Neale and Oltmanns, 1980; Rieder, 1979).

The research strategy is typically longitudinal and developmental. Most frequently, but not exclusively, subjects are selected based on schizophrenic pathology in a biological parent. The weakness inherent in this criterion is its restrictedness. Approximately 10 percent of such children are likely to develop the disorder, but a more substantial proportion (up to 50 percent) would be expected to develop other forms of psychopathology. However, there are discrepancies among the projections (cf. H. Schulsinger, 1976, and Bleuler, 1978), and subject sampling may account for some of the variations in outcome data. For example, the Mednick-Schulsinger project reported high rates of deviancy in the offspring of schizophrenic mothers (Mednick et al., 1971). Their parent cohort included mothers whose onset of schizophrenia had occurred at an early age, as had the birth of their children. In a substantial number of cases, mother and infant were separated following birth of the child, and offspring were subsequently placed in a foster home or institution. In addition, the index group had experienced a number of birth and pregnancy difficulties.

A study conducted by Rodnick and Goldstein (1974) is particularly significant toward understanding some of the processes possibly underlying the enhanced risk to children of young schizophrenic mothers. An interesting parallel to this research exists in the studies that Weissman, Paykel, and Klerman have conducted on infants and young children of severely depressed mothers (Weissman et al., 1972; Weissman, 1979). Rodnick and Goldstein studied the recovery of the caretaking function among good premorbid (reactive) and poor premorbid (process) schizophrenic mothers who had required hospitalization in a community mental health center. The median stay in the hospital was ten days, a brief period due to the closing of many California state mental hospitals. Upon the mothers' return from the hospital, the investigators observed mother-child interactions at home, and they later made follow-up observations, at thirty days, six months, and one year following discharge. Interviews and home visits served as the basis for ratings of caretaking in the two groups of mothers. The poor premorbid mothers were considerably younger than their good premorbid counterparts. Their youngest child typically was a recently born infant, whereas the youngest offspring of the good premorbid mothers was approaching middle childhood. Results revealed that six months were required before the good premorbid mothers returned to an adequate level of caretaking, while one year was required for the poor premorbid group.

One can speculate about the nature of a gene-environment interaction in such cases. Process cases typically show evidence of a strong genetic substrate, and this may be reflected in a predisposition to schizophrenia among the offspring of mothers whose premorbid history is poor and whose disorder has an early onset. When an infant is at home without adequate caretaking for one year, the attachment process is threatened significantly. Inadequate nurturance and genetic predisposition may well interact to heighten vulnerability in such infants. This combination of attributes is not unlike that observed in the Mednick-Schulsinger cohort of schizophrenic mothers.

As for the reactive group (now more likely to be diagnosed as having a schizophreniform disorder), the mothers tended to break down in their late twenties when their children were older, so the offspring have had at least normal child care for a significant time span. This combination of reduced genetic risk and more adequate caretaking may reduce the risk for a schizophrenic disorder in the offspring of good premorbid mothers.

Poor caretaking is not the exclusive province of schizophrenic mothers. Weissman (1979) has reported the powerful impact that a seriously depressed mother has on her offspring, whether they are infants, children, or adolescents. The depressed women she described were "only moderately involved in their children's daily lives, reported difficult communications, lessened affection, and considerable friction with their children," and this contrasted with the experience of normal women, who had "relatively harmonious, involved and affectionate relations . . . with their children" (Weissman, 1979, 100).

CENTRAL VARIABLES The central variables of the various programs on risk for schizophrenia are so numerous that summarizing them has required an extensive multipaged table (see Garmezy, 1975, 186–191; also republished in Rieder, 1979, 252–259). Many of these variables have failed to differentiate between index children and their attendant comparison groups. Those which do have some degree of discriminatory power include the variables discussed below.

Many studies give evidence of *deviant attentional* functioning in children at risk for schizophrenia (Asarnow et al., 1977; Cohler et al., 1977; Rutschmann et al., 1977; Garmezy, 1978). Nuechterlein (1983) has applied signal detection theory to a vigilance task with children of schizophrenic mothers and hyperactive children. The former showed a lower perceptual sensitivity than normal controls, while the hyperactive children's attentional deficits were reflected in a lack of caution in responding.

There is some evidence that children at risk who are clinically deviant show *deficits on neurological tests* (Rieder and Nichols, 1979), but the deficits are not specific to either parental or child psychopathology.

Earlier findings of *deviant psychophysiological functioning* in children at risk have not proved to be robust. Recent studies report diminished P300 amplitude, a late component of the human average evoked potential, in adult schizophrenic patients (Morstyn et al., 1983) and in children at risk for schizophrenia (Friedman et al., 1982). It is hypothesized that this late positive waveform may be associated with the processing of signals, the orienting response, and cognitive processes, particularly the brain's responses to changes in stimuli and to discrepancies in the environment.

Replications of such findings are needed to establish the reliability of this possible neurophysiological indicator.

Perinatal *obstetrical complications* with infants at risk have been reported by numerous investigators (Mednick et al., 1971; Fish, 1960; McNeil and Kaij, 1978). Other researchers have questioned whether this variable is specific to schizophrenia or is more a function of the severity of a mother's illness, irrespective of her type of disorder (Sameroff et al., 1982).

A small subset of infants born to schizophrenic mothers are reported to show *neurological deviations* (Marcus, 1974; Marcus et al., 1981). These deficits, too, may occur in children who are at risk for other forms of psychopathology.

School performance of index children is variable, with some research programs reporting that motivation and emotional stability are lowered.

Temperament differences in infants at risk tend to be small and nonsignificant.

Intellectual test performance in some instances may be depressed, but such deficits are relatively insignificant.

Deviant family interactions, measured by patterns of communication deviance and high levels of EE, have been reported, as noted earlier (Rodnick et al., 1982). Families at risk also lack a positive affective climate when parent and child are engaged in play (Baldwin et al., 1982).

Psychiatric casualties among the index children are now beginning to appear, but current samples are too small and patterns of clinical symptoms are too diverse and highly variable to make the observations definitive (Watt, 1984). This picture can be expected to stabilize somewhat as the index children enter the age period of heightened risk for schizophrenia (age 20 and older).

METHODOLOGICAL ISSUES IN RISK RESEARCH

Risk researchers have been their own strongest critics (Garmezy, 1977; Rieder, 1979; Lewine et al., 1981). Many problems and shortcomings are now evident to risk researchers. Although the points that follow are cast in the context of schizophrenia risk research, many of them are also applicable to research on the risk for other forms of mental disorder.

1. *The limitation inherent in selecting children on the basis of parental illness.* In schizophrenia, as noted previously, this selection method raises the base rate of the likely incidence of the disorder from 1 percent in the general population to 10 to 12 percent, a marked increment but one that leaves almost 90 percent of diagnosed schizophrenics unaccounted for by the method of selection.

2. *Parental sex bias.* Parental cohorts have consisted primarily of schizophrenic mothers rather than schizophrenic fathers. Compared with women, male schizophrenics typically are characterized by earlier onset of the disorder and lower competence, as indicated by their poorer premorbid histories. Thus, the selection of mothers heightens the likelihood that more competent parents, more likely to be diagnosed as schizoaffective, will be selected. With the publication of DSM-III, risk researchers in schizophrenia have had to rediagnose their parent groups; consequently, some projects have reported a substantial diagnostic shift toward the affective disorders in the parent cohorts and a reduction in the numbers diagnosed as schizophrenic.

3. *The difficulties inherent in longitudinal research.* The problem of main-

taining families in long-term research programs is a difficult one. Heavy attrition over time is usual, more so if the sample comprises persons of greater instability, reduced competence, and low levels of motivation and commitment. Longitudinal investigators, too, are eroded by the fact that investigations must stretch over decades in order to obtain data on final outcome dispositions.

4. *The problem of sample size.* Sample size in risk investigations is inevitably limited by the low base rates for children born to schizophrenic parents. Control for variations in age, social class, ethnic and racial composition, parental age, family structure, and intactness further attenuates the sizes of cohort samples.

5. *The problem of diagnosis.* The general problem of obtaining reliable diagnoses that typifies most research on psychopathology also applies in risk research. Although DSM-III offers improved specificity in the diagnosis of schizophrenia, the stringent diagnostic requirements will also reduce the pool of patients available for participation in risk studies.

6. *The problem of selecting variables in research.* The wide range of dependent variables used by risk groups attests to the uncertainty that surrounds the selection of variables. The search for predictors or precursors of the disorder is inherently a very difficult task.

A related task, and one which further justifies risk research, is to trace the development of children who are at risk by virtue of their parents' disordered status, irrespective of the ultimate outcome for the child at risk. Tracing the developmental course of subgroups with varying outcomes would yield information about the operation of both risk factors *and* protective factors in children reared under deleterious circumstances. Such information could prove valuable in constructing rationally based programs of preventive psychiatry.

THE SEARCH FOR PROTECTIVE FACTORS

The numerous studies cited for the three major mental disorders indicate that both the concept and the investigation of risk status in children now has a strong foothold in psychiatric research. In contrast, the collateral area, the study of protective factors that inhibit pathogenic processes, has been almost entirely neglected.

The reasons for this deficiency are not at all clear. Part of it may stem from our preoccupation with deviance. Rutter (1979) has noted that we have a "regrettable tendency" to focus on ills and shortcomings rather than on the factors that support and protect children reared in deprivation and that ameliorate their conditions. On the other hand, we have focused our attention on factors underlying the marked individual differences in people's adaptation under stress. Were we to systematize and expand such observations, we might begin to understand the nature of the "inoculants" which attenuate the damaging effects of deprivation and disadvantage, and in doing so provide a more adequate rationale for intervention programs in preventive psychiatry.

In a recent publication, the author has reviewed some of the protective factors suggested in the research literature (Garmezy, 1983). Rutter and his colleagues have identified a number of risk-reducing factors for children living in disadvantaged environments. The factors include positive temperament factors and the presence in the home of a parent whose relationship to the child is one of warmth, affection, supportiveness, and the absence of criticism. Also important is the socializing influence of a school where teachers and administrators have concern for the growth and well-being of the child and actualize their concern by making realistic demands of the child and by providing a setting in which learning can take place (Rutter, 1979). Three broad categories of protective variables are thus suggested: individual personality dispositions, a supportive family milieu, and a support system that encourages and reinforces the child's efforts to cope with adversity by strengthening the child's positive attributes and values.

A recently completed long-term longitudinal study by Werner and Smith (1982) is appropriately titled *Vulnerable but Invincible: A Study of Resilient Children*, and it reaffirms the importance of these three categories of variables. The study examined the adaptation of young adults who had been exposed as infants to perinatal stress and as children to poverty, parental mental health problems, family instability, limited parent education, and the like. At a dispositional level, children who were adaptive under stress revealed better health histories and behavioral patterns marked by activity, social responsiveness, autonomy, and a positive orientation to self and others. These attributes were complemented by a family milieu marked by family closeness, parental support, and a respect for a child's individuality. External supports from peers, older friends, teachers, and so forth also accompanied adaptation.

Kauffman et al. (1979), describing the competent children of psychotic mothers, also emphasized the quality of relationships within the nuclear family and in the outside world with peers and adults. The children exhibited age-appropriate social skills, manifested a degree of unusual competence, demonstrated mastery, and maintained high levels of motivation, attention, and intelligence. They also enjoyed success, enhancing their sense of self-esteem. In sum, personal dispositions, warm relationships with their mothers, and external supports from peers and other adults seemed to mark these highly adaptive children.

The study of children at risk offers a natural laboratory for comparing children who show successful adaptation with those who fail to meet environmental demands. Although relatively sparse, the literature on protective factors can help to ensure that personality, family, and environmental milieu variables will be included in future studies of children at risk for the major mental disorders. Rutter has suggested some of the variables for differentiating between children who move along paths of maladaptation toward mental disorder and those who move toward maturity and competence: "the patterning of stresses, individual differences caused by both constitutional and experiential factors, compensating experiences outside the home, the development of self-esteem, the scope and range of available opportunities, an appropriate degree of environmental structure and control, the availability of personal bonds and intimate relationships, and the acquisition of coping skills" (Rutter, 1979, 70).

These and other factors reviewed in this chapter suggest the magnitude of the scientific task that faces those who elect to study children who are at risk for mental disorder. The ultimate value of such studies will be to enhance psychiatric knowledge about the developmental forces that influence adaptation and maladaptation, not only in children, but in adults as well.

Chapter 8

Children at Acute Risk:
Psychic Trauma
by Lenore Cagen Terr, M.D.

> *"I have two very early childhood memories: of my father being
> mentally ill and of waking up in a hospital room and being strapped
> in a bed. Pneumonia my mother tells me. But I have always been
> fighting a hysteria that plagued me as a child."*
> *"What activates it?"*
> *"The old fear of extinction and I don't mean dying. I mean the
> fear of being reduced to nothing, of being crushed."*

—Excerpt from a *Newsweek* interview
with the author, V.S. Naipaul,
16 November 1981

Common as is the expression "he was traumatized as a child," psychiatric studies of psychic trauma in childhood were rare and of relatively
poor quality until very recent times. Little direct observation of psychically traumatized youngsters was conducted, and those few observa-
tional studies which were attempted did not yield specific data regarding the immediate and long-term manifestations of psychic trauma in
childhood. This chapter reviews the literature, with a particular emphasis on new research, discusses several upcoming areas of study, and
examines various approaches to intervention.

REVIEW OF THE LITERATURE

Retrospective Psychoanalytic Case Reports of Adults

Many of the works on "traumatized children" published before the 1970s
consisted of retrospective single case reconstructions from adult psy-
choanalyses in which childhood trauma was inferred from adult behavior, free associations, therapeutic transferences, and dreams (e.g., Bonaparte, 1945; Greenacre, 1949; Katan, 1973). Occasionally, psychoanalysts
searched for old psychic traumas in the lives or works of artists, rather
than from actual patients (Steinberg and Weiss, 1954; Niederland, 1976).
In an extreme example of this type of writing, Katan (1962) proposed,
after simply reading *The Turn of the Screw*, that the 5-year-old Henry James
had traumatically witnessed "the primal scene." This reconstruction of
an early psychic trauma was based solely upon the fictional story itself.
When challenged, Katan (1966) found little, if any, convincing evidence
of this trauma from James's personal memoirs, remarks to friends, or
notes. Such reconstructive journeys into the childhood frights of artistic
or literary figures, fascinating as they are to read, do little to promote
an accurate understanding of real overwhelming events as they affect
children. "Adultomorphic," entirely retrospective approaches to childhood have recently been criticized within psychoanalysis itself by Emanuel
Peterfreund (1978; 1982).

Another psychoanalytic trend which for many years discouraged acquisition of knowledge about early trauma was the generally held belief

that adults and older children describing gruesome past incidents may have mistakenly remembered their fantasies as real and convinced themselves that their nightmares had actually taken place. Horror stories from childhood were more often than not psychoanalyzed as vivid inner conflicts rather than as actualities. Freud himself contributed to this trend, and a recent psychoanalytic controversy publicized in the lay press has revolved about Freud's personal reasons for ignoring psychic trauma after making such initially exciting contributions to its understanding (see Gelman's 1981 article in *Newsweek*).

Since ancient times, however, children *have* been abused, sexually misused, kidnapped, snatched, and subjected to terrible frights. When real occurrences like these are recalled later in life, they may take the form of "screen memories" (Freud, 1899). Countering the trend to overlook psychic trauma, a small minority of analysts tried to urge their colleagues to watch screen memories closely for real trauma. Hansi Kennedy, for instance, after prospectively following the memories of one little girl she had known at the Hampstead Nurseries during the war, stated that children's memories "are much nearer the surface and distortions much less elaborate and complicated than in the case of an adult" (1950, 280). Twenty-one years later, Kennedy (1971) criticized the psychoanalytic tendency to discount real psychic trauma. She said that the analysis of children at times leads "into analyzing what the child is experiencing predominantly in terms of his defenses and his projections of wishes, fantasies, and conflicts without acknowledging sufficiently that, in certain cases, what the child brings is shaped by the fact that he lived in a 'crazy world' which has become internalized" (391). Greenacre (1981) also contributed greatly to this minority view in psychoanalysis, insisting that adult screen memories often represent real traumas. She asserted that psychoanalysts "did not always deal adequately with the emotional nature of the actual, historically true part of an early traumatic impression, unless it was specifically repeated in the transference or otherwise acted out in some detail. Such patients might sometimes gain equilibrium through a defensive intellectualization, but be vulnerable if new stress was experienced" (36).

Because of its preferred emphasis on fantasy over actuality, its frequent failure to consider screen memories as posttraumatic memory traces, and its tendency to "adultomorphise" its approach to early childhood, the retrospective psychoanalytic study of adults did not provide as many crucial insights into childhood trauma as might have seemed possible. A full understanding of childhood psychic trauma would have to depend upon direct observations of the youngsters themselves.

World War II Observations

Those early behavioral scientists who did observe children directly for answers to the puzzles of childhood fright and shock often considered the children's parents to be the most important factor in the youngster's reactions. Anna Freud's wartime work at Hampstead, England, is an example of this emphasis. Her poignant case descriptions of war-traumatized children are classics to this day. (See "Bertie," Freud, A., and Burlingham, 1942, 197, or the notes on the little Holocaust survivors, Freud, A., and Dann, 1951). Anna Freud and her colleagues concluded that the presence or absence of parents was more a crucial determinant for how a child would fare during the war than were the bombings themselves. The Hampstead group did not concentrate upon psychically traumatic effects per se. For instance, in the case of the obviously war-traumatized child, Bertie, they barely discussed the effect on him of a devastating air attack. Separation, not trauma, commanded Anna Freud's group's wartime attention.

Other wartime researchers in the United States, France, and England gave similar emphasis to parent-child relationships. Discussing children's reactions to a San Francisco air raid shortly after Pearl Harbor, Solomon (1942) saw the youngsters' behaviors as reflections of how calm or how panicky their guardians had been. Among children living in a residential treatment center, he found that only the youngsters whose houseparents or teachers panicked became frightened themselves. Carey-Trefzer (1949) studied London children who survived the blitz and concluded that both exposure to bombing(s) and evacuation from home (separation from mothers) created immediate and long-term disturbances. She also pointed out that a "nervous mother" could harmfully influence her child. "A mother's neurosis not only aggravated the reaction of the child at the time of the damaging experience, but also . . . her emotional instability prevented the child from settling down later" (Carey-Trefzer, 1949, 540). Mercier observed a few French families during the time of war anticipation and/or immediately following the German invasion of France (Mercier and Despert, 1943). This report also concluded that children "temporarily reflect the attitudes of the surrounding adults." (The report is particularly detailed and can be reread today from the perspective of what is currently known about childhood trauma.)

Long-term separations from parents during wartime did damage youngsters. Separations led to prolonged grief reactions and in some instances to new psychological dependencies upon parent substitutes (Freud, A., and Burlingham, 1942; Mercier and Despert, 1943). But most such separations probably would not suddenly and intensively overwhelm the child's coping and defensive operations as would a bombing or a hostile encounter with the Nazis. The long-term effects of wartime separations could be observed in children's personality characteristics, their regressions to earlier behaviors, and their chronic lack of pleasure. Excellent works have been written since the war about childhood grief and enforced separations from parents (e.g., Bowlby, 1951; Barnes, 1964; Bowlby, 1973; Solnit, 1973; Anthony, 1973; Goldstein, Freud, A., and Solnit, 1973). These more recent works imply that childhood separations and classical psychic trauma are not identical conditions. The symptomatologies and the long-term effects of grief and of psychic trauma do differ significantly, although the two conditions may of course exist side by side.

Peacetime Observations and Confusions (1945–1967)

One child psychiatrist of the 1940s and 1950s focused his observations directly upon the traumatized children themselves. David Levy (1945) considered children's reactions to their hospitalizations to be similar to traumatized soldiers' wartime mental problems. Levy's young child patients had been "traumatized" in hospitals, by surgical operations which had been insufficiently explained, or by procedures which were carried out with no regard for the young patients' levels of emotional and cognitive development. Levy drew the very important conclusion that children could suffer psychic traumas themselves much the same as adults do. He suggested a form of uninterpreted play therapy that was nondirective, sometimes "wild," and messy (Levy, 1939). Levy's "abreactive therapy" appeared somewhat analogous to the abreactions traumatized soldiers experienced under hypnosis (Grinker and Spiegel, 1945). Levy's recommended abreactive play therapy understandably never achieved widespread popularity among therapists. But his ideas about the origin of psychic traumas in the operating room eventually became a focus for further research (e.g., Jessner et al., 1952), as well as an inspiration for a new humanism in pediatric inpatient care.

The first large-scale study of children's reactions to peacetime disasters was conducted in 1953 and 1954 (Bloch et al., 1956). The research group was invited as representatives of the National Institute of Mental Health to interview the survivors of a tornado that had hit Vicksburg, Mississippi. When the tornado struck, a large number of children were watching a Saturday matinee movie. The investigators provided questionnaires to the children at one Vicksburg school, and they personally interviewed 88 of the parents. Though the children were the focus of their research, the investigators did not interview the youngsters themselves. They stated, "One could not approach parents for information about their children unless one was prepared to deal with the parents' problems first" (Bloch et al., 1956, 421). From their study, Bloch et al. concluded that children who were physically injured, children who were present in the impact zone, and children who either lost a family member or who had a family member injured were most likely to suffer "overt anxiety, anxiety equivalents, symptom formation, or intensification of pathological character traits" (418). The Vicksburg report emphasized the parents' role in the child's responses as did most of the other childhood trauma literature of the 1940s and 1950s. Bloch et al. observed that those children whose parents underwent "dissociative-demanding" reactions after the tornado became anxious themselves, and the investigators also found "a relationship between a history of parental psychopathology and the child's emotional disturbance" (420). Vicarious experiences with death or injury to friends did not seem to create emotional disturbance in these youngsters. (For opposite viewpoints on "vicarious trauma," see Lifton, 1979, or Beardslee and Mack, 1982.)

A curious inactivity fell upon the childhood trauma field over the next 25 years. It appeared to some child psychiatrists that the War had presented such a unique opportunity to observe childhood psychic trauma that there was little to be gained by studying the effects of peacetime disaster. An even more potent deterrent to further research was the fact that the psychic trauma field in general had become fuzzy and undefined. So many conditions entirely unrelated to shock, surprise, or intense external stimuli had become classified as traumas that the term psychic trauma was no longer meaningful.

The concept of psychic trauma began its long journey into nebulousness when psychiatrists, including Freud himself, began to overlook its original definitions. In 1920 Freud had defined traumatic as "any excitations *from outside* which are powerful enough to break through the protective shield. . . . There is no longer any possibility of preventing the mental apparatus from being flooded with large amounts of stimulus . . . which have broken in and of . . . binding them" (29–30, emphasis added). In 1926, Freud added that the essence of a traumatic situation was "the experience of helplessness." To reword Freud's original definitions in the terms of the 1980s, psychic trauma "occurs when sudden, intense, unexpected anxiety overwhelms the individual's abilities to cope and to defend" (Terr, 1981a, 741). Although the "stimulus barrier" or "protective shield" concept has recently come under question (Peterfreund, 1978; Shapiro and Stern, 1980; Esman, 1983), Freud's 1920 definition requires that the traumatic event be external, intense, and overwhelming.* This definition is clear and strict enough to eliminate conditions which are not associated with repetitive symptomatologies such as nightmares, reenactment, and play.

The confusion began in the middle of this century when psychoanalysts and dynamic psychiatrists put forth some additional theories about psychic trauma. One was the idea that psychic trauma could originate entirely from internal stimulations (Fenichel, 1945; Rangell, 1967). Another was the idea of retrospective trauma, that a seemingly benign event could, as cognitive development progressed, be later recognized as traumatically intense (Freud, 1937). A third concept contributing to the confusion was the idea of retroactive trauma, that "an event might acquire its traumatic quality at a subsequent maturational phase when susceptibility to the particular past event has been achieved" (Rangell, 1967, 64). Fourth was the idea of strain trauma (Kris, 1956; Sandler, 1967) or cumulative trauma (Khan, 1963), that a series of stressful events (or long-lasting situation), not psychically shocking per se, could generate accumulating tensions which might lead to trauma. A fifth concept was the idea of screen trauma, that one posttraumatic memory could "screen" for another traumatic experience buried deep in repression (Glover, 1929). Finally, there was the idea of constructive trauma, that some good could come to the child from a psychic trauma (Waelder, 1967). The result of these cumbersome terminologies and subtheories was that by the middle 1960s the true "psychic trauma" became almost lost among a rash of additions.

In 1967, Anna Freud recognized the widespread misuse of psychic trauma terminologies and literally rescued the concept. At a meeting on psychic trauma, she commented, "I welcome this opportunity to inquire more closely into the current usage of the term 'trauma' and, perhaps, to rescue it from the widening and overuse that are the present-day fate of many other technical terms in psychoanalysis and, in the course of time, lead inevitably to a blurring of meaning and finally to the abandonment and loss of valuable concepts" (235). She strongly urged a return to Freud's 1920 definition. In 1968, in an otherwise unrelated paper, she insisted that an external event must take place, in order for there to be a posttraumatic reaction, and she discarded much of the terminology which had blurred the trauma field for so long. Since then, although the old words still pop up in the literature (e.g., cumulative trauma applied to child abuse, Green, 1983), it has become more pos-

*Editor's note: Dr. Daniel N. Stern reviews the recent findings concerning the stimulus barrier and their theoretical implications in Part I of *Psychiatry Update: Volume II* (pages 9–11, 15).

sible to develop clear research objectives by using the narrower definition.

The Stress Literature (1960s–1980s)

Although most of the psychiatric literature on stress does not deal with children, Lois Murphy's early studies of coping patterns in preschoolers (1962) set the tone for a generation of "coping" studies which followed. Murphy (1974) continued to study her sample of children into adulthood and recognized, as they developed, "a circular relation between vulnerability and stress experience." Shortly after John F. Kennedy's assassination, Murphy's associate, Moriarty, sent questionnaires to teenagers whom they had been following. The adolescents' statements regarding this shocking occurrence were in total agreement with the character assessments made of them much earlier as children (Moriarty, 1976).

One important theme in the stress literature is that anyone may develop stress-related coping patterns, given unexpected, unsolvable, and intense enough conditions. This will occur regardless of the person's prior vulnerabilities, parenting, and so forth. Janis (1958; 1962) conceptualized that an intense threat creates "reflective fear," which in turn may lead to any of three adjustment modes: need for vigilance, need for reassurance, or compromise formation. Lazarus et al. (1974) showed that in stressful situations in which there seems to be no way out, individuals tend to manipulate the stress intrapsychically. Aylon (1982) demonstrated these interior manipulations in her study of Israeli children who survived terrorist attacks, but she did not describe her methodologies or study group.

After reviewing several studies of coping and stress, Hamburg and Adams (1967) noted that following stress, phasic waves of denial and numbing alternate with compulsive thoughts and emotional pangs. Horowitz (1976) expanded upon these points, demonstrating how psychiatrists may treat the cycles of denial and intrusive thoughts in stressed patients with hysterical, obsessional, or narcissistic personality patterns, but he was particularly careful to disclaim any applicability of this work to children. In the author's work, school-aged children have not shown such phasic alternations between denial and intrusive symptoms (Terr, 1981b; 1983b). The most likely reason that this cycling does not occur in children is that during traumatic events children apparently do not massively deny external reality.

In a thorough review of the literature on adult sensory deprivation and psychic trauma, Hocking made a convincing point which has influenced subsequent studies of children and of adults: "As the degree of stress is increased, predisposing factors become less important, and the stressful situation itself more important, until extreme degrees of stress produce symptoms of psychologic disability in all who are exposed to them" (Hocking, 1970, 23). A new importance was placed upon the intensity of the stressor, as opposed to degrees of prior vulnerability, or in the case of children degrees of parents' contributions and perhaps even the child's own level of development. This emphasis on the stressor has supplanted earlier points of view regarding psychic trauma, and it is reflected in the American Psychiatric Association's DSM-III (1980).

In its definition of Posttraumatic Stress Disorder, DSM-III states that a traumatic event is "generally outside the range of usual human experience." It goes on to explain that the stressor must be of sufficient magnitude that it would be expected to produce "significant symptoms of distress in most people and is generally outside the range of such common experiences as simple bereavement, chronic illness, business losses, or marital conflict" (American Psychiatric Association, 1980, 236). For children, one could now almost always infer that such previously designated traumas as the birth of a sibling, a frightening threat from a parent (Solnit and Kris, 1967), a bad case of chicken pox, or a cold, harsh upbringing would not qualify as traumatic events, except in the most unusual circumstances.

A finding in the adult stress literature which seems particularly applicable to children is the demonstrated tendency of stress and fear to spread throughout a population. Washburn and Hamburg (1965) reported that fear spread among African baboons after a local scientist shot two animals. Even though the entire band of baboons had not witnessed the shooting, the fearful behavior of some dominant animals led others to act afraid for eight months. This spreading effect was later demonstrated in adult human beings following the Buffalo Creek flood. Relatives of victims and community members far distant from Buffalo Creek at the time of the disaster suffered serious emotional distress after the flood (Stern, 1976). "Contagion" was also demonstrated in the Chowchilla, California, group (Terr, 1979), but the "spread" through this population carried with it a unique and ironic twist. Panic spread from the kidnapped children of Chowchilla to their parents, not vice versa. This finding was at 180° variance from the World War II findings which had emphasized parent-to-child contagion. Posttraumatic anxiety in fact could spread in any direction between the generations, and within peer groups as well (Terr, 1981a). For example, the childhood game, "Ring around the rosie, A pocket full of posies, Ashes, Ashes, We all fall down," originated in the horrors of the medieval plagues and spread from one generation of children to the next.

Studies of Massive Disaster and Degradation (1960s–1980s)

The Holocaust literature demonstrates that massive, prolonged psychic trauma, human degradation, and reduction to animal status create syndromes heretofore unrecognized in individual traumas: chronic lifelong depressions, chronic psychophysiological reactions, psychic numbing, and guilt (Chodoff, 1959; de Wind, 1968; Krystal and Niederland, 1968; Sterba, E., 1968; Krystal, 1978). These studies do not directly apply to childhood trauma because such stressors are so extreme, so long lasting, and so dehumanizing. Recent studies do seem to indicate that the children of Holocaust survivors are also prone to chronic depression and guilt (Borocas and Borocas, 1973; Sonnenberg, 1974; Epstein, 1979). The professional literature regarding the spreading of anxiety and guilt to the second generation of Holocaust survivors generally does indicate that such contagion exists. However, these studies of the second generation have recently been criticized for their prejudice, methodological inadequacies, and misinterpretations (Solkoff, 1981). Solkoff has suggested that any new studies employ more carefully selected samples, better matched control groups, more careful descriptions of intrafamilial interactions, and more easily duplicated research designs.

The atomic bombing of Hiroshima occasioned the very important disaster study by Lifton (1967). Lifton poignantly showed how the survivors experienced a loss of the sense of invulnerability, a profound psychic numbing, and survivors' guilt. A few of the persons Lifton interviewed at Hiroshima had been children when the atomic bomb exploded in 1945. When Lifton interviewed them in the 1960s, they were still suffering the resultant emotional effects. Lifton thus demonstrated that massive psychic trauma in childhood could be long lasting and devastating to the personality. He also showed that the traumatic event could be recollected in its entirety much later in life. Very recently, Lifton has gone on to theorize that all inhabitants of today's world are nuclear survivors and as such experience survivors' guilt and psychic numbing (Lifton, 1979; 1982). This controversial point of view requires further data to support it. Recent studies of children's reactions to the threat of nuclear disaster will be discussed later in this chapter.

RECENT RESEARCH

The Aberfan and Buffalo Creek Studies

The first onsite studies devoted exclusively to interviews with traumatized children occurred following the Aberfan and Buffalo Creek disasters. Both projects provided important new descriptive findings. At Aberfan, Wales, a tip mine precariously sitting above the town roared down a nearby mountainside, engulfing a primary school. Five teachers and 107 schoolchildren were killed. Lacey (1972), a child psychiatrist at the local child guidance center, over the next four years evaluated 56 children who came to him with various emotional complaints. His study group therefore consisted of self-designated or parent-designated psychiatric patients. Lacey determined that the most severely affected children were those who had "anxiety-creating situations in their backgrounds." He found that many of the most anxious youngsters had experienced "a striking number of grief situations" in the past, making them and their parents "more vulnerable" to the trauma. Since Lacey's study sample was skewed toward chronic family and childhood disturbances, his data did not reflect the actual incidence of, and preexisting conditions for, childhood psychiatric disturbances following disasters.

The 1972 West Virginia Buffalo Creek disaster was studied by a number of researchers from Yale University and the University of Cincinnati (see "Disaster at Buffalo Creek," 1976; Erikson, 1976; Lifton and Olson, 1976). The catastrophe occurred when a coal-mining slag dam broke unexpectedly, flooding the valley and killing a great many people. Newman (1976) a Cincinnati child psychiatrist, personally interviewed 11 of the child survivors. She employed such projective techniques as requesting that the youngsters draw pictures and later asking them to explain their art work. She also inquired about their wishes and asked them to make up stories. Newman found that the child survivors at Buffalo Creek "shared a modified sense of reality, increased vulnerability to future stresses, altered senses of the power of the self, and early awareness of fragmentation and death" (Newman, 1976, 312). The two youngest children (ages 26 months and 3 years) condensed together two separate symbols which had related to their traumas. Newman did not follow the children over an extended period of time, nor did she conclude what symptoms, signs, and psychodynamic mechanisms would be expected in childhood trauma. Nonetheless, her work has greatly influenced subsequent studies, particularly those relying on traumatized children's art works as expressions of posttraumatic fantasies. For example, Galante (1982) uses drawings in her art-therapeutic work with groups of child survivors of the recent Italian earthquake, and Pynoos and Eth (in press[b]) have incorporated children's art work into their ninety-minute psychiatric interviews of children who have witnessed extreme acts of violence.

The Chowchilla Kidnapping Studies

In July of 1976, 26 California schoolchildren, ages 5 to 14, and their bus driver were kidnapped at gunpoint and subjected to 27 hours of terror. The kidnappers drove the school bus into a dry creek bed, loaded the children into vans, and drove them about for 11 hours in total darkness without any food, water, or bathroom stops. At 2:00 or 3:00 A.M., the kidnappers took each child's name and demanded a personal object from each one of them. They then demanded that the children descend into "the hole," which was in reality a buried truck trailer. The youngsters remained buried alive for 16 hours until 2 of the older boys dug the group out. The entire group emerged physically unharmed. (The bus driver had been unfamiliar to many of the children and behaved rather passively throughout the experience, according to the children's accounts.) This event presented an ideal opportunity to study the effects of a pure peacetime trauma upon a previously "normal" group of children who had been entirely removed from their parents during the experience.

Five months after the kidnapping, the Chowchilla parents issued a plea in a newspaper article for someone to help their children (Miller and Tompkins, 1976). The author initiated two psychiatric studies, each consisting of personal interviews of the children and interviews with the parents. The first project involved all 23 youngsters who had remained in Chowchilla and took about eight months to complete (Terr, 1979). The second study was a four- to five-year follow-up of 25 of the 26 kidnapped children and of one child who had gotten off the bus just before the kidnapping (Terr, 1983b). Simultaneously, ongoing clinical psychiatric work took place with individually traumatized youngsters.

The first-year Chowchilla study demonstrated several phenomena which had not been described or explained previously in the medical-psychological literature. Upon the initial surprise of the kidnapping, each child feared separation from parent(s), death, and/or further fear (fear itself). During the ordeal, the children balked at any change in circumstances, and afterwards they were particularly cautious when confronted with new situations. Many children misperceived visual or sound cues, and some even hallucinated. A few experienced immediate time distortions, and many more later exhibited serious disturbances in time sense, mispositioning sequences and believing in their own psychic and prophetic powers. Each one of the youngsters remembered the details from their experiences, almost as if the memories had been burned into consciousness. As soon as they were kidnapped, many of the youngsters retrospectively discovered omens or turning points from some time before the trauma and, as it later turned out, from events or dreams which closely followed the trauma. These omens remained powerful influences on later symptomatologies and personality patterns.

Shortly after the trauma, the children began to show fears, repetitions, and personality alterations. Each of the victims feared kidnapping or experienced "fears of the mundane" (the dark, vehicles, being alone, being outside, strangers). Several children continued to experience perceptual distortions which fed these fears. Some had panic attacks when they unexpectedly confronted a feared object, and a few became more fearful around the anniversary of the kidnapping.

Repetitive phenomena included posttraumatic dreams, posttraumatic play, reenactment, and psychophysiological reenactments. The children experienced four types of posttraumatic repetitive dreams: (1) unremembered terror dreams, often including newly developed sleep talk or sleepwalking, (2) exactly repeated dreams depicting the traumatic event, (3) modified repetition dreams, and (4) deeply disguised dreams of kidnapping. Two types of nonrepetitive dreams also were described for the first time: (1) dreams of the child's own death and (2) dreams which the child believed to be predictive. The author has also found these dream types in a study in which several "normal" control children matched for age, sex, and ethnicity with the Chowchilla group turned out also to have been traumatized (Terr, 1983c).

"Posttraumatic play," a very commonly occurring posttraumatic repetitive phenomenon, was reported for the first time in the literature in two of the author's papers, one relating to the Chowchilla children (Terr, 1979) and one relating to a separately traumatized group of individuals (Terr, 1981a). This special type of play has 11 features: incessant repetition; unconscious linkage to the trauma; literalness; wide age range affected; varying lag times between the event and commencement of the play; contagiousness to nontraumatized youngsters and to entirely new generations of children; dangerousness; use of art, storytelling, and audioduplication; secretiveness; and failure of the play to relieve anxiety (Terr, 1981a). Reenactment is a phenomenon which has previously been alluded to, but not thoroughly described clinically in relation to psychic trauma. This phenomenon accounted for serious and bizarre behaviors by the Chowchilla children, as they unconsciously repeated segments of their kidnapping experience. Some reenactments occurred so frequently that they evolved into personality changes, whereas others took place dramatically, suddenly, and only once every few months or years. Some reenactments were psychophysiological. For instance, one child hit in the stomach by a kidnapper's gun butt experienced stomachaches for years afterwards, never consciously associating the original blow with the subsequent pains. Within one year of the Chowchilla kidnapping, 19 children had undergone personality changes. Several of these changes were regressions to earlier behaviors or exaggerations of previous traits, but many of them came about because of repeated reenactments.

The four- to five-year Chowchilla follow-up study (Terr, 1983b) indicated that many of the personality changes, fears, perceptual distortions, omens, and repetitive physical, mental, and behavioral phenomena had continued. As a matter of fact, posttraumatic play, omens, memories of misperceptions, and death dreams had come to involve even more kidnapped children. Several youngsters reported that some of their fears had subsided, particularly their fears of things with which they had to interact continually, such as fears of buses, vans, and strangers. Thus, with a mechanism similar to that which allows for relief following a combat-fatigued soldier's early return to the battlefield (George Hexter, personal communication), the Chowchilla children extinguished some of their fears. Every child, however, at four to five years after the kidnapping remained highly fearful of certain things. Two of the most striking findings in the long-term follow-up of the Chowchilla kidnapping were the horrible death nightmares that 14 children dreamed and the pessimistic and foreshortened future views held by 23 of the 25 youngsters.

When the author interviewed a "normal" control group of 25 about their futures, dreams, and any terrible events they had experienced, 8 of them reported death dreams, 6 of which were connected with past fright or unconsciousness (Terr, 1983c). Of those control children who reported limited personal future expectations, death dreams, or repeated nightmares, 10 exhibited the effects of past severe frights. Five described enough confirmatory repetitive phenomena or fears for the author to conclude that they had been psychically traumatized. This high prevalence of fear and psychic trauma in a "normal" group suggests that psychically traumatic events and their psychological aftermaths are far more common than might have been expected. Furthermore, this control study confirmed the importance of a foreshortened future view and death dreams among the long-term effects of childhood trauma.

Several of the psychiatric findings from the Chowchilla studies have recently been confirmed in studies of traumatized adults. Adults may play posttraumatically (Terr, 1981b). They may exhibit time distortions including omen formation, time skew, condensation of events, durational distortion, reliance upon rhythms during stress, and foreshortening of the future (Terr, 1983e; 1984). Also like children, adults may misperceive or hallucinate during traumas, and they often fear fear itself. On the other hand, school-aged children exhibit some differences from adults after traumatic events. Children experience no amnesia, they do not deny external reality, alternating with intrusive repetitive phenomena, and they experience no sudden, intrusive, unbidden flashbacks. Children do play out or reenact their trauma more than adults, and they exhibit more extensive cognitive and perceptual malfunctions under traumatic circumstances than adults (Terr, 1979).

All of the Chowchilla children, regardless of parental responses, past vulnerabilities, or family psychopathology, exhibited posttraumatic symptoms at both the one-year and the four- to five-year follow-up. Although there were some differences in the longer-term severity of clinical symptoms, depending on past physical or mental vulnerabilities, family-community bonding, or serious family problems, each Chowchilla child was affected by the traumatic event long afterward. While the oedipal, latency, and adolescent stages of development were all represented in the group, responses to the traumatic event were relatively uniform across the ages, contrary to what might have been expected. A future study of traumatized infants, toddlers, and preschoolers might clarify whether this uniformity of posttraumatic response also exists at the very earliest levels of emotional and cognitive development.

Research Issues Related to Trauma

CROSS-CULTURAL PERSPECTIVES At the end of World War II, Tulchin and Levy (1945) conducted a Rorschach study of 22 British and 22 Spanish refugee youngsters who had survived the war. The Spanish children had been subjected to greater wartime stresses, although both groups had suffered. The Rorschach test results highlighted Spanish versus Anglo-Saxon temperamental differences, but the authors also postulated that "the more intense and more traumatic experience of the Spanish group of refugee children has made its mark, and plays a part in the dynamic personality structure, as disclosed in the Rorschach findings" (Tulchin and Levy, 1945, 368).

Unfortunately, studies of psychic trauma in the culturally dispossessed child are few. However, *The Basic Handbook on Psychiatry* contains an excellent section on cultural differences among children (Noshpitz, 1979, 239–327) and includes a chapter by Carlin about "catastrophically uprooted" Vietnamese, Cambodian, Korean, and Laotian children. In this chapter, Carlin (1979) described a Korean child who had been adopted by Americans at 1 year and who at age 13 still had "indescribable night terrors." Carlin reported that in all other aspects of the girl's life the young Korean had adjusted very well. At age 2½, a Vietnamese boy, one year after his evacuation, believed that the sudden loud sounds he heard were Vietcong soldiers coming to get him in America. Carlin stressed that the full acquisition of the English language and the achievement of a stable home life in America were crucial factors in Southeast Asian children's later adjustment.

INJURY, RAPE, ABUSE, AND SUICIDE Childhood surgery or injury, sexual or physical assault, and parental suicide include major emotional complications which may partly mask their psychically traumatic effects. The posttraumatic symptoms may be overridden by such psychological necessities as handling radical changes in body image, accommodating to adult-demanded sexual behaviors, coping with diminished physiological capacities, facing repeated surgeries, expecting repeated parental attacks and rejection, and undergoing profound grief and mourning. The child may not mention nightmares or omens, and clinicians must be aware that unrecognized and untreated posttraumatic effects may partly block the child's eventual physical and emotional recovery from the injury or event.

Psychic trauma is not a major focus in the literature that deals with childhood injuries, assaults, and victimizations. Excellent articles, however, deal with the more specific psychological problems of children experiencing burns (Galdston, 1972; Bernstein, 1979), amputations (Schechter and Holter, 1979), mutilating surgeries (Earle, 1979), rape by a stranger (Lipton and Roth, 1969), and parental suicide (Cain and Fast, 1972). Green (1983), Wasserman et al. (1983), Yates (1981), Fraiberg (1975), and the author (Terr, 1970) have written about children's psychological adjustments to abuse by parents.

TRAUMATIZED CHILDREN AND THE LAW One newly emerging area of research in childhood trauma considers how traumatized children function as police and courtroom witnesses following incest, rape, kidnapping, attack, and homicide. While the perceptual distortions of psychically traumatic experiences may limit any child or adult victim's accuracy in the courtroom, the child's failure to deny or repress may make him or her a more credible or complete reporter than the adult who has undergone similar stresses. Because of posttraumatic mental changes, courts must evaluate each potential child witness separately, rather than arbitrarily deciding that certain ages, levels of intelligence, or beliefs in concepts of "the truth" qualify or disqualify a child as a witness (Terr, 1980). Pynoos and Eth (in press[a]) have described how children of various ages may function as witnesses in the criminal process following parental homicide. From their work with the Los Angeles Police Department, they demonstrated that while children want to talk about what has happened and wish to see justice done, they experience terrible loyalty conflicts when one parent murders another. These child witnesses suffer posttraumatic symptoms.

Serious problems can arise when family issues involving frightened youngsters come directly to the courts. In their fervor to prosecute and jail errant parents, court workers and attorneys must not forget the needs of young children. One study demonstrated what harm solely punitive legal approaches could do to battered children (Terr and Watson, 1968). Rosenfeld (1979) drew from 100 incest cases he had evaluated to caution that the primarily criminal handling of such cases may bypass treatment for the child-victim and therapeutic planning for the family.

Several new areas at the interface between law and the psychology of trauma await investigation. For instance, child snatching by parents often entails psychic trauma or grief and mourning in the child (Senior et al., 1982; Terr, 1983a; Shetky and Haller, 1983). Child pornography participants (Burgess et al., 1981), child hostages, and child victims of rape and other sexual assaults require further study and more intervention that combines psychiatric and legal efforts.

THE QUESTION OF VICARIOUS TRAUMA Escalona (1965) administered questionnaires to 311 schoolchildren aged 10 to 17 and asked them to predict what lay ahead for the world over the next ten years; 70 percent spontaneously raised the possibility of a nuclear war. Schwebel (1965) published a poll of 3,000 students questioned during the cold war escalation around the Cuban missile crisis; 44 percent predicted nuclear war. When so many children predict nuclear catastrophe, does this indicate that they were indirectly traumatized following Hiroshima? Shortly after the Three Mile Island nuclear plant accident Schwebel and Schwebel (1981) distributed questionnaires to 368 students in grades 4 through 12 from ten New Jersey school districts, asking them for their predictions about nuclear disasters. Of this large group, 70 percent predicted that there would be a serious nuclear plant accident, but these children did not appear as intensely worried about such accidents as Schwebel's earlier (1965) study group had been about nuclear war. Though a greater percentage of students predicted catastrophe in the 1981 study, the students believed that the federal government would step in to help or that a nuclear accident could be contained in some way.

The nuclear disarmament movement of late 1981 and 1982 inspired new studies designed to demonstrate children's attitudes about nuclear war. Beardslee and Mack (1982) conducted a large survey of Boston schoolchildren regarding their expectations of nuclear war, and Mack (1982) reported in a series of anecdotes that some children hesitated to plan too much or to work especially hard at school because they felt it would all become futile once a war occurred. Some of Beardslee and Mack's youngsters did not believe that they would live to grow up. These Boston schoolchildren appeared quite frightened, and perhaps some were even vicariously traumatized, but Beardslee and Mack did not prove this conclusively. One of the problems in this work, as well as in that of the Schwebels, was that the surveys immediately followed large public outcries about nuclear war and nuclear plant catastrophes. It would be interesting to know how schoolchildren would respond during a more settled period.

During a relatively quiet historical period just before the worldwide antinuclear demonstrations, the author interviewed 25 normal schoolchildren, ages 9 to 17, from McFarland and Porterville, California (Terr, 1983c). Each child was asked how he or she envisioned the world's future as well as his or her own personal future. Although the interviews included no specific questions about nuclear war, pollution, the economy, and so forth, several children spontaneously brought up these issues. Seven children were worried about worldwide nuclear war, 2 were frightened about the economy, 2 were concerned about crime, and 3 voiced concern about world population and food shortages. None of the children had thought of altering personal life plans because of these concerns, even though the child's life planning was the central theme of each interview. Although some of this California valley group were deeply concerned about worldwide catastrophe, they still went on, steadily making their own future plans and tacitly believing in their own personal safety. There was no evidence of "vicarious traumatization" in these youngsters.

INTERVENTIONS

As in any new area of study in psychiatry, treatments have lagged behind descriptive and field studies. Early intervention was demonstrated to be successful in wartime work with traumatized soldiers (Grinker and Spiegel, 1945). More recent long-term studies of survivors of a marine accident (Leopold and Dillon, 1963), miners ten years after a cave-in (Ploeger, 1972), and the Buffalo Creek survivors six years later (Gleser et al., 1981) indicate that the psychic trauma may often exert its effects many years after the precipitating event. There may also be significant lag periods before the onset of symptoms (Terr, 1981a; 1983b). Thus, although prompt intervention is to be strongly encouraged, longer-term follow-up work with individual patients is necessary to determine its effectiveness.

Several books suggest methods of working with communities following disasters (Grosser et al., 1964; Barton, 1969; Luchterhand, 1971; Parad et al., 1976; Tierney, 1979). Direct work with children following community catastrophe has not been a major focus in these writings, but the National Institute of Mental Health has recently published a disaster manual for workers dealing with children (Farberow and Gordon, 1981). One social agency developed the novel idea of setting up a radio talk show on the day of a devastating earthquake to answer questions from bystanders and victims of all ages (Blaufarb and Levine, 1972).

Unfortunately, the agency did not provide much follow-up counseling after its unusual early intervention. A research and treatment group set up a community storefront clinic after the Beverly Hills Supper Club disaster, but most victims and their families did not come for help (Lindy et al., 1981). Clearly, traumatized individuals, both adults and children, do not like to think of themselves as sick or neurotic. Mental health professionals must therefore go out directly to frightened children and their parents, rather than expecting the children and parents to seek their services.

At this time, the treatment of choice for psychic trauma in children is psychodynamic group, family, and individual psychotherapy. While propranolol may have a place in treating the panic symptoms of posttraumatic syndromes in children, no adequate data have yet been published. Behavioral modification techniques have been effective in controlling posttraumatic fears in some adults, but the entire posttraumatic stress syndrome cannot be relieved by behavioral modification alone.

Group Interventions

Fixed groupings cannot be forced upon trauma victims, nor do groups always need to be established immediately. Traumatized individuals tend to become angry at their co-victims and at their own communities (Erikson, 1976), because they cannot directly vent their rage at the perpetrators, at the negligent parties, or at the gods themselves. If a waiting period precedes the release of victims, mental health workers should contact the families then and wait with them, forming relationships prior to the relief or despair which will come with knowledge of the victims' outcomes (Terr, 1979). Children should be included in these early efforts. Schoolchildren cluster easily into classroom or special interest groups, which mental health professionals can treat in case of disaster. Galante worked with classroom groups following the Italian earthquake catastrophe (1982). Such clusters may also be employed to help children ventilate their feelings about the death of a peer or a similarly unexpected occurrence.

Zimmerman (1983), a consultant to the United States State Department, has offered suggestions for intervening when large groups of hostages are taken, as in the Pakistani or Iranian terrorist actions. He has advised that groups of recovered hostages be kept together and away from home for a few days in order to form small, informal, and spontaneous groupings. Then after a day or two, they should attend a large, professionally run "minimarathon" lasting three or four hours. Affected children may also attend these marathon sessions. Zimmerman believes that released hostages must be enabled to move into their own spontaneous voluntary groupings and that they should therefore be buffered from immediate family contact and protected, without being restricted, from the press. During this buffer period, the returning hostages may be individually examined both physically and psychiatrically. Although these suggestions have not been scientifically studied, some appear applicable to community catastrophes as well as to terrorist actions.

Interventions with the Family

Bloch et al. (1956) pointed out years ago that under posttraumatic conditions the investigator or therapist often has to deal first with parents' problems before gaining access to the child. One way to do this quickly is to allow the parents to organize spontaneous small groups in which they have natural affinities and then to arrange for these parent groups to work with a professional. For instance, in Chowchilla one such parent group worked weekly for about seven months, sharing concerns about families and marriages, as well as developing techniques for dealing with their children's posttraumatic play reenactments and fears (Terr, 1979).

Given proper information and suggestions from a psychiatrist, parents can perform the role of auxiliary therapists following Furman's principles of parent guidance (1957; 1969). Because posttraumatic symptoms are so repetitive, a parent will have ample opportunities to explain or interpret the child's dreams, play, or behaviors to the child. This may provide great relief to the traumatized child. Feeling that the parents understand, hearing that their seemingly weird behaviors are connected to the horrible event, and learning that the parents have enough emotional energy to focus on them after a catastrophe provides the children with some solace and symptom relief. Furthermore, given that posttraumatic fears and play are so contagious, training parents to deal with these issues may spare siblings or peers from acquiring transmitted symptoms.

The traumatized child may be treated in conjunction with the whole family or the parents. This is especially appropriate where the entire family has been traumatized in the same way. The problem with this approach is that even if the trauma is the same for each family member, the child's interpretation of the dangers, the meanings, and the personal turning points is an individual one, depending on history, cognitive capacities, vulnerabilities, and stage of development. If available, individual psychotherapy for the child would be the treatment of choice. Moreover, when the family is usually seen as a group, some individual sessions for each member must be provided.

Individual Psychotherapy

The psychiatrist working with the traumatized child may employ several treatment options: abreaction, suggestion, clarification, and interpretation. Hypnosis and amobarbital interviews, so frequently employed with soldiers evacuated from World War II battlefields (Grinker and Spiegel, 1945), probably do not have a place in the treatment of traumatized children. Because youngsters' control, cognitive, and defensive mechanisms are relatively immature, taking away their tenuous personal control through hypnosis may represent a second ego assault rather than a helpful treatment modality. The treatment of choice for the child over 8, depending upon verbal skills, is insight-directed psychodynamic psychotherapy. Even a child younger than 8, if he or she is verbal enough to express emotions entirely in words, may enter into verbal psychotherapy without the play techniques. (See Katan, 1961, for comments on the significance of early verbalizations in toddlers).

Play techniques for childhood trauma are still evolving and are as yet not entirely established. Levy's (1939) nondirective, noninterpretive play has fallen from favor, although it did effectively relieve childhood frights. Shapiro (1973) has suggested that the therapist set up a doll scene that looks like the traumatic one. For a child who had traumatically witnessed her mother's spontaneous delivery of a stillborn baby, Shapiro left paper towels full of red paint and a baby doll lying alongside his other play equipment. MacLean (1977) also used this kind of play technique, providing a leopard doll for a very young boy who had actually been attacked by a leopard. If a child already has spontaneous posttraumatic play, he or she can be observed and eventually treated through this play, particularly if the child lives in an institutional setting or if he or she willingly shares secrets with the therapist (Terr, 1983d). The therapist may also plan a corrective dénouement for the traumatized child's play. This type of play reassurance is occasionally effective because it defuses an omen or proves to the child that no action that he or she knew of could have helped, i.e., that he or she was not responsible for the events (Terr, 1983d). Gardner (1971) imposed new endings for children's stories in his "mutual storytelling technique," a method which appears particularly applicable to childhood trauma. Poetry therapy (Lerner, 1978), although not yet worked out for psychic trauma, may allow for the strong abreactions and interpretations which would relieve traumatized children. Art work, of course, may be employed much like child's play, particularly to bring out children's wishes that events had never taken place. Audio or video duplication can also be applied to the treatment of childhood trauma.

Simple repetition in therapy, however, will not permanently defuse posttraumatic states. The child's helplessness, the bad luck of the experience, the randomness of its occurrence, and the parent's inability to do anything about it must all be fully explored with the child. The child thus can learn to isolate the event as something extreme and unusual and go on to face the future, free to love, work, and play effectively.

SUMMARY

Psychic trauma in childhood is a relatively new field in psychiatric research and theory, and it has been more thoroughly researched with youngsters in latency and adolescence than with preschoolers. Treatment modalities are not yet well delineated, but many therapeutic possibilities have been suggested. Treatment-effectiveness studies will be required before we know what types of therapy work best for each situation. Longer-term follow-up studies into adulthood may eventually reveal whether children spontaneously overcome real traumas or whether they carry them into adulthood, forever bearing special vulnerabilities to stress.

Chapter 9 # Children with Mental Retardation
by Irving Philips, M.D.

INTRODUCTION

Definition

Mentally retarded and brain damaged children are a neglected group at risk for mental illness. Three percent of the population are considered retarded. DSM-III defines Mental Retardation as "(1) significantly subaverage general intellectual functioning, (2) resulting in, or associated with, deficits or impairments in adaptive behavior, (3) with onset before age 18" (American Psychiatric Association, 1980, 36). Significantly subaverage intellectual functioning is defined as two standard deviations from the norm, so that children or adults with an IQ below 70 are considered to be mentally retarded.

Retarded individuals may be divided into two groups on the basis of etiologic factors: 85 percent are mildly retarded, with primarily psychosocial etiologies, and 15 percent have severe to moderate deficits associated with primarily organic etiologies. Organic etiologies include injuries, microcephaly, mongolism, phenylketonuria, and cerebral agenesis. Disorders in this group are usually diagnosed early in life, often at birth. These children have various stigmata that distinguish them from other children, and they readily appear different to parents, peers, teachers, and community.

Developmental Considerations

The child whose retardation is diagnosed early in life often presents great difficulty to his or her family. Human infancy is normally characterized by a long period of dependence on other persons, and interpersonal reactions during this period influence the infant's development. A warm, tender relationship experienced by the infant with the mother can foster a sense of confidence and trust in the world. There is probably no more tragic experience for parents than to be told that their child is mentally defective. Faced with this disappointment, parents may react to the child in a variety of ways, from withdrawal to guilty oversolicitude. If the parents are depressed and disappointed, inconsistent in their care, hostile and angry, or inhibited and frightened, the infant may react with symptoms indicating distortions of personality development. The child may view the world with a sense of distrust and suspicion, becoming too frightened to try new tasks or growing angry in retaliation.

During the first year of life, the retarded child exhibits a delay in reaching developmental landmarks, showing retarded development in skills such as locomotion, language, and adaptive behavior. Although the retarded child may be similar to peers in physical size, he or she may not have the motor control necessary to compete. While other children are engaging in parallel and later in cooperative play, the retarded child has difficulty keeping up with age mates. By the time the child is physically ready to play, he or she may have outgrown in age and size those children with whom playing might be profitable, and the younger children find it hard to play with the older retarded child. This difficulty in play may be a further crippling factor, intensifying the child's sense of inferiority. Self-isolation and an inhibition from attempting new or competitive tasks may result.

The child may have to remain at home and may need continuous parental supervision, which further intensifies parental disappointment and causes the child to feel increasingly more isolated and unworthy. The experience of entering school presents difficulties to any child who has had earlier problems in life, and the retarded child may be more vulnerable in this situation. With the feeling of being different and unwanted, the child may stay apart from others. Thus, he or she may be shunned and teased by peers, be called names and taunted, and be the fall guy for the class bully and the victim of jokes. In reaction to the inability to solve environmental and internal conflicts, the retarded child may develop a variety of symptoms of emotional disorder. These run the gamut from simple transient behavior problems to severe neurotic, delinquent, and schizophrenic disorders.

The larger group of retarded children to be considered are those who are mildly retarded, the 85 percent whose retardation is related primarily to psychosocial factors. Families often are broken and dysfunctional, and parents or parent surrogates are concerned largely with the harsh economic realities of staying alive or subsisting; their energies are not devoted to verbal communication and learning endeavors. Problems in this group come from parental indifference and apathy, distrust and suspicion, and social isolation. These factors often result in poor and inhibited school performance.

Children in this group are not diagnosed as mentally retarded at birth, and they may or may not manifest slow development. They are usually diagnosed as retarded by the schools. They learn slowly, show little interest, and are poor in language and communication skills. When tasks of reading, writing, and arithmetic are demanded, they fall behind. They usually have much absenteeism for repeated minor illnesses. These youngsters manifest inattention to school tasks, immaturity in school behavior and personality development, slowed language development, and low achievement scores. They fall behind in school subjects, and each term their academic distance from their peers increases. On standard achievement tests, they score in the mildly retarded range and sometimes are placed in special classes. Their discouragement increases, apathy becomes more apparent, and learning is increasingly more difficult. They may present a variety of behavior problems in reaction to their indifference. In adolescence, they may become school dropouts, ill prepared in either academic or vocational skills. They may become chronically unemployable or exhibit delinquent antisocial behavior (Philips, 1966).

Policy Issues

Children with intelligence below the norm are generally avoided by mental health workers in their everyday practice. Children with mental retardation are considered to be helpless and hopeless, as if little could be done for them. They are rarely seen in mental health clinics. All too many believe that they belong in institutions. Little differentiation is made about levels of retardation and potentialities; all retarded individuals are considered to be alike, a homogeneous group. They are believed to be subject to delinquency and promiscuity with impulsive and hyperactive behavior. Although these common misconceptions are changing, they are changing ever too slowly. Children with mental retardation exhibit emotional signs and symptoms which inhibit and limit their development, and yet few integrated facilities are available to meet their mental health needs (Philips, 1967).

Public policy dictates movement toward deinstitutionalization, normalization, and mainstreaming and has brought retarded children and adults into our towns and cities in greater numbers. In California, the institutional population decreased from 11,483 in 1970 to 7,656 in 1980 (State of California Department of Health, in press). The institutional population is for the most part severely retarded and multiply handicapped, with IQs below 30 and generally in need of custodial lifetime care. These people account for only 5 to 10 percent of the retarded population. The remainder are generally in the community. Continued efforts are underway to place retarded children in the least restrictive environments and as close to their homes as possible, in settings that approach the normal living arrangements that would be expected for all children. This effort is the dictate of P.L. 94–142 (Education for all Handicapped Children Act, 1975), which has been interpreted and judicially upheld as meaning that retarded children must be included in mainstream society and its services. The provision of public education is no exception: it is required, or an alternative must be provided.

Skodiak (1968), Skeels (1966), and Skeels and Harms (1948) demonstrated that children adopted into families from institutional care fared better than those of control populations that remained in custodial care. They achieved greater skills and IQ attainment and maintained their progress into adulthood, as demonstrated by their increased competence and vocational achievement. Yet the major difficulty precluding successful community placement for retarded children is psychiatric disorder and behavioral deviation. This population has increased vulnerability and is truly at risk for emotional disorder.

EPIDEMIOLOGY OF EMOTIONAL DISORDER

At the Mental Retardation Program of the University of California at San Francisco (UCSF), an analysis of 100 consecutive intake interviews revealed that only 13 percent of the retarded children had normal psychosocial adaptation (Philips and Williams, 1975; see Table 1). Psychiatric problems of psychotic proportions appeared in 38 of the 100 children. Their behavior was so disturbed and distorted that psychotic disorganization was readily apparent. In a control population of 79 children with normal intelligence during the same period, 18 percent had evidence of psychotic maldevelopment.) In the group of 38 psychotic retarded children, 21 (55 percent) showed evidence of central nervous system pathology. In contrast, among the 62 who were nonpsychotic, 27 (43.5

Table 1. Psychiatric Diagnosis Among 100 Mentally Retarded Children

Psychiatric Diagnosis	Number	Degree of Retardation Among 62 Nonpsychotic Children		
		Borderline/ Mild	Moderate	Severe
Psychotic symptoms	38	—	—	—
No psychiatric disorder	13	5	6	2
Neuroses	5	3	2	0
Personality disorders and certain other nonpsychiatric disorders	16	13	3	0
Behavioral disorders	26	18	5	3
Transient situational disorders	2	2	0	0

Source: Philips and Williams (1975), Table 4.

percent) showed evidence of organic disease. Forty-nine of the 100 children were diagnosed as having personality, neurotic, behavioral, or situational disorders. The category with the largest number of children was behavioral disorders, followed closely by personality disorders. Cytryn and Lourie (1980) cited studies that assigned a risk of psychotic illness in retarded children as high as 40 percent. The findings of a Nebraska study indicated that approximately 25 percent of retarded patients with emotional disorder had evidence of psychosis (Menolascino, 1969; 1970).

Other studies substantiate a high rate of emotional disorder among retarded individuals. In an excellent review of the subject, Corbett (1976) noted that Chazan (1964) found that emotional disorders were twice as frequent in retarded subjects compared with controls. Tizard and Grad's (1961) epidemiologic study of severely retarded children found 43 percent with emotional difficulty. In the Isle of Wight study by Rutter et al. (1970), 30 percent were rated as disturbed by parents and 42 percent by teachers. This compared with 5.6 percent in the general population.

In the UCSF study, the type of emotional disorder was similar to that of disturbed children with normal intelligence. The author and his colleagues believe that the mental deficiency or disease is a contributing stress, but that the child's emotional disorder is probably not an organically inevitable concomitant of the defect. Such disordered behavior in retarded children is probably a function of the same kinds of processes that give rise to emotional disorder in children who have no definable disease. Nonetheless, the more retarded the individual, the more frequent and intense the psychopathology. Corbett (1976) made a similar observation based on his review of epidemiologic studies. "Although . . . psychiatric disorders in mentally retarded children are as heterogeneous as in any other group of children, this particularly holds for the mildly retarded group. . . . There are certain disorders (namely psychosis and the hyperkinetic syndrome) and certain items of deviant behaviour (particularly stereotyped movements) which are more common in the retarded, particularly in the more severely handicapped, than amongst children of normal intelligence" (832).

The UCSF study found that psychosocial adversity further intensifies the risk for emotional disorder (Philips and Williams, 1975; see Table 2). This finding was confirmed by the studies of Rutter (1983), who noted that "adverse effects not only summated but rather that they potentiated one another so that the combined effect of the two together was greater than the sum of the two considered separately."

In summary, a profile of the psychopathological manifestations of mentally retarded children would show a high incidence of psychotic disorganization. Children who have organic findings tend to come to the clinic earlier in their lives. Those with no organic findings would come to the clinic after entering school. The presence or absence of organicity would have little relationship to the symptom presented. A major portion of referrals would be children with borderline or mild retardation, and they would tend to be referred after they were admitted to school. Generally, the group seen would include more people from the lower socioeconomic classes than would be found in the general clinic population because of a higher incidence of psychosocial etiologies.

Children with mental retardation have a higher frequency of emotional disorder, but their symptoms are no different from those found

Table 2.   Social Class and Etiology of Retardation Among 62 Nonpsychotic Mentally Retarded Children

| Social Class[1] | Number of Children by Etiology of Retardation | |
	Organic	Psychosocial
I and II	6	3
III	7	6
IV and V	14	26
Total	27	35

Source: Philips and Williams (1975), Table 3.
[1] According to Hollingshead's two-factor index of social position

in a general clinic population. There is no evidence that the symptoms of mentally retarded children fit into a special category related to the retardation. The development of emotional disorder in retarded children often begins with transient situational problems that become more fixed as the child's development is distorted. Such difficulties, coupled with negative social attitudes, may intensify less acute problems as the child encounters each developmental level. In addition, the birth of a retarded child obviously arouses reactive problems in the family, and these problems will result in difficulties caring for the offspring. This has been noted in many studies (Bernstein, 1970; Szymanski and Tanguay, 1980; Solnit and Stak, 1961; Ende and Brown, 1978), and it may account for the high incidence of behavioral and personality disorders among retarded children.

INTERVENTION AND PREVENTION

Prevention of mental retardation entails a variety of approaches, depending on etiology, severity, intensity, and duration. The general principles governing these preventive efforts differ little from those used with children who are favored with normal intelligence.

Primary Prevention

In primary prevention, efforts are directed toward averting the defect that increases the likelihood of a disorder. It is obvious that reducing the incidence of mental retardation in the general population will provide the greatest good in this area of concern. In the global sense, social reform will be the most effective intervention toward primary prevention. Adequate nutrition, housing, employment, and education will improve the environments of children in families which are themselves at a greater risk for dysfunction and disruption. In their concept of "parental casualty," Sameroff and Chandler (1975) have postulated that as environmental difficulty increases, families become increasingly dysfunctional over time, with a particularly disruptive effect upon offspring. To strengthen families wherever possible, to provide proper placement, temporary or permanent, when indicated, and to effect relinquishment when necessary are basic measures for supporting the cognitive, physical, and emotional development of children.

Early education and intervention programs like Head Start and Follow Through are effective for children at risk, especially for those from deprived backgrounds. In his Milwaukee study, Heber selected a group of children who came from deprived slum areas and whose parents' IQs were below 80 (Heber and Garber, 1975). The Milwaukee study demonstrated that intensive work with the offspring of such families could lead to wide shifts in performance and significant changes in skill development. Although Head Start and similar efforts have been limited in scope and outcome (Brieter and Englemann, 1966; Bronfenbrenner, 1975), educational intervention is basic and necessary to insure the realization of untapped potential. P.L. 94–142 has increased pressure on the schools to provide an educational experience for all children, especially those whose intellectual and emotional development lags behind the majority. Many behavioral techniques have been developed to help children remain in school and in regular classes (Schiefelbusch, 1979; Bijou, 1983; Bijou and Dunitz-Johnson, 1981). Methods have also been developed to teach parents how to instruct their moderately and severely handicapped children (Sherer and Sherer, 1976).

Genetic counseling is an effective tool for advising parents who are at risk of having children with certain disorders. For instance, for parents who have had a child with Down's syndrome, the risk of having another is far greater with cases of translocation than with those with trisomy. Dominant autosomal conditions are highly predictable as is specific enzymatic defect. Counseling and mass screening are helpful in such conditions, but a word of caution should be noted. Genetic management and sterilization for intelligence control are not only questionable, but to be condemned.

Medical management can also help to reduce reproductive casualties. Parent education, prevention of prematurity, adequate nutrition, and treatment for alcohol- and drug-abusing mothers are all basic to good care. Pregnant teenagers are a risk group for having infants with Down's syndrome and other forms of mental retardation. Good obstetrical care and pediatric management are essential for prevention. Recent advances in immunization have been effective in reducing the incidence of mental retardation resulting from the complications of rubella and measles encephalitis. The combination of good prenatal and perinatal care, regular well-baby visits, proper nutrition, and immunization are essential to any care, but vital to the prevention of mental retardation in populations at risk.

For retardation which has organic etiologies, new primary preventive efforts can be expected to emerge from scientific breakthroughs in biological marker research, and this will help to reduce the incidence of the population born with defects. Nonetheless, to prevent the development of retardation with nonorganic etiology, children from deprived backgrounds will continue to need intervention that entails medical care, education, and rehabilitation efforts. Social change is evolutionary and a process slow in coming, but we have the means to achieve these ends and should strive for their attainment.

Secondary Prevention

Secondary prevention refers to the treatment of an acute illness to avoid complication and chronicity. In the case of mental retardation, secondary prevention begins with prompt intervention in those factors that are contributing to the retardation and involves the treatment of those processes that lead to dysfunction. Since an interaction of impersonal (biological), personal (psychological), and environmental (cultural) factors is always present in mental retardation, intervention in any of these three areas may benefit the individual and his or her family.

Early recognition of several specific disorders, before retarded functioning occurs, is essential to the secondary prevention of mental retardation. These disorders, defined by Garrard and Richmond (1965), include (1) hyperbilirubinemia and bilirubin encephalopathy; (2) phenylketonuria; (3) galactosemia; (4) hypothyroidism of various metabolic types; (5) idiopathic hypercalcemia; (6) hypoglycemia of various metabolic types; (7) hydrocephalus; (8) premature synostosis of cranial sutures; (9) subdural hematomas; (10) lead poisoning; (11) bacterial meningitides; (12) congenital syphilis; (13) acute intracranial hypertension due to encephalitis, glomerulonephritis, or other causes; and (14) pyridoxine deficiency. This list should grow as the primary mechanisms for disease processes are better understood.

An infant with an untreated metabolic disorder (e.g., phenylketonuria or lead encephalopathy) may succumb to such associated sequelae as frequent convulsions or progressive deterioration. Early intervention can prevent these effects as well as the associated mental retardation that is secondary to a primary biological predisposing defect. Phenylketonuria, an inborn error of metabolism, is often cited as an example of the necessity for prompt early intervention and prevention. Reliable and valid tests are available, and mass screening in the early days of life is now a prerequisite in most of the United States. Dietary management, with a diet low in phenylalanine started early in life, may prevent manifestations of severe deterioration and subsequent mental deficiency. In many of these conditions, medical or surgical treatment can prevent serious problems from developing later in childhood. Untreated, children with these conditions will be counted among those with severe and moderate retardation.

A second and larger group with associated mental retardation is the broad category of children with perceptual-motor dysfunction, with or without hyperkinesis. Even though the etiology remains in question, appropriate intervention using psychoeducational techniques does prevent subsequent retardation. Sensory defects such as hearing loss or partial blindness may be factors in associated mental retardation. Proper evaluation and treatment of these defects will result in marked improvements in social and educational performance.

A third category amenable to secondary prevention is defined broadly as psychosocial retardation. This category includes defective mother-child relationships and disturbed attachment, inadequate emotional interaction in institutional settings, insufficient enrichment at home for social, intellectual, and emotional growth, and severe emotional disorder with impairment of affectional learning. These conditions are due to interactional or environmental factors which may accentuate biological etiologies or which may themselves be primarily etiologic.

Early enrichment through child care, developmental centers, and preschool programs may reverse some of the negative effects of these forces. In these situations, the child psychiatrist can play a significant role toward alleviating developmental retardation. As a consultant to well-baby clinics, schools, and social welfare agencies, and as an advocate with others in city, state, and federal agencies, the psychiatrist may help initiate services that will enrich life for children of the urban and rural poor.

Secondary prevention is a challenge calling both for direct service to the child and family and for collaborative efforts between professionals and laymen to awaken the conscience of the community. The community must be made to consider that its priorities include a delivery system which provides services to foster the optimal development of all children.

Tertiary Prevention

Tertiary prevention is amelioration of the disorder once it occurs. In the case of children with mental retardation, efforts are directed toward limiting the disability and enhancing their innate potential. With some retarded children, tertiary prevention begins at the time of birth. The toll on parents is considerable once they learn that their child is mentally retarded. Dreams are shattered, and priorities and expectations are altered. Counseling with parents to help them begin to recognize their "loss" may help them to deal more constructively with the child's limited development. Parents who have been helped at these crucial moments in the child's development usually return for questions at critical periods, seeking advice and counsel. Community and volunteer agencies such as Associations for Retarded Citizens may be beneficial.

Many experiments have focused on helping parents learn how to train their retarded children to achieve developmental skills. Such efforts have aided considerably in the child's development (Sherer and Sherer, 1976). Although attainment of normal skills may not be expectable, emotional difficulty may be reduced and social adaptation may be enhanced. It is not the level of intellectual attainment that determines outcome, but psychosocial adaptation.

If the child must be placed out of the home, the environment should be normalized to approach that of his or her own home. This will entail developing small therapeutic units rather than large institutions. The doctrine of the least restrictive environment is essential in such care.

Bowlby (1969) and Ainsworth (1973) have described how inadequate or anxious attachment may distort development. Direct treatment of the child and the family has been shown to temper such defects in development and to initiate a return to normal developmental pathways. Fraiberg et al. (1975) have demonstrated the reversibility of severe developmental difficulties through direct treatment with the primary caretaker.

Inadequate institutional settings reinforce difficult situations. Programs that provide environmental enrichment foster development. Provence and Lipton (1962) demonstrated in prospective studies the negative effects of poor institutions on developing children. Kugel and Wolfensberger (1969) showed how normalization of institutionalized children's environments led to marked functional improvements in all areas of the children's lives.

Many children who have problems of retardation also have difficulty in behavior. Psychiatric problems are considerably more prevalent among the mentally retarded children than among their more favored peers. Professionals, however, often have inhibitions and prejudice regarding psychiatric care for the mentally retarded. Countertransference problems are significant barriers to successful psychiatric intervention. On the other hand, many case reports and research efforts have indicated the efficacy of psychotherapeutic intervention with retarded individuals (Szurek and Philips, 1966; Szymanski, 1980). Behavior modification techniques have also been reported effective and should be used where appropriate (Bornstein et al., 1982). Psychopharmacologic substances have been used to control behavior (Freeman, 1970), and these interventions should be used judiciously when there are clear-cut indications. Recreational and vocational rehabilitation should be provided as integral parts of helping retarded persons to achieve psychosocial adaptation.

In summary, intervention must be directed toward primary, secondary, and tertiary prevention. A panoply of services must be provided, from birth to adulthood, and whenever possible within the mainstream of society.

Chapter 10 # Parenting and Children at Risk [†]
by Henry Grunebaum, M.D.

INTRODUCTION

Jeremiah 31:29 says, "If the Fathers have eaten sour grapes, the children's teeth shall be set on edge." The Bible does not tell us whether anything can be done to prevent this unfortunate outcome, nor does it say whether the children have inherited a tendency to malocclusions or if they have learned that sour grapes are the diet of choice. These are much like the questions confronted in the risk research that studies and seeks interventions for the children of parents who are psychiatrically disturbed.

This chapter begins with a review of what is known about the children of schizophrenic and depressed parents, with a particular emphasis on aspects of their parenting. Taking a broader perspective, the chapter then discusses problems in parenting more generally and next considers the stress which all parents encounter, emphasizing the risk to children.

The findings about children at risk because a parent is mentally ill lead naturally to intervention strategies targeted at diagnostic groups of parents. The chapter discusses some of those which can easily be carried out by mental health professionals in clinical practice and in mental hospitals. Finally, the chapter delineates the advantages of extending interventions beyond diagnosed groups to offer community-based programs for parents and children more generally, where there is evidence of problems in parenting. Since the family is, however, embedded in a societal context, a brief epilogue considers the family from the perspectives of systems theory and social justice.

The phrase *children at risk* has had two meanings. To clinicians it means children who are likely to have difficulties in the future. To researchers it has meant children of mentally ill parents, particularly those with schizophrenia. Researchers have studied these children primarily be-

†The author wishes to thank his colleagues and friends, Bert Cohler and Karlen Lyons-Ruth for their careful review of this manuscript, and Norman Watt for graciously providing prepublished manuscripts of a book reviewing recent research on high-risk children.

cause of the light they may shed on the etiology of the illness. Less often have they been studied with a primary goal of identifying practical and immediate preventive efforts. This chapter attempts to show the value of both research and intervention with children at risk, using both definitions of children at risk.

CHILDREN WITH MENTALLY ILL PARENTS

Basic Studies

Children of psychotic parents have been of great research interest over the past 25 years. Studying the children, researchers can explore the precursors of mental illness before the illness is altered by hospitalizations and medication. Usually the illness studied has been schizophrenia, and usually the ill parent has been the mother.*

The studies are usually of the follow-back type or of the follow-up type. In the follow-back studies, a group of currently mentally ill adults is located, and school records or earlier research data are reviewed in retrospect (Watt, 1974). These studies have the disadvantages that the desired information is often not available and that the findings, while statistically differentiating future patients from controls, have little predictive power due to large numbers of both false positives and false negatives. Follow-up studies have the disadvantages of taking many years with consequent sample attrition, of changes in diagnostic criteria, of developing measures for variables which are applicable over a wide range of ages, and of ethical constraints (such as when the investigator encounters children in difficulty who require assistance) (Wynne, 1968).

Furthermore, the high-risk samples of children of mentally ill parents consist of a small and probably atypical group of children. Only 10 percent of the total range of schizophrenic individuals have schizophrenic parents, and children selected because they have a schizophrenic parent therefore have a high genetic load which is not typical of most adult schizophrenics. Finally, as Kagan (1980) has pointed out, the Western belief in developmental continuity, which he contrasts with the Eastern belief in the possibility of drastic change, is probably misplaced and leads the investigator to look for psychological deviations in childhood which are similar to the manifestations of the condition in adulthood. In fact, the relevant variables may be quite different in childhood. The search for continuities may also lead the investigator to ignore the discontinuities that arise from such unpredictable childhood events as a devoted teacher taking an interest or a caring grandmother dying.

Early clinical studies of the children of schizophrenic mothers include those by Sobel (1961), who described the impaired mother-child relationship, and by Fish (1957; 1984), who found that the children manifested "pandevelopmental retardation." The first to study these children intensively were Mednick and his colleagues in Copenhagen (Mednick, 1970; Mednick and Schulsinger, 1973) and the author's own group (Grunebaum et al., 1963). Mednick found that the children of schizophrenics presented problems in school, had poorer performance

---

*Preceptor's note: In his discussion of methodological issues in this research, Dr. Garmezy points out the bias inherent in studying only the children of schizophrenic mothers and not including the children of schizophrenic fathers.

on the continuous-association test, and showed an abnormal electrodermal response and that their mothers' pregnancies and their immediate postnatal periods were characterized by greater difficulties. The author's group, beginning in 1961, found that while the children of schizophrenic mothers did have impaired ability to attend continuously (Gamer et al., 1977b), the children of depressed mothers were particularly likely to be impaired (Grunebaum et al., 1978). The findings held true for both three- and five-year-old children of psychotic mothers (Cohler et al., 1977). These children had greater intratest scatter and lower developmental quotients on the Wechsler scales and greater impairment in deploying attention than the children of schizophrenics. It seemed that the depressed mothers' apathetic withdrawal had exerted a profound effect on their children (Cohler et al., 1983).

Recent Findings

In the early 1970s, a large number of research groups began to investigate children of psychotic mothers, and their findings have recently been reported in the book, *Children at Risk for Schizophrenia: A Longitudinal Perspective* (Watt et al., 1984). Many of the early research findings have been supported and amplified by these studies, and much in addition has been learned.

DEVELOPMENTAL DATA   Psychotic mothers are less likely than controls to wish to become pregnant or to be happy while pregnant, and they have fewer social supports during their pregnancies (McNeil and Kaij, 1984). There is some evidence that the pregnancies of schizophrenics are more stressful and difficult (Mednick et al., 1984; Cudeck et al., 1984; McNeil and Kaij, 1984) and that the children have lower birth weights and more neurological difficulties. Sameroff et al. (1984), however, suggest that many of these differences can be explained by the stress of the mothers' socioeconomic situation rather than their diagnosis of schizophrenia. Children of the mentally ill are far more likely to be given up for adoption, particularly if their mothers are lower class, unmarried, socially incompetent, and severely disturbed. The children of these mothers are more likely to be premature and developmentally deviant than the children of psychotic mothers who keep them. This, it should be noted, may skew the population of adoptees.

During infancy, the children show poor motor functioning, poorer sensorimotor coordination, and increased frequency of neurological abnormalities (Marcus et al., 1984; McNeil and Kaij, 1984). It is important to acknowledge the pioneering research of Fish, who has since 1952 followed a group of children selected for risk on the basis of having schizophrenic mothers. The findings in infancy and early childhood of "pandevelopmental retardation" and disorganization of neurological maturation, characterized by "soft neurological signs," erratic functioning, decreased vestibular responses, and unusual quiet periods, appeared to correlate with later psychosis (Fish, 1984).

In childhood, although most of the children are not grossly deviant (Rolf et al., 1984), they are as a group less competent, both cognitively and socially, according to teacher and peer ratings (Weintraub and Neale, 1984; Wynne, 1984; Kokes et al., 1984; Yu et al., 1984). Cognitive impairments are manifest in the IQ, the Bender-Gestalt, the continuous-performance test, the object-sorting test, and focused attention, and they are more easily distracted (Weintraub and Neale, 1984; Cornblatt and Erlenmeyer-Kimling, 1984; Erlenmeyer-Kimling et al., 1984). The children are also more likely to be socially deviant, showing differences in the direction of increased aggression and disruption (Weintraub and Neale, 1984).

In adolescence, the offspring show increased interpersonal disharmony, less scholastic motivation, increased emotional instability, and lower intelligence on teacher ratings (Jones et al., 1984; Watt, 1984). On the basis of an extended follow-up, Anthony and his colleagues concluded that for many of the children their parent's mental illness was the crucial event in their lives (Worland et al., 1984). Anthony (1984) noted that with physical emancipation the children had more detachment and more objectivity, but that they continued to be both exasperated and ashamed. The parent seemed "less frightening, less peculiar, and mellowing," and the now adult children often recommended separation or divorce as a relief for the nonpsychotic parent.

FAMILY INTERACTION   Early studies by Gamer et al. (1977a; 1977b) found that ill mothers showed less positive affect and were more likely to be either too directive or too diffuse. Confirming these findings in a free-play situation, Baldwin et al. (1984) found that the schizophrenic spouses interacted less than the healthy spouses and less than psychoneurotic depressives, who in turn interacted less than patients with affective disorder. They found that either censure or praise from a mentally ill parent was disruptive to the child (Klein and Salzman, 1984). Unfortunately, the Baldwin et al. study lacked a normal control group. Looking at interaction from a different point of view, Wynne (1984) has reported that the transactional style and warmth, as well as active, warm, and balanced communication among family members, predicted good teacher and peer ratings of children's competence, while communication deviance predicted poor competence ratings. These findings are similar to what Rodnick et al. (1984) found with a sample of troubled adolescents.

Marital adjustment was generally worst in couples with a schizophrenic spouse, next worst in the patient control group, and best in the normal controls (Weintraub and Neale, 1984). Couples with an ill spouse were less conciliatory, less happy, and less involved in outside activities, and the depressed patients gave their marriages particularly poor ratings. Family solidarity was adversely affected and divorce was common; as might be expected, financial security was impaired. The schizophrenic mothers were more child centered. Schizophrenic fathers were perceived more negatively than normals, while depressed fathers were seen as no different from normals. Since clinical interventions with the healthy spouse are likely to be considered, it is of particular interest that the "healthy" husbands of mentally ill mothers often controlled their children through inducing guilt or anxiety. Clearly these are very troubled families.

OUTCOMES AND KEY VARIABLES   Some of the children of psychotic parents become psychotically disturbed. Mednick et al. (1984) found that those children who became psychotic tended to have low IQs and prior attentional difficulties and to have mothers with a severe course of illness and pregnancy and birth complications. If they were boys, they were likely to be anxious, lonely, and disturbing in school, while girls were anhedonic, withdrawn, and isolated.

While the diagnosis of the parent is significant, what makes the most impact is their level of functioning. In general, the most adversely affected children of psychotics had depressed parents, the next most had schizophrenic parents, and the least affected had parents with manic-depressive diagnoses (Rolf et al., 1984; Cole et al., 1984), confirming the findings of the author's group (Grunebaum et al., 1978). Accumulating evidence, recently reviewed by Beardslee et al. (1983), indicates that the children of depressed parents are also at risk for cognitive impairment and for difficulties with peers, in school, and with parents. As many as 40 percent of these children may have diagnosable illness themselves, and they may be particularly vulnerable in early infancy and adolescence. Chronic parental impairment has been found to be more pathogenic than acute episodes, and intercurrent level of functioning to have great influence, particularly when associated with a narrow range of affective responsivity (Fisher et al., 1980).

Family difficulties appear to be worse when the mother is the patient rather than the father (Kokes et al., 1980). Sex of the affected parent also contributes to the impact of the illness upon the offspring. Since courtship and marriage involve some degree of social assertiveness, a chronically mentally ill man is not likely to have the social skills requisite for a sustained relationship or steady employment (Phillips, 1968). Women, who are traditionally somewhat less active in the courtship process, may marry, have children, and then succumb to mental illness during the first years after childbirth, due, perhaps, to the role strain which accompanies the transition to parenthood and which leads nearly one-fourth of all women with children of preschool age to feel depressed (Campbell et al., 1976; Weissman and Myers, 1978; Brown and Harris, 1975; Cohler and Geyer, 1982). Thus, in contemporary society, the affected parent tends to be the mother rather than the father.

When the father is impaired and hospitalized, he is likely to be extruded from the home, particularly if his behavior has been abusive. Although his family may go on welfare, his wife is still in the role of housekeeper and mother. When the mother is hospitalized, the burdens on the father and husband are severe. Holding down a job, caring for the children, maintaining continuing contact with the hospitalized wife and mother, and arranging for baby-sitting and help from the extended family—all require considerable redefinition of the father's traditional role. After an initial period of trying to hold the family together and to manage all expected household tasks, these fathers may become depressed and often seek divorce (Grunebaum et al., 1983).

Musick and her colleagues (1979) found that it was not the quantity of "overtly negative or hostile behavior," but rather the lack of "joie de vivre," playful enthusiasm, consistency, and connectedness, which distinguished the psychotic mothers' interactions with their children from those of normal mothers. Only the mentally ill mothers acted inappropriately and expressed no positive emotions to their children. The lack of pleasant dialogue most clearly characterized their interactions with the children. It is not the absolute quantity of what parents give children (counts of this or that behavior), but rather the quality of the dialogue between them that matters.

It is vital here to note that Bleuler (1978; 1984) found in his mixed sample of children of schizophrenic parents that 84 percent were married and had a higher social status than their parents; others have pointed out that only a small subset of the children are deviant (11 to 44 percent), depending on the study and measure (Watt, 1984). A variety of studies suggest that the offspring of mentally ill parents are likely to be creative adults (Karlsson, 1968), and Kauffman et al. (1979) found that precursors of this could be found during childhood in children who were called "superkids."

This brief review of many years of devoted work by large groups of collaborating researchers hardly does justice to their findings much less their efforts.

SUMMARY As high-risk research has progressed, the model employed has evolved to include both genetic diathesis and environmental stress. However, there are no certain criteria which infallibly diagnose nonrelapsing schizophrenics. Strauss (1984) has pointed out that the belief "once a schizophrenic, always a schizophrenic" is false. The schizophrenic parent, as he so aptly states, is thus "a moving target."

Not only is there the problem of diagnosis, but some workers have noted that chronicity, the degree to which the psychosis is involving of the child, and lack of affective reactivity may be more important features than diagnosis (Wynne, 1984). In addition, all studies which have compared psychotics with different diagnoses have found that all the children tend to differ from controls, and in the same directions. According to Lewine (1984), these findings are consistent with the idea that while a general vulnerability to psychosis is genetically transmitted, the particular form is a function of environmental factors. Furthermore, Sameroff et al. (1984) believe that some environmental factors, particularly poverty, may be more significant than the genetic factors.

The implications of high-risk studies for the etiology of schizophrenia more generally must take into account the overrepresentation of females among the parents (Lewine et al., 1984). Also, the children being studied are unrepresentative in that, unlike most individuals who become schizophrenic, they have a schizophrenic parent.

Wynne (1984) in particular has emphasized the contribution of family variables to the final outcome, citing the findings of B. R. Mednick (1973). In this study, a child who had breakdowns as an adult tended also to have a deviant father; some effects of separation on the children were ameliorated if a grandparent or other relative took over the rearing; and separation appeared to have more adverse effects on males than females. The importance of the family for all children at risk is supported by the magnificent longitudinal study of Werner and Smith (1982). In this study of 698 poor children on the rural island of Kauai, the presence of alternate care givers in the family and support from grandparents, siblings, and kin distinguished those who thrived from those who succumbed to the chronic poverty, perinatal stress, and family psychopathology that characterized the entire sample.

In summary, children with a psychotic parent are likely to have social and cognitive deficits, and they also clearly tend to have educational, economic, and social disadvantages. Although parental psychiatric symptoms generally have not yet been shown to add specific elements of risk to the risk stemming from marital conflict, inadequate parental role performance, and low socioeconomic status, the severity and chronicity of parental mental illness apparently do affect children adversely. Similarly, while schizophrenia may have specific effects, they have not yet been found, and severe depression seems at least as damaging, if not more so, to the children. Some of them are at risk themselves for psychosis, some will be "superkids," and the vast majority will have to deal all their lives with the experience of having a psychotic parent. (Recently, investigators have begun to study other groups of children at risk by virtue of specific parental pathology, such as alcoholism [see recent review by el-Guebaly, 1983] and incarceration [Weintraub, 1983; Fishman, 1983].)

CHILDREN WITH PARENTS UNDER STRESS

An entirely different perspective on children at risk by virtue of parental psychiatric disability becomes apparent if we view parenting as a stressful activity that demands new competencies and requires new emotional capacities. Cohler and Musick (1982) have recently reviewed the data which document the developmental task of becoming a parent. Particularly for the woman, this task involves assuming a new social role since most couples, according to Gutmann (1975), respond to the "chronic emergency" of being a parent with the man assuming the economic and the woman the child-care responsibilities. This pattern continues today, even though sex-role stereotypes are increasingly challenged. Insofar as the earliest role allocations influence identifications most powerfully, the parent most present early will have the most impact; for most adults today, this parent was the mother (Dinnerstein, 1977). Many studies have demonstrated that women report greater psychological impairment, even controlling for response styles (Kessler et al., 1981; Phillips and Seagal, 1969) and that married women are probably more unhappy than single women (Radloff, 1975; Radloff and Rae, 1979). Employment may or may not increase a woman's sense of well-being (Stewart and Salt, 1981), for even when women work, they remain the parent principally responsible for child care (Cohler and Grunebaum, 1981).

Given the stress of parenting, it is no surprise that surveys find between 20 and 25 percent of women in the community with untreated marked depressive symptoms (Weissman and Myers, 1978). Depression is related to the number of children under five, to the extent of economic hardship, and to the availability of the husband as a confidant (Brown and Harris, 1975). The fact that these women may be alone as parents in oppressive situations may explain the frequency of depression (Reid and Morrison, 1983). Investigations of psychiatric symptoms in parents may accurately reflect women's response to motherhood but may not reflect men's response to fatherhood; in fact, far less is known about men's response to parenting, particularly the psychopathology of fatherhood. Clinical experience suggests that men respond more to the lessened availability of their wives than to the stresses of fathering. Insofar as men actually do share the work of parenting, their responses to parenting require studies comparable to the studies of mothering, rather than the unquestioning approval that the popular press has hitherto given to these pioneering parents. From another perspective, data also suggest that parental behavior is influenced by the temperament and characteristics of the child. The "difficult-to-comfort" child, the "fragile" child, and the retarded child are clearly stressful to parents.

In contrast to the extensive research on risk to children of parents with defined psychopathology, few studies are available on risk to children of parents under stress without psychiatric hospitalization. From those studies that are available, however, the evidence suggests that parental mental illness itself is not the major source of risk for such children. Instead, severe marital discord, lax discipline, large family size, paternal criminality, and poor maternal functioning are more commonly associated with childhood behavior disorders (Rutter, 1980).

Children with behavior disorders (externalizing children) are at highest risk for later difficulty. Rutter and colleagues studied a large cohort of British school children at 10 and 14 years of age and found that the majority of behavior disorders were present early in the child's school career and were stable over time (Rutter et al., 1975a; 1975b; Rutter, 1979). A follow-up study in Minneapolis (Garmezy and Devine, 1984) found that it was the externalizing children, rather than the children of psychotic mothers, who were the most deviant and about whom the "horror stories" were told. Robins (1966; 1972) followed up a large sample of children referred for child guidance and found that 70 percent of those referred as children for severe behavior disorders later showed major psychopathology or sociopathology as adults, including psychosis, drug addiction, alcoholism, and sociopathy.

Rutter (1980) has emphasized that risk does not result from a single factor, but from a combination of stressors. The child's potential interacts with the familial variables, which interact with the larger support network of the family as it is embedded in the society, and these interactions lead to the final outcome. Lyons-Ruth, the author, and their colleagues are currently following a group of infants from low-income, multirisk environments (Lyons-Ruth et al., 1983). Only 16 percent of the mothers of these infants had ever received psychiatric treatment. These low-income women, whose infants were referred to a special parenting support service, reported levels of depression equal to that of depressed psychiatric outpatients, while a matched group of low-income women who related adequately to their infants reported low levels of depression similar to the general population. Clearly, matched groups of low-income women with infants can differ dramatically in the degree of depression they experience. The highly depressed women in this study reported family histories characterized by less parental warmth, fewer peer friendships, and poorer family organization and supervision (Lyons-Ruth et al., 1983). On a final note, we must recognize a more global source of stress for parents. An interactional systems view of the family would also take into account the extent to which society values parenting and the status which society accords to parenting. An adequate understanding of parenting behavior and its impact on children today would have to recognize that parents value their children despite, rather than because of, the status that society accords to parenting.

ISSUES IN PREVENTIVE INTERVENTION

Preventive intervention with children at risk is a relatively new undertaking and has taken several directions: (1) informed clinical practice with mental patients; (2) family planning services for patients; (3) special programs for the children of parents with a particular diagnosis, usually schizophrenia; and (4) generic programs for children from a catchment area referred because of health care provider concerns about the quality of parenting.

Two major problems arise in preventive intervention with children whose parents are impaired in their ability to rear them. The first is the problem of case finding. In the course of their daily work, mental health professionals are natural case finders. As clinicians encounter cases of mentally ill parents, they also find cases of children at risk, and they can help these children if they are informed and motivated. Efforts have been made to gather a group of children of mentally ill parents and to provide them with specially designed interventions. These efforts may be viewed as attempts at true primary prevention. One difficulty that arises here is that children of a given age can be located only from a large geographic area. Rolf and Hasazi (1977), for example, found it difficult to locate enough cases in Vermont. Another difficulty here is that the intervention strategies seem to bear only a modest relationship to what one is attempting to prevent and that the assessment of long-term effects is next to impossible. As an alternative strategy, cases can be gathered from a broad range of referral sources, with the only common features being that clinicians are concerned about the quality of parenting which a child is receiving, regardless of its cause, and that the children are of approximately similar ages. Advantages of this generic approach, which draws children from a smaller geographic area, are that coordination with other service providers can be enhanced and social networking among parents can be facilitated. Disadvantages are that pathology-specific interventions cannot be studied, and long-term assessment is again next to impossible.

A second major problem in preventive intervention is specifying the goal of prevention and the nature of the preventive efforts. Some believe that the only appropriate goal of prevention is to lower the incidence of a specific illness, such as schizophrenia, in the target population (Lamb and Zusman, 1981). At present, however, no projects are endeavoring to lower the incidence of schizophrenia; indeed, no one has proposed a plausible intervention strategy.

One goal which does appear feasible is to improve the lives of the children of mentally ill parents and perhaps thereby to lower the incidence of the milder, but much more frequent, forms of psychopathology in this population. Bleuler (1984) has quoted one functioning adult from this population as saying, "One cannot laugh as other people laugh after having gone through this misery." Interventions directed toward this goal generally include various forms of support and guidance to the parents, specific education in child-care practices, enrichment programs for the children, and interventions at times of familial crisis.

Related to this goal are the often ignored children of schizophrenic parents who emerge unscathed or only relatively impaired by the experience. In one of the first reports focusing on the issue of invulnerability in children, Kauffman et al. (1979) reviewed the cases of a number of children who showed superior competence at home, at school, and with peers; the more resilient children were better able to use adults' attention, were more appealing to adults, and were better able to involve adults, other than their sick parent, in their lives as a kind of substitute parent. Cohler and Musick (1982) made similar observations on the competent children in their sample, but they stressed the mother's contribution. The mothers of competent children were able to facilitate outside social contacts for their children and maintained a positive view of those experiences, while the mothers of less competent children involved the child in their own social isolation and in their fears and suspicions regarding social contact.

These findings suggest the utility of giving the children of mentally ill parents a wide range of community supports. On the other hand, Erlenmeyer-Kimling et al. (1984) and others who have a strongly genetic view of etiology believe that only a very specific and focused intervention will be of any value. Many others, such as Sameroff et al. (1984) and Bleuler (1984), clearly imply that among the variety of interventions some may be useful to some children, but not to others.

INTERVENTIONS AND THEIR OUTCOMES

Informed Clinical Practice

The psychiatrist during the course of clinical practice has perhaps the most important opportunities for preventive intervention (Philips, 1983). At admission an assessment of the patient's family and children and of their well-being is vital. All too often when parents are admitted to mental hospitals, detailed histories are obtained of their childhoods and their sibling relationships, but no more than cursory attention is paid to the well-being and care afforded their children. Only rarely do mental health professionals become involved in ensuring the provision of adequate foster care for the children of hospitalized patients, a task which is usually left to the family. Not surprisingly, Ekdahl et al. (1962) and Fasman et al. (1967) found that the children of psychiatrically hospitalized patients suffered far more disruptions of their lives and more abuse and neglect than did the children of parents hospitalized for tuberculosis, particularly when the mother was the hospitalized parent.

Attention to the children of mentally ill parents requires that the healthier spouse be supported in parenting (Grunebaum et al., 1983). Laboring with the burden of a mentally ill partner is not easy, and the obligations of child care require added effort. In such families, children commonly take on some of the burden, assuming parental roles and sometimes moving toward the role of spouse. Support for the spouse left at home should not be limited to psychological support, but should also endeavor to mobilize the appropriate community support systems. Families are often woefully ignorant of the services potentially available, and they may also require guidance to overcome the shame, guilt, and fear which can prevent them from using services. Finally, it is vital that the clinician discuss directly with the patient and the spouse the importance of contraception. Interestingly, the profession which once thought that sexual impulses were at the root of all mental problems now often hesitates to ask directly, "Are you taking adequate precautions now to prevent your getting pregnant?"

Family Planning Services

Family planning services, including both counseling and contraception of mental patients, particularly female patients, is probably the single most effective form of primary prevention known today (Grunebaum et al., 1971; Abernethy and Grunebaum, 1972; 1973; Grunebaum and Abernethy, 1975; Grunebaum et al., 1975; Clough et al., 1976). The fact that these services are not routine has a twofold basis: mental health professionals do not view family planning as their responsibility, and family planners do not view mental patients as an important population at risk.

Family planning services for mental patients have a sound rationale that goes well beyond the obvious benefit of risk reduction for children. In the first place, the vast majority of mentally ill hospitalized women desire such services. Furthermore, these services, usually unavailable to women in mental hospitals, are today part of good medical care for all fertile women. In the hospital, these services can be provided with appropriate attention to informed consent and freedom of choice.

Mentally ill women tend to have disproportionate numbers of unwanted pregnancies and unwanted births, and they sometimes even become pregnant in the mental hospital, often using contraception sporadically or ineffectively. The effect on the patient of unwanted children cannot be estimated, but clearly it is not in her best interest. Once these patients receive counseling, though, follow-up demonstrates that they tend to continue the regime they decided to use in the hospital.

Finally, family planning is probably cost-effective. To provide a family planning counselor and a weekly gynecological clinic in a mental hospital costs about $15,000 to $20,000 per year. Foster placement and care for one child in the community today costs at least $5,000 per year (Massachusetts figure).

Unfortunately, these interventions for mental patients and children have no lobby. To the author's knowledge, only metropolitan Boston has mental health facilities which routinely offer family planning services. Facilities offering these services include community mental health centers, urban and rural state mental hospitals, and various geographically dispersed day hospitals and inpatient units. In all of these settings, patients have welcomed and used the services. More than 80 percent of all female admissions are counseled and given adequate gynecological care. A large proportion of the patients decide that during and immediately after a psychiatric hospitalization is not the time to become pregnant and have a child (Grunebaum et al., 1971; Abernethy and Grunebaum, 1972; Grunebaum and Abernethy, 1975).

Programs for Children and Their Mentally Ill Parents

JOINT ADMISSION   Joint admissions to mental hospitals for infants and young children along with their mentally ill mothers was first pioneered by Main (1958) at the Cassel Hospital in England with neurotic patients, and in the United States by the author's group with psychotic patients at the Massachusetts Mental Health Center (Grunebaum et al., 1963). The rationale was that having both mother and child on the ward offered a unique opportunity to observe, support, and intervene therapeutically in their relationship. The programs focused the staff's attention on the patient *qua* mother. For the joint admission to proceed optimally, a period of adjustment on the ward was necessary before the baby or child would join its mother. During this period, the staff could get to know the patient, and an agreement was developed among the mother, her husband, the ward staff, and the treating psychiatrist

(Grunebaum et al., 1963). Of particular importance for a successful joint admission was paying sufficient attention to the relationship of the woman and her husband both as a couple and as parents. This program was subsequently repeated in a large state mental hospital (Van der Walde et al., 1968).

Results of the Massachusetts Mental Health Center joint admission program were assessed by comparing the children in the program with the children of normal controls and with the children of mentally ill mothers who did not participate in the program. (Neither of the comparison groups were random, and both were to a considerable extent biased, the latter in the direction of increased severity of psychopathology.) The children in the joint admission program showed somewhat less positive affect than the normal controls, but they were superior to the nonparticipants in interpersonal relationships and language use and on developmental tests (Gallant, 1975). These findings suggest that the children are not harmed by their stay on the wards and may perhaps benefit from it.

With today's increasing pressure for shorter hospitalizations and lessened emphasis on psychotherapeutic intervention during hospitalization, joint admissions are less commonly contemplated. Nonetheless, it appears useful therapeutically and underlines some important principles. Therapists treating mentally ill parents should not only talk to them about their children, but should also observe the parents with their children in the office, perhaps in the ward, and also at home. Observation will reveal much that is not otherwise reported.

INTENSIVE NURSING AFTERCARE PROGRAM The first project providing assistance after discharge to psychiatrically ill women with young children was the Intensive Nursing Aftercare Project (INAC), begun in 1967 (Grunebaum and Cohler, 1983; Cohler and Grunebaum, 1983; Cohler and Grunebaum, 1981). The twin goals of the project were to prevent readmission and to foster a better mother-child relationship. Fifty psychotic women with children 5 years old and under were recruited from state mental hospitals, enlisted in the project, and then randomly assigned to an intensive (90 minutes/week) and a minimal treatment group. Fifty normal control subjects were obtained through advertisements and carefully matched with the patients and the children on a case-by-case basis. The intensive and minimal treatment groups were quite similar in terms of diagnoses and severity of illness, and the control group was well matched on demographic and child variables. At termination few differences were found between the two treatment groups, either in the mothers' readmissions or psychopathology or in the children. The mothers who benefited from the interventions appeared to have better interpersonal relationships, better premorbid adjustment, and less chronicity. While the mothers felt that the intervention was valuable, their husbands noticed no change.

A more recent advance over the INAC is the Thresholds Study (Musick et al., 1979; 1981) in which Cohler also participated. This program attempted to integrate a social rehabilitation approach with the psychodynamic and social psychiatric orientation of the INAC. Interventions included psychotherapy, medication, education and work rehabilitation, and child development education groups for the mothers, and a therapeutic nursery for the children, as well as videotaping of mother-child interactions followed by discussion, coaching, and repetition. Mothers who received this broad-based program were compared with randomly assigned mothers who received home visits from a mental health professional. The two groups showed few differences after 18 to 24 months. Readmission rates for mothers were the same, and children in both groups seemed to improve in their developmental quotients. (The most deviant children improved the most, a finding which may represent regression to the mean.) Of clinical importance is the fact that program attendance increased dramatically when a van picked up the mother and child and delivered them home. This suggests that making services readily available may be of great importance, particularly when coupled with active outreach.

Anthony (1984) has attempted an intervention program largely focused on the children in his sample. His program has offered compensatory support for school-aged and adolescent children, including extra-familial community resources, enhanced reality testing, exercises aimed at increasing their understanding of the parent's psychiatric illness, and individual, group, and family psychotherapy. These efforts have apparently reduced maladjustment somewhat, but since cases were neither randomly assigned to different treatments nor matched with controls, drawing conclusions about the success of the intervention is difficult.

Generic Programs

While research may profit from interventions with populations defined by diagnosis, other advantages accrue from community-based programs which use difficulties in the mother-child relationship as entry criteria. The fact that multiple risk factors and breakdown in family relationships are so directly related to childhood psychopathology offers a strong rationale for basing prevention programs on the more general criteria. For instance, less than 10 percent of child protection cases involve parents with a major psychiatric disorder. Special efforts can be made to ensure that these generic programs also include psychiatrically hospitalized parents from the community catchment area.

Case finding for generic programs is facilitated by the broad range of care givers who encounter mother-child relationship problems. Visiting nurses, welfare and protective service social workers, and well-baby clinic pediatricians, as well as pediatric inpatient staff serving nonorganic failure-to-thrive cases, can all make referrals based on their observations of mother-child difficulties or families in trouble.

In the current Family Support Project of Lyons-Ruth, the author, and colleagues (Lyons-Ruth et al., 1983), the twin acceptance criteria of very low income and dysfunctional parenting resulted in a caseload with a high incidence of the parental risk factors identified by large-scale studies. Of the families referred to the project, 42 percent had at least one minority parent, 60 percent were single-parent families, 80 percent were on AFDC, 45 percent of the mothers had not graduated from high school, and 42 percent were found to have abused or neglected their children. Among the fathers, 30 percent had been imprisoned, and over 50 percent were violent, substance abusing, or both. Only 16 percent of the mothers had experienced psychiatric hospitalization, and only 23 percent had ever received psychiatric treatment. However, and most significantly, 60 percent of the mothers reported levels of depression identified in previous studies as indicating a need for psychiatric treatment. Among the remaining 40 percent, 8 percent had had recent hospitalizations for depression, and 8 percent had had their children remanded into state custody for severe neglect. Thus, absence of a psychiatric history, or even absence of reported depressions, does not preclude the presence of severe behavorial pathology.

Women with young children, inadequate financial resources, and poor communication, with or without a spouse, were more likely to be depressed, and the children of these depressed mothers were at risk. They scored lower on the mental and motor scales of the Bayley than controls, and this correlated with maternal depression and poor family health. On the Ainsworth Strange Situation (Ainsworth et al., 1978), the children of mothers followed by protective services were a distinct group: they were more avoidant with their mothers, who in turn appeared most likely in interviews to deny personal problems. Given that only 16 percent of these parents had had a psychiatric illness, these findings support this chapter's general thrust that stress and deprivation pile up, problem parenting develops, and thus adverse outcomes ensue for children.

The content of these generic intervention programs can include day care, consultation with teachers and/or parents, referral, direct contact with child, parent, and family, and advocacy follow-up. In Vermont, for instance, Rolf and Hasazi (1977) provided enrichment programs focusing on nutrition, gross and fine motor, cognitive, and sensory activities, structured and unstructured play for children with and without adults, and self-care and skill-training sessions. They found that 80 percent of their subjects had improved on a variety of measures by the end of the intervention (an average of 9.5 months). Of particular interest is that the project accepted and worked with externalizing children with behavior disorders, who have the poorest prognosis, and that the most change occurred in measures of this factor. This project was unable to find untreated control subjects as deviant as their intervention group, and it would have been unethical to leave the less deviant children untreated.

PROGRAMMATIC CHALLENGES   Rolf and Hasazi (1977) have delineated more clearly than others the difficulties of working with this population. The parents are often very difficult to work with. They may avoid treatment, threaten project staff, neglect and abuse their children, and so forth. Consequently, the project staff is caught between the needs of the parents and the needs of the child. Other cautions are that such parents may be acutely sensitive to feelings of being "labeled" and that working with children in a group runs the danger of the contagion of symptoms from the more disturbed.

As to interventions, with parents who seem to deny or minimize the child's problem ("He is just like I was"), it is best to deal with them directly to help them develop appropriate concern. While Rolf and Hasazi found group sessions of little value, Lyons-Ruth et al. (1983) found them exceedingly popular and useful. Rolf and Hasazi found, as did the author (Grunebaum, 1977), that supporting and counseling the healthier spouse when possible is the wisest use of treatment resources.

The problem of taking sides in an adversary situation is a real dilemma for the clinician.

The staff of such centers are working under considerable stress, of frustration at meager results, or improvement undone at home, of choosing sides between child and parent, and sometimes of physical or legal threat. Rolf and Hasazi (1977) describe some of the daily problems staff encounter with these parents: "inability to get up on time to get the children to the center . . . giving the children barbiturates or marijuana, subjecting the children to sexual or assaultive experiences, and resisting the center's efforts to teach the children new social skills" (117). Anthony (1984) has commented on the exasperating difficulties these families present in keeping appointments, giving usable directions, being there at the agreed-upon times, and holding deep suspicions of professionals. Work with these high-risk families is clearly not for the faint at heart.

Two currently ongoing projects deliver services in the home, those of Lyons-Ruth et al. (1983) and Goodman (1983). These projects are finding that families who remain in the program for a month are likely to remain for a year or more of treatment. Although erratic in keeping appointments and slow to trust the worker, these families nevertheless developed deep investments when there was outreach to the home, pragmatic help in securing needed services, and a focus on the mother as well as the child.

Like the joint admission and INAC projects, these projects have found most success in working with the moderately disturbed families, rather than the most disturbed. All of these endeavors have found it important to have a contract with the parents and to terminate care if the contract is grossly violated. The Family Planning Project found it impossible to succeed with psychotic women who were delusionally determined to get pregnant, even when previous pregnancies had been terminated or a child had been removed from their care.

Ultimately, it may be most efficient to aim at cases where there is some hope of effecting change. Where this does not exist, placement or adoption must be seriously considered before it is too late.

EPILOGUE

A comprehensive approach to children at risk must take a systems view. Neither the child nor the parents act independently of one another. They act as an interlocking unit in a dynamic relationship which itself is not isolated, but is a part of the larger society, a society which in many ways is unsupportive of parenting and of children's needs (Grunebaum, J., 1983). The largest proportion of children at risk includes those who have single parents, poor parents, minority parents, uneducated parents, too young parents, and too many siblings. Thus, they have parents who are caring for them under stress. Because of the inadequate health care and nutrition their mothers receive during pregnancy, they are likely to be premature or to have developmental difficulties. They live in deprived neighborhoods and go to inferior schools, and thus they are likely to be hard to parent.

A society which valued children would value parenting by both parents. (According to the Labor Department, "parent" ranks in prestige with "parking-garage attendant.") A society which valued children would support the parent-child relationship more adequately. Such a policy of social justice would be the single most significant preventive intervention for children at risk.

This chapter has perforce discussed only a small part of the complex system of people and events which impinge on children, namely, those children at risk by virtue of parental psychiatric disability and because of parenting under stress. Mindful of the conclusion for which considerable evidence has been cited, that depression in mothers is probably the single greatest psychiatric disability affecting children, each reader must judge the contribution of sexism and socioeconomic factors to the genesis and maintenance of that condition. And it is probable that adequate economic support for parenting, for schools, and for health services would be the greatest single contribution to family health and healthy child development.

Chapter 11 # Children of Divorce: The Dilemma of a Decade†
by Judith S. Wallerstein, Ph.D.

INCIDENCE AND SOCIAL IMPACTS OF DIVORCE

The experience of growing up in the United States has changed within the past decade. The startling prediction made in the middle 1970s (Bane, 1976) that 30 to 40 percent of children born in the 1970s would experience their parents' divorce has been overtaken by reality. Current trends translate into even more startling expectations. It is now estimated that 45 percent of all children born in 1983 will experience their parents' divorce, 35 percent will experience a remarriage, and 20 percent will experience a second divorce (personal communication, Arthur J. Norton [Assistant Chief of the Population Division of the United States Bureau of the Census], 1983). In 1981, approximately 22.5 million young people, or 36 percent of all children under 18, were living in a family other than the traditional two-parent family. This group included 11.4 million children living with their mothers only; 1.2 million living with fathers only; 6.4 million living with one biological parent and one stepparent; and the remainder living with adoptive parents, grandparents, or in foster homes. For black children, living with two parents is already less common than living with one parent (Zill, 1983).

While the incidence of divorce has increased across all age groups, the most dramatic rise has occurred among young adults (Norton, 1983). As a result, children in divorcing families are younger than in previous years and include more preschool children. In 1981, 31 percent of the country's children aged 5 or younger lived with their mothers only (United States Bureau of the Census, 1982b). A recent study of California couples divorcing between the years 1966 and 1977 found that mari-

†The Center for the Family in Transition, of which the author is the Executive Director, is supported by a grant from the San Francisco Foundation. The Zellerbach Family Fund supported the author's research in the California Children of Divorce Project, one of the sources of data for this chapter.

tal dissolution was associated with the presence in the family of a child aged 2 or under (Rankin and Maneker, 1983). There is also evidence that very young children are predominant among those whose custody and visitation is in contest. Jessica Pearson has reported on a tally of children involved in mediated cases in four widely separated court systems: 44 percent of the children in dispute were 5 years old or younger (personal communication, Jessica Pearson [Principal Investigator of the Divorce Mediation Research Project, Denver, Colorado], 1982).

Although many children weather the stress of marital discord and family breakup without psychopathological sequelae, a significant number falter along the way. Children of divorce are significantly overrepresented in outpatient psychiatric, family agency, and private practice populations compared with children of divorce in the general population (Gardner, 1976; Kalter, 1977; Tessman, 1977; Tooley, 1976). The best predictors of mental health referrals for school-aged children are parental divorce or parental loss as a result of death (Felner et al., 1975). A national survey of adolescents whose parents had separated and divorced by the time the children were 7 years old found that 30 percent of these children had received psychiatric or psychological therapy by the time they reached adolescence, compared with 10 percent of adolescents in intact families (Zill, 1983).

A longitudinal study in northern California followed 131 children who were ages 3 to 18 at the decisive separation. At the five-year mark, the investigators found that more than one-third were suffering from moderate to severe depression (Wallerstein and Kelly, 1980a). These findings are especially striking since the children were drawn from a non-clinical population and were accepted into the study only if they had never been identified before the divorce as needing psychological treatment and only if they were performing at age-appropriate levels in school. Therefore, the deterioration observed in these children's adjustment occurred largely following the family breakup.

Finally, several studies suggest that children of divorce show lower achievement and experience greater difficulty in learning than their classmates from two-parent families. One national survey reported a higher incidence of disrupted learning, erratic attendance, higher dropout rates, increased tardiness, and deteriorated social behavior among youngsters from single-parent families (Brown, 1980). Another survey revealed that 15 percent of teenagers living with divorced mothers had been expelled or suspended from school at some time between elementary school and high school, whereas only 3 percent of teenagers from low-conflict, intact families had sustained a similar experience (Zill, 1983). Also relevant to the children's experience is the fact that divorced adults use inpatient and outpatient mental health services at a significantly higher rate than adults in intact marriages (Bloom et al., 1979).

Divorce differs from many other stressful childhood experiences in that its immediate impact is not confined to children in the divorcing family, or even to those in the immediate social or psychological vicinity. Teachers in widely separated communities report that after a family quarrel children from intact families come to school asking anxiously, "Will my parents divorce?" The high proportion of young adults who are postponing marriage today may well reflect anxieties associated with the accelerated breakup of marital relationships (Cherlin, 1981). The long-range consequences of the widespread pattern of conjugal succession (Furstenberg, 1982) for society and for future forms of the family are, of course, unknown. Some researchers have cautiously reported "a real, although small, amount of intergenerational transmission of marital instability" (Pope and Mueller, 1979, 109). Other recent research has revealed an unexpectedly powerful commitment to ideals of fidelity and lifelong monogamy among children of divorce as they enter young adulthood many years after the family crisis (Wallerstein, in press[a]).

The many divorced families in our midst and the burdens imposed on parent and child are familiar aspects of the social scene and have become part of our national consciousness. Surely it is no accident that the widely acclaimed 1982 film, E.T., depicts both the central character, Elliott, a sober, sensitive child, and his alter ego, E.T., a funny-looking extraterrestrial child with super coping skills, as lonely children who are cut off from home base and who must fend for themselves in a world where adults are unsympathetic and sometimes hostile and dangerous. Also no accident, the film notes almost casually that Elliott's father has run off to Mexico with another woman, while his unhappy mother careens her way through work, child care, and household chores with little time or capacity left for pleasure in her children. As the author has noted elsewhere, E.T. captures and offers, almost en passant, some essential truths about today's family (Wallerstein, 1982). In a great many American homes today, the overburdened and unhappy single parents can provide only limited nurturance to their children, and a great many children, especially young children, feel cut off and lonely, estranged from parents whose behavior they find incomprehensible or frightening.

Still another aspect of divorce distinguishes it from other stresses of childhood. Divorce is inextricably intertwined with family law and family policy. Marital dissolution occurs within a public forum in which the conflicting rights and complementary roles and responsibilities of men, women, and children are basic issues. At stake is the capacity of the family following divorce to carry out its child-rearing functions adequately. Accordingly, a lively debate has focused on how to safeguard the child's interests subsequent to marital rupture.

Much of the recent debate within the political arena and the courts has been passionate and shrill, infused with the private angers and public indignation of men and women who are engaged in struggles with each other over real or imagined wrongs, over power, and over money. The various parties have generally agreed with the principle that the complex issues should be decided carefully, with full regard to the available knowledge, the grave issues at stake, and the best interests of the child. However, the specific policies that have emerged have too often reflected political expediencies and compromises. Major policy changes are often too readily adopted, radically altering the lives of thousands of children, without a searching examination of the issues, without adequate knowledge, and without building in methods for evaluating the consequences of these changes. When this occurs, significant numbers of children can be placed at even greater risk, and the system, the law, or both may end up adding substantially to children's suffering.

Although policy makers, legislators, and judges have increasingly sought support from the findings of behavioral science and guidance from the mental health profession, the accumulation of psychological knowledge has not kept up with the rapid pace of family law. Knowledge is fragmentary and insufficient to address the many changes proposed for family policy. Despite the wide acknowledgment given to the law and mental health interface, the major task of building cooperation and mutual understanding lies ahead. The subtleties of psychological thinking and the shadings of individual differences that are so critical to the clinical process translate poorly in the arenas of courts and legislatures. Moreover, the several years of follow-up required to assess the impacts of changed circumstances or family arrangements are ill suited to the pressured agendas of the political and judicial process.

THE NATURE OF DIVORCE

We have within the past decade begun to acquire solid knowledge in many critical areas: the nature of the divorcing process; the responses of children and adolescents by age and sex; the immediate and long-lasting impacts of divorce on children and adults and on parent-child relationships; factors in good and poor outcome in the short- and long-term perspective; custody and visitation; the role of the father and the role of the visiting parent; and the staying power of anger and the dangers of continued interparental conflict to the child. We have also begun to develop a range of intervention methods and strategies aimed specifically at this population. Many methodological issues remain, however, related to sample sizes and sampling techniques, the need for more extensive cross-sectional and longitudinal studies, the need for appropriate comparison groups, and the need to study divorce within diverse social and cultural contexts and to examine different custodial and visitation arrangements. There also remains the major issue of translating the broad goals of primary and secondary prevention into intervention theory and program. In neither research nor treatment has it been easy to maintain in focus the many complex issues that converge in the divorcing family. The unfortunate tendency, as Richards (1982) has suggested in a recent overview of the field, is to collapse all of the varieties of divorce into a single category, as if divorce were a single event occurring at a precise moment.

Perhaps even more important than recognizing these issues is that we acknowledge that the examination of divorce leads us into an uncharted terrain in our understanding of child development, of parent-child relationships, and of the complex interrelationships of the child and both parents, whether they live together or separately. What is striking overall is that the entire pattern of conscious and unconscious psychological needs, wishes, and expectations which parents and children bring to each other is profoundly altered under the impact of marital rupture and its many ripple effects. Yet neither developmental nor clinical theory has incorporated the new observations which have come out of the work with separation, divorce, and remarriage.

The Process of Divorce

Divorce is a long, drawn-out process of radically changing family relationships that has several stages, beginning with the marital rupture and its immediate aftermath, continuing over several years of disequilibrium, and finally coming to rest with the stabilization of a new postdivorce or remarried family unit. Various complicated changes, many of them unanticipated and unforeseeable, are set into motion by the marital rupture and are likely to occupy a significant portion of the child or adolescent's growing years. As the author and her colleague have reported elsewhere, women in the California Children of Divorce study required three to three-and-a-half years following the decisive separation before they achieved a sense of order and predictability in their lives (Wallerstein and Kelly, 1980a). This figure probably underestimates the actual time trajectory of the child's experience of divorce. A prospective study reported that parent-child relationships began to deteriorate many years prior to the divorce decision and that the adjustment of many children in these families began to fail long before the decisive separation (Morrison, 1982). This view of the divorcing process as long lasting accords with the perspective of a group of young people who reported at a ten-year follow-up that their entire childhood or adolescence had been dominated by the family crisis and its extended aftermath (Wallerstein, in press[a]).

Stages in the Process

The three broad successive stages in the divorcing process, while they overlap, are nevertheless clinically distinguishable. *The acute phase* is precipitated by the decisive separation and the decision to divorce. This stage is often marked by steeply escalating conflict between the adults, physical violence, severe distress, depression accompanied by suicidal ideation, and a range of behaviors reflecting a spilling of aggressive and sexual impulses. The adults frequently react with severe ego regression and not unusually behave at odds with their more customary demeanor. Sharp disagreement in the wish to end the marriage is very common. The narcissistic injury to the person who feels rejected sets the stage for rage, sexual jealousy, and depression. Children are generally not shielded from this parental conflict or distress. Confronted by a marked discrepancy in images of their parents, children do not have the assurance that the bizarre or depressed behaviors and moods will subside. As a result, they are likely to be terrified by the very figures they usually rely on for nurturance and protection.

As the acute phase comes to a close, usually within the first two years of the divorce decision, the marital partners gradually disengage from each other and pick up the new tasks of reestablishing their separate lives. *The transitional phase* is characterized by ventures into new, more committed relationships, new work, school, and friendship groups, and sometimes new settings, new life-styles, and new geographical locations. This phase is marked by alternating success and failure, encouragement and discouragement, and it may also last for several years. Children observe and participate in the many changes of this period. They share the trials and errors and the fluctuations in mood. For several years, life may be unstable and home may be unsettled.

Finally, *the postdivorce phase* ensues with the establishment of a fairly stable single-parent or remarried household. Eventually three out of four divorced women and four out of five divorced men reenter wedlock (Cherlin, 1981). Unfortunately, though, remarriage does not bring immediate tranquility into the lives of the family members. The early years of the remarriage are often encumbered by ghostly presences from the earlier failed marriages and by the actual presences of children and visiting parents from the prior marriage or marriages. Several studies suggest widespread upset among children and adolescents following remarriage (Goldstein, 1974; Kalter, 1977; Crohn et al., 1981). A large-scale investigation that is still in process reports long-lasting friction around visitation (Jacobson, 1983).

Changes in Parent-Child Relationships

DIMINISHED CAPACITY TO PARENT Parents experience a diminished capacity to parent their children during the acute phase of the divorcing process and often during the transitional phase as well (Wallerstein and Kelly, 1980a). This phenomenon is widespread and can be considered an expectable divorce-specific change in parent-child relationships. At its simplest level, this diminished parenting capacity appears in the household disorder that prevails in the aftermath of divorce, in the rising tempers of custodial parent and child, in reduced competence and a greater sense of helplessness in the custodial parent, and in lower expectations of the child for appropriate social behavior (Hetherington et al., 1978; 1982). Diminished parenting also entails a sharp decline in emotional sensitivity and support for the child, decreased pleasure in the relationship, decreased attentiveness to the child's needs and wishes, less talk, play, and interaction with the child, and a steep escalation in inappropriate expression of anger. One not uncommon component of the parent-child relationship coincident with the marital breakup is the adult's conscious or unconscious wish to abandon the child and thus to erase the unhappy marriage in its entirety. Child neglect can be a serious hazard.

PARENTAL DEPENDENCE ON THE CHILD In counterpoint to the temporary emotional withdrawal from the child, the parent may develop a dependent, sometimes passionate, attachment to the child or adolescent, beginning with the breakup and lasting throughout the lonely postseparation years (Wallerstein, in press[b]). Parents are likely to lean on the child and to turn to the child for help, placing the child in a wide range of roles such as confidante, advisor, mentor, sibling, parent, caretaker, lover, concubine, extended conscience or ego control, ally within the marital conflict, or pivotal supportive presence in staving off depression or even suicide. This expectation that children should not only take much greater responsibility for themselves, but should also provide psychological and social support for the distressed parent, is sufficiently widespread to be considered a divorce-specific response, along with that of diminished parenting. Such relationships frequently develop with an only child or with a very young, even a preschool, child. Not accidentally, issues of custody and visitation often arise with regard to the younger children. While such disputes of course reflect the generally unresolved anger of the marriage and the divorce, they may also reflect the intense emotional need of one or both parents for the young child's constant presence (Wallerstein, in press[b]).

Parents may also lean more appropriately on the older child or adolescent. Many youngsters become proud helpers, confidantes, and allies in facing the difficult postdivorce period (Weiss, 1979). Other youngsters draw away from close involvement due to their fears of engulfment, and they move precipitously out of the family orbit, sometimes before they are developmentally ready.

THE VISITING RELATIONSHIP The visiting relationship has no real counterpart in the intact family. Insufficient recognition has been given to the difficulty involved with transplanting a parent-child relationship that has developed within the rich soil of family life into the relatively impoverished, strange, and limited ground of the visit. A great many close parent-child relationships fail to take root outside of the family, but many parent-child relationships that were failing within the unhappy marriage take on new life within the narrow constraints of the visit (Wallerstein and Kelly, 1980b). Although the tensions stirred by the visits are likely in many, if not most, families to be very intense, these tensions tend to diminish over time. The extent of the father's visiting depends less on the relationship between the divorcing couple than on his feelings about the divorce, on the children's ages and responsiveness, on his and their capacity to overcome the inherent difficulties in the visiting relationship, on the presence or absence of children within the remarriage, and on his own psychological stability (Kelly and Wallerstein, 1977; Kelly, 1981). In a national survey of children between the ages of 11 and 16 from divorced families, close to half the children had had no contact with their outside parent, customarily the father, during the five preceding years (Furstenberg, 1982). There is encouraging evidence that a brief intervention immediately after the decisive separation can turn this around and significantly reduce the incidence of disrupted contact between father and child. For example, less than 10 percent of the children in the California Children of Divorce Project had not had any contact with their fathers at the five-year mark (Wallerstein and Kelly, 1980a).

The emotional importance to children of their relationships with both parents does not become any less following divorce. Although the mother's caretaking and psychological roles become increasingly central in families where the mother has custody, there is no evidence that the father's psychological significance declines correspondingly. The children's yearning for the father is poignantly evident following divorce. The visiting relationship remains centrally important to children and their well-being long after the parents' separation, divorce, or remarriage. The self-image of a child reared in a two-parent family prior to a divorce appears tied to both biological parents, regardless of the parent's subsequent physical presence within the family (Wallerstein and Kelly, 1980a; Kelly, 1981).

CHILDREN'S REACTIONS TO DIVORCE

Initial Responses

Children and adolescents experience the separation and its aftermath as the most stressful period of their lives. The family rupture evokes an acute sense of shock, intense anxiety, and profound sorrow. Many children are relatively content and even well-parented in families where one or both parents are unhappy. Few youngsters experience any relief with the divorce decision, and those who do are usually older and have witnessed physical violence or open conflict between their parents. The child's early responses are governed neither by an understanding of issues leading to the divorce nor by the fact that divorce has a high incidence in the community. To the child, divorce signifies the collapse of the structure that provides support and protection. The child reacts as to the cutting of his or her lifeline.

The initial suffering of children and adolescents in response to a marital separation is compounded by realistic fears and by fantasies about catastrophes which the divorce will bring in its wake. Children suffer with a pervasive sense of vulnerability as they feel that the protective and nurturant function of the family has given way. They grieve over the loss of the noncustodial parent, over the loss of the intact family, and often over the multiple losses of neighborhood, friends, and school. Children also worry about their distressed parents. They are concerned about who will take care of the parent who has left and whether the custodial parent will be able to manage alone. They experience intense anger toward one or both parents whom they hold responsible for disrupting the family. Some of their anger is reactive and defends them against their own feelings of powerlessness, their concern about being lost in the shuffle, and their fear that their own needs will be disregarded as the parents give priority to their wishes and needs. Some children, especially young children, suffer with guilt over fantasied misdeeds which they feel may have contributed to the family quarrels and led to the divorce. Others feel that it is their responsibility to mend the broken marriage (Wallerstein and Kelly, 1980a).

The responses of the child must also be considered within the social context of the divorce and in particular within the loneliness and social isolation that so many children experience. Children face the tensions and sorrows of divorce with little help from anybody else. Fewer than 10 percent of children in the California Children of Divorce study had any help at the time of the crisis from adults outside the family, although many people, including neighbors, pediatricians, ministers, rabbis, and family friends, knew the family and the children (Wallerstein and Kelly, 1980a). Thus, another striking feature of divorce as a childhood stress is that it occurs in the absence of or falling away of customary support.

DEVELOPMENTAL FACTORS Developmental factors are critical in the responses of children and adolescents at the time of the marital rupture. Despite significant individual differences in the child, in the family, and in parent-child relations, the child's age and developmental stage appear to be the most important factors governing the initial response. The child's dominant needs, his or her capacity to perceive and understand family events, the central psychological preoccupation and conflict, the available repertoire of defense and coping strategies, and the dominant patterning of relationships and expectations all reflect the child's age and developmental stage.

A major finding in divorce research has been the common patterns of response within different age groups (Wallerstein and Kelly, 1980a). The age groups which share significant commonalities in perceptions, responses, underlying fantasies, and behaviors are the preschool ages 3 to 5, early school age or early latency ages 5½ to 8, later school age or latency ages 8 to 11, and, finally, adolescent ages 12 to 18 (Kelly and

Wallerstein, 1976; Wallerstein and Kelly, 1974; 1975; 1976; 1980a; Wallerstein, 1977). These responses, falling as they do into age-related groupings, may reflect children's responses to acute stress generally, not only their responses to marital rupture.

Observations about preschool children derived from longitudinal studies in two widely different regions, namely, Virginia and northern California, are remarkably similar in their findings (Hetherington, 1979; Hetherington et al., 1978; 1982; Wallerstein and Kelly, 1975; 1980a). Preschool children are likely to show regression following one parent's departure from the household. The regression usually occurs in the most recent developmental achievement of the child. Intensified fears are frequent and are evoked by routine separations from the custodial parent during the day and at bedtime. Sleep disturbances are also frequent. The preoccupying fantasy of many of the little children is fear of abandonment by both parents. Yearning for the departed parent is intense. Young children are likely to become irritable and demanding and to behave aggressively with parents, with younger siblings, and with peers.

Children in the 5- to 8-year-old group are likely to show open grieving. They are preoccupied with feelings of concern and longing for the departed parent. Many share the terrifying fantasy of replacement. "Will my daddy get a new dog, a new mommy, a new little boy?" were the comments of several boys in this age group. Little girls wove elaborate Madame Butterfly fantasies, asserting that the departed father would some day return to them, that he loved them "the best." Many of the children in this age group could not believe that the divorce would endure. About half suffered a precipitous decline in their schoolwork (Kelly and Wallerstein, 1976).

In the 8- to 12-year-old group, the central response often seems to be intense anger at one or both parents for causing the divorce. In addition, these children suffer with grief over the loss of the intact family, with anxiety, loneliness, and the humiliating sense of their own powerlessness. Youngsters in this age group often see one parent as the "good" parent and the other as "bad," and they appear especially vulnerable to the blandishments of one or the other parent to engage in marital battles. Children in later latency also have a high potential for assuming a helpful and empathic role in the care of a needy parent. School performance and peer relationships suffered a decline in approximately one-half of these children (Wallerstein and Kelly, 1976).

Adolescents are very vulnerable to their parents' divorce. The precipitation of acute depression, accompanied by suicidal preoccupation and acting out, is frequent enough to be alarming. Anger can be intense. Several instances have been reported of direct violent attacks on custodial parents by young adolescents who had not previously shown such behavior (Springer and Wallerstein, 1983). Preoccupied with issues of morality, adolescents may judge the parents' conduct during the marriage and the divorce, and they may identify with one parent and do battle against the other. A good number become anxious about their own future entry into adulthood, concerned that they may experience marital failure like their parents (Wallerstein and Kelly, 1974). Researchers have also called attention to the adolescents' impressive capacity to grow in maturity and independence as they respond to the family crisis and the parents' need for help (Weiss, 1979).

SEX DIFFERENCES In the preschool and latency ages, boys are reported to be more vulnerable than girls to the acute stress of the marital rupture, as well as to the more chronic stresses of the transitional phase. Major differences between preschool boys and girls in a wide range of cognitive, social, and developmental measures have been reported (Hetherington et al., 1982). While divorce did not appear to disrupt traditional sex-role typing for girls, two years after the divorce boys were scoring lower on male preference and higher on female preference on the sex-role preference tests. The boys were also spending more time playing with girls and with younger children. They showed an affective narrowness and a constriction in fantasy and social play and were more socially isolated than their female peers.

Sex differences also emerged in the California Children of Divorce study. While boys and girls did not differ in their overall psychological adjustment at the time of the marital breakup, at 18 months later the boys' psychological adjustment had deteriorated markedly, whereas that of the girls had greatly improved, making for a significant gap between the two groups (Wallerstein and Kelly, 1980a). Other evidence further suggests that marital turmoil has a greater impact on boys than on girls both in divorced families and in intact, discordant families (Emery and O'Leary, 1982; Rutter, 1970; Block et al., 1981).

How much of this differential effect between the sexes is mediated by the mother having custody is unknown. The Texas custody research project compared a small group of latency-aged children in the custody of the same-sex parent with a matched group in the custody of the opposite-sex parent and with a matched group of children in intact families. Again, the results suggested that the sex of the custodial parent has a direct bearing on the child's social adjustment. Children in the custody of the same-sex parent showed more maturity, greater sociability, more independence, and less demanding behavior than did children in the custody of the opposite-sex parent (Santrock and Warshak, 1979; Warshak and Santrock, 1983).

Finally, a confounding set of observations is reported from the 10-year follow-up study of the California Children of Divorce Project. Findings here suggest that girls from divorced families may have a more stormy adolescence and a more conflict-ridden entry into young adulthood than their male counterparts. A significant number of the young women were caught up in a web of short-lived sexual relationships, and they described themselves as fearful of commitment, anticipating infidelity and betrayal (Wallerstein, in press[a]). It may be that boys, especially young boys, have a more difficult time immediately following the divorce, but that girls find adolescence a particularly hazardous time. An important research agenda resides in the questions of whether and how and at what ages the development of boys and girls is mediated by custodial and visitation arrangements.

Long-Range Outcomes

The child's response to divorce must be distinguished from his or her long-range development and psychological adjustment. No single theme appears among all of those children who enhance, consolidate, or continue their good development after the divorce crisis has finally ended. Nor is there a single theme which appears among all of those who deteriorate either moderately or markedly. Instead, the author and her colleague (Wallerstein and Kelly, 1980a) have found a set of complex configurations in which the relevant components appear to include (1) the extent to which the parent has been able to resolve and put aside conflict and angers and to make use of the relief from conflict provided by the divorce (Emery, 1982; Jacobson, 1978); (2) the course of the custodial parent's handling of the child and the resumption or improvement of parenting within the home (Hess and Camara, 1979); (3) the extent to which the child does not feel rejected by the noncustodial or visiting parent and the extent to which this relationship has continued regularly and kept pace with the child's growth; (4) the extent to which the divorce has helped to attenuate or dilute a psychopathological parent-child relationship; (5) the range of personality assets and deficits which the child brought to the divorce, including both the child's history in the predivorce family and his or her capacities in the present, particularly intelligence, the capacity for fantasy, social maturity, and the ability to turn to peers and adults; (6) the availability to the child of a supportive human network (Tessman, 1977); (7) the absence in the child of continued anger and depression; and (8) the sex and age of the child.

The central hazards which divorce poses to children's psychological health and development are the diminished or disrupted parenting and the interparental conflict which so often follow and which can become consolidated within the postdivorce family. When parents undertake the divorce thoughtfully after careful consideration of alternatives, when they have anticipated the psychological, social, and economic consequences for all involved, when they have provided comfort and appropriate understanding to the children, and when they have arranged to maintain good parent-child relationships, then the children are not likely to suffer developmental interference or enduring psychological distress. Alternatively, if the divorce is undertaken in ways that humiliate or enrage a partner, if anger and unhappiness dominate the postdivorce relationship, if the children are poorly supported or informed, coopted as allies, fought over, or viewed as extensions of the adults, if the child's relationship with one or both parents is impoverished and disrupted, and if the child feels rejected, then the most likely outcome for the children is developmental interference, depression, or both (Wallerstein and Kelly, 1980a).

Another way to conceptualize outcome in divorce is to consider whether the child him- or herself has been able to master successfully the tasks posed by the divorce. Although the child's long-range adjustment is significantly related to many factors in the postdivorce family, his or her own capacity and efforts at mastery are also significant in the ultimate outcome. In order to maintain psychic integrity and development, the child engages in mastery efforts which can be seen as a series of six coping tasks, beginning with the time of the marital rupture and culminating with the close of adolescence. These tasks represent a substantial addition to the usual tasks of growing up (Wallerstein, 1983).

DISPUTED CUSTODY AND VISITATION

Aptly described as "children of Armageddon" (Watson, 1969), the most stressed children of divorce are those who are the objects of continuing acrimonious legal battles between their divorcing parents. Approximately 10 percent of divorcing families with children go on to full-scale legal battles, and one-third return to court for modification of the original orders (Freed and Foster, 1974). Most families make custody and visitation arrangements without recourse to the courts. Even these private arrangements occur under the shadow of the law, and in contested cases they are very much influenced by the court's decision making (Mnookin and Kornhauser, 1979).

While those adults who engage in continuous conflict over their children have been insufficiently studied, some evidence suggests a clustering of severe psychiatric disorder among them (Tall and Johnston, 1982). The causes of continued legal contests between divorcing spouses are complex and multidetermined. A history of repeated unmourned losses in one or both adults is not uncommon and may go hand in hand with a pathological dependence on the constant presence of the child to ward off depression. In addition, the severe narcissistic injury of the divorce may trigger a rage against the divorcing spouse which continues via the conflict over the children, undimmed by the passage of years and binding the partners to each other.

The experiences of the past decade have cast increasing doubt on the appropriateness of the court as a forum for the resolution of these issues. Not only is it acknowledged that the adversarial system is poorly suited to resolving family conflict, but it is also recognized that the adversarial system adds significantly to the already overwhelming stress of the children and adults.

Mediation

Mediation has taken hold quickly as an intervention for divorcing families in dispute (Coogler, 1978; Haynes, 1981). Some programmatic issues are unresolved, however: whether mediation falls within the domain of the attorney, the mental health professional, or both, working separately or in tandem, and what should be required in the way of licensing, professional standards, and training. A more important issue is whether mediation will live up to its early promise. An important concern is that the mediator's role may leave the child's interests without adequate protection. The mediation process makes the assumption that the child's interests will be protected by the parents, but this may prove to be unwarranted, considering the impaired judgment of parents who are in intense conflict (Huntington, 1982).

In January of 1981, California enacted mandatory mediation for divorcing families who are disputing custody, visitation, or both. Since California has been a leader in family law, other states are likely to follow suit in the near future. Mandatory mediation has to date achieved a high settlement rate, ranging from 55 to 85 percent of the disputing families in the different counties. Preliminary reports from a study of mediation in four court systems (Hartford, Denver, Minneapolis, and Los Angeles) indicate that families who use mediation are pleased with the process and the outcome, but that a significant number reject mediation (Pearson et al., 1982).

Another reflection of the trend away from the adversarial system has been mental health professionals' increasing conviction that mental health experts should serve the court in its decision-making process rather than act as partisan for one party to the dispute (Derdeyn, 1975; 1976; 1978;

Solow and Adams, 1977). The growing conviction among practitioners is that "the adversarial system is ill suited to deal optimally with custody conflicts, causes psychopathology in parents who resort to it to settle custody conflicts, is psychically detrimental to children, and is therefore antithetical to good psychiatric practice" (Gardner, 1982, 11). The Group for the Advancement of Psychiatry (1980) recognized the impact of the entire family's interrelationships during the postdivorce years and argued that the whole family should be examined before a custody or visitation decision.

Custody

The changing roles of men and women are mirrored in the courts and in legislation regarding custody and visitation. Our society has moved away from the expectation that single-parent custody, combined with reasonable visitation with the noncustodial parent, is the expectable legacy of divorce. Early in this decade, the courts relied extensively on the concept of "the psychological parent" (Goldstein et al., 1973), assuming that except under unusual circumstances or for older children the mother would fulfill this role. Recent attention has focused on the contribution of the father as parent and as potential primary parent (Jacobs, 1982; Santrock and Warshak, 1979; Warshak and Santrock, 1983). Actually, custodial arrangements have changed little throughout the nation over the past ten years, and approximately 90 percent of children of divorce remain in their mother's custody (United States Bureau of the Census, 1982b). At the same time, however, approximately one-half of the states have enacted legislation that permits joint custody. The push in some states, notably California, is toward joint custody as the presumptive preference for all divorcing families, including families in dispute. Community attitudes and social policy are in flux.

Many custodial arrangements fall under the rubric of joint custody. These include joint legal custody, in which the child resides with one parent but both parents share decision making in areas yet unclarified, and joint physical custody, in which the child may divide his or her time in varying combinations between each parent's home.

Joint physical custody selected by both parents can be regarded as a new family form or structure. Under the appropriate circumstances, it may have advantages for the divorcing family, especially perhaps in the transition from divorce to remarriage. Some research suggests that children in latency can benefit greatly from joint physical custody when the arrangement is accompanied by cooperation between parents, by strong, steadfast commitment to the parenting role, and by genuine love and respect for the children (Steinman, 1981). In a comprehensive review of the literature on joint custody, Clingembeel and Reppucci (1982) propose a detailed research agenda that would encompass, along with the characteristics of child, parent, and community, the expectable changes in the family life cycle, notably remarriage, and the changing developmental needs of child and parent.

Since parents in most places are free to select joint physical or legal custody for their children without recourse to the courts, subject only to fairly routine court approval, the sticking point has been whether the law should award joint custody in the face of one parent's strong opposition. Except for one admittedly very limited tally of court returns of such families (Ilfeld et al., 1982), no research findings bear directly on this issue. By and large, experts in psychiatry and law have opposed joint physical custody unless the parents agree fully on the arrangement (Benedek and Benedek, 1979; Goldzband, 1980; Gardner, 1982).

FUTURE DIRECTIONS

Despite the accumulating reports of the difficulties that many children in divorced families experience, society has on the whole been reluctant to regard children of divorce as a special group at risk. Notwithstanding the magnitude of the population affected and widespread implications for public policy and law, community attention has been very limited, research has been poorly supported, and appropriate social, psychological, economic, or preventive measures have hardly begun to develop. Recently, the alarm has been sounded in the national press about the tragically unprotected and foreshortened childhoods of children of divorce and their subsequent difficulties in reaching maturity (Winn, 1983). Perhaps this reflects a long overdue awakening of community concern.

The agenda for research on marital breakdown, separation, divorce, and remarriage, and the roads that families travel between each of these way stations is long and has been cited repeatedly in this chapter. The knowledge that we have acquired is considerable. But the knowledge that we still lack is critical. More knowledge is essential in order to provide responsible advice to parents, to consult effectively with the wide range of other professionals whose daily work brings them in contact with these families, to design and mount education, treatment, or prevention programs, and to provide guidelines for informed social policy.

The research priority should be to examine the many issues on the interface of marital breakdown and social policy, since the social hazards of uninformed legislative and judicial decisions are grave. Priority in the development of interventions should be given to special high-risk groups. These groups include adolescents and children living in families where divorce represents the first step in the deterioration or disintegration of the family and children who are experiencing a second divorce. Very young children are also at high risk. They represent an entirely unexamined group, and they are likely at the time of the marital breakdown to experience disruption of their relationship with both parents at the same time. A final high-risk group includes those children in postdivorce families where the custodial and visitation arrangements are fragile and where the divorcing process itself fails to reach closure or resolution.

Although children of divorce have been identified as a major group for preventive intervention, few programs have been developed (Philips, 1983). A major obstacle to designing and implementing preventive programs is the paucity of appropriate intervention theory and clinical knowledge. The vast body of theory and clinical wisdom accumulated over the decades of practicing psychotherapy still has no counterpart in preventive intervention. The dominant paradigm of crisis theory and crisis intervention, based on the early work of Lindemann (1944) and Caplan (1955), may be more applicable to acute stress and bereavement than to the chain of events in marital breakdown and the extended time trajectory of the divorce process. What are critically needed are prevention programs aimed specifically at divorcing families and based on the considerable knowledge we already have regarding the stages in the divorcing process, the expectable changes in parent-child relationships, and the configurations of factors associated with good and poor outcomes.

Finally, we must recognize that almost all of the divorce research and interventions have dealt with predominantly white, middle-class children in communities where the two-parent nuclear family is the dominant family structure. The usefulness of our observations could therefore be limited to these communities. On the other hand, more extensive research could show that the responses to major life experiences of loss, death, and divorce are rooted in developmental factors that span broad social, economic, racial, and ethnic differences.

References for the Introduction

Garmezy N: Children at risk: The search for the antecedents of schizophrenia. Part I. Conceptual models and research methods. Schizophr Bull 8:14–90, 1974

Philips I: Opportunities for prevention in the practice of psychiatry. Am J Psychiatry 140:389–395, 1983

Sameroff AJ, Chandler MJ: Reproductive risk and the continuum of caretaking casualty, in Review of Child Development Research, vol 4. Edited by Horowitz FD, Hetherington M, Scarr-Salapatek S, Spiegel G. Chicago, University of Chicago Press, 1975

Swain DB, Hawkins RC II, Walker LO, Penticuff JH (eds): Preface, in Exceptional Infant. Vol 4. New York, Brunner/Mazel, 1980a

Swain DB, Hawkins RC II, Walker LO, Penticuff JH (eds): A taxonomy of psychosocial risk factors in infancy: A guide to recent research, in Exceptional Infant, vol 4. New York, Brunner/Mazel, 1980b

Werner EE, Smith RS: Vulnerable but Invincible. A Longitudinal Study of Resilient Children and Youth. New York, McGraw-Hill, 1982

References for Chapter 7

Children Vulnerable to Major Mental Disorders: Risk and Protective Factors

Asarnow RF, Steffy RA, MacCrimmon DJ, Cleghorn JM: An attentional assessment of foster children at risk for schizophrenia. J Abnorm Psychol 86:267–275, 1977

Baldwin AL, Cole RE, Baldwin CP: Parental pathology, family interaction, and the competence of the child in school. Monogr Soc Res Child Dev 47:197 (5), 1982

Beardslee WR, Bemporad J, Keller MB, Klerman GL: Children of parents with major affective disorder: A review. Am J Psychiatry 140:825–832, 1983

Bender L: Behavior problems in the children of psychotic and criminal parents. Genet Psychol Monogr 19:229–339, 1937

Bennett I: Delinquent and Neurotic Children. New York, Basic Books, 1960

Birley JLT, Brown GW: Crises and life changes preceding the onset or relapse of acute schizophrenia: Clinical aspects. Br J Psychiatry 116:327–333, 1970

Bleuler M: The Schizophrenic Disorders: Long-term Patient and Family Studies. New Haven, Yale University Press, 1978

Brown GW, Birley JLT, Wing JK: Influence of family life on the course of schizophrenic disorders: A replication. Br J Psychiatry 121:241–258, 1972

Cadoret R, Winokur G: Genetic studies of affective disorders, in The Nature and Treatment of Depression. Edited by Flach FF, Draghi SC. New York, John Wiley & Sons, 1975

Cloninger CR, Reich T, Guze SB: Genetic-environmental interactions and anti-social behaviour, in Psychopathic Behaviour: Approaches to Research. Edited by Hare RD, Schalling D. Chichester, John Wiley & Sons, 1978

Coddington RD: The significance of life events as etiologic factors in the diseases of children. I. A survey of professional workers. J Psychosom Res 16:7–18, 1972a

Coddington RD: The significance of life events as etiologic factors in the diseases of children. II. A study of a normal population. J Psychosom Res 16:205–213, 1972b

Cohler BJ, Grunebaum HU, Weiss JL, Gamer E, Gallant DH: Disturbance of attention among schizophrenic, depressed and well mothers and their children. J Child Psychol Psychiatry 18:115–135, 1977

Conger JJ, Miller WC: Personality, Social Class, and Delinquency. New York, John Wiley & Sons, 1966

Dohrenwend BS, Dohrenwend BP (eds): Stressful Life Events. New York, Wiley Interscience, 1974

Fish B: The detection of schizophrenia in infancy. J Nerv Ment Dis 125:1–24, 1957

Fish B: Involvement of the central nervous system in infants with schizophrenia. Arch Neurol 2:115–121, 1960

Friedman D, Vaughn HGJ, Erlenmeyer-Kimling L: Cognitive brain potentials in children at risk for schizophrenia. Schizophr Bull 8:514–531, 1982

Garmezy N: Children at risk: The search for the antecedents to schizophrenia. Part II. Ongoing research programs, issues and intervention. Schizophr Bull 9:55–125, 1974

Garmezy N: The experimental study of children vulnerable to psychopathology, in Child Personality and Psychopathology, vol. 2. Edited by Davids A. New York, John Wiley & Sons, 1975

Garmezy N: On some risks in risk research. Editorial. Psychol Med 7:1–6, 1977

Garmezy N: Attentional processes in adult schizophrenia and children at risk. J Psychiatr Res 14:3–34, 1978

Garmezy N: The current status of research with children at risk for schizophrenia and other forms of psychopathology, in Risk Factor Research in the Major Mental Disorders. Edited by Regier DA, Allen G. Washington DC, U. S. Government Printing Office. Department of Health and Human Services Publication No. (ADM) 81-1068, 1981

Garmezy N: Stress-resistant children: The search for protective factors. Proceedings of the 10th International Congress of the International Association for Child and Adolescent Psychiatry and Allied Professions, July 1983. (In press, Elmsford NY, Pergamon Press, edited by Rutter M, Hersov L.).

Garmezy N, Streitman S: Children at risk: the search for the antecedents of schizophrenia. Part 1. Conceptual models and research methods. Schizophr Bull 9:55–125, 1974

Gershon ES: The genetics of affective disorders, in Psychiatry Update: Vol II. Edited by Grinspoon L. Washington DC, American Psychiatric Press, 1983

Gershon ES, Hamovit JR, Guroff JJ, Dibble E, Leckman JF, Sceery W, Targum SD, Nurnberger JI Jr, Goldin LR, Bunney WE Jr: A family study of schizoaffective, bipolar I, bipolar II, unipolar and normal control probands. Arch Gen Psychiatry 39:1157–1167, 1982

Glueck S, Glueck E: Delinquents and Non-Delinquents in Perspective. Cambridge MA, Harvard University Press, 1968

Gruenberg EM: Risk factor research methods, in Risk Factor Research in the Major Mental Disorders. Edited by Regier DA, Allen G. Washington DC, U.S. Government Printing Office, Department of Health and Human Services Publication No. (ADM) 81-1068, 1981

Guze SB: Criminality and Psychiatric Disorders. New York, Oxford University Press, 1976

Hersov LA, Berger M, Shaffer D (eds): Aggression and Anti-Social Behaviour in Childhood and Adolescence. Oxford, Pergamon Press, 1978

Hirschfeld RMA, Cross CK: Psychosocial risk factors in depression, in Risk Factor Research in the Major Mental Disorders. Edited by Regier DA, Allen G. Washington DC, U. S. Government Printing Office, Department of Health and Human Services Publication No. (ADM) 81-1068, 1981

Hirschfeld RMA, Cross CK: Epidemiology of affective disorders: Psychosocial risk factors. Arch Gen Psychiatry 39:35–46, 1982

Hirschfeld RMA, Cross CK: Personality, life events and social factors in depression, in Psychiatry Update: Vol II. Edited by Grinspoon L. Washington DC, American Psychiatric Press, 1983

Holmes TH, Rahe RH: The social readjustment rating scale. J Psychosom Res 11:213–218, 1967

Holzman PS: The search for a biological marker of the functional psychoses, in Preventive Intervention in Schizophrenia: Are We Ready? Edited by Goldstein MJ. Washington DC, Department of Health and Human Services Publication No. (ADM) 82-1111, 1982

Hutchings B, Mednick SA: Registered criminality in the adoptive and biological parents of registered male adoptees, in Genetics, Environment and Psychopathology. Edited by Mednick SA, Schulsinger F, Higgins J, Bell B. Amsterdam, North Holland Publishing Co, 1974

Kashani JH, Husain A, Shekim WO, Hodges KK, Cytryn L, McKnew DH: Current perspectives on childhood depression: An overview. Am J Psychiatry 138:143–153, 1981

Kauffman C, Grunebaum H, Cohler B, Gamer E: Superkids: Competent children of psychotic mothers. Am J Psychiatry 136:1398–1402, 1979

Kraepelin E: Dementia Praecox and Paraphrenia. Edinburgh, ES Livingston, 1919

Leff JP: Schizophrenia and sensitivity to the family environment. Schizophr Bull 2:566–574, 1976

Lewine RRJ, Watt NF, Grubb TW: High-risk-for-schizophrenia research: Sampling bias and its implications. Schizophr Bull 7:273–280, 1981

Lewis JM, Rodnick EH, Goldstein MJ: Intrafamilial interactive behavior, parental communication deviance, and risk for schizophrenia. J Abnorm Psychol 90:448–457, 1981

McCord W, McCord J: Origins of Crime. New York, Columbia University Press, 1959

McKnew DH, Cytryn L, Efron AM, Gershon ES, Bunney WE Jr: Offspring of patients with affective disorders. Br J Psychiatry 134:148–152, 1979

McNeil TF, Kaij L: Obstetric factors in the development of schizophrenia: Complications in the births of preschizophrenics and in reproduction by schizophrenic parents, in The Nature of Schizophrenia: New Approaches to Research and Treatment. Edited by Wynne LC, Cromwell RL, Matthysse S. New York, John Wiley & Sons, 1978

Marcus J: Cerebral functioning in offspring of schizophrenics. Int J Ment Health 3:57–73, 1974

Marcus J, Auerbach J, Wilkinson L, Burack CM: Infants at risk for schizophrenia: The Jerusalem infant development study. Arch Gen Psychiatry 38:703–713, 1981

Mednick SA, Mura E, Schulsinger F, Mednick B: Perinatal conditions and infant development in children with schizophrenic parents. Soc Biol 18:103–113, 1971

Meyer A: The life-chart, in Contributions to Medical and Biological Research. New York, Paul B Hoeber, 1919

Morstyn R, Duffy FH, McCarley RW: Altered P300 topography in schizophrenia. Arch Gen Psychiatry 40:729–734, 1983

Neale JM, Oltmanns TF: Schizophrenia. New York, John Wiley & Sons, 1980

Nuechterlein KH: Signal detection in vigilance tasks and behavioral attributes among offspring of schizophrenic mothers and among hyperactive children. J Abnorm Psychol 92:4–28, 1983

Nurnberger JI, Gershon ES: Genetics, in Handbook of Affective Disorders. Edited by Paykel ES. New York, Guilford Press, 1982

Olweus D: Aggression in the Schools: Bullies and Whipping Boys. Washington DC, Hemisphere Publishing Co, 1978

Patterson GR: Coercive Family Process. Eugene OR, Castalia Publishing Co, 1982

Prange AJ Jr, Loosen PT: Somatic findings in affective disorders: Their status as risk factors, in Risk Factor Research in the Major Mental Disorders. Edited by Regier DA, Allen G. Washington DC, U. S. Government Printing Office, Department of Health and Human Services Publication No. (ADM) 81-1068, 1981

Puig-Antich J, Gittelman R: Depression in childhood and adolescence, in Handbook of Affective Disorders. Edited by Paykel ES. New York, Guilford Press, 1982

Regier DA: Statement of objectives, in Risk Factor Research in the Major Mental Disorders. Edited by Regier DA, Allen G. Washington DC, U. S. Government Printing Office, Department of Health and Human Services Publication No. (ADM) 81-1068, 1981

Reid WH: Genetic correlates of antisocial syndromes, in The Psychopath. Edited by Reid WH. New York, Brunner/Mazel, 1978

Rieder RO: Children at risk, in Disorders of the Schizophrenic Syndrome. Edited by Bellak L. New York, Basic Books, 1979

Rieder RO, Nichols PL: Offspring of schizophrenics. III. Hyperactivity and neurological soft signs. Arch Gen Psychiatry 36:665–674, 1979

Robins LN: Deviant Children Grown Up. Baltimore, Williams & Wilkins, 1966

Robins LN: Sturdy childhood predictors of adult antisocial behavior: Replications from longitudinal studies. Psychol Med 8:611–622, 1978

Rodnick EH, Goldstein MJ: Premorbid adjustment and the recovery of the mothering function in acute schizophrenic women. J Abnorm Psychol 83:623–628, 1974

Rodnick EH, Goldstein MJ, Doane JA, Lewis JM: Association between parent-child transactions and risk for schizophrenia: Implications for early intervention, in Preventive Intervention in Schizophrenia: Are We Ready? Edited by Goldstein MJ. Washington DC, Department of Health and Human Services Publication No. (ADM) 82-1111, 1982

Rosenthal D: Genetic Theory and Abnormal Behavior. New York, McGraw-Hill, 1970

Rutschmann J, Cornblatt B, Erlenmeyer-Kimling L: Sustained attention in children at risk for schizophrenia. Arch Gen Psychiatry 34:571–574, 1977

Rutter M: Relationship between child and adult psychiatric disorders. Acta Psychiatr Scand 48:3–21, 1972

Rutter M: Protective factors in children's responses to stress and disadvantage, in Primary Prevention of Psychopathology, vol 3, Social Competence in Children. Edited by Kent MW, Rolf JE. Hanover NH, University Press of New England, 1979

Sameroff AJ, Seifer R, Zax M: Early development of children at risk for emotional disorder. Monogr Soc Res Child Dev 47:199(7), 1982

Schulsinger H: A ten-year follow-up of children of schizophrenic mothers: Clinical assessment. Acta Psychiatr Scand 53:371–386, 1976

Slater E, Cowie V: The Genetics of Mental Disorder. London, Oxford University Press, 1971

Vaughn CE, Leff JP: The influence of family and social factors on the course of psychiatric illness. Br J Psychiatry 129:125–137, 1976a

Vaughn CE, Leff JP: The measurement of expressed emotion in the families of psychiatric patients. Br J Soc Clin Psychol 15 (Part 2):157–165, 1976b

Vaughn CE, Snyder KS, Freeman W, Jones S, Falloon IRH, Liberman RP: Family factors in schizophrenic relapse: A replication. Schizophr Bull 8:425–426, 1982

Watt NF: In a nutshell, in Children at Risk for Schizophrenia: A Longitudinal Perspective. Edited by Watt NF, Anthony EJ, Wynne LC, Rolf J. New York, Cambridge University Press, 1984

Watt NF, Anthony EJ, Wynne LC, Rolf J (eds): Children at Risk for Schizophrenia: A Longitudinal Perspective. New York, Cambridge University Press, 1984

Weissman MM: Depressed parents and their children: Implications for prevention, in Basic Handbook of Child Psychiatry, vol 4. Edited by Noshpitz JD. New York, Basic Books, 1979

Weissman MM, Paykel ES, Klerman GL: The depressed woman as a mother. Soc Psychiatry 7:98–108, 1972

Werner EE, Smith RS: Vulnerable but Invincible: A Study of Resilient Children. New York, McGraw-Hill, 1982

West DJ: The Young Offender. New York, International Universities Press, 1967

West DJ, Farrington DP: Who Becomes Delinquent? London, Heinemann Educational Books Ltd, 1973

Winokur G, Clayton P, Reich T: Manic-Depressive Illness. St. Louis, CV Mosby, 1969

Wynne LC, Cromwell RL, Matthysse S (eds): The Nature of Schizophrenia: New Approaches to Research and Treatment. New York, John Wiley & Sons, 1978

References for Chapter 8

Children at Acute Risk: Psychic Trauma

American Psychiatric Association: Diagnostic and Statistical Manual of Mental Disorders, 3rd ed. Washington DC, American Psychiatric Association, 1980

Anthony EJ: Mourning and the psychic loss of the parent, in The Child and his Family, vol 2. Edited by Anthony EJ, Koupernick C. New York, John Wiley & Sons, 1973

Aylon O: Children as hostages. The Practitioner 226:1773–1781, 1982

Barnes M: Reactions to the death of a mother. Psychoanal Study Child 19:339–357, 1964

Barton A: Communities in Disaster. Garden City NY, Doubleday, 1969

Beardslee W, Mack J: The impact on children and adolescents of nuclear development, in Psychosocial Aspects of Nuclear Development, Task Force Report #20. Washington DC, American Psychiatric Association, 1982

Bernstein N: The child with severe burns, in The Basic Handbook of Child Psychiatry, vol 1. Edited by Noshpitz J. New York, Basic Books, 1979

Blaufarb H, Levine J: Crisis intervention in an earthquake. Soc Work 17:16–19, 1972

Bloch D, Silber E, Perry S: Some factors in the emotional reaction of children to disaster. Am J Psychiatry 113:416–422, 1956

Bonaparte M: Notes on the analytic discovery of a primal scene. Psychoanal Study Child 1:119–125, 1945

Borocas C, Borocas H: Manifestations of concentration camp effects on the second generation. Am J Psychiatry 130:820–821, 1973

Bowlby J: Maternal Care and Mental Health. Geneva, World Health Organization, 1951

Bowlby J: Attachment and Loss, vol 2, Separation. New York, Basic Books, 1973

Burgess A, Groth A, McCausland M: Child sex initiation rings. Am J Orthopsychiatry 51:110–119, 1981

Cain A, Fast I: Children's disturbed reactions to parent suicide: Distortions of guilt, communication, and identification, in Survivors of Suicide. Edited by Cain A, Fast I. Springfield IL, Charles C Thomas, 1972

Carey-Trefzer C: The results of a clinical study of war-damaged children who attended the Child Guidance Clinic, the Hospital for Sick Children, Great Ormand Street, London. J Ment Sci 95:535–559, 1949

Carlin J: The catastrophically uprooted child: Southeast Asian refugee children, in The Basic Handbook of Child Psychiatry, vol 1. Edited by Noshpitz J. New York, Basic Books, 1979

Chodoff P: The German concentration camp as a psychological stress. Arch Gen Psychiatry 22:78–87, 1959

de Wind E: The confrontation with death. Int J Psychoanal 49:302–305, 1968

Disaster at Buffalo Creek. Special Section, Am J Psychiatry 133:295–316, 1976

Earle E: The psychological effects of mutilating surgery in children and adolescents. Psychoanal Study Child 34:527–546, 1979

Epstein H: Children of the Holocaust. New York, GP Putnam's Sons, 1979

Erikson K: Everything in Its Path. New York, Simon & Schuster, 1976

Escalona S: Children and the threat of nuclear war, in Behavioral Science and Human Survival. Edited by Schwebel M. Palo Alto CA, Behavioral Science Press, 1965

Esman A: The "stimulus barrier"—a review and reconsideration. Psychoanal Study Child 38:193–207, 1983

Farberow N, Gordon N: Manual for Child Health Workers in Major Disasters. Rockville MD, National Institute of Mental Health, 1981

Fenichel O: The Psychoanalytic Theory of Neurosis. New York, WW Norton & Co, 1945

Fraiberg S: Ghosts in the nursery: A psychoanalytic approach to the problems of impaired infant-mother relationships. J Am Acad Child Psychiatry 14:387–422, 1975

Freud A: Comments on trauma, in Psychic Trauma. Edited by Furst S. New York, Basic Books, 1967

Freud A: Acting out. Int J Psychoanal 49:165–170, 1968

Freud A, Burlingham D: Report 12. (1942), in The Writings of Anna Freud, vol 3. New York, International Universities Press, 1973

Freud A, Dann S: An experiment in group upbringing. Psychoanal Study Child 6:127–168, 1951

Freud S: Screen memories (1899), in Complete Psychological Works, standard ed, vol 3. London, Hogarth Press, 1962

Freud S: Beyond the pleasure principle (1920), in Complete Psychological Works, standard ed, vol 18. London, Hogarth Press, 1955

Freud S: Inhibitions, symptoms, and anxiety (1926), in Complete Psychological Works, standard ed, vol 20. London, Hogarth Press, 1959

Freud S: Moses and monotheism (1937), in Complete Psychological Works, standard ed, vol 23. London, Hogarth Press, 1964

Furman E: Treatment of under-fives by way of parents. Psychoanal Study Child 12:250–262, 1957

Furman E: Treatment via the mother, in The Therapeutic Nursery School. Edited by Furman R, Katan A. New York, International Universities Press, 1969

Galante R: Presentation on the treatment of the child earthquake victims in Italy. Part of the Abramson Fund Symposium: Children of Disaster. Presented at the American Academy of Child Psychiatry Annual Meeting, Washington DC, 1982

Galdston R: The burning and healing of children. Psychiatry 35:57–66, 1972

Gardner R: Therapeutic Communication With Children: The Mutual Storytelling Technique. New York, Science House, 1971

Gelman D: Of finding the hidden Freud. Newsweek, 30 November 1981, 64–70

Gleser G, Green B, Winget C: Prolonged Psychological Effects of Disaster. New York, Academic Press, 1981

Glover E: The screening function of traumatic memories. Int J Psychoanal 10:90–93, 1929

Goldstein J, Freud A, Solnit A: Beyond the Best Interests of the Child. New York, Free Press, 1973

Green A: Dimension of psychological trauma in abused children. J Am Acad Child Psychiatry 22:231–237, 1983

Greenacre P: A contribution to the study of screen memories. Psychoanal Study Child 3/4:73–84, 1949

Greenacre P: Reconstruction: Its nature and therapeutic value. J Am Psychoanal Assoc 29:386–402, 1981

Grinker R, Spiegel J: Men Under Stress. Philadelphia, Blakiston, 1945

Grosser G, Wechsler H, Greenblatt M (eds): The Threat of Impending Disaster. Cambridge MA, MIT Press, 1964

Hamburg D, Adams J: A perspective on coping: Seeking and utilizing information in major transitions. Arch Gen Psychiatry 17:277–284, 1967

Hocking F: Extreme environmental stress and its significance for psychopathology. Am J Psychother 24:4–26, 1970

Horowitz M: Stress Response Syndromes. New York, Jason Aronson, 1976

Janis I: Psychological Stress: Psychoanalytic and Behavioral Studies of Surgical Patients. New York, John Wiley & Sons, 1958

Janis I: Psychological effects of warnings, in Man and Society in Disaster. Edited by Baker C, Chapman D. New York, Basic Books, 1962

Jessner L, Blom G, Waldfogel S: Emotional implications of tonsillectomy and adenoidectomy on children. Psychoanal Study Child 7:126–169, 1952

Katan A: Some thoughts about the role of verbalization in early childhood. Psychoanal Study Child 16:184–188, 1961

Katan A: Children who were raped. Psychoanal Study Child 28:208–224, 1973

Katan M: A causerie on Henry James's The Turn of the Screw. Psychoanal Study Child 17:473–493, 1962

Katan M: The origin of The Turn of the Screw. Psychoanal Study Child 21:583–635, 1966

Kennedy H: Cover memories in formation. Psychoanal Study Child 5:275–284, 1950

Kennedy H: Problems in reconstruction in child analysis. Psychoanal Study Child 26:386–402, 1971

Khan M: The concept of cumulative trauma. Psychoanal Study Child 18:286–306, 1963

Kris E: The recovery of childhood memories in psychoanalysis. Psychoanal Study Child 11:54–88, 1956

Krystal H: Trauma and effects. Psychoanal Study Child 33:81–116, 1978

Krystal H, Niederland W: Clinical observations on the survivor syndrome, in Massive Psychic Trauma. Edited by Krystal H. New York, International Universities Press, 1968

Lacey G: Observations on Aberfan. J Psychosom Res 16:257–260, 1972

Lazarus R, Averill J, Opton E: The psychology of coping: Issues of research and assessment, in Coping and Adaptation. Edited by Coelho G, Hamburg D, Adams J. New York, Basic Books, 1974

Leopold R, Dillon H: The psycho-anatomy of a disaster: A longtime study of post-traumatic neuroses in survivors of a maritime explosion. Am J Psychiatry 119:913–921, 1963

Lerner A: Poetry in the Therapeutic Experience. Elmsford NY, Pergamon Press, 1978

Levy D: Release therapy. Am J Orthopsychiatry 9:713–736, 1939

Levy D: Psychic trauma of operations in children. Am J Dis Children 69:7–25, 1945

Lifton RJ: Death in Life. New York, Random House, 1967

Lifton RJ: The Broken Connection. New York, Simon & Schuster, 1979

Lifton RJ: Beyond psychic numbing: A call to awareness. Am J Orthopsychiatry 52:619–629, 1982

Lifton RJ, Olson E: The human meaning of total disaster. Psychiatry 39:1–18, 1976

Lindy J, Grace M, Green B: Survivors: Outreach to a reluctant population. Am J Orthopsychiatry 51:468–478, 1981

Lipton G, Roth E: Rape: A complex management problem in the pediatric emergency room. J Pediatr 75:859–866, 1969

Luchterhand E: Sociological approaches to massive stress in natural and man-made disasters. Int Psychiatr Clinics 8:29–53, 1971

Mack J: The perceptions of US-Soviet intentions and other psychological dimensions of the nuclear arms race. Am J Orthopsychiatry 52:590–599, 1982

MacLean G: Psychic trauma and traumatic neurosis: Play with a four-year-old boy. Can Psychiatr Assoc J 22:71–76, 1977

Mercier M, Despert J: Effects of war on French children. Psychosom Med 5:266–272, 1943

Miller G, Tompkins S: Chowchilla: The bitterness lingers. Fresno Bee, 14 November, 1976

Moriarty A: Reactions to the assassination of a president, in Vulnerability, Coping and Growth. Edited by Murphy L, Moriarty A. New Haven CT, Yale University Press, 1976

Murphy L: The Widening World of Childhood: Paths Towards Mastery. New York, Basic Books, 1962

Murphy L: Coping, vulnerability, and resilience in childhood, in Coping and Adaptation. Edited by Coelho G, Hamburg D, Adams J. New York, Basic Books, 1974

Newman CJ: Children of disaster: Clinical observations at Buffalo Creek. Am J Psychiatry 133:316–312, 1976

Niederland W: Psychoanalytic approaches to artistic creativity. Psychoanal Q 45:185–212, 1976

Noshpitz J (ed): The Basic Handbook of Child Psychiatry, vol 1. New York, Basic Books, 1979

Parad H, Resnik H, Parad L (eds): Emergency and Disaster Management. Bowie MD, Charles Press Publishers, 1976

Peterfreund E: Some critical comments on psychoanalytic conceptualizations of infancy. Int J Psychoanal 59:427–441, 1978

Peterfreund E: The Process of Psychoanalytic Therapy: Models and Strategies. Hillsdale NJ, Lawrence Erlbaum Associates, 1982

Ploeger A: A ten year follow-up of miners trapped for two weeks under threatening circumstances, in Stress and Anxiety. Edited by Spielberger C, Sarason J. Washington DC, Hemisphere, 1972

Pynoos R, Eth S: The child as criminal witness to homicide. J Soc Issues in press[a]

Pynoos R, Eth S: Witness to violence: The child interview. J Am Acad Child Psychiatry in press[b]

Rangell L: The metapsychology of psychic trauma, in Psychic Trauma. Edited by Furst S. New York, Basic Books, 1967

Rosenfeld AA: Endogamic incest and the victim-perpetrator model. Am J Dis Children 133:406–410, 1979

Sandler J: Trauma, strain, and development, in Psychic Trauma. Edited by Furst S. New York, Basic Books, 1967

Schechter M, Holter F: The child amputee, in The Basic Handbook of Child Psychiatry, vol 1. Edited by Noshpitz J. New York, Basic Books, 1979

Schwebel M: Nuclear cold war: Student opinion and professional responsibility, in Behavioral Science and Human Survival. Edited by Schwebel M. Palo Alto, CA, Behavioral Science Press, 1965

Schwebel M, Schwebel B: Children's reactions to the threat of nuclear plant accidents. Am J Orthopsychiatry 51:260–270, 1981

Senior N, Gladstone T, Nurcombe B: Child snatching: A case report. J Am Acad Child Psychiatry 20:579–583, 1982

Shapiro S: Preventive analysis following a trauma: A four-and-a-half-year-old girl witnesses a stillbirth. Psychoanal Study Child 28:279–285, 1973

Shapiro T, Stern D: Psychoanalytic perspectives on the first year of life: The establishment of the object in an affective field, in The Course of Life, vol 1. Edited by Greenspan S, Pollock G. Rockville MD, National Institute of Mental Health, 1980

Shetky D, Haller L: Parental kidnapping. J Am Acad Child Psychiatry 22:279–285, 1983

Solkoff N: Children of survivors of the nazi holocaust: A critical review of the literature. Am J Orthopsychiatry 51:29–42, 1981

Solnit A: Child placement—on whose time? J Am Acad Child Psychiatry 12:385–392, 1973

Solnit A, Kris M: Trauma and infantile experiences: A longitudinal perspective, in Psychic Trauma. Edited by Furst S. New York, Basic Books, 1967

Solomon J: Reactions of children to black-outs. Am J Orthopsychiatry 12:361–362, 1942

Sonnenberg S: Workshop report: Children of survivors. J Am Psychoanal Assoc 22:200–204, 1974

Steinberg E, Weiss J: The art of Edvard Munch and its function in his mental life. Psychoanal Q 23:408–423, 1954

Sterba E: The effects of persecutions on adolescents, in Massive Psychic Trauma. Edited by Krystal H. New York, International Universities Press, 1968

Stern G: The Buffalo Creek Disaster. New York, Random House, 1976

Terr L: A family study of child abuse. Am J Psychiatry 127:665–671, 1970

Terr L: Children of Chowchilla: A study of psychic trauma. Psychoanal Study Child 34:547–623, 1979

Terr L: The child as a witness, in Child Psychiatry and the Law. Edited by Shetky D, Benedek E. New York, Brunner/Mazel, 1980

Terr L: Forbidden games: Post-traumatic child's play. J Am Acad Child Psychiatry 20:741–760, 1981a

Terr L: Psychic trauma in children: Observations following the Chowchilla schoolbus kidnapping. Am J Psychiatry 138:14–19, 1981b

Terr L: Child snatching: A new epidemic of an ancient malady. J Pediatr in press, 1983a

Terr L: Chowchilla revisited: The effects of psychic trauma four years after a schoolbus kidnapping. Am J Psychiatry in press, 1983b

Terr L: Life attitudes, dreams, and psychic trauma in a group of normal children. J Am Acad Child Psychiatry 22:221–230, 1983c

Terr L: Play therapy and psychic trauma: A preliminary report, in Handbook of Play Therapy. Edited by Schaefer C, O'Connor K. New York, Wiley Interscience, 1983d

Terr L: Time sense following psychic trauma: A clinical study of ten adults and twenty children. Am J Orthopsychiatry 53:244–261, 1983e

Terr L: Time and trauma. Psychoanal Study Child 39, Fall, 1984

Terr L, Watson A: The battered child rebrutalized: Ten cases of medical/legal confusion. Am J Psychiatry 124:126–133, 1968

Tierney K: Crisis Intervention Programs for Disaster Victims: A Source Manual for Smaller Communities. United States Department of Health, Education, and Welfare (ADM), 1979

Tulchin S, Levy D: Rorschach test differences in a group of Spanish and English refugee children. Am J Orthopsychiatry 15:361–368, 1945

Waelder R: Trauma and the variety of extraordinary challenges, in Psychic Trauma. Edited by Furst S. New York, Basic Books, 1967

Washburn S, Hamburg D: The study of primate behavior, in Primate Behavior. Edited by DeVore I. New York, Holt Rinehart & Winston, 1965

Wasserman G, Green A, Allen R: Going beyond abuse: Maladaptive patterns of interaction in abusing mother-infant pairs. J Am Acad Child Psychiatry 22:245–252, 1983

Yates A: Narcissistic traits in certain abused children. Am J Orthopsychiatry 51:55–62, 1981

Zimmerman I: Adaptation to terrorism and political violence. Presented at the Los Angeles Group Psychotherapy Society Annual Meeting, Los Angeles CA, June 1983

References for Chapter 9

Children with Mental Retardation

Ainsworth MDS: The development of infant-mother attachment, in Review of Child Development Research. Edited by Caldwell BM, Ricciuti HN. Chicago, University of Chicago Press, 1973

American Psychiatric Association: Diagnostic and Statistical Manual of Mental Disorders, 3rd ed. Washington DC, American Psychiatric Association, 1980

Bernstein N: Diminished People. Boston, Little Brown & Co, 1970

Bijou SW: The prevention of mild and moderate retarded development, in Curative Aspects of Mental Retardation: Biomedical and Behavioral Advances. Edited by Menolascino FJ, Neman R, Stark JA. Baltimore, Paul Brookes Publishing Co, 1983

Bijou SW, Dunitz-Johnson E: Interbehavior analysis of developmental retardation. Psychol Rev 31:305–329, 1981

Bornstein PH, Bach P, Anton B: Behavioral treatment of psychopathological disorders, in Psychopathology in the Mentally Retarded. Edited by Matson JL, Barrett RP. New York, Grune & Stratton, 1982

Bowlby J: Attachment and Loss, vol 1. Attachment. New York, Basic Books, 1969

Brieter C, Englemann S: Teaching Disadvantaged Children in Preschool. Englewood Cliffs NJ, Prentice Hall, 1966

Bronfenbrenner U: Is early intervention effective, in Exceptional Infant, vol 3. Edited by Friedlander BZ, Sterritt GM, Kirk GE. New York, Brunner/Mazel, 1975

Chazan M: The incidence and nature of maladjustment among children in schools for the educationally subnormal. Br J Educat Psychol 34:292–304, 1964

Corbett J: Mental retardation: Psychiatric aspects, in Child Psychiatry. Modern Approaches. Edited by Rutter M, Hersov L. Oxford, Blackwell Scientific Publications, 1976

Cytryn L, Lourie R: Mental retardation, in Textbook of Psychiatry. Edited by Kaplan HI, Freedman AM, Sadock BJ. Baltimore, Williams & Wilkins Co, 1980

Education for All Handicapped Children Act. P.L. 94-142. Washington DC, United States Printing Office, 1975

Ende RN, Brown C: Adaptation to the birth of a Down's syndrome infant: Grieving and maternal attachment. J Am Acad Child Psychiatry 17:299–323, 1978

Fraiberg S, Adelson E, Shapiro V: Ghosts in the nursery: A psychoanalytic approach to the problems of impaired infant-mother relationships. J Am Acad Child Psychiatry 14:387–421, 1975

Freeman R: Psychopharmacology and the retarded child, in Psychiatric Approaches to the Mentally Retarded Child. Edited by Menolascino F. New York, Basic Books, 1970

Garrard SD, Richmond JB: Diagnosis in mental retardation, in Medical Aspects of Mental Retardation. Edited by Carter CH. Springfield IL, Charles C Thomas, 1965

Heber R, Garber H: The Milwaukee project: A study of the use of family intervention to prevent cultural family retardation, in Exceptional Infant, vol 3. Edited by Friedlander BZ, Garritt GM, Kirk GE. New York, Brunner/Mazel, 1975

Kugel RB, Wolfensberger W: Changing Patterns in Residential Services for the Mentally Retarded. Washington DC, President's Committee on Mental Retardation, 1969

Menolascino F: Emotional disturbances in mentally retarded children. Am J Psychiatry 126:168–176, 1969

Menolascino F: Psychiatric Approaches to Mental Retardation. New York, Basic Books, 1970

Philips I: Prevention and Treatment of Mental Retardation. New York, Basic Books, 1966

Philips I: Psychopathology and mental retardation. Am J Psychiatry 124:29–35, 1967

Philips I, Williams N: Psychopathology and mental retardation. I. Psychopathology. Am J Psychiatry 132:1265–1271, 1975

Provence S, Lipton RC: Infants in Institutions. New York, International Universities Press, 1962

Rutter M: Stress, coping, and development: Some issues and some questions, in Stress, Coping and Development. Edited by Garmezy N, Rutter M. New York, McGraw Hill, 1983, in press

Rutter M, Tizard J, Whitmore K (eds): Education, Health and Behavior. London, Longman, 1970

Sameroff AJ, Chandler MJ: Reproductive risk and the continuum of caretaking casualty, in Review of Child Development Research, vol 4. Edited by Horowitz FD. Chicago, University of Chicago Press, 1975

Schiefelbusch RL: Advances in school and classroom learning, in Behavioral Systems for the Developmentally Disabled. Edited by Hammerlyn LAH. New York, Brunner/Mazel, 1979

Sherer DE, Sherer MS: A model for early childhood intervention, in Intervention Strategies for High Risk Infants and Young Children. Edited by Tjossem RD. Baltimore, University Park Press, 1976

Skeels HM: Adult states of children with contrasting early life experiences. Monogr Soc Res Child Dev 31:1–65, 1966

Skeels HM, Harms I: Children with inferior social histories: Their mental development in adoptive homes. J Genet Psychol 72:283–294, 1948

Skodiak M: Adult states of individuals who experience early intervention, in Proceedings of the First Congress, International Association Scientific Study of Mental Deficiency, 1968

Solnit AJ, Stak MH: Mourning and the birth of a defective child. Psychoanal Study Child 16:523–537, 1961

State of California Department of Health: State Hospital Populations 1982. Sacramento CA, State of California Department of Health, in press

Szurek SA, Philips I: Mental retardation and psychotherapy, in Prevention and Treatment of Mental Retardation. Edited by Philips I. New York, Basic Books, 1966

Szymanski LS: Individual psychotherapy with retarded persons, in Emotional Disorders of Mentally Retarded Persons. Edited by Szymanski LS, Tanguay PE. Baltimore, University Park Press, 1980

Szymanski LS, Tanguay PE (eds): Emotional Disorders of Mentally Retarded Persons. Baltimore, University Park Press, 1980

Tizard J, Grad JC: The Mentally Handicapped and Their Families: A Social Survey. London, Oxford Press, 1961

References for Chapter 10

Parenting and Children at Risk

Abernethy V, Grunebaum H: Toward a family planning program in psychiatric hospitals. Am J Public Health 62:1638–1646, 1972

Abernethy V, Grunebaum H: Family planning in two psychiatric hospitals: A preliminary report. Fam Plann Perspect 5:94–99, 1973

Ainsworth MDS, Blehar MC, Waters E, Wall S: Patterns of Attachment: A Psychological Study of the Strange Situation. Hillsdale NJ, Lawrence Erlbaum Associates, 1978

Anthony EJ: Neonatal and early development of children at risk for schizophrenia, in Children at Risk for Schizophrenia: A Longitudinal Perspective. Edited by Watt NF, Anthony EJ, Wynne LC, Rolf JE. New York, Cambridge University Press, 1984

Baldwin CP, Baldwin AL, Cole RE, Kokes RF: Free play family interaction and the behavior of the patient in free play, in Children at Risk for Schizophrenia: A Longitudinal Perspective. Edited by Watt NF, Anthony EJ, Wynne LC, Rolf JE. New York, Cambridge University Press, 1984

Beardslee WR, Bemporad J, Keller MB, Klerman GL: Children of parents with major affective disorder: A review. Am J Psychiatry 140:825–832, 1983

Bleuler M: Die Schizophrenen Geistesstörungen im Lichte Langjähriger Kranken und Familiengeschichten. Stuttgart, Verlag, GT 1972. In translation: The Schizophrenic Disorders: Long-Term Patients and Family Studies. Translated by Clemens S. New Haven CT, Yale University Press, 1978

Bleuler M: Different forms of childhood stress and patterns of adult psychiatric outcome, in Children at Risk for Schizophrenia: A Longitudinal Perspective. Edited by Watt NF, Anthony EJ, Wynne LC, Rolf JE. New York, Cambridge University Press, 1984, in press

Boyd J, Weissman MM: Epidemiology of affective disorders: A reexamination and future directions. Arch Gen Psychiatry 38:1039–1046, 1981

Brown G, Harris T: Social Origins of Depression: A Study of Psychiatric Disorder in Women. New York, Free Press, 1975

Campbell A, Converse P, Rodgers W: The Quality of American Life: Perceptions, Evaluations, and Satisfactions. New York, Russell-Sage, 1976

Clough L, Abernethy V, Grunebaum H: Contraception for the severely psychiatrically disturbed: Confusion, control, and contraindication. Compr Psychiatry 17:601–606, 1976

Cohler BJ, Geyer S: Psychological autonomy and interdependence within the family of adulthood, in Normal Family Processes: Implications for Clinical Practice. Edited by Walsh F. New York, Guilford Press, 1982

Cohler BJ, Grunebaum H: Mothers, Grandmothers, and Daughters: Personality and Child Care in Three-Generation Families. New York, John Wiley & Sons, 1981

Cohler BJ, Grunebaum H: Children of parents hospitalized for mental illness: II. The evaluation of an intervention program for mentally ill mothers of young children. J of Children in Contemporary Society, Vol. 15, No. 1, Feb. 1983

Cohler BJ, Musick J: Psychopathology of parenthood: Implications for mental health of children. Paper presented at the sixth Annual Meeting of the Michigan Association for Infant Mental Health, Ann Arbor, March 1982

Cohler BJ, Gallant DH, Grunebaum H, Weiss J, Gamer E: Attention dysfunction and childcare attitudes among mentally ill and well mothers and their young children, in Social Context of Learning and Development. Edited by Glidewell JC. New York, Gardner-Wiley, 1977

Cohler BJ, Gallant DH, Grunebaum HU, Kauffman C: Social adjustment among schizophrenic, depressed, and well mothers and their school-aged children, in Children of Depressed Parents: Risk, Identification and Intervention. Edited by Morrison HL. New York, Grune & Stratton, 1983

Cole RE, Al-Khayyal M, Baldwin AL, Baldwin CP, Fisher L, Wynne LC: A cross-setting assessment of family interaction and the prediction of school competence in children at risk, in Children at Risk for Schizophrenia: A Longitudinal Perspective. Edited by Watt NF, Anthony EJ, Wynne LC, Rolf JE. New York, Cambridge University Press, 1984

Cornblatt B, Erlenmeyer-Kimling L: Early attentional predictors of adolescent behavioral disturbances in children at risk for schizophrenia, in Children at Risk for Schizophrenia: A Longitudinal Perspective. Edited by Watt NF, Anthony EJ, Wynne LC, Rolf JE. New York, Cambridge University Press, 1984

Cudeck R, Mednick SA, Schulsinger F, Schulsinger H: A multidimensional approach to the identification of schizophrenia, in Children at Risk for Schizophrenia: A Longitudinal Perspective. Edited by Watt NF, Anthony EJ, Wynne LC, Rolf JE. New York, Cambridge University Press, 1984

Decina P, Kestenbaum CJ, Farber S, Kron L, Gargan M, Sackeim HA, Fieve RR: Clinical and psychological assessment of children of bipolar probands. Am J Psychiatry 140:548–553, 1983

Dinnerstein D: The Mermaid and the Minotaur: Sexual Arrangements and Human Malaise. New York, Harper & Row, 1977

Ekdahl MC, Rice EP, Schmidt WM: Children of parents hospitalized for mental illness. Am J Public Health 52:428–435, 1962

Erlenmeyer-Kimling L, Marcuse Y, Cornblatt B, Friedman D, Rainer JD, Rutschmann J: The New York high-risk project, in Children at Risk for Schizophrenia: A Longitudinal Perspective. Edited by Watt NF, Anthony EJ, Wynne LC, Rolf JE. New York, Cambridge University Press, 1984

Fasman J, Grunebaum H, Weiss J: Who cares for the children of psychotic mothers? Br J Psychiatry, 9:84–99, 1967

Fish B: The detection of schizophrenia in infancy. J Nerv Ment Dis 125:1–24, 1957

Fish B: Characteristics and sequelae of the neurointegrative disorder in infants at risk for schizophrenia (1952–1982), in Children at Risk for Schizophrenia: A Longitudinal Perspective. Edited by Watt NF, Anthony EJ, Wynne LC, Rolf JE. New York, Cambridge University Press, 1984

Fisher L, Kokes RF, Harder DW, Jones JE: Child competence and psychiatric risk: VI. Summary and integration of findings. J Nerv Ment Dis 168:353–355, 1980

Fishman SH: The impact of incarceration on children of offenders, in Children of Exceptional Parents. Edited by Frank M. New York, Haworth Press, 1983

Gallant D: Children of mentally ill mothers, in Mentally Ill Mothers and Their Children. Edited by Grunebaum H, Weiss J, Cohler BJ, Hartman C, Gallant D. Chicago, University of Chicago Press, 1975

Gamer E, Gallant D, Grunebaum H, Cohler BJ: Children of psychotic mothers. Arch Gen Psychiatry 34:592–597, 1977a

Gamer E, Grunebaum H, Cohler BJ, Gallant D: Children at risk: Performance of three-year-olds and their mentally ill and well mothers on an interaction task. Child Psychiatry Hum Dev 8:102–114, 1977b

Garmezy N, Devine V: Project competence: The Minnesota studies of children vulnerable to psychopathology, in Children at Risk for Schizophrenia: A Longitudinal Perspective. Edited by Watt NF, Anthony EJ, Wynne LC, Rolf JE. New York, Cambridge University Press, 1984

Goodman S: Young children of severely emotionally disturbed mothers. Paper presented at the Biennial Meeting of the Society for Research in Children's Development. Detroit, April 1983

Grunebaum H: Children at risk for psychosis and their families: Approaches to prevention, in Child Psychiatry, Treatment and Research. Edited by McMillan MF, Henao S. New York, Brunner/Mazel, 1977

Grunebaum H, Abernethy V: Ethical issues in family planning for hospitalized psychiatric patients. Am J Psychiatry 132:236–240, 1975

Grunebaum H, Cohler BJ: Children of parents hospitalized for mental illness: I. Attentional and interactional studies. J of Children in Contemporary Society vol 15, No 1, February 1983

Grunebaum H, Gamer E, Cohler BJ: The spouse in depressed families, in Children of Depressed Parents: Risk, Identification and Intervention. Edited by Morrison HL. New York, Grune & Stratton, 1983

Grunebaum H, Weiss J, Hirsch L, Barrett J: The baby on the ward. Psychiatry 26:29–53, 1963

Grunebaum H, Abernethy V, Rofman S, Weiss J: Family planning attitudes, practices and motivations of mental patients. Am J Psychiatry 128:740–744, 1971

Grunebaum H, Weiss J, Gallant D, Cohler BJ: Attention in young children of psychotic mothers. Am J Psychiatry 131:887–891, 1974

Grunebaum H, Abernethy V, Clough L, Groover B: Staff attitudes toward a family planning service in the mental hospital. Community Ment Health J 11:280–285, 1975

Grunebaum H, Cohler BJ, Kauffman C, Gallant D: Children of depressed and schizophrenic mothers. Child Psychiatry Hum Dev 8:219–229, 1978

Grunebaum J: The place of parenting in (our) society and "woman's place." Unpublished manuscript, 1983

el-Guebaly N: The offspring of alcoholics: Outcome predictors, in Children of Exceptional Parents. Edited by Frank M. New York, Haworth Press, 1983

Gutman D: Parenthood: A comparative key to the lifecycle, in Life-Span Developmental Psychology: Normative Crises. Edited by Datan N, Ginsberg L. New York, Academic Press, 1975

Holzman IR: Fetal Alcohol Syndrome (FAS)—A review, in Children of Exceptional Parents. Edited by Frank M. New York, Haworth Press, 1983

Jones JE, Wynne LC, Al-Khayyal M, Doane JA, Ritzler B, Singer MT, Fisher L: Predicting current school competence of high-risk children with a composite cross-situational measure of parental communication, in Children at Risk for Schizophrenia: A Longitudinal Perspective. Edited by Watt NF, Anthony EJ, Wynne LC, Rolf JE. New York, Cambridge University Press, 1984

Kagan J: Perspectives on continuity, in Constancy and Change in Human Development. Edited by Brim OG Jr, Kagan J. Cambridge MA, Harvard University Press, 1980

Karlsson JL: Genealogic studies of schizophrenia, in The Transmission of Schizophrenia. Edited by Rosenthal D, Kety S. New York, Pergamon Press, 1968

Kauffman C, Grunebaum H, Cohler BJ, Gamer E: Superkids: Competent children of psychotic mothers. Am J Psychiatry 136:1398–1402, 1979

Kessler R, Brown R, Broman C: Sex differences in psychiatric help seeking: Evidence from four large-scale surveys. J Health Soc Behav 22:49–64, 1981

Klein RH, Salzman LF: Response-contingent learning in children at risk, in Children at Risk for Schizophrenia: A Longitudinal Perspective. Edited by Watt NF, Anthony EJ, Wynne LC, Rolf JE. New York, Cambridge University Press, 1984

Kokes RF, Harder DW, Fisher L, Strauss JS: Child competence and psychiatry risk: V. Sex of patient and dimensions of psychopathology. J Nerv Ment Dis 168:348–352, 1980

Kokes FR, Harder DW, Perkins P, Strauss JS: Diagnostic, symptomatic and descriptive characteristics of parents in the University of Rochester child and family study, in Children at Risk for Schizophrenia: A Longitudinal Perspective. Edited by Watt NF, Anthony EJ, Wynne LC, Rolf JE. New York, Cambridge University Press, 1984

Lamb HR, Zusman J: A new look at primary prevention. Hosp Community Psychiatry 32:843–848, 1981

Lewine RRJ: Stalking the schizophrenia marker: Evidence for a general vulnerability model of psychopathology, in Children at Risk for Schizophrenia: A Longitudinal Perspective. Edited by Watt NF, Anthony EJ, Wynne LC, Rolf JE. New York, Cambridge University Press, 1984

Lewine RRJ, Watt NF, Grubb TW: High-risk-for-schizophrenia research: Sampling bias and its implications, in Children at Risk for Schizophrenia: A Longitudinal Perspective. Edited by Watt NF, Anthony EJ, Wynne LC, Rolf JE. New York, Cambridge University Press, 1984

Lyons-Ruth K, Connell D, Botein S, Grunebaum H, Bumagin S: Maternal family history, maternal caretaking, and infant attachment in multiproblem families. J Preventive Psychiatry, 1983, in press

McNeil TF, Kaij L: Offspring of women with nonorganic psychoses, in Children at Risk for Schizophrenia: A Longitudinal Perspective. Edited by Watt NF, Anthony EJ, Wynne LC, Rolf JE. New York, Cambridge University Press, 1984

Main TF: Mothers with children in a psychiatric hospital. Lancet 2:845–847, 1958

Marcus J, Auerbach J, Wilkinson L, Burack GM: Infants at risk for schizophrenia: The Jerusalem infant development study, in Children at Risk for Schizophrenia: A Longitudinal Perspective. Edited by Watt NF, Anthony EJ, Wynne LC, Rolf JE. New York, Cambridge University Press, 1984

Mednick BR: Breakdown in high-risk subjects: Familial and early environmental factors. J Abnorm Psychol 82:469–475, 1973

Mednick SA: Breakdown in individuals at high risk for schizophrenia: Possible predispositional perinatal factors. Ment Hygiene 54:50–63, 1970

Mednick SA, Schulsinger F: Studies of children at high risk for schizophrenia, in Schizophrenia: The First Ten Dean Award Lectures. Edited by Dean SR. New York, MSS Information Corp, 1973

Mednick SA, Cudeck R, Griffith JJ, Talovic SA, Schulsinger F: The Danish high-risk project: Recent methods and findings, in Children at Risk for Schizophrenia: A Longitudinal Perspective. Edited by Watt NF, Anthony EJ,

Wynne LC, Rolf JE. New York, Cambridge University Press, 1984

Munson S, Baldwin AL, Yu P, Baldwin CP, Greenwald D: A clinical research approach to the assessment of adaptive function in children at risk, in Children at Risk for Schizophrenia: A Longitudinal Perspective. Edited by Watt NF, Anthony EJ, Wynne LC, Rolf JE. New York, Cambridge University Press, 1984

Musick J, Clark R, Cohler BJ: The mothers' project: A program for mentally ill mothers of young children, in Infants: Their Social Environments. Edited by Weissbourd B, Musick J. Washington DC, National Association for the Education of Young Children, 1981

Musick J, Clark R, Cohler BJ, Dincin J: Interactional patterns of schizophrenic, depressed and well mothers and their young children. Paper presented at Annual Meeting, American Psychological Association, New York, 1979

Neale JM, Winters KC, Weintraub S: Information processing deficits in children at high risk for schizophrenia, in Children at Risk for Schizophrenia: A Longitudinal Perspective. Edited by Watt NF, Anthony EJ, Wynne LC, Rolf JE. New York, Cambridge University Press, 1984

Philips I: Opportunities for prevention in the practice of psychiatry. Am J Psychiatry 140:389–395, 1983

Phillips D, Seagal B: Sexual status and psychiatric symptoms. Am Sociol Rev 34:58–72, 1969

Phillips L: Human Adaptation and Its Failures. New York, Academic Press, 1968

Radloff L: Sex differences in mental health: The effects of marital and occupational status. Sex Roles 3:249–265, 1975

Radloff L, Rae D: Susceptibility and precipitating factors in depression: Sex differences and similarities. J Abnorm Psychol 88:174–181, 1979

Reid WH, Morrison HL: Risk factors in children of depressed parents, in Children of Depressed Parents: Risk, Identification, and Intervention. Edited by Morrison HL. New York, Grune & Stratton, 1983

Robins LN: Deviant Children Grown Up. Baltimore, Williams & Wilkins, 1966

Robins LN: Followup studies of behavior disorders in children, in Psychopathological Disorders of Childhood. Edited by Quay HC, Werry JS. New York, Wiley Interscience 1972

Rodnick EH, Goldstein MJ, Lewis JM, Doane JA: Parental communication style, affect and role as precursors of offspring schizophrenia-spectrum disorders, in Children at Risk for Schizophrenia: A Longitudinal Perspective. Edited by Watt NF, Anthony EJ, Wynne LC, Rolf JE. New York, Cambridge University Press, 1984

Rolf JE, Hasazi J: Identification of preschool children at risk and some guidelines for primary intervention, in The Issues: The Primary Prevention of Psychopathology, vol 1. Edited by Joffe J, Albee G. Hanover NH, University of New England Press, 1977

Rolf JE, Crowther J, Teri L, Bond L: Contrasting developmental risks in preschool children of psychiatrically hospitalized parents, in Children at Risk for Schizophrenia: A Longitudinal Perspective. Edited by Watt NF, Anthony EJ, Wynne LC, Rolf JE. New York, Cambridge University Press, 1984

Rutter M: Protective factors in children's responses to stress and disadvantage, in Social Competence in Children. Edited by Kent M, Rolf JE. Hanover NH, University of New England Press, 1979

Rutter M (ed): Scientific Foundations of Developmental Psychiatry. London, William Heinemann Medical Books, 1980

Rutter M, Cox A, Tupling C, Berger M, Yule W: Attachment and adjustment in two geographical areas. I. The prevalence of psychiatric disorder. Br J Psychiatry 126:493–509 1975a

Rutter M, Yule B, Quinton D, Rowlands O, Yule W, Berger M: Attainment and adjustment in two geographical areas. III. Some factors accounting for area differences. Br J Psychiatry 126:520–533, 1975b

Sameroff AJ, Barocas R, Seifer R: The early development of children born to mentally ill women, in Children at Risk for Schizophrenia: A Longitudinal Perspective. Edited by Watt NF, Anthony EJ, Wynne LC, Rolf JE. New York, Cambridge University Press, 1984

Sobel D: Children of schizophrenic patients: Preliminary observations of early development. Am J Psychiatry 118:512–517, 1961

Stewart A, Salt P: Life-stress, life-styles, and illness in adult women. J Pers Soc Psychol 40:1063–1069, 1981

Strauss JS: Overview: Adult diagnosis in the study of vulnerability to schizophrenia, in Children at Risk for Schizophrenia: A Longitudinal Perspective. Edited by Watt NF, Anthony EJ, Wynne LC, Rolf JE. New York, Cambridge University Press, 1984

Van der Walde P, Meeks D, Grunebaum H, Weiss J: Joint admission of mothers and children to a state hospital. Arch Gen Psychiatry 18:706–711, 1968

Watt NF: Childhood and adolescent routes to schizophrenia, in Life History Research in Psychopathology, vol 3. Edited by Ricks DF, Thomas A, Roff M. Minneapolis, University of Minnesota Press, 1974

Watt NF: In a nutshell: The first two decades of high-risk research in schizophrenia, in Children at Risk for Schizophrenia: A Longitudinal Perspective. Edited by Watt NF, Anthony EJ, Wynne LC, Rolf JE. New York, Cambridge University Press, 1984

Watt NF, Anthony EJ, Wynne LC, Rolf JE (eds): Children at Risk for Schizophrenia: A Longitudinal Perspective. New York, Cambridge University Press, 1984

Weintraub JF: The offender as parent, in Children of Exceptional Parents. Edited by Frank M. New York, Haworth Press, 1983

Weintraub S, Neale JM: The Stony Brook high-risk project, in Children at Risk for Schizophrenia: A Longitudinal Perspective. Edited by Watt NF, Anthony EJ, Wynne LC, Rolf JE. New York, Cambridge University Press, 1984

Weintraub S, Neale JM: Social behavior of children at risk for schizophrenia, in Children at Risk for Schizophrenia: A Longitudinal Perspective. Edited by Watt NF, Anthony EJ, Wynne LC, Rolf JE. New York, Cambridge University Press, 1984

Weissman MM, Myers JK: Rates and risks of depressive symptoms in a United States urban community. Acta Psychiatr Scand 57:219–231, 1978

Werner EE, Smith RS: Vulnerable but Invincible: A Longitudinal Study of Resilient Children and Youth. New York, McGraw Hill, 1982

Worland J, Janes CL, Anthony EJ, McGinnis M, Cass L: St. Louis risk research project: Comprehensive progress report of experimental studies, in Children at Risk for Schizophrenia: A Longitudinal Perspective. Edited by Watt NF, Anthony EJ, Wynne LC, Rolf JE. New York, Cambridge University Press, 1984

Wynne LC: Methodologic and conceptual issues in the study of schizophrenics and their families, in The Transmission of Schizophrenia. Edited by Rosenthal D, Kety SS. Oxford, Pergamon Press, 1968

Wynne LC: The University of Rochester child and family study: Overview of research plan, in Children at Risk for Schizophrenia: A Longitudinal Perspective. Edited by Watt NF, Anthony EJ, Wynne LC, Rolf JE. New York, Cambridge University Press, 1984

Yu P, Prentky R, Fisher L, Baldwin AL, Greenwald D, Munson S, Baldwin CP: Child competence as assessed by clinicians, parents, teachers, and peers, in Children at Risk for Schizophrenia: A Longitudinal Perspective. Edited by Watt NF, Anthony EJ, Wynne LC, Rolf JE. New York, Cambridge University Press, 1984

References for Chapter 11

Children of Divorce: The Dilemma of a Decade

Bane MJ: Marital disruption and the lives of children. J Soc Issues 32:103–117, 1976

Benedek EP, Benedek RS: Joint custody: Solution or illusion? Am J Psychiatry 136:1540–1544, 1979

Block JH, Block J, Morrison A: Parental agreement-disagreement on child rearing orientations and gender-related personality correlates in children. Child Dev 52:965–974, 1981

Bloom BL, White SW, Asher SJ: Marital disruption as a stressful life event, in Divorce and Separation: Context, Causes, and Consequences. Edited by Levinger G, Moles OC. New York, Basic Books, 1979

Brown BF: A study of the school needs of children in one-parent families. The Phi Delta Kappa (April) 537–540, 1980

Caplan G (ed): Emotional Problems of Early Childhood. New York, Basic Books, 1955

Cherlin AJ: Marriage, Divorce, Remarriage. Cambridge, Harvard University Press, 1981

Clingempeel WG, Reppucci ND: Joint custody after divorce: Major issues and goals for research. Psychol Bull 91:102–127, 1982

Coogler OJ: Structural Mediation in Divorce Settlement. Lexington MA, Lexington Books, 1978

Crohn H, Brown H, Walker L, Beir J: Understanding and treating the child in the remarried family, in Children of Separation and Divorce: Management and Treatment. Edited by Stuart IR, Abt LE. New York, Van Nostrand Reinhold Co, 1981

Derdeyn AP: Child custody consultation. Am J Orthopsychiatry 45: 791–801, 1975

Derdeyn AP: Child custody contests in historical perspective. Am J Psychiatry 133:1369–1376, 1976

Derdeyn AP: Child custody: A reflection of cultural change. J Clin Child Psychol 7:169–173, 1978

Emery RE: Interparental conflict and children of discord and divorce. Psychol Bull 92:310–330, 1982

Emery RE, O'Leary KD: Children's perceptions of marital discord and behavior problems of boys and girls. J Abnorm Child Psychol 10:11–24, 1982

Felner RD, Stolberg AL, Cowen EL: Crisis events and school mental health referral patterns of young children. J Consult Clin Psychol 43:305–310, 1975

Freed DJ, Foster HH: The shuffled child and divorce court. Trial 10:26–41, 1974

Furstenberg FF Jr: Conjugal succession: Reentering marriage after divorce, in Life-Span Development and Behavior, vol 4. Edited by Baltes PB, Brim OG. New York, Academic Press, 1982

Gardner RA: Psychotherapy and Children of Divorce. New York, Jason Aronson, 1976

Gardner RA: Family Evaluation in Child Custody Litigation. Cresskill NJ, Creative Therapeutics, 1982

Goldstein HS: Reconstructed families: The second marriage and its children. Psychiatr Q 48:433–440, 1974

Goldstein J, Freud A, Solnit A: Beyond the Best Interests of the Child. New York, Free Press, 1973

Goldzband MG: Custody Cases and Expert Witnesses: A Manual for Attorneys. New York, Harcourt Brace Jovanovich, 1980

Group for the Advancement of Psychiatry: Divorce, Child Custody and the Family. New York, Mental Health Materials Center, 1980

Haynes J: Divorce Mediation. New York, Springer Publishing Co, 1981

Hess RD, Camara KA: Post-divorce relationships as mediating factors in the consequences of divorce for children. J Soc Issues 35:79–96, 1979

Hetherington E: Divorce: A child's perspective. Am Psychol 34:851–858, 1979

Hetherington E, Cox M, Cox R: The aftermath of divorce, in Mother-Child Relations. Edited by Stevens H, Mathews M. Washington DC, National Association for Education of Young Children, 1978

Hetherington EM, Cox M, Cox R: Effects of divorce on parents and children, in Nontraditional Families: Parenting and Child Development. Edited by Lamb ME. Hillsdale NJ, Lawrence Erlbaum Associates, 1982

Huntington DS: Divorce and the developmental needs of children, in Mediation of Child Custody and Visitation Disputes. California Chapter, Association of Family and Conciliation Courts, Institute for Training and Research, 1982.

Ilfeld FW Jr, Ilfeld HZ, Alexander JR: Does joint custody work? A first look at outcome data of relitigation. Am J Psychiatry 139:62–66, 1982

Jacobs J: The effect of divorce on father: An overview of the literature. Am J Psychiatry 139:1235–1244, 1982

Jacobson DS: The impact of marital separation/divorce on children: II. Interparental hostility and child adjustment. J Divorce 2:3–20, 1978

Jacobson DS: Conflict, visiting and child adjustment in the stepfamily: A linked family system. Paper presented at Annual Meeting of the American Orthopsychiatric Association, Boston, 1983

Kalter N: Children of divorce in an outpatient psychiatric population. Am J Orthopsychiatry 47:40–51, 1977

Kelly JB: The visiting relationship after divorce: Research findings and clinical implications, in Children of Separation and Divorce: Management and Treatment. Edited by Stuart IR, Abt LE. New York, Van Nostrand Reinhold Co, 1981

Kelly JB, Wallerstein JS: The effects of parental divorce: Experiences of the child in early latency. Am J Orthopsychiatry 46:20–32, 1976

Kelly JB, Wallerstein JS: Part-time parent, part-time child: Visiting after divorce. J Clin Child Psychol 6:51–55, 1977

Kelly JB, Wallerstein JS: The divorced child in the school. National Principal 59:51–58, 1979

Lindemann E: Symptomatology and management of acute grief. Am J Psychiatry 101:141–148, 1944

Mnookin RH, Kornhauser L: Bargaining in the shadow of the law: The case of divorce. Yale Law J 88:950–997, 1979

Morrison AL: A prospective study of divorce: Its relation to children's development and parental functioning. Unpublished dissertation, University of California at Berkeley, 1982

Norton AJ: Family life cycle: 1980. J Marriage Fam 45:267–275, 1983

Pearson J, Thoennes N, Vanderkooi L: The decision to mediate: Profiles of individuals who accept and reject the opportunity to mediate contested child custody and visitation issues, in Therapists, Lawyers, and Divorcing Spouses. Edited by Fisher EO, Fisher MS. New York, Haworth Press, 1982

Philips I: Opportunities for prevention in the practice of psychiatry. Am J Psychiatry 140:389–395, 1983

Pope H, Mueller CW: The intergenerational transmission of marital instability: Comparisons of race and sex, in Divorce and Separation: Context, Causes, and Consequences. Edited by Levinger G, Moles OC. New York, Basic Books, 1979

Rankin RP, Maneker JS: The duration of marriage in a divorcing population: The impact of children. Unpublished manuscript, 1983

Richards MPM: Marital separation and children: Some problems of method and theory. Paper presented at Fourth Rugby Research Seminar of the National Marriage Guidance Council, April 1982

Rutter M: Sex differences in children's response to family stress, in The Child in His Family. Edited by Anthony EJ, Koupernik C. New York, John Wiley & Sons, 1970

Santrock JW, Warshak RA: Father custody and social development in boys and girls. J Soc Issues 35:112–125, 1979

Solow RA, Adams PL: Custody by agreement: Child psychiatrist as child advocate. J Psychiatry Law 5:77–100, 1977

Springer C, Wallerstein JS: Young adolescents' responses to their parents' divorces, in Children and Divorce. Edited by Kurdek LA. San Francisco, Jossey-Bass, 1983

Steinman S: The experience of children in a joint custody arrangement: A report of a study. Am J Orthopsychiatry 51:403–414, 1981

Tall J, Johnston J: Mandatory mediation within a court setting. Paper presented at Annual Meeting of the American Orthopsychiatric Association, San Francisco, 1982

Tessman LH: Children of Parting Parents. New York, Jason Aronson, 1977

Tooley K: Antisocial behavior and social alienation post divorce: The "man of the house" and his mother. Am J Orthopsychiatry 46:33–42, 1976

United States Bureau of the Census, Current Population Reports, P-23, No 114: Characteristics of American Children and Youth: 1980. Washington DC, US Government Printing Office, 1982a

United States Bureau of the Census, Current Population Reports, Series P-20, No 372: Marital Status and Living Arrangements: March 1981. Washington DC, US Government Printing Office, 1982b

Wallerstein JS: Responses of the pre-school child to divorce: Those who cope, in Child Psychiatry: Treatment and Research. Edited by McMillan MF, Henao S. New York, Brunner/Mazel, 1977

Wallerstein JS: Current environments for young children in separating and divorced families. Presented at the MacArthur Conference on Child Care: Growth Fostering Environments for Young Children (to be published in conference proceedings), Chicago, 1982

Wallerstein JS: Children of divorce: The psychological tasks of the child. Am J Orthopsychiatry 53:230–243, 1983

Wallerstein JS: Children of divorce: Preliminary report of a ten-year follow-up, in The Child in His Family, vol 5. Edited by Anthony EJ, Chilland C. New York, John Wiley & Sons, in press[a]

Wallerstein JS: Parent-child relationships following divorce, in Clinical Aspects of Parenthood. Edited by Anthony EJ, Pollock G. Boston, Little Brown & Co, in press[b]

Wallerstein JS, Kelly JB: The effects of parental divorce: The adolescent experience, in The Child in His Family: Children at Psychiatric Risk, vol 3. Edited by Anthony EJ, Koupernik C. New York, John Wiley & Sons, 1974

Wallerstein JS, Kelly JB: The effects of parental divorce: The experiences of the preschool child. J Am Acad Child Psychiatry 14:600–616, 1975

Wallerstein JS, Kelly JB: The effects of parental divorce: Experiences of the child in later latency. Am J Orthopsychiatry 46:256–269, 1976

Wallerstein JS, Kelly JB: Divorce counseling: A community service for families in the midst of divorce. Am J Orthopsychiatry 47:4–22, 1977

Wallerstein JS, Kelly JB: Surviving the Breakup: How Children and Parents Cope With Divorce. New York, Basic Books, 1980a

Wallerstein JS, Kelly JB: Effects of divorce on the father-child relationship. Am J Psychiatry 137:1534–1539, 1980b

Warshak RA, Santrock JW: The impact of divorce in father-custody and mother-custody homes: The child's perspective, in Children and Divorce. Edited by Kurdek LA. San Francisco, Jossey-Bass, 1983

Watson A: The children of Armageddon: Problems of children following divorce. Syracuse Law Rev 21:231–239, 1969

Weiss RS: Growing up a little faster. J Soc Issues 35:97–111, 1979

Winn M: The loss of childhood. The New York Times Magazine, 8 May 1983

Zill N: Divorce, marital conflict, and children's mental health: Research findings and policy recommendations. Testimony before Subcommittee on Family and Human Services, United States Senate Subcommittee on Labor and Human Resources, 22 March 1983

III

Consultation-Liaison Psychiatry

Part III

Consultation-Liaison Psychiatry

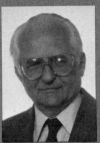

Zbigniew J. Lipowski, M.D.,
Preceptor

Professor of Psychiatry
University of Toronto at the
  Clarke Institute of Psychiatry

Authors for Part III

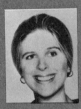

Stephanie Cavanaugh, M.D.
Chief, Consultation-Liaison Service
Associate Professor of Psychiatry
Rush-Presbyterian-St. Luke's
  Medical Center

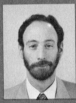

Robert M. Wettstein, M.D.
Assistant Professor of Psychiatry
Rush-Presbyterian-St. Luke's
  Medical Center

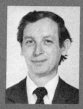

Harvey Moldofsky, M.D.

Professor of Psychiatry
and of Medicine
University of Toronto
Psychiatrist-in-Chief
Toronto Western Hospital

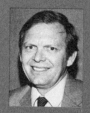

Charles V. Ford, M.D.

Professor of Psychiatry
Director, Consultation-
Liaison Service
Vanderbilt University
School of Medicine
Vanderbilt Medical Center

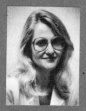

Mary Jane Massie, M.D.

Assistant Attending Psychiatrist
Psychiatry Service
Memorial Sloan-Kettering
Cancer College
Assistant Professor of Psychiatry
Cornell University
Medical Center

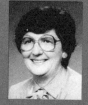

Jimmie C. Holland, M.D.

Chief
Psychiatry Service
Memorial Sloan-Kettering
Cancer College
Professor of Psychiatry
Cornell University
Medical Center

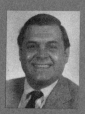

Michael R. Milano, M.D.

Assistant Clinical Professor
of Psychiatry
Columbia Presbyterian
Medical Center

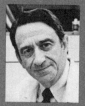

Donald S. Kornfeld, M.D.

Professor of Clinical
Psychiatry
Columbia Presbyterian
Medical Center

Consultation-Liaison Psychiatry

	Page
Introduction to Part Three *Zbigniew J. Lipowski, M.D.*	177
Chapter 12	179
History, Definition, and Scope of Consultation-Liaison Psychiatry *Zbigniew J. Lipowski, M.D.*	
History	179
Current Definition and Scope	183
Conclusions	186
Chapter 13	187
Prevalence of Psychiatric Morbidity in Medical Populations *Stephanie Cavanaugh, M.D.,* *Robert M. Wettstein, M.D.*	
Introduction	187
Mental Disorders in Outpatient Populations	189
Mental Disorders in Inpatient Populations	198
Specific Psychiatric Disorders	203
Conclusions	213
Chapter 14	215
Clinical Research at the Interface of Medicine and Psychiatry *Harvey Moldofsky, M.D.*	
Mechanisms of Illness	215
Therapeutic Studies	226
Conclusions	230
Chapter 15	231
Psychiatry and Geriatric Medicine *Charles V. Ford, M.D.*	
Patterns of Consultation	231
Psychiatric Diagnosis	231
Roles of the Consultation-Liaison Psychiatrist	236
Conclusion	238

Chapter 16   *239*
Psychiatry and Oncology
  Mary Jane Massie, M.D.,
  Jimmie C. Holland, M.D.
Risk Factors and Management Issues
  in Cancer   239
Psychiatric Disorders in Cancer Patients   245
Nausea and Vomiting   254
Psychological Sequelae in Cured and
  Long-Surviving Patients   254
Summary   256

Chapter 17   *256*
Psychiatry and Surgery
  Michael R. Milano, M.D.,
  Donald S. Kornfeld, M.D.
The Preoperative Phase   256
The Perioperative Phase   260
The Postoperative Phase   262
Psychiatric Aspects of Specific
  Procedures and Fields   262
Psychiatric Liaison with Surgery   276

References for Part Three   *278*

Introduction
by Zbigniew J. Lipowski, M.D.

The reciprocal relations between the mental or psychological and the somatic or physiological aspects of man's functioning in health and disease have been key themes in Western thought and medicine for 2,500 years. From the time of Hippocrates until the seventeenth century, Western medicine was both somatically and holistically oriented. All illness was considered to be disordered somatic function, and the patient was seen as a psychophysiological whole. Then Descartes split asunder the concepts of mind and body, and the mental aspects of man became the concern of philosophers and theologians, while the body became the province of scientists and physicians. Despite this split, the role of emotions in health and disease remained a strong interest of medicine until the second half of the nineteenth century. Virchow's theory of cellular pathology and the subsequent bacteriological discoveries of Pasteur and Koch then propelled medicine toward a mechanistic approach and away from any regard for psychosocial factors in human health and disease (Lipowski, in press).

In the United States, Benjamin Rush, the father of American psychiatry, in the late eighteenth century established a tradition of a truly holistic approach to medicine (Lipowski, 1981). That tradition, however, was soon eclipsed, and psychiatry and medicine separated from each other conceptually, clinically, and geographically. Attempts to bring them back together began in the second half of the nineteenth century but encountered entrenched opposition. At the turn of the century, though, Adolf Meyer and other psychobiologically oriented psychiatrists succeeded in attaining a measure of collaboration. By the 1920s, general hospital psychiatric units were developing on a growing scale. These units served as a vehicle for the teaching of clinical psychiatry and for collaborative clinical work between psychiatrists and nonpsychiatric physicians. The trend received added impetus from the emergence of psychosomatic medicine in the early 1930s (Lipowski, 1981; in press).

Consultation-liaison psychiatry emerged around 1930 as an effort to apply psychosomatic conceptions to medical practice and to provide psychiatric consultations to medical and surgical patients in the general hospitals (see the Preceptor's chapter in this Part). In the past decade, consultation-liaison psychiatry has shown unprecedented growth and has become a subspeciality of psychiatry. This rapid growth has created a need to update it.

Each of the chapters in this Part covers a major aspect of consultation-liaison psychiatry, and all are authored by colleagues who have actively contributed to its growth in at least one of its core areas: conceptual, clinical, investigative, or educational.

In the first chapter, the Preceptor reviews the history and defines the scope of consultation-liaison psychiatry, highlighting its present state.

In the second chapter, Drs. Stephanie Cavanaugh and Robert M. Wettstein survey the studies of the prevalence of psychiatric disorder in medical patient populations, and they also discuss the methodological problems that stem from difficulties in reliable case finding. These problems have challenged psychiatric epidemiology generally, but they are especially formidable in medical settings. As Drs. Cavanaugh and Wettstein discuss, medical patients tend to display overlapping symptoms of both physical and psychiatric illness, which complicates the diagnosis of psychopathology. Furthermore, DSM-III has not elaborated a diagnostic schema and nosology that is sufficiently applicable to such a mixed patient population. A reliable estimate of the frequency of psychiatric morbidity in medical settings is a pressing need, however, if we are to formulate guidelines for staffing consultation-liaison services, for teaching, and for planning specific research projects.

Dr. Harvey Moldofsky undertakes the difficult task of surveying recent research at the interface of medicine and psychiatry. To review this research in detail and to include all its diverse aspects would be impossible in the space allotted, and some relevant studies are discussed in the other chapters. As Dr. Moldofsky demonstrates, psychosomatic research has recently moved away from studies of the putative role of psychological factors in the etiology of the so-called psychosomatic disorders. The focus today is much broader and includes the psychophysiological mechanisms and processes which mediate between life events and their subjective appraisal by the individual, on the one hand, and the development, course, and outcome of subsequent physical illness, on the other. Furthermore, the impact of physical illness or injury on various aspects of psychological functioning has attracted growing research interest lately, as the chapters on oncology and surgery illustrate.

The remaining three chapters deal primarily with three clinical areas that concern consultation-liaison psychiatrists: geriatrics, oncology, and surgery. Dr. Charles V. Ford discusses the psychiatric problems of elderly patients encountered in medical settings. The aging of the population in general and the high prevalence and incidence of both physical and psychiatric morbidity among older people converge to make this a very timely topic. Its growing importance has only begun to gain the appreciation of consultation-liaison psychiatrists. (This chapter complements the Part on geriatric psychiatry in Volume II of *Psychiatry Update*.)

Drs. Mary Jane Massie and Jimmie C. Holland focus their chapter on the fast-developing area of psychiatric oncology. Their chapter and its subject illustrate clearly how involved consultation-liaison psychiatrists have become in clinical work and research with one of the most important diseases. Yet, only two decades ago, cancer was thought to be too "organic" a disease to call for psychosomatic research or for psychiatric care.

Finally, Drs. Michael R. Milano and Donald S. Kornfeld explore the interface of psychiatry and surgery. Advances in surgical techniques have helped to save lives, but they have also given rise to a range of psychiatric complications and psychosocial problems that consultation-liaison psychiatrists are called upon to diagnose, treat, and, if possible, prevent. The work of Dr. Kornfeld and his associates on cardiac surgery exemplifies the complexity and clinical relevance of this aspect of consultation-liaison psychiatry.

Many subjects that concern consultation-liaison psychiatry could not be covered within the space limits of this Part. Hemodialysis, cardiac rehabilitation, somatoform disorders, pediatrics, and the use of psychotropic drugs in the physically ill are among these relevant topics. The Preceptor is responsible for choosing the subjects that are included and believes that they are representative of the focal concerns of consultation-liaison psychiatry today.

Chapter 12

History, Definition, and Scope of Consultation-Liaison Psychiatry
by Zbigniew J. Lipowski, M.D.

HISTORY

Beginnings: 1930–1945

Efforts to bring psychiatry into the general hospital and to provide psychiatric consultations for medical and surgical patients began around the turn of this century (Sweeney, 1962). At the forefront of those efforts were the leaders of the influential psychobiological school of psychiatry, such as Meyer and White, who advocated a holistic approach to both medicine and psychiatry (Lipowski, 1981a). In 1929 one of Meyer's students, George W. Henry, wrote a pioneering paper on the work of a psychiatric consultant attached to the medical wards of a general hospital. Another of Meyer's followers, Helen Flanders Dunbar, began in 1930 to work as such a consultant at the Columbia Medical Center. She launched a large-scale psychosomatic study of medical and surgical patients and became one of the founders of psychosomatic medicine. Consultation-liaison psychiatry thus emerged as an outgrowth of general hospital psychiatry, psychobiology, and psychosomatic medicine (Lipowski, 1981a).

Between 1934 and 1940, the Rockefeller Foundation granted funds to six university hospitals for the creation of psychiatric departments which would do collaborative clinical work and teaching (Greenhill, 1977). At the Colorado General Hospital in Denver, one of those new departments was named the Psychiatric Liaison Department, and it functioned de facto as a general hospital psychiatric unit without beds (Billings, 1941). This department's director, Edward G. Billings, was probably the first writer to introduce the term *liaison psychiatry* into the literature (Billings, 1939). In an enthusiastic report on the progress of his department, he claimed that the integration of psychiatry and medicine in the general hospital had raised diagnostic and therapeutic effectiveness, shortened hospital stays of patients, and resulted in considerable savings (Billings, 1941). A few other hospitals organized distinct psychiatric consultation services based in their psychiatric units (Ripley, 1940). Liaison teaching was hailed as an effective means of breaking down the barriers between medicine and psychiatry (Ebaugh and Rymer, 1942). By the middle 1940s the Rockefeller grants had been phased out, and consultation-liaison services entered a period of slowed but continued growth.

Conceptual Development: 1945–1970

Between 1946 and 1957, consultation-liaison services were established in a number of teaching hospitals, including the Mount Sinai Hospital in New York, the Johns Hopkins Hospital, the Strong Memorial Hospital in Rochester, NY, and the Massachusetts General Hospital (Greenhill, 1977). These new services attracted individuals to work at the borderland between medicine and psychiatry, and they in turn began to formulate objectives, operational models, and procedural methods for consultation-liaison psychiatry. The first comprehensive review of this conceptual work appeared in 1967 (Lipowski, 1967a; 1967b), and the first handbook was published in 1968 (Schwab, 1968).

The main functions proposed for consultation-liaison psychiatrists included delivering clinical service in the form of psychiatric consultations to nonpsychiatric physicians, teaching the psychosocial and psychiatric aspects of medicine, and conducting research at the interface of medicine and psychiatry (Lipowski, 1967a; 1967b). The professed objectives of the field itself were to raise patient care standards in the general hospitals by increasing attention to the neglected psychosocial dimension, to help prevent, diagnose, and manage psychiatric morbidity in medical settings, and to build working and conceptual bridges between medicine and psychiatry. The crucial question, one that elicited diverse answers, was how best to attain those objectives. Consultation-liaison psychiatrists developed several strategies. Some centered on the provision and proper conduct of the consultations, and others centered on teaching psychosocial aspects of medicine and psychosomatic concepts to medical students and nonpsychiatric physicians. The approaches which evolved reflected the predominant trends in psychiatry, notably psychodynamics, social psychiatry, crisis theory, and the biopsychosocial conceptions of disease and medical care that are based on general systems theory.

The conduct and process of psychiatric consultation received much attention. In its traditional form, consultation had entailed a diagnostic assessment and management advice concerning a patient referred by a nonpsychiatric physician. The consultation tended to follow the usual medical model, involved neither therapy with the patient nor contact with the consultee, and was not concerned with interpersonal issues or teaching. In the 1950s and 1960s consultation-liaison psychiatrists proposed several new and broader models which substantially modified the conduct of the psychiatric consultation in medical settings. The five new models were

1. a patient-oriented consultation which included not only a formal diagnostic assessment but also, as a basis for psychological management, a psychodynamic evaluation of the patient's personality and reaction to illness (Kahana and Bibring, 1964);
2. a crisis-oriented, therapeutic consultation involving a rapid assessment of the patient's predicament and coping style, along with psychotherapeutic intervention by the consultant (Weisman and Hackett, 1960);
3. a consultee-oriented consultation, in which the main target was the consultee and his or her problem with a given patient (Schiff and Pilot, 1959);

4. a situation-oriented consultation focused on the interaction between the patient and the clinical team (Greenberg, 1960); and
5. an expanded psychiatric consultation concerned with the patient as a central figure in an operational group that included him or her, the clinical staff, and the patient's family (Meyer and Mendelson, 1961).

These models went far beyond the traditional medical format and constituted a practically important advance. They highlighted the need for psychodynamic understanding of the patient's attitude and behavior, of his or her interactions with concerned others, and of the needs of the consultee. The consultant was expected to play an expanded role, one that included therapy, mediation in interpersonal conflicts, and teaching.

Further conceptual developments focused on the communicational and ethical aspects of the consultation process itself. The process usually includes a series of communications, beginning with the request for a consultation, followed by a comprehensive diagnostic interview with the patient, and entailing various verbal and written communications with the consultee and other members of the clinical staff (Lipowski, 1967a). The field began to recognize that these communications need to clarify the issues involved and must be practically useful. The linguistic and ethical aspects of consultation must be taken into account, that is, the manner in which participants use language and bring their respective values to bear on the conduct and outcome of consultation (Sandt and Leifer, 1964).

A major conceptual development involved the formulation of two related, yet distinct, operational models for consultation-liaison services: the consultation model and the liaison model. According to the former, the primary concern of consultation-liaison psychiatrists should be to deliver clinical service to patients and consultees in the form of prompt, competent, and practically useful psychiatric consultations, and, where indicated, therapy for the patient. Teaching was considered secondary.

In contrast, the liaison model emphasized sustained, regular contact between the psychiatrist and one or more divisions of a general hospital for the purpose of teaching, case finding, crisis prevention and intervention, and consulting (Bernstein and Kaufman, 1962; Beigler et al., 1959). The liaison psychiatrist was expected to become a member of the medical team and to be free to interview any patient without a formal referral (Bernstein and Kaufman, 1962).

Kaufman (1953) stressed that the liaison psychiatrist should make his or her contribution to the medical team explicitly as a psychiatrist. On the other hand, Engel et al. (1957) of the University of Rochester (NY) insisted that the physician doing liaison work should be trained both in medicine or one of its subspecialities and in psychiatry, since such a person would be most able to offer a professional role model of a psychosocially oriented doctor to nonpsychiatrists and medical students. Provision of psychiatric consultation was not a matter of concern to the liaison staff. The Rochester model was idiosyncratic in its emphasis on teaching and on the dual training of the liaison physician. It really represented psychosocial medicine, not consultation-liaison, a point which has often been overlooked in discussions of its merits and its alleged superiority over the other approaches to consultation-liaison work.

Another proposed organizational model was that of a consultation-liaison team which would include nonmedical liaison workers such as nurses, social workers, and psychologists, as well as psychiatrists (Greenhill, 1977; Lipowski, 1967a). The addition of nonmedical personnel was expected to increase the scope and effectiveness of a consultation-liaison service, provided that the tasks of the individual members were clearly delineated and that their work was coordinated by a liaison psychiatrist in charge.

By 1970, consultation-liaison psychiatry had thus emerged as a distinct area of special interest in psychiatry, one with reasonably well-defined goals, scope, and organizational and work models. What lagged behind were the spread of the services beyond the prestigious teaching hospitals, training in consultation-liaison psychiatry, and research on the outcomes of consultation-liaison work.

Growth: 1970 to Present

Consultation-liaison psychiatry began to grow rapidly in the early 1970s, thanks largely to a decision by the National Institute of Mental Health to sponsor the expansion of existing services and the establishment of new ones and to fund fellowships for trainees in consultation-liaison work (Eaton et al., 1977). As a result, the number and size of consultation-liaison services have increased markedly, and many young psychiatrists have been attracted to the field. Consultation-liaison psychiatry has become an integral part of psychiatric residency training (Schubert and McKegney, 1976). Its scope has expanded to include the whole range of medical subspecialities and settings such as critical care units, neurology, pediatrics, obstetrics, and so forth (Faguet et al., 1978; Pasnau, 1975). Concurrently, the literature has grown in volume and diversity of topics. Two new journals, largely devoted to consultation-liaison subjects, have been founded, *Psychiatry in Medicine* (now the *International Journal of Psychiatry in Medicine*) and *General Hospital Psychiatry*. Several handbooks have been published (Glickman, 1980; Pasnau, 1975; Strain and Grossman, 1975), and several reviews have appeared (Greenhill, 1977; Lipowski, 1974; 1979). Theoretical articles have focused on such issues as the application of a systems approach to psychiatric consultation (Glazer and Astrachan, 1978–79; Tarnow and Guttstein, 1982–83), the importance of group dynamics in medical settings (Wise and Goldberg, 1981), the social role and status of the liaison psychiatrist (Mohl, 1979), and the stresses of consultation-liaison work (Wise and Berlin, 1981). Some writers have addressed the ethical problems facing the consultation-liaison psychiatrist who is asked to legitimate medical or surgical treatment for a patient who refuses it (Perl and Shelp, 1982; Starkman and Youngs, 1974). Last but not least, much-needed reports on the outcomes of consultation-liaison clinical work and teaching have begun to appear and have recently been reviewed (McKegney and Beckhardt, 1982). Research at the interface of medicine and psychiatry has attracted a growing number of consultation-liaison psychiatrists and shows increasing methodological sophistication (Lipowski, 1983a).

The unprecedented recent growth of consultation-liaison psychiatry has fostered diverse viewpoints on what its main objectives should be and how to attain them. Sharp controversy has arisen between the proponents of the liaison model, on the one hand, and those of the consultation model, on the other. Advocates for the former model assert that intensive liaison and a social systems approach are superior by virtue of their high educational and preventive efficacy (Strain and Grossman, 1975). Their opponents argue that the consultation-liaison psychiatrist's overriding concern should be the patient and the delivery of clinical service, while social issues and efforts to convert consultees to the biopsychosocial model are better left alone (Cassem, 1983). These polemics have at times been acrimonious and needlessly divisive. Some consultation-liaison psychiatrists have gone so far as to speak of consultation psychiatry and liaison psychiatry as two separate domains (Glickman, 1980; Strain and Grossman, 1975). In the author's opinion, such a sharp dichotomy is false and serves to undermine the subspeciality as a whole (Lipowski, 1981b; 1983c). Both consultation and liaison are integral components of the work, as the very designation *consultation-liaison* underscores. The controversy really pertains to what is the best strategy toward better psychosocial patient care, and it must be resolved by rational debate, outcome studies, and compromise, if consultation-liaison psychiatry is to develop further and to achieve its goals.

Over the past 15 years or so, consultation-liaison psychiatry has been transformed from a marginal area of special interest into a full-fledged subspeciality of psychiatry, one with a defined scope, objectives, and procedures. As advances in medical treatment have brought with them a new crop of psychosocial and psychiatric problems and complications, consultation-liaison psychiatry has itself become more complex, and its practitioners now need to possess a considerable body of specialized knowledge and skills.

CURRENT DEFINITION AND SCOPE

Consultation-liaison may now be defined as a subspeciality of psychiatry concerned with (1) the diagnosis, treatment, study, and prevention of psychiatric morbidity among physically ill and somatizing patients (those who communicate their emotional distress in the form of somatic symptoms) and (2) the provision of psychiatric consultations, liaison, and teaching for nonpsychiatric health workers in all types of clinical settings, but especially in general hospitals (Lipowski, 1983a). This definition of consultation-liaison psychiatry delimits the scope of the field in terms of the nature of the target patient population, the clinical settings in which consultation-liaison psychiatrists work, and the functions which they perform.

Confusion has surrounded the term *liaison* in this context, and the ambiguity of the term has contributed to the controversy referred to earlier. The term has been used in three main senses: first, as a shorter synonym for consultation-liaison psychiatry, second, to refer to regular contacts by a liaison psychiatrist with members of a particular medical or surgical ward or special unit, and, third, to express one's predilection for the liaison model of consultation-liaison psychiatry. As the meaning of liaison itself is imprecise and the term is often used loosely, futile arguments over the place of liaison in consultation-liaison have arisen readily.

The Patients

The two main groups of patients with whom consultation-liaison psychiatrists work are the physically ill and the somatizers. The physically ill constitute about 70 to 80 percent of the patients referred (Lipowski and Wolston, 1981), and they present a wide range of diagnostic and therapeutic problems. First, they display psychosocial reactions to their illnesses or injuries, reactions which often add to the burden of the illness for both the patient and his or her family. Consultation-liaison psychiatrists need to be familiar with the cognitive, emotional, behavioral, and interpersonal dimensions of these reactions and be ready to intervene in preventing and managing those which are maladaptive (Lipowski, 1983c). Second, the physically ill may develop one or both of two basic sets of psychiatric complications related to their illnesses, those which result from cerebral dysfunction and constitute the organic brain syndromes and those which represent reactions to the personal meaning of the illness and its social and economic consequences (Lipowski, 1975). The most common psychiatric disorders encountered in this patient population include depressive and anxiety disorders and the organic brain syndromes (Lipowski and Wolston, 1981). Third, a physically ill patient may present a diagnostic problem because psychopathological symptoms replace or mask the strictly physical ones (Hall, 1980; Lipowski, 1967b). Fourth, a patient may develop a psychiatric disorder as a side effect of medical drugs (Shader, 1972) or in response to hospitalization or a nonpharmacologic medical or surgical treatment. As well as saving lives, medical advances such as open heart surgery, renal hemodialysis, intravenous hyperalimentation, critical care medicine, surgery for obesity, and many others have resulted in an array of psychiatric problems with which a consultation-liaison psychiatrist must be familiar.

The second large group of patients are the somatizing patients, those who fear or believe themselves to be physically ill because they are experiencing somatic symptoms and those who for some reason communicate their needs or distress in terms of bodily discomfort (Barsky and Klerman, 1983; Ford, 1983). This ill-defined and insufficiently studied group accounts for 20 to 30 percent of consultation-liaison psychiatrists' case loads on medical and surgical wards, and the patients pose a formidable diagnostic and therapeutic challenge. They present with pain or some other physical symptom which, even after exhaustive investigations, cannot be explained in terms of demonstrable pathophysiology. They also tend to seek medical care persistently, to be resented by physicians, and to overuse health care resources.

Aside from and transcending these two groupings, since elderly people account for about a third of the general hospital population, consultation-liaison psychiatrists must be familiar with the whole range of geropsychiatric problems (Lipowski, 1983b).

The Settings

The most common and important settings for consultation-liaison work are the medical and surgical wards and the specialized units of the general hospital. Some consultation-liaison psychiatrists work full- or part-time in outpatient clinics, rehabilitation centers, nursing homes, and primary care. Each clinical setting offers specific problems related to its own social and physical features and to the characteristics of the patients treated in it. The consultation-liaison worker must be familiar with the specifics of each milieu, be it an oncology or dermatology ward, a coronary or burn unit, or a rehabilitation division for cardiac or stroke patients.

Functions of Consultation-Liaison Psychiatrists

Clinical work, teaching, and research are the main functions of consultation-liaison psychiatrists. The clinical work includes consulting, liaison, and therapy.

CLINICAL WORK: CONSULTATION   Psychiatric consultation is the cornerstone of consultation-liaison clinical activities. Consultations are primarily patient centered in that the consultant's overriding concerns are the patient's welfare, psychological state, distress, behavior, complaints, and therapeutic needs. At the same time, the consultant must consider the consultee's concerns and expectations regarding the patient's diagnosis, behavior, and management. The several models of consultation described earlier are applied flexibly as the situation demands. At a very minimum, however, a properly conducted consultation should include (1) a comprehensive biopsychosocial evaluation of the patient; (2) adequate communication with the consultee and, if indicated, other members of the clinical team; (3) an interview with a key member of the patient's family; (4) follow-up of the patient throughout his or her hospitalization; and (5) appropriate referral of the patient for subsequent psychiatric care if needed (Lipowski, 1967a). Such a comprehensive consultation features a measure of liaison with the clinical staff concerned with the patient's care and has teaching potential for all concerned.

CLINICAL WORK: LIAISON   A properly conducted consultation, as noted, contains a measure of liaison with the consultee and may involve efforts to enhance communication, trust, and cooperation between patients and staff. Liaison may thus be viewed as an integral component of psychiatric consultation in medical settings (Lipowski, 1967a; 1981b). More intensive liaison, entailing regular contacts with a given clinical team, is usually employed in those hospital areas where there is a high incidence of psychiatric morbidity and psychosocial problems such as psychological stress for the clinical staff. Intensive liaison tends to concentrate on critical care medicine, hemodialysis and burn units, oncology, rehabilitation, and pediatrics (Greenhill, 1977; Lipowski, 1974). A consultation-liaison psychiatrist attached to such an area is concerned not only with individual patients, but also with the ward or unit as a social milieu whose dynamics influence patient care for better or worse. The extent to which a given consultation-liaison service focuses on liaison depends on its ideological orientation, its human and financial resources, and the medical staff's receptiveness. Intensive liaison must not be regarded as appropriate for all situations and settings, but must be applied with discrimination and flexibility.

CLINICAL WORK: THERAPY   A third clinical activity of consultation-liaison work is therapy. The consultation-liaison psychiatrist functions as a therapist both directly and indirectly. Directly, he or she provides brief psychotherapy at the patient's bedside where indicated, as a means of crisis intervention and to help the patient cope adaptively with the illness and its consequences (Weisman and Hackett, 1960). Indirectly, the consultation-liaison psychiatrist functions as a therapist by offering specific advice to the consultee. Advice may be psychological, psychopharmacologic, or both. Psychological advice to the consultee or other members of the medical team may focus on how to approach a given patient psychologically. Other interventions, direct or indirect, may include application of behavioral medicine or relaxation techniques (Goldiamond, 1979), hypnosis (Wain, 1979), counseling on alcoholism-related problems (Beresford, 1979), and family therapy (Lipsitt and Lipsitt, 1981). Advice on the use of psychotropic drugs is frequently involved in consultation-liaison work (Lipowski and Wolston, 1981), and the psychiatrist must be thoroughly familiar with the indications for and the hazards of the various psychotropic drugs with medical patients (Solow, 1975).

TEACHING   Teaching the psychosocial aspects of medicine and medical psychiatry has been a key function of consultation-liaison psychiatrists from the beginning. Educational efforts have involved medical students, nonpsychiatric physicians, psychiatric residents, consultation-liaison fellows, and others. Some consultation-liaison psychiatrists view teaching as their primary responsibility, while others regard it as a relatively secondary function, subordinate to and largely focused on the clinical work.

RESEARCH   Beginning with Dunbar in 1930, consultation-liaison psychiatrists have been involved in studies at the interface of medicine and psychiatry. A second major research interest of consultation-liaison psychiatry is still in its beginnings, evaluation of the clinical and teaching aspects of consultation-liaison work (McKegney and Beckhardt, 1982). Evaluation studies have explored a variety of issues, including the benefits of psychiatric consultation for the patient and the consultee, the consultee's compliance with the consultant's recommendations, and the outcome of consultation-liaison teaching in terms of medical students' and physicians' attitudes toward patients. The least-explored evaluation issue has been the cost-effectiveness of consultation-liaison interventions (Levitan and Kornfeld, 1981). A third group of research studies has examined the types, prevalence, and incidence of psychiatric morbidity among medical patients.

CONCLUSIONS

Although fifty years old, consultation-liaison psychiatry has only recently emerged as a major psychiatric subspeciality concerned with the psychosocial and psychiatric problems of medical patients. As the scope and complexity of the field have increased, proper specialized training has become necessary. The field now incorporates a body of knowledge, techniques, and theoretical formulations regarding the characteristics of the patients and the clinical settings that are of special concern. Efforts to integrate psychiatry and medicine have encountered formidable obstacles (Brown and Zinberg, 1982) and have had only modest success. The success that has been achieved, however, has resulted largely from the clinical work and teaching efforts of consultation-liaison psychiatrists.

Chapter 13

Prevalence of Psychiatric Morbidity in Medical Populations

by Stephanie Cavanaugh, M.D. and Robert M. Wettstein, M.D.

INTRODUCTION

The considerable prevalence of emotional disturbances in the general medical population is well established (Hankin and Oktay, 1979). The nature of the relationship between emotional disturbance and physical illness is, however, complex (Lipowski, 1975; 1979). When one encounters an emotional disturbance in a general medical patient, the following questions come to mind. First, to what extent was the emotional disorder present prior to the onset of the physical illness? Second, to what degree is the emotional disturbance related to issues other than the physical illness? Third, are the behavioral disturbances influenced by organic brain disease, i.e., structural or functional alterations of brain tissue? Finally, how did or how will the patient's emotional status affect the onset, course, or outcome of the medical illness? Such questions are clearly difficult to answer, since illness, both psychiatric and physical, is a final common pathway of a number of complex variables.

Considerable methodological difficulties surround prevalence studies. A patient with demonstrable physical illness and emotional dysfunction may have either "normal" emotional distress or a psychiatric illness. For example, a patient hospitalized on a medical ward with terminal cancer may complain of sadness, anxiety, inability to think and concentrate, loss of energy, initial and terminal insomnia, anorexia, and weight loss. A patient with these symptoms would be identified as a probable psychiatric case by a screening test such as the General Health Questionnaire (GHQ). Nevertheless, the patient's internist might state that his or her symptoms were "understandable" given the stressors of illness and hospitalization (Klerman, 1981). A psychiatrist, on the other hand, might see the patient as having distress of sufficient intensity to warrant intervention. Although not exactly comparable to the patient with a physical illness, the bereaved patient is an example of a patient presenting with a "psychiatric syndrome," but demonstrating a "normal" reaction to loss. Clayton et al. (1972) reported that 35 percent of widows fulfilled criteria for a major depressive disorder at one month following bereavement, and certainly bereaved patients suffer considerable anguish. Furthermore, recent studies relevant to the topic of this chapter show that bereaved and depressed patients are immunosuppressed and may be more vulnerable to physical illness (Ostfeld et al., 1983; Schleifer et al., 1983).

Because of the methodological variations and flaws in studies assessing the prevalence of emotional or psychiatric disturbance in medical populations, much of the data have limited general application. Psychiatric nomenclature and diagnostic criteria have changed significantly over the years that this research has been conducted, and generally accepted diagnoses have rarely been used. Furthermore, little research has been done to delineate psychiatric illness or to standardize psychiatric measures in medical populations. Consequently, the diagnostic criteria applicable to psychiatric populations are used in medical populations; for example, the vegetative symptoms used to make the diagnosis of a psychiatric illness can also be caused by physical illness (Kathol and Petty, 1981). DSM-III is of little assistance to the clinician attempting to diagnose psychiatric disorders in medically ill populations (Strain, 1981).

Psychiatric prevalence rates are affected by demographic characteristics, referral patterns, and the chronicity, severity, and type of medical illness of the patients attending the site studied. Private practice, office-based physicians may well encounter a greater proportion of patients without established or documented medical disease than hospital-based, outpatient referral clinics or inpatient medical units. The medically healthier sample will include more patients with functional disease than with concurrent medical and psychiatric disorders. Some studies carefully assess the presence and extent of physical illness while others do not. Thus, patients with somatic complaints unexplained by a physical illness are combined with those with demonstrable organic illness. High prevalence rates may result from including patient samples with minor rather than major psychiatric disorders, psychosomatic disorders (e.g., colitis, peptic ulcer disease), and patients without diagnosable medical disease who report somatic or functional symptoms. Prevalence data may be obtained retrospectively from medical charts, or prospectively with self-report questionnaires, or with diagnostic interviews. The diagnostic interview may be conducted by the general practitioner during a regular 15-minute clinic visit, by a research assistant skilled in interviewing psychiatric but not medical populations, or by psychiatrists experienced with patients in medical populations. Point prevalence and period prevalence are sometimes confused; incidence data are rarely reported. Furthermore, sampling biases arise in assessing the presence of psychiatric morbidity in a medical population which is confined to those actively seeking medical care and which excludes those who are not currently using medical services.

A final set of preliminary considerations relates to the use of screening tests for both clinical and research purposes. Clinically, screening tests have been shown to be valuable in detecting "hidden psychiatric disorders" in medical populations (Johnstone and Goldberg, 1976). This is particularly important given the underrecognition of emotional disorders by primary care physicians which has been reported by many authors (Goldberg and Blackwell, 1970; Cavanaugh, 1983; Nielsen and Williams, 1980). Failure to recognize psychiatric morbidity can result in unnecessary or risky specialized investigations, referrals, or intervention. Strain (1979) has suggested that a battery of screening tests can be given on admission, along with other routine medical diagnostic tests, to obtain a "psychological CBC." Such tests can help to determine the severity of dysfunction and provide a standardized measure of change over time. Johnstone and Goldberg (1976) found that detection by screening tests of hidden psychiatric disorder in a family practice setting had a beneficial outcome when the disorder was treated. In this study, 1,093 patients were given the GHQ, and those with hidden disorders were assigned to a treatment or control group. Treated patients had a shorter duration for the episode than those who were not treated, and patients with more severe disorders continued to show significant improvement over the control group.

Psychiatric screening instruments commonly used to detect general psychopathology in medical populations have been the Hopkins Symptom Checklist (HSCL) and the Cornell Medical Index (CMI), as well as the GHQ. The GHQ has been used in a number of populations and for the most part has been found to be fairly sensitive (.85) and specific (.80) in detecting emotional dysfunction (Goldberg, 1972). The GHQ score has been found to correlate well with severity ratings made by independent psychiatric interviews (Goldberg, 1972). Likewise, the CMI has been helpful in estimating the prevalence and severity of emotional morbidity (Shepherd et al., 1966). Other studies have shown the screening tests not to be useful in identifying psychiatric dysfunction. Glass et al. (1978), for example, found the HSCL did not distinguish psychiatric patients with and without psychiatric disease.

Screening tests for specific psychiatric disorders include the Beck Depression Inventory (BDI), the Zung, the Center for Epidemiological Studies Depression Scale (CES-D), and the Taylor Manifest Anxiety Scale. For the most part, these have not been standardized in medical populations. Standardization is essential because several of the items in these instruments are modified by physical illness. Screening instruments which detect organic brain dysfunction such as the Mini Mental Status Examination (MMSE) are presently being standardized for both inpatient and outpatient populations. It would appear that after standardization of screening tests is accomplished, a battery of relevant screening tests could be developed for different medical populations. One of the authors, for example, believes that the BDI, GHQ, and MMSE best measure the parameters of particular interest to the internist in inpatient medical populations: cognitive dysfunction, nonpsychotic psychiatric disturbance, and depression (Cavanaugh, 1983).

The remainder of the chapter reviews the research surveying the spectrum of psychiatric morbidity in outpatient and inpatient general medical populations and then presents work on several individual psychiatric disorders in these populations.

MENTAL DISORDERS IN OUTPATIENT POPULATIONS

Regier et al. (1978), in an extensive review of available epidemiologic data and recent mental health services research, estimated the one-year prevalence of mental disorder in the United States population to be at least 15 percent. Only one-fifth of these were identified in the mental health sector, while three-fifths were in the primary medical care sector. The authors stated that "based on multiple special surveys of general practice populations, 15 percent of a primary care physician's patients are estimated to have a mental disorder" (Regier et al., 1978, 689). A World Health Organization report reviewing studies of psychiatric disorder in general practice patients stated, "Since many of the relevant psychological variables are continuously distributed in populations, psychiatric case reporting will depend largely on what is accepted as the threshold of clinical abnormality. By current standards of what justifies medical intervention, between 10 and 20 percent of the general population present in any one year as psychiatric cases; about one-third of these can be classed as new cases" (World Health Organization, 1973, 18). Hankin and Oktay (1979), in the most comprehensive review of the literature on the identification and prevalence of psychiatric morbidity in medical settings, reviewed approximately seventy studies of medical outpatients between 1959 and 1975. They also concluded that the majority of studies found a rate of disorder between 10 and 20 percent.

According to the Hankin and Oktay (1979) review, the period prevalence rates of mental disorder for British general practice studies varied from under 1 percent to 25 percent, depending on several factors: (1) broader definitions of mental disorder resulted in higher reported psychiatric morbidity; (2) use of psychiatrist diagnoses or self-report symptom questionnaires resulted in higher rates than use of general practitioner diagnoses or rates of referral to a psychiatrist; (3) psychiatric morbidity of patients attending a practitioner's office exceeded that of patients who were only registered to the practice; and (4) age and sex distribution of the patients in the general practice altered prevalence rates, as people aged 25 to 44 and women in general were reported to be at higher risk for mental disorder. Studies at British outpatient clinics have reported rates of psychiatric disorder ranging from 21 to 77 percent. These studies frequently used self-report symptom questionnaires; different cutting points, as well as the other variables noted earlier, alter the rates obtained. Several British follow-up studies found that 27 to 73 percent of all patients studied remained psychologically impaired, depending on the length of follow-up.

Similar findings were obtained in surveys of North American populations. Prepaid group practice rates have varied from 4 to 15 percent, and private general practice rates from 4 to 29 percent. Hospital outpatient rates have ranged from 53 to 88 percent for women and 21 to 79 percent for men. As with the British studies, rates vary with research setting, sampling method, case identification method, and the demographic characteristics of the population.

For purposes of illustration and clarification, several representative reports are discussed briefly below and summarized in Table 1. Published reports subsequent to 1975, many of which incorporate contemporary psychiatric nomenclature and structured psychiatric research interviews, are also discussed.

In his important general practice study, Kessel (1960) prospectively surveyed 911 adult patients registered to a four-physician group general practice in London. An illness which reflected "an important psychiatric component" to the general practitioner was designated as "conspicuous psychiatric morbidity" (CPM). ICD-6 criteria were also used, though the general practitioners usually made symptomatic diagnoses. Nine percent of the registered study population had CPM, while 5 percent of the sample were diagnosed as "mental, psychoneurotic, or personality disorder" on ICD-6. An additional 5 percent had further personality problems which were unrelated to their presenting illnesses. Higher rates of psychiatric morbidity among women were noted, but age had no effect on the prevalence of CPM. Kessel noted a marked variation among physicians in the rate of diagnosing psychiatric cases. He concluded that the use of the ICD-6 classification led to an underestimated prevalence of psychiatric morbidity in this population.

Typical of the earlier British studies is the one by Shepherd et al. (1966). They used the CMI and general practitioners to assess 14,697 patients in fifty London general practices. One-fourth of the patients had a CMI of 10 or more. The practitioners assessed the patients during routine ten-minute visits. Patients were grouped into those with a formal psychiatric disorder using ICD-6 criteria and those with psychiatric conditions associated with the onset or course of the physical illness. The prevalence of the former was 10.2 percent and the latter 4.9 percent, with a total prevalence of 13.9 percent.

Johnstone and Goldberg (1976) evaluated 1,093 consecutive new attendees at a general practice office, using the GHQ and general practitioner assessments. They reported that 32 percent of the population had "conspicuous psychiatric illness," as assessed by the general practitioner. An additional 11.5 percent had "hidden psychiatric illness," detected by the GHQ but not by the general practitioner.

Finn and Huston's study (1966) is typical of American studies using general practitioner assessment. They surveyed 29,400 patients of 291 full-time private practice physicians in Iowa, using nonpsychiatric physician interviews and no specific diagnostic criteria. An "emotional component" was identified by the primary physician as an important factor in the patient's illness in 18.5 percent of the patients. In 3.3 percent of the sample, the emotional component was judged the "major factor," while in 15.5 percent the emotional component was one of the important factors in the patient's presenting illness. An emotional component was most prevalent in women in general and in people aged 45 to 64. The patients were also evaluated with regard to specific major psychiatric diagnoses, and the authors concluded that while the prevalence of minor emotional disturbance in medical patients is high, the prevalence of major psychiatric disorder is low.

Locke and Gardner (1969) used a similar approach to study the prevalence of psychiatric problems in the practices of 58 internists and general practitioners in New York State. Each physician was asked to report on all patients seen during a one-month period, and a total of 11,144 adult white patients were studied. The authors used no psychiatric interviews or standardized diagnostic criteria. They reported that 17 percent of their sample had "psychiatric problems;" women in general and people aged 35 to 54 suffered maximum morbidity. Eleven percent suffered from "psychoneurosis," 3 percent from "personality disorder," 1 percent from a "psychosis," and 1 percent from a "brain syndrome." Only 35 percent of the patients reported a psychiatric problem as their chief complaint. Patients with gastrointestinal disease or diseases related to "senility" had the highest rates of psychiatric problems, and the authors also reported an increased risk of psychiatric problems for any patients who had seen their primary care physician at least once in the twelve months prior to the study.

Characteristic of research using current nosology, Glass and his colleagues (1978) administered the HSCL and a life-events questionnaire to 124 consecutive admissions to general medical clinics. Eighty-two of these patients were then seen for a diagnostic psychiatric interview, and the interviewer rated each patient on common symptoms of anxiety and depression. Using the Feighner criteria, 83 percent of the 82 were then diagnosed as having a psychiatric disorder: anxiety neurosis 28 percent, primary depression 19 percent, secondary depression 12 percent, organic brain syndrome 7 percent, and schizophrenia 1 percent. The au-

Table 1. Outpatient General Medical Studies

Source	# Pts.	Population	Assessment Technique	Diagnostic Criteria	Overall Results		Results by Diagnoses	
Roberts and Norton (1952)	50	Consecutive new patients, Yale U Medical Clinic; New Haven, CT	Psychiatric interviews by psychiatrist and social worker	None reported	TOTAL with "positive" diagnosis of "psychiatric illness"	72%	Schiz. reaction	2%
							Anxiety reaction	2%
							Character reaction	2%
							Alcoholism	2%
					Functional somatic complaints without medical disease	44%		
					Psychosomatic medical disease	16%		
Kessel (1960)	911	Registered adults at group general practice; London	Prospective assessment by primary physician	ICD-6	TOTAL with "conspicuous psychiatric morbidity" (CPM) (Registered)	9%	Hysteria Anxiety, Depression, Hypochondriasis	1% 5%
					Mental, psychoneurotic, or pers. disorder	5%		
					Men with CPM	7%		
					Women with CPM	11%		
					TOTAL with CPM (Attending)	14%		
					Mental, psychoneurotic, or pers. disorder	8%		

Study	N	Sample	Instrument	Criterion	Results
Culpan et al. (1960)	322	Hospital outpatients (100 medical controls, 104 normal controls, 118 neurotic); London	Cornell Medical Index (CMI)	>10 yes responses to questions M through R = "emotional disturbance"	TOTAL with "emotional disturbance": Medical clinic — Women 36%, Men 15%; Normal controls — Women 25%, Men 8%; Neurotic outpatients — Women 77%, Men 67%; Without org. illness 38%; With organic illness 13%
Culpan and Davies (1960)	100	Consecutive new referrals to hospital medical outpatient department; London	Brief psychiatric interview; CMI	None reported	TOTAL with psychiatric illness 51%; Women 56%; Men 42% (CMI scores greater for those with psych illness and no org illness than those with org illness and no psych illness)
Shepherd et al. (1966)	14,697	Patients in fifty general practices; London	CMI; private practitioner interviews	CMI≥10 ICD-6	TOTAL 25%; TOTAL psychiatric morbidity 13.9%[1]; Formal psychiatric disorder 10.2%[1] — Psychosis 0.6%, Mental subnorm 0.2%, Neurosis 8.9%, Pers. disorder 0.6%; Psychiatric associated conditions 4.9%[1] — Psychosomatic 3.0%, Org illness w. psych overlay 1.5%, Psychosocial problems 0.8%; Peak ages 45–65; Higher in women

Table 1. Continued

Source	# Pts.	Population	Assessment Technique	Diagnostic Criteria	Overall Results	Results by Diagnosis
Finn and Huston (1966)	29,400	Patients of 291 general practitioners and nonpsychiatric specialists; Iowa	Primary care physicians' evaluations	None reported	TOTAL with "emotional component" to their physical illness 18.5% Women 22% Men 14% Maximum prevalence ages 45–64 Depression increased with increasing age	Anxiety symptoms 29% Depression symptoms 10% Hypochondriasis 7% Psychosom. disorders 10% Brain disease 4%
Locke and Gardner (1969)	11,144	Universal report on all white adult patients of 58 general practitioners and internists during one month; Monroe County, NY	No standard technique	None reported	TOTAL with "psychiatric problems" 17% Women 21% Men 11% Maximum prevalence ages 35–54 Gastrointestinal and senile patients had highest prevalence of psychiatric problems	Psychoneurosis 11% Pers. disorder 3% Psychosis 1% Brain syndrome 1%

Study	N	Population	Assessment		Findings
Rosen et al. (1972)	1,413	Adults attending outpatient hospital general medical clinics; Monroe County, NY	General practitioner assessment	None reported	TOTAL with "emotional disorder" 22% Severe impairment 3% Moderate impairment 11% Mild impairment 8% Women 25% Maximum rates at ages 35–44 Men 16% Maximum rates at ages 45–64
Johnstone and Goldberg (1976)	1,093	Consecutive new attendees at general practitioner's office; England	Assessment by general practitioner; General Health Questionnaire (GHQ)	None reported	TOTAL "conspicuous psychiatric illness" by practitioner 32% TOTAL additional "hidden psychiatric illness" detected by GHQ but not by practitioner 11.5%
Meyer et al. (1978)	698	Consecutive new referrals to hospital outpatient general medical clinic; Baltimore, MD	Brief structured interview; Hopkins Symptom Checklist (HSCL)	None reported	TOTAL who required psychiatric treatment 47% Those requiring treatment more likely to be female, single, and young, and have poor psychosocial functioning

Table 1. Continued

Source	# Pts.	Population	Assessment Technique	Diagnostic Criteria	Overall Results		Results by Diagnosis	
Glass et al. (1978)	82	Consecutive new university hospital medical outpatients; Chicago, IL	Psychiatric interview; HSCL; Life-events questionnaire	Feighner	TOTAL with psychiatric illness	83%	Schizophrenia	1%
							Prim. depression	19%
							Sec. depression	12%
							Anxiety neurosis	28%
							Alcoholism	2%
							Org. brain syndrome	7%
							Undiagnosed psychiatric illness	12%
					No psychiatric illness	17%		
Hoeper et al. (1979)	247	Adults at primary care outpatient clinic, no emergencies; Wisconsin	GHQ-30; SADS-L	RDC	TOTAL with psychiatric illness	26.7%	Major depression	5.8%
							Minor depression	3.4%
							Intermittent dep.	5.0%
							Cyclothymic pers.	2.0%
							Labile pers.	3.7%
							Phobic disorders	5.8%
							Generalized anxiety	1.6%
Marks et al. (1979)	4,098	Outpatients attending 91 general practitioners; Manchester, England	GHQ-60; General practitioner assessment of CPM	None reported	TOTAL with CPM as assessed by general practitioner	31%		
					TOTAL probable prevalence by GHQ	40%		
					TOTAL identified by both GHQ and general practitioner	19%		
					Maximum prevalence: Ages 40–60 Unemployed Married but living apart Least education			

Study	N	Setting	Instrument	Classification	Diagnosis	Rate
Harding et al. (1980)	1,624	Primary medical care outpatient clinics; Four developing countries	Self-reporting Questionnaire (SRQ); Present State Exam (PSE)	ICD-8	Definite cases: Depressive neurosis Anxiety neurosis Schizophrenia Affective psychosis	6.8% 4.3% 0.43% 0.24%
Dhadphale et al. (1983)	388	Random outpatient hospital clinic patients, ages 18–55, no emergencies, no acute illness; Kenya	SRQ; Standardized Psychiatric Interview (SPI)	ICD-8	TOTAL with psychiatric morbidity — 29% Depression 10% Anxiety 9% Schizophrenia 2% Manic-depressive psychosis 5% Women 31% Men (n.s.) 26% Maximum prevalence ages 36–55	

[1] "These totals cannot be obtained by adding the rates for the relevant diagnostic groups, because while a patient may be included in more than one diagnostic group, he will be included only once in the total" (Shepherd et al., 1966, 81).

thors noted, however, that the HSCL self-report ratings did not assist in separating the psychiatric cases from those who were without psychiatric diagnosis.

Hoeper et al. (1979) used the GHQ-30 and the SADS-L to assess the prevalence of RDC mental disorders in nonemergency adult patients at a primary care clinic in Wisconsin. First, they administered the GHQ-30, and then, using SADS-L, they interviewed a sample made up of those who were GHQ-positive (cutting score 4) and those who were GHQ-negative. Finally, RDC diagnoses were made, without knowledge of the GHQ-30 results. The weighted prevalence of RDC disorder was 26.7 percent: major depressive disorder 5.8 percent, minor depression 3.4 percent, intermittent depression 5.0 percent, cyclothymic personality 2.0 percent, labile personality 3.7 percent, phobic disorder 5.8 percent, and generalized anxiety 1.6 percent. The authors concluded that the GHQ-30 appeared to detect "general distress or demoralization rather than specific psychopathologies," but that mental illness is overrepresented in primary care users compared with the general population.

In recent work done outside Britain or the United States, Dhadphale et al. (1983) studied the prevalence of psychiatric disorders among 388 randomly selected adult patients at an outpatient hospital clinic in Kenya. Patients were screened with the Self-Reporting Questionnaire followed by the Standardized Psychiatric Interview (Goldberg et al., 1970). A total of 29 percent of the population had psychiatric morbidity by ICD-8 criteria, with a nonsignificant difference between sexes. The absence of a significant sex difference in psychiatric morbidity in this population contrasts with the Western studies' findings of a higher prevalence among women. The maximum prevalence of psychiatric morbidity was in the group between the ages of 36 and 55. The authors suggested that the higher prevalence of psychiatric morbidity among older patients could have been due to the cumulative effect on point prevalence of a chronic disease. They also reported that most patients with psychiatric morbidity presented with somatic symptoms, though psychiatric symptoms were readily elicited when patients were specifically questioned about their emotional states.

MENTAL DISORDERS IN INPATIENT POPULATIONS

In contrast to the large numbers of outpatient studies, studies of the prevalence of the psychiatric disorders among medical inpatients are few.

Kaufman et al. (1959) evaluated the "incidence" of emotional illness among 253 medical ward admissions to Mt. Sinai Hospital in New York over one year. Liaison psychiatrists interviewed each patient using DSM-I criteria. Of the 253 patients studied, 66.8 percent were diagnosed as suffering from some psychiatric condition: 13.7 percent had character disorder, 7.5 percent functional psychosis, 5.1 percent "senility" with or without psychosis, and 13.1 percent organic brain disease with or without psychosis. Thirty-six percent of the sample were diagnosed as having a "psychoneurosis," 16.2 percent with "neurotic depression," 6.0 percent with "anxiety reaction," 5.1 percent with "hysteria" (conversion and phobic), and 1.6 percent with obsessive-compulsive disorder. Of those who were diagnosed as having a "psychosomatic" medical diagnosis (diabetes mellitus, peptic ulcer disease, ulcerative colitis, allergic reactions, and hypertension), 82.3 percent were also diagnosed with a

Table 2. Inpatient General Medical Studies

Source	# Pts.	Population	Assessment Technique	Diagnostic Criteria	Overall Results	Results by Diagnoses	
Querido (1959)	1,630	General hospital inpatients; Amsterdam	Group evaluation by psychiatrist, social worker, physician	None reported	TOTAL "distress"	47%	
Kaufman et al. (1959)	253	Medical ward admissions, Mt. Sinai Hospital; New York, NY	Psychiatric interview	DSM-I	TOTAL psychiatric disease	66.8%	
					Depression increased with age and female sex	Character dis	13.7%
						Psychoneurotic	36.0%
						Neurotic dep.	16.2%
						Anx reaction	6.0%
						Hysteria	5.1%
						Mixed	6.3%
						Obs-Compulsive	1.6%
					Psychiatric disease increased if medical diagnosis was "functional" or "psychosomatic"	Other	0.8%
						Functional psychosis	7.5%
						Psychotic dep.	0.8%
						Invol psychosis	0.8%
						Schizophrenia	5.5%
						Other	0.4%
						Senile	5.1%
						Organic brain syndrome	3.1%

Table 2. Continued

Source	# Pts.	Population	Assessment Technique	Diagnostic Criteria	Overall Results	Results by Diagnoses
Denney et al. (1966)	39	Consecutive admissions to medical ward of county hospital; Oregon	CMI; Mental Status Schedule (MSS)	CMI>32.6, MSS>13.25 = "psychiatric disorder"	TOTAL "psychiatric disorder" CMI (N = 39; median: 47.5)	72%
					TOTAL "psychiatric disorder" MSS (N = 25; median: 17.0)	68%
	54	Consecutive admissions to medical ward of university hospital; Oregon	CMI; MSS	See above	TOTAL "psychiatric disorder"CMI (N = 54; median: 24.0)	32%
					TOTAL "psychiatric disorder" MSS (N = 34; median: 11.7)	35%
Kurland and Hammer (1968)	97	Male patients on general medical ward of veterans hospital; Chicago, IL	MMPI; Patients' ratings; Physicians' ratings	None reported	MMPI HS, D, HY scales related to patients' ratings of illness severity and pain/discomfort and physicians' ratings of illness severity	
					Greater emotional reaction to illness in young patients	
Johns (1972)	234	Medical and surgical inpatients of public hospital; Australia	CMI	CMI>30	TOTAL serious emotional disturbance	53%
					Women	65%
					Men	35%

Study	N	Setting	Instrument	Criteria		%	By category	%
Maguire et al. (1974)	170	Medical ward admissions; England	SPI; GHQ-60	None reported	TOTAL psychiatric illness by GHQ	26%	By SPI: Depressed	15%
					Mild	15%	Anxiety	6%
					Moderate	7%	Org psychosis	4%
					Severe	4%		
Cheah et al. (1979)	136	Consecutive geriatric admissions upon transfer from med/surg wards in veterans hospital (primary problems medical, not psychiatric); Arkansas	Psychiatric evaluation	DSM-II	No psychiatric symptoms	19%	Org brain syn	54%
							Mild	41%
							Moderate	16%
							Severe	43%
							"Depression/dysphoria"	37%
							Mild	74%
							Moderate	20%
							Severe	6%
							Paranoid	4%
							Alcohol-related	8%
Cavanaugh (1983)	335	Medical admissions, tertiary care hospital; Chicago, IL	GHQ-30; Mini Mental Status Examination (MMSE); Beck Depression Inventory (BDI)	GHQ≥5	TOTAL	61.1%	Total Depressed	32%
				MMSE≤23	TOTAL	27.7%	Mild	18%
				BDI≥14			Moderate and severe	14%
				BDI = 14–20				
				BDI≥21				

psychiatric disorder. Of those for whom a firm medical diagnosis could be reached, 89.5 percent were diagnosed with a psychiatric disorder.

Denney et al. (1966) studied consecutive admissions to a medical ward at a county hospital in Oregon and at the University of Oregon Medical School Hospital. They administered the 195-item CMI to all patients in the sample in conjunction with the Mental Status Schedule (MSS), an 82-question, standardized mental status examination. The authors concluded that the county hospital sample had twice as many "disturbed patients" than the university hospital sample and closely resembled a true psychiatric sample. Psychosocial disability was considerably greater in the county hospital population where the patients were older and less well educated, had lower social status, and were more often divorced or widowed. County hospital patients also appeared to be more severely medically ill than the medical school hospital patients; three times as many of them died.

Kurland and Hammer (1968) prospectively administered the MMPI to 97 men on a general medical ward of a veterans hospital. In addition, the patients rated the nature, duration, and degree of seriousness of their illness, pain, discomfort, and worry about their illnesses, and their physicians also rated the seriousness of their illness. Scores on the HS, D, and HY scales of the MMPI were significantly related to the patients' ratings of the seriousness of their illnesses and their ratings of the severity of their pain and discomfort and to the physicians' ratings of the patients' illnesses. Younger patients were more likely to interpret their illnesses as serious and showed "greater emotional reaction to actual serious illness."

Johns (1972) administered the CMI to 234 medical and surgical patients in a general ward of a public hospital in Australia. Fifty-three percent of the sample had a score of 30 or greater, indicating serious emotional disturbance. The author concluded that "though the CMI probably overestimates the degree of emotional disturbance in women when a cutoff total score of 30 is used," women had "more neurotic illness" than men: approximately one-fifth of men and one-half of women had significant emotional disturbances (Johns, 1972, 43).

Maguire et al. (1974) prospectively evaluated the psychiatric morbidity of 170 consecutive admissions to general medical wards in Oxford, England. The patients were initially administered the GHQ-60 and, if they scored over 11, were then administered the Standardized Psychiatric Interview (Goldberg et al., 1970). Seventy-seven of the 170 patients scored over 11 on the GHQ, and the interview identified 45 patients as psychiatrically ill. Of the 45, 25 reportedly had "mild" psychiatric illness, 13 "moderate," and 7 "severe." Fifteen percent of the total sample were diagnosed by the interview as "depressed," 6 percent as having "anxiety," and 4 percent as having an "organic psychosis." Affective disorders accounted for 80 percent of psychiatric disorders. But in 38 percent of this group, the authors believed that the mood disturbance represented an "adverse psychologic response to physical illness." Patients who were diagnosed as having a "psychosomatic" disease (asthma, chronic peptic ulcer, irritable colon, ulcerative colitis, ileitis, essential hypertension, rheumatoid arthritis, and skin disease) had significantly more psychiatric disturbance than those diagnosed as having metabolic disease, neoplastic disease, or no medical disease.

One of the authors (Cavanaugh, 1983) assessed 335 randomly selected medical patients with the GHQ-30, the MMSE, and the BDI. In this study, 61.1 percent had a GHQ of 5 or more, and 34.5 percent had a GHQ of 10 or more. Age, race, sex, and socioeconomic group did not affect GHQ scores. Probable psychiatric dysfunction defined by a GHQ score of 5 or more was also analyzed by type of medical illness: cancer 78 percent, renal insufficiency 72 percent, genitourinary 70 percent, autoimmune 67 percent, hematologic 65 percent, gastrointestinal 64 percent, respiratory 56 percent, cardiovascular 56 percent, and endocrine 29 percent. Evidence of cognitive dysfunction, defined by an MMSE score of 23 or less, was found in 27.7 percent. The study found more cognitive dysfunction in those who were older, black, or of lower socioeconomic status. The BDI identified 18 percent with "mild" depression and 14 percent with "moderate" or "severe" depression.

Medical inpatient studies to date permit few inferences about the prevalence of psychiatric distress, symptoms, or diagnoses. The inpatient studies have not used contemporary psychiatric nomenclature and structured interviews, and the influence of demographic variables on emotional dysfunction remains unclear.

SPECIFIC PSYCHIATRIC DISORDERS

Estimating the prevalence of specific psychiatric disorders in various medical populations is difficult, given that no consistent diagnostic criteria have been used. Nevertheless, anxiety and depressive disorders appear to be the most prevalent in medical populations. For example, these disorders have accounted for 44 to 87 percent of emotional dysfunction in several major studies: 50 percent in the study by Finn and Huston (1966), 83 percent in the one by Glass et al. (1978), 87 percent in that of Hoeper et al. (1979), 73 percent in that of Dhadphale et al. (1983), and 44 percent in the study by Kaufman et al. (1959). Although not necessarily generalizable to a general medical population, a recent study of cancer patients by Derogatis et al. (1983) provides some insight into the distribution of specific psychiatric disorders in medical settings. In a multicenter study, the point prevalence of DSM-III diagnoses in 215 cancer patients was assessed by psychiatric interview. Forty-seven percent of patients received a DSM-III diagnosis on Axis I or II: 2 percent of the total sample had Anxiety Disorders, 6 percent Major Affective Disorders, 4 percent Organic Mental Disorders, and 32 percent Adjustment Disorders. Eighty-five percent of the psychiatric diagnoses consisted of anxiety or depressive disorders.

Depressive Disorders

The prevalence of depressive symptomatology in the outpatient medical population varies from 5.5 percent to 48 percent when assessed by self-report rating scales (BDI, Zung, CES-D). (See Table 3.) The lower the cutting score of the test, the less specific it is for depressive symptoms, and the more likely it is that the symptomatology of other disorders is recorded. Hankin and Locke (1983) screened 1,921 clinic patients in the departments of medicine and obstetrics and gynecology and found that 21 percent had a cutting score of 16 or more on the CES-D, while physician interviews identified only 4.8 percent of the population as having depressive symptomatology. Linn and Yager (1980) used the Zung and

Table 3. Depressive Disorders in Medical Outpatient Populations

Source	# Pts.	Population	Assessment Technique	Diagnostic Criteria	Results	
Finn and Huston (1966)	29,400	Medical outpatients; Iowa	Primary care physicians' evaluations	None reported	10%	
Salkind (1969)	80	General practices; England	BDI	BDI≥11 BDI≥13 BDI≥17	48% 36% 25%	
Glass et al. (1978)	82	New university hospital medical outpatients; Chicago, IL	Psychiatric interview	Feighner	19% 12%	Primary depression Secondary depression
Hoeper et al. (1979)	247	Adults at primary care outpatient clinic, no emergencies; Wisconsin	SADS-L	RDC	5.8% 3.4% 5.0% 2.0%	Major depression Minor depression Intermittent depression Cyclothymic personality
Linn and Yager (1980)	100	Outpatient medical clinic; Los Angeles, CA	Zung	Z≥50 Z≥60	42% 21%	
Nielsen and Williams (1980)	526	Medical private practice group; Washington, DC	BDI	BDI≥13 BDI≥17	12.2% 5.5%	

Study	N	Setting	Instrument	Criteria	Prevalence	Findings
Wright et al. (1980)	199	Family practice clinic patients; Louisville, KY	Zung; Psychiatric interview	Z≥50; Feighner	41%; 17%; 24%	(24% mild; 13% moderate; 4% severe); Depressive disorder; Significant depressive symptoms; No relationship for age, sex; positive relationship for low SES, marital status, severity of medical illness, stressful life events
Harding et al. (1980)	1,624	Primary medical care outpatient clinics; four developing countries	SRQ; PSE	ICD-8	6.8%; 0.24%	Depressive neurosis; Affective psychosis
Seller et al. (1981)	222	Family practice clinic; Buffalo, NY	BDI	BDI = 11–20; BDI≥21	20%; 15%	
Hankin and Locke (1983)	1,921	Adults attending pre-paid group practice, internal medicine and ob-gyn; Columbia, MD	Center for Epidemiological Studies Depression Scale (CES-D); Physician interview	CES-D≥16	21%; 4.8%	
Zung et al. (1983)	1,086	Outpatient family medicine clinic; North Carolina	Zung	Z≥55	13.2%	
Dhadphale et al. (1983)	388	Adult outpatient hospital clinic; Kenya	SPI	ICD-8	10%	

found that 42 percent of medical outpatients had evidence of depressive symptomatology with a cutting score of 50 or more, and Wright et al. (1980) found a prevalence of 41 percent using the Zung and the same cutting score. Zung et al. (1983) found that 13.2 percent had a Zung of 55 or more in a family practice setting. Nielsen and Williams (1980) used psychiatric interviews and DSM-II criteria to standardize the BDI in a private practice group; 12.2 percent had evidence of mild depression (BDI 13 or more), and 5.5 percent had moderate to severe depression (BDI 17 or more). Salkind (1969) found that 48 percent of British private practice patients had a BDI of 11 or more and 25 percent had a BDI of 17 or more. Finally, Seller et al. (1981) found that 35 percent had a BDI of 11 or more, and 15 percent had a BDI of 21 or greater.

These prevalence rates for depressive symptomatology, determined through screening tests, exceed the rates for depressive disorders obtained through physician interviews. Finn and Huston (1966) found that 10 percent of medical outpatients were believed to be depressed by the primary care physician. Increase in age correlated with increased prevalence of depression, with 25 percent of the patients over age 65 experiencing depressive symptoms. Using standardized psychiatric interviews and Feighner criteria in hospital outpatients, Glass et al. (1978) found that 19 percent had a primary depressive disorder and 12 percent had a secondary depressive disorder. Wright et al. (1980) found that 17 percent of family practice clinic patients had a depressive disorder by Feighner criteria, while 24 percent more had significant depressive symptoms. Hoeper et al. (1979) used the SADS-L and RDC criteria and found the prevalence of major depressive disorder to be 5.8 percent, minor depressive disorder 3.4 percent, intermittent depressive disorder 5.0 percent, and cyclothymic personality disorder 2.0 percent. Using the Standardized Psychiatric Interview and ICD-8 criteria, Dhadphale et al. (1983) found a 10 percent prevalence rate of depressive disorder in Kenya. Harding et al. (1980) used different instruments, but also used ICD-8 criteria, and they obtained a 6.8 percent rate at medical clinics in four developing countries.

In summary, much of the reported depressive symptomatology in outpatient medical populations appears to be mild and would probably be classified in DSM-III under Adjustment Disorder with Depressed Mood. If, however, one uses higher cutting scores on screening tests or structured interviews and diagnostic criteria, rates of significant depressive symptoms or major depressive disorder range from 5 to 25 percent. It also appears that point prevalence rates of depressive symptoms and major depressive disorders in outpatient medical samples exceed those in community populations (Weissman and Boyd, 1983). All medical outpatient studies show women to have a higher prevalence of depressive symptoms than men. Age does not appear to affect rates of depressive symptomatology among medical outpatients (Zung et al., 1983; Nielsen and Williams, 1980). Depressive symptomatology is higher in medical outpatients who are single, divorced, widowed, from lower socioeconomic groups, or recently stressed, and who have serious physical illnesses (Zung et al., 1983; Wright et al., 1980).

In medical inpatient populations, Schwab et al. (1967a), Moffic and Paykel (1975), and one of the authors (Cavanaugh, 1983) all used a BDI cutting score of 14 or more and found the prevalence of depressive symptoms to be 22, 24, and 32 percent respectively (see Table 4). All

Table 4. Depressive Disorders in Medical Inpatient Populations

Source	# Pts.	Population	Assessment Technique	Diagnostic Criteria	Results	
Kaufman et al. (1959)	253	Medical ward admissions, Mt. Sinai Hospital; New York, NY	Psychiatric interview	DSM-I	16.2% 0.8% 0.8%	Neurotic depression Psychotic depression Involutional psychosis
Schwab et al. (1967a)	153	Consecutive inpatient admissions, U of Florida; Gainesville, FL	BDI; Hamilton Rating Scale for Depression (HAM-D)	BDI≥14	22%	
Maguire et al. (1974)	170	Medical ward admissions; England	GHQ-60; SPI	None reported	15%	
Moffic and Paykel (1975)	150	General medical inpatients, New Haven Hospital; New Haven, CT	BDI; Psychiatric interview	BDI≥14	24% 29%	At admission Later
Cheah et al. (1979)	136	Consecutive geriatric admissions, veterans hospital; Arkansas	Psychiatric interview	DSM-II	27% 7% 2%	Depression/dysphoria Mild Moderate Severe
Fava et al. (1982)	85	General medical inpatients; Italy	CES-D	None reported	19.6 Mean 21 Mean 14 Mean	Men and women Women Men
Cavanaugh (1983)	335	Medical admissions, tertiary care hospital; Chicago, IL	BDI	BDI≥14 BDI = 14–20 BDI≥21	32% 18% 14%	Total depressed Mild Moderate and severe

three reported that most of the symptomatology was mild. The third study (Cavanaugh, 1983) found that only 14 percent of patients had a BDI of 21 or more, indicating moderate to severe depressive symptomatology. As did Schwab et al. (1967a), this study (Cavanaugh, 1983) also found that depressive symptoms were higher in young black men and in middle- and upper-class women. Both studies also found that patients with cancer, gastrointestinal disease, renal insufficiency, and autoimmune disease had more depressive symptomatology. Similarly, Moffic and Paykel (1975) found that depressive symptomatology was higher in those more seriously ill, in pain, or with prolonged hospitalization. Fava et al. (1982), using the CES-D, found that women and older patients had more depressive symptomatology. Kaufman et al. (1959) used psychiatric interviews and DSM-I criteria with medical inpatients and found that 16.2 percent had neurotic depression, 0.8 percent had psychotic depression, and 0.8 percent had involutional psychosis. Women had more "psychoneurotic" depression than men. These authors also found an age-related increase in depression in men over 50, but not in women.

Anxiety Disorders

Prevalence rates of anxiety disorders in outpatient medical populations range from 1.6 to 29 percent, as shown in Table 5. The prevalence appears lower when strict diagnostic criteria for anxiety disorders are used and higher when anxiety symptoms or anxiety neuroses are recorded. The milder symptomatology would probably be termed Adjustment Disorder with Anxious Mood in DSM-III.

Both Kaufman et al. (1959) and Maguire et al. (1974) reported a 6 percent prevalence of anxiety disorders in inpatient populations. Lucente and Fleck (1972) studied the prevalence of anxiety symptoms in 408 consecutive admissions to medical and surgical wards of four general hospitals. Using the Taylor Manifest Anxiety Scale and the Hospitalization Anxiety Scale, they found that 21 percent of the population scored in the "high" range, 46 percent in the "moderate" range, and 34 percent in the "low" range. Anxiety symptoms increased with the number of past medical hospitalizations, with female sex, and with decreased age. Black patients were significantly more anxious than white patients, and Catholic patients were more anxious than Protestant patients. The authors found no consistent correlation between the patients' anxiety levels and their types of medical illness, except that cancer patients were more anxious than others.

Other Disorders

SCHIZOPHRENIA The prevalence of schizophrenia in outpatient medical populations appears to be low, reportedly 0.4 to 2.0 percent in four studies (see Table 6). Kaufman et al. (1959) found a point prevalence of 5.5 percent in their inpatient population. These rates are comparable to those obtained in the general population (Taylor and Abrams, 1978).

SOMATOFORM DISORDERS Assessing the prevalence of somatoform disorders in medical populations is particularly confounded by

Table 5. Anxiety Disorders in Medical Populations

Source	# Pts.	Population	Assessment Technique	Diagnostic Criteria	Results	
			OUTPATIENTS			
Roberts and Norton (1952)	50	New patients, Yale U Medical Clinic; New Haven, CT	Psychiatric interview	None reported	2%	Anxiety reaction
Finn and Huston (1966)	29,400	Medical outpatients; Iowa	Primary medical physician evaluation	None reported	29%	Anxiety symptoms
Glass et al. (1978)	82	New outpatients, university medical clinic; Chicago, IL	Psychiatric interview; HSCL	Feighner	28%	Anxiety neurosis
Hoeper et al. (1979)	247	Adults at primary care outpatient clinic, no emergencies; Wisconsin	GHQ-30; SADS-L	RDC	1.6% 5.8%	Generalized anxiety Phobic disorder
Harding et al. (1980)	1,624	Primary medical care outpatient clinics; Four developing countries	SRQ; PSE	ICD-8	4.3%	Anxiety neurosis definite cases
Dhadphale et al. (1983)	388	Adults, outpatient clinic; Kenya	SRQ; SPI	ICD-8	9%	Anxiety

Table 5. Continued

Source	# Pts.	Population	Assessment Technique	Diagnostic Criteria	Results	
			INPATIENTS			
Kaufman et al. (1959)	253	Medical ward admissions, Mt. Sinai Hospital; New York, NY	Psychiatric interview	DSM-I	6%	Anxiety reaction
Lucente and Fleck (1972)	408	Consecutive medical and surgical admissions, four general hospitals; USA	Taylor Manifest Anxiety Scale; Hospitalization Anxiety Scale; Physician, nursing ratings; Self-report ratings	None reported	21% 46% 34%	High anxiety Moderate anxiety Low anxiety
Maguire et al. (1974)	170	Medical ward admissions; England	SPI; GHQ-60	None reported	6%	Anxiety

Table 6. Schizophrenic Disorders in Medical Populations

Source	# Pts.	Population	Assessment Technique	Diagnostic Criteria	Results
		OUTPATIENTS			
Roberts and Norton (1952)	50	New patients, Yale U Medical clinic; New Haven, CT	Psychiatric interview	None reported	2%
Glass et al. (1978)	82	New consecutive university hospital medical outpatients; Chicago, IL	Psychiatric interview	Feighner	2%
Harding et al. (1980)	1,624	Primary medical care outpatient clinics; Four developing countries	PSE	ICD-8	0.43%
Dhadphale et al. (1983)	388	Random outpatient clinic patients; Kenya	SPI	ICD-8	2%
		INPATIENTS			
Kaufman et al. (1959)	253	Medical ward admissions, Mt. Sinai Hospital; New York, NY	Psychiatric interview	DSM-I	5.5%

changes in psychiatric nomenclature over time. While DSM-III distinguishes among Somatization Disorder, Conversion Disorder, Psychogenic Pain Disorder, and Hypochondriasis, available research data, with few notable exceptions, are much less clear in this regard. Studies with the most clearly defined diagnostic criteria indicate that "hysteria" (Somatization Disorder) ranges from 0 to 5 percent in medical inpatients and outpatients, while Conversion Disorder occurs in as many as 33 percent of patients in medical populations (see Table 7).

PSYCHOLOGICAL FACTORS AFFECTING PHYSICAL CONDITION From the available literature, it is virtually impossible to estimate the prevalence of Psychological Factors Affecting Physical Condition (DSM-III). The prevalence of the classical psychosomatic diseases (e.g., asthma, peptic ulcer, colitis) can be readily obtained in medical populations. An accurate assessment of psychological factors relating to the onset, course, and outcome of physical illness is, however, much more difficult. The older British studies often combined these two categories. Shepherd et al. (1966) found that 4.9 percent of 14,697 general practice patients had psychosomatic or psychiatric conditions associated with physical illness (Table 1). In an American study, Finn and Huston

Table 7. Somatoform Disorders in Medical Populations

Source	# Pts.	Population	Assessment Technique	Diagnostic Criteria	Results	
			OUTPATIENTS			
Kessel (1960)	911	Registered adults at group general practice center; London	General practitioner assessment	ICD-6	1%	Hysteria
Finn and Huston (1966)	29,400	Patients of 291 general practice nonpsychiatric specialists; Iowa	Primary care physicians' evaluations	None reported	7%	Hypochondriasis
			INPATIENTS			
Purtell et al. (1951)	2,274	General hospital admissions for psychiatric evaluation; Massachusetts	Psychiatric interview	Purtell criteria for hysteria	4.0% 0.0%	Hysteria in women Hysteria in men
Kaufman et al. (1959)	253	Medical ward admissions, Mt. Sinai Hospital; New York, NY	Psychiatric interview	DSM-I	5.1%	Hysteria
Majerus et al. (1960)	66	Postpartum women on maternity ward; St. Louis, MO	Structured psychiatric interview	Purtell criteria for hysteria	3%	Hysteria
Murphy et al. (1962)	101	Postpartum women on maternity ward; St. Louis, MO	Structured psychiatric interview	Purtell criteria for hysteria	1%	Hysteria
Lewis and Berman (1965)	16,000	Retrospective survey of all discharges from Wisconsin General Hospital, 1953–1963; Wisconsin	Medical record review	Attending physician's diagnosis	0.36% 0.8%	Conversion reaction Hysterical pers. Women four times more likely to be diagnosed with hysteria than men
Woodruff (1967)	295	Consecutive admissions of women to medical ward; St. Louis, MO	Structured psychiatric interview	Perley-Guze criteria for hysteria	0.3%	Hysteria
Farley et al. (1968)	100	Postpartum women on second postpartum day; St. Louis, MO	Structured psychiatric interview	Perley-Guze criteria for hysteria	1% 33%	Hysteria Conversion symptoms

(1966) reported an "emotional component" in 18.5 percent of their patients. As noted, this component was judged to be the major factor in the patient's illness in 3.3 percent of the total sample and one of the important factors in the patient's illness in 15.5 percent.

ALCOHOL-RELATED DISORDERS McIntosh (1982) reviewed 53 studies of alcohol-related diagnoses among medical inpatients.* He reported that the prevalence rates for current alcohol dependence syndromes ranged from 13 to 48 percent. Surveys which measured both current and past alcohol dependence syndromes reported prevalence rates ranging from 7 to 20 percent. Alcohol-related disabilities were present in 7 percent of medical inpatients. Considering both past or present alcohol dependence and alcohol-related disabilities, the rates ranged from 24 to 51 percent. The studies also showed that men received alcohol-related diagnoses three times more frequently than women and that rates were significantly higher in veterans or public hospital populations than among other inpatients. McIntosh concluded that routine use of screening instruments such as the Michigan Alcohol Screening Test, along with quantification of alcohol use as part of the usual medical history, would help to establish credible prevalence estimates.

PERSONALITY DISORDERS Criteria for "psychoneurotic disorders" (i.e., conversion, obsessive-compulsive, phobic, hysterical, dissociative, anxiety, depressive) have been loosely defined in the past and have often overlapped with personality or character pathology. Reviewing the prevalence of personality disorders in older studies would therefore be meaningless. From the few studies that do distinguish them, rates of character pathology range from 2 to 6 percent in outpatient populations. Roberts and Norton (1952) reported a prevalence of 2 percent, Locke and Gardner (1969) 3 percent, and Hoeper et al. (1979) 5.7 percent (Table 1). One inpatient study by Kaufman (1959) showed the prevalence to be 13.7 percent (Table 2).

CONCLUSIONS

Current research suggests a number of relationships between medical and emotional or psychiatric disorders. First, physical and emotional illnesses tend to cluster together (Eastwood, 1975; Lipowski, 1975; Kessler et al., 1983). Second, significant life stressors may be associated with the onset of medical illness (Rahe and Arthur, 1978; Cohen, 1981). Third, emotional distress may be associated with increased medical morbidity and mortality (Kimball, 1969; Sime, 1976). Fourth, patients with emotional distress or psychiatric disorders use medical care services more frequently than patients without such disorders (Hankin et al., 1982; Widmer and Cadoret, 1978; Hankin and Oktay, 1979). And finally, psychological intervention may reduce medical morbidity and mortality (Mumford et al., 1982) and medical care utilization (Schlesinger et al., 1983; Jones and Vischi, 1979).

Emotional distress, psychiatric symptoms, and psychiatric disorders are prevalent to various degrees in general medical populations. The

*Editor's note: In Part IV of this volume, Robins describes the seven alcohol-related diagnoses in DSM-III and compares the criteria with the RDC and Feighner criteria.

prevalence rate in outpatient medical populations appears to range from 10 to 20 percent, but the prevalence among inpatients is difficult to ascertain due to a paucity of data. Although medical outpatient studies show that women in general and people aged 35 to 55 are at greater risk for emotional or psychiatric disturbance, the inpatient studies report conflicting data. Moreover, the types of medical illness which present a high risk for emotional disorders have been poorly studied. Anxiety and depressive disorders account for the majority of emotional distress or psychiatric disorders among medical patients, and emotional distress or adjustment disorders appear to be more frequent than the major psychiatric disorders. Furthermore, emotional distress or psychiatric symptomatology appears more prevalent in medical populations than in community samples (Finlay-Jones and Burvill, 1977). The major psychiatric disorders, particularly major depression, may also be more prevalent in medical settings than in the community (Weissman and Boyd, 1983).

Future research in this area and practical conclusions from research to date must be guided by an understanding of the purpose of epidemiologic studies (Weissman and Boyd, 1983). These studies aim to define the prevalence of a particular illness in the population and to identify contributing risk factors and etiologies. Screening tests are devised to evaluate large numbers of patients, particularly those in high-risk groups. Then, depending upon the particular etiologic factors, programs are designed for primary, secondary, or tertiary prevention. Finally, the prevalence of the illness is reassessed to evaluate the efficacy of prevention and treatment. In the past two decades, epidemiologic research in psychiatry has been greatly enhanced by the development of standardized diagnostic criteria. Psychiatric raters have been trained to collect data reliably, using structured psychiatric interviews. Reliable or valid diagnostic criteria, however, are as yet unestablished for medical populations.

The outcome of emotional or psychiatric disturbance in medical populations remains uncertain. Much of the psychiatric disturbance in medical populations is mild and remits as the illness resolves or as the psychosocial stressor or loss is relieved or integrated by the patient (Goldberg and Blackwell, 1970). Nevertheless, some medical patients will develop chronic, disabling psychiatric illnesses which will prevent their returning to previous levels of social functioning (Stern et al., 1977). Lloyd and Cawley (1982), for example, found that myocardial infarction patients who had been psychiatrically ill before their infarction had prolonged psychiatric morbidity, compared with those whose psychiatric conditions had been precipitated by infarction. Risk factors for developing a chronic or severe psychiatric disorder need to be more carefully delineated for medical populations. Conceivably, the risk factors include demographic variables, premorbid personality traits, personal or family psychiatric history, and recent or previous life events or social supports. Similarly, while increased medical morbidity and health care utilization are sometimes characteristic of medical patients with emotional dysfunction (Hankin et al., 1982; Kessler et al., 1983), the frequency of these characteristics remains undetermined. The risk factors for these sequelae also remain poorly defined. Identification of such antecedents would be helpful in designing intervention efforts for these high-risk groups.

Theoretically, the identification and appropriate treatment of emotional dysfunction in medical populations would lead to a decrease in psychiatric and medical morbidity and a decrease in utilization of health care services. At the present time, however, and most importantly in the next decade, psychiatrists alone will be unable to respond to major, much less minor, psychiatric illnesses (Gardner, 1970; Graduate Medical Education National Advisory Committee, 1981). Consequently, the burden of dealing with most of the emotional dysfunction in medical populations will continue to fall on the physicians and nurses who care for patients in primary care settings.

With the rising cost of hospital care and diminished federal funding, less money will be available for consultation-liaison programs to provide education for primary care personnel (Pincus et al., 1983). Nonetheless, the data presented in this chapter mandate psychosocial training programs for physicians and nurses in these settings. This should occur at a medical student, resident, and postgraduate level. Specific treatment programs, using cost-efficient interventions, need to be developed for medical patients with emotional dysfunction. Certainly, social workers, psychologists, and nurse practitioners can provide much of this care in both outpatient and inpatient settings under the supervision of psychiatrists and primary care physicians. Nevertheless, consultation-liaison psychiatrists will in the future be challenged to provide leadership in planning educational programs for primary care personnel and in designing treatment programs to meet the psychiatric and psychosocial needs of medically ill patients.

Chapter 14 Clinical Research at the Interface of Medicine and Psychiatry
by Harvey Moldofsky, M.D.

Psychosomatic research at the interface of medicine and psychiatry is devoted to answering two fundamental questions. (1) How does the interaction of biological, psychological, and social factors influence the onset and the course of disease? (2) What is the role of psychological and social interventions in the prevention and treatment of disease? This chapter reviews the recent studies bearing on these questions.

MECHANISMS OF ILLNESS

The studies relating to the first question are concerned with the mechanisms of illness, and they employ three different approaches: psychological, psychobiological, and psychosocial. Psychological studies are concerned with personality, mood, and cognition. Psychobiological studies use novel instruments and techniques for studying specific populations of sick people or experimental animals. From these studies have evolved the research disciplines of psychophysiology, psychoendocrinology, psychoimmunology (or behavioral immunology), and developmental psychobiology. Psychosocial studies examine the role of family and sociocultural factors in initiating or perpetuating illness.

Psychological Studies

PERSONALITY Early psychosomatic researchers tended to overemphasize the etiologic role of personality aspects in certain diseases. The notion that specific personality characteristics correlate with specific diseases (Dunbar, 1943) later gave way to an interest in the etiologic role of specific emotional conflicts in specific diseases, such as hypertension, asthma, peptic ulcer, rheumatoid arthritis, ulcerative colitis, Graves' disease, and neurodermatitis (Alexander et al., 1968). A more recent formulation purports that specific psychodynamic constellations alone are insufficient to account for these diseases, but rather that multiple biological, psychological, and social factors contribute in a variable fashion to the etiology of disease (Weiner, 1977; Engel, 1977; Leigh and Reiser, 1980). Such multifactorial theories of etiology have had considerable currency lately. Yet for practical reasons researchers are adopting models of investigation that are much less complex and are focusing on specific questions. The studies use specialized techniques that have been tested for reliability and validity to discover answers by sophisticated statistical methods. Such an approach is evident in the studies of a specific constellation of personality traits that appears to correlate with coronary heart disease.

Over the past ten years, researchers have directed much attention to persons exhibiting competitiveness, aggressive and hostile strivings, a sense of time urgency, drive, and ambition (Friedman and Rosenman, 1959). This constellation of personality traits, known as *Type A behavior*, has been shown to be predictive of coronary heart disease (Schucker and Jacobs, 1977; Scherwitz et al., 1977). Type A behavior is now a well-established independent risk factor for coronary heart disease (Review Panel on Coronary-Prone Behavior and Coronary Heart Disease, 1981). The evidence is compelling. Type A behavior has been shown to be related to coronary atherogenesis and disease severity as assessed by autopsy (Friedman et al., 1968), by coronary angiography (Frank et al., 1978; Blumenthal et al., 1978; Zyzanski et al., 1978), and by the thallium-201 stress test (Kahn et al., 1982). But the findings are not always consistent. In three ethnic groups—Irish Catholic, Italian Catholic, and white Anglo-Saxon Protestant—angiographic evidence for coronary artery disease was found to be unrelated to Type A, depression, or stress (Dimsdale et al., 1980). On the other hand, blood pressure and heart rate responses in Type A personalities were heightened under challenging experimental conditions, still suggesting that this behavior may promote coronary heart disease (Corse et al., 1982). Research must therefore address the following topics: the nature of the association between Type A behavior and other risk factors for coronary heart disease, the specificity of the Type A behavioral pattern to the disease (Type A subjects have also been shown to be at particular risk for accidents, suicide, and homicide) (Jenkins et al., 1974), the interrelationship of Type A behavior and depression in influencing the disease, and the validity of the association across various populations (Review Panel on Coronary-Prone Behavior and Coronary Heart Disease, 1981).

MOOD   The scientific study of the link between dysphoric states and psychosomatic disorders dates back to the pioneering work of Cannon, who demonstrated the influence of emotions on body functions (Cannon, 1920). Recently, attention has focused on the role of specific affective disturbances in human morbidity. Examples of this research focus include the studies of bereavement, depression, and "alexithymia" (a condition where there is an inability to express emotional experiences in words).

The studies of *bereavement* fall into two categories, the epidemiologic investigations of the frequency of physical illness among the bereaved and research on mortality among bereaved persons. Some authors have claimed that young bereaved persons have more physical distress and take more tranquilizers and hypnotics than young married control subjects (Parkes and Brown, 1972; Clayton, 1974). Except for those already ill, older widows and widowers differ little from married persons in their need for medical or psychiatric care (Clayton, 1979). Research in England and Sweden, on the other hand, has shown increased mortality for older widowers during the first six months of bereavement (Young et al., 1963; Rees and Lutkins, 1967; Parkes et al., 1969; Ward, 1976; Mellstrom et al., 1982). The recent Swedish study showed excess mortality of about 25 percent among widowers aged 70 to 74 years compared with married men of similar age (Mellstrom et al., 1982). This was due mainly to cancer, cardiovascular disease, accidents, suicide, and cirrhosis of the liver. The authors therefore suggested that life-style factors, i.e., the increased use of alcohol and tobacco by the widowers, might account for the difference in mortality rates.

Psychoanalytic theory has influenced research on the role of *depression* in the onset of disease. Members of the medical-psychiatric liaison group of the University of Rochester Medical Center have studied the influence of real or fantasied object loss on depression and the onset of disease (Schmale, 1958; Engel, 1967; Schmale et al., 1970). They have suggested that the unresolvable object loss, accompanied by affects of helplessness or hopelessness, results in a reaction of giving up. This cognitive-affective pattern appeared to facilitate the onset of a wide variety of medical, psychosomatic, and psychiatric diseases (Schmale and Engel, 1967; Adamson and Schmale, 1965; Ader and Schmale, 1980).

Subsequent epidemiologic and clinical studies have shown inconsistent results. Two follow-up studies of patients with depressive illness showed cancer deaths to be higher than expected in males (Kerr et al., 1969; Whitlock and Siskind, 1979). Other epidemiologic studies, however, have found that those with unipolar or bipolar depressive illness have no increase in death, either from cancer (Evans et al., 1974; Niemi and Jaaskelainen, 1978) or from any "natural" cause (Eastwood et al., 1982).

Furthermore, systematic attempts to assess the significance of depression for medical illness, severity of disease, and course of illness have also resulted in differing findings. Clinical self-ratings of hopelessness by a group of hospitalized physically ill patients were low and did not differ from assessments in the general population (Greene et al., 1982).

In addition, no relationship was found between depression and either the severity of illness or subjective illness beliefs among medical patients in a general hospital (Wise and Rosenthal, 1982). However, in a prospective study of the relationship of a specific mood pattern and articular pain to prognosis, rheumatoid arthritic patients who showed an inverse association of hopelessness with pain had an unfavorable outcome. Those rheumatoid arthritic patients for whom anxiety or hostility was associated with pain demonstrated a favorable prognosis over the two-year study period (Moldofsky and Chester, 1970). Similar observations were made in a prospective study of women who had early breast cancer and were treated with simple mastectomy with or without radiotherapy. Those patients who showed stoicism-acceptance or helplessness-hopelessness three months after surgery had a less favorable outcome after five years compared with those who showed denial or a fighting spirit (Greer et al., 1979). The reasons for the conflicting clinical observations relate to the differing methods of study, to the role of denial as a psychological defense mechanism in the face of life-threatening or disabling disease, or to the presence of an "alexithymic" state (Sifneos, 1973).

The term alexithymia was coined by Sifneos (1973). Literally *alexithymia* means "no words for mood." The concept stems from the clinical observations of patients with psychosomatic diseases by the French psychoanalysts Marty and de M'Uzan (1963). The patients had an impoverished fantasy life associated with concrete, present-oriented thinking called the "pensée opératoire" (operative thinking). Such patients are unable to find appropriate words to describe feelings, are preoccupied with physical complaints, use detailed, repetitive content of speech, have rare recollection of dreams, and have interpersonal relationships marked by dependency or aloofness. They are found to be dull and boring in psychotherapy (Apfel and Sifneos, 1979).

The alexithymia concept has been recently reviewed by Lesser (1981). Much of the literature is theoretical, anecdotal, and speculative. There are no reliable and valid instruments to measure the phenomenon. While possibly pathological in Western culture, alexithymia might not be pathological in Eastern cultures or specific to patients with psychosomatic illness. A recent experimental study obtained self-ratings of emotional distress and physiological responses of normal subjects and patients with headache, hypertension, and rheumatoid arthritis when they were exposed to stressful stimulation. The study showed a negative correlation between physiological activity and subjective ratings of stressfulness for both groups (Anderson, 1981). Thus, an absence of emotional responsivity was not specific to patients with psychosomatic disorders. Clearly, further well-controlled studies using reliable psychological and physiological measurements are required.*

COGNITION The mode of body perception and the personal significance of body experience are important in the evolution of disorders where body image disturbances are primary clinical features. Distor-

*Editor's note: In his chapter in Part V of this volume, Nemiah explores the alexithymia concept further, with a particular emphasis on its possible relationship to panic anxiety as a psychosomatic symptom.

tions of body image are especially characteristic of the eating disorders anorexia nervosa and obesity (Garfinkel and Garner, 1982).

Over the past 25 years, anorexia nervosa has become more prevalent, and it is most often identified in young women in Western society. Bruch (1973) suggested that perceptual and conceptual disturbances were fundamental to the relentless pursuit of thinness. Numerous studies of visual self-image have shown that anorectic women overestimate their overall bodily width or selected parts such as their shoulders, waist, hips (Slade and Russell, 1973; Crisp and Kalucy, 1974; Garner et al., 1976; Pierloot and Houben, 1978; Garfinkel et al., 1979; Casper et al., 1979). This overestimation of body size is also related to distortion of satiety (Garfinkel et al., 1979), to body dissatisfaction and poor self-esteem (Garner and Garfinkel, 1981), and to poor prognosis (Slade and Russell, 1973; Crisp and Kalucy, 1974; Garfinkel et al., 1977b; Goldberg et al., 1977; Casper et al., 1979; Garfinkel et al., 1979).

Overestimation of body size is also found with obesity, so that the type of body image distortion is not specific to thinness or fatness (Slade and Russell, 1973; Garner et al., 1976). Faulty perception of internal and external signals influences obese people to eat excessively. Overweight persons are overresponsive to the sight, smell, and taste of food (Rodin, 1976), but are underresponsive to satiety cues (Schachter, 1971) and to gastric contractions associated with hunger (Stunkard and Koch, 1964). They show regulatory disturbances in dieting (Herman, 1978), but they do not necessarily select more to eat in public eating places (Coll et al., 1979). Following intestinal bypass surgery for excessive obesity, subjects reduce their intake of high-calorie foods (Halmi et al., 1981; Sclafani, 1981) and revise their estimate of physical size in accordance with their weight loss. However, their sense of unattractiveness persists (Schiebel and Castelnuovo-Tedesco, 1978), and marital discord may ensue (Neill et al., 1978).

Psychobiological Studies

PSYCHOPHYSIOLOGY Two fundamental approaches have been employed to investigate the relationship of psychological and physiological mechanisms in disease. The first involves studying physiological responses to specific stimuli during wakefulness; the second involves studying physiological changes during sleep when changes are presumably the function of specific natural states, not of external stimuli. The first method dates back 150 years to Beaumont's 1833 observations through a fistulous opening of how stressful events affected the function of Alexis St. Martin's stomach. Just over 100 years later, clinical observations of patients with gastric fistulae confirmed the importance of emotional stimuli for changes in gastric physiology (Wolf and Wolff, 1947; Engel et al., 1956). Today's sophisticated physiological methods permit more detailed inquiry into the interrelationship of mind and body in disease. Recent publications offer excellent reviews of the literature on the psychophysiological aspects of a wide range of diseases (Weiner, 1977; Weiner, 1982) and on such selected topics as asthma (Stein, 1982; Kinsman et al., 1980; Knapp et al., 1976), hypertension (Weiner, 1979), and cardiovascular disorders (Verrier and Lown, 1981; Steptoe, 1981). Contemporary concepts about psychophysiological mechanisms in disease onset depart from the earlier notion of linear causation that postulated an external stressful stimulus, a cognitive and affective response to it, and the consequent dysfunction of a peripheral organ. The idea of a linear chain linking social or external stimuli to physiological responses is too simplistic. Furthermore, this transactional model did not explain how psychological experience is transformed by the brain into physiological activity and disease involving a selected organ (Weiner, 1977).

A variant of the transactional model, one involving arousal or activation, emphasizes a specific biological response or pattern of responses (Engel, 1960; Lader, 1972; Roessler and Engel, 1977). The response may be specific to the evocative stimulus. For example, a psychologically stressful stimulus induces anxiety and hyperventilation in normal subjects (Suess et al., 1980). Another possibility, however, is that the response may be specific or idiosyncratic to selected individuals. This conception has practical application to the study of persons at risk for a specific disease or already ill with that disease. For example, Type A coronary-prone men respond with greater heart rate, or higher systolic blood pressure, or both than do Type B men when they are exposed to challenging cognitive, psychomotor, and physical performance tasks (Dembrowski et al., 1978; Manuck and Garland, 1979; Van Egeren, 1979; Glass et al., 1980; Goldhand, 1980; Pittner and Houston, 1980; Corse et al., 1982). Furthermore, patients with coronary heart disease show greater blood pressure response to frustrating cognitive tasks than those without heart disease (Corse et al., 1982). But how these observations link to other risk factors for heart disease, or how they are transformed into heart disease, requires a more complex model of disease.

In many chronic diseases, genetic, neurochemical, neurohormonal, and immunological systems carry varying degrees of causal importance. To account for the variable influence of these diverse regulating biological operations, Weiner (1976) suggested the notion of heterogeneity among etiologic factors in a specific disease. He pointed to the diversity of biological predispositions that have been shown to be associated with a common disease outcome. For example, a variety of physiological regulatory disturbances are found with peptic duodenal ulcer, essential hypertension, rheumatoid arthritis, anorexia nervosa, obesity, bronchial asthma, Graves' disease, and coronary artery disease (Weiner, 1982).

The brain's waking state is implicit in the transduction into specific physiological disorders of such psychological factors as personality, dysphoric states, and cognitive disturbances. Yet some illnesses have been shown to involve not only waking experiences but also the circadian sleep-wake cycle, and recently certain features of sleep physiology or circadian rhythm have been related to the emergence of disease.

A new era in psychobiological research followed the discovery that distinct physiological and psychological features defined two states of sleep—rapid eye movement (REM) sleep and non–rapid eye movement (NREM) sleep. Specific physiological disturbances, evident only during sleep or particular sleep states, provoke certain medical and behavioral disorders. Physiologically, for example, sleep apnea that occurs in NREM and REM sleep is associated with hypertension, right heart failure, secondary polycythemia, and nocturnal cardiac arrhythmias and may be associated with sudden, unexplained nocturnal deaths (Guilleminault et al., 1978). Psychologically, sleep apnea is associated with excessive daytime somnolence and impaired intellectual functioning. Successful treatment of sleep apnea usually reverses both the physiological and the psychological symptoms. Similarly, periodic involuntary leg movements during NREM sleep (nocturnal myoclonus) and disruption of sleep continuity are associated with excessive daytime somnolence in some people. These sleep-related, periodic involuntary leg movements and an α-frequency EEG sleep anomaly accompany the widespread musculoskeletal pain and chronic fatigue in the "fibrositis" syndrome, or rheumatic pain modulation disorder (RPMD) (Moldofsky et al., in press). This α-frequency EEG sleep anomaly, characteristic of patients with the RPMD, has been induced experimentally by disrupting stage 4 (deep) NREM sleep with noise, and the resulting sleep disturbance was followed by similar musculoskeletal complaints in healthy subjects (Moldofsky et al., 1975; Moldofsky and Scarisbrick, 1976). Such nonrestorative sleep features are also associated with the morning symptoms of generalized aching, stiffness, and fatigue in acutely ill rheumatoid arthritis patients (Moldofsky et al., 1983).

Some physical disorders interrupt the continuity of sleep or are associated with specific sleep states. Studies have sought to determine whether the physiological features of REM or NREM sleep trigger a nocturnal attack of angina, peptic ulcer pain, asthma, or migraine (Moldofsky, 1982). Only in the case of nocturnal migraine is there a consistent association with REM sleep (Dexter and Weitzman, 1970; Hsu et al., 1977; Kayed et al., 1978). The literature is sparse on the relative contributions of physiological changes and psychological state to these nocturnal symptoms. However, men whose impotence is associated with medical pathology have shown failure of REM-related penile tumescence, while men with psychogenic impotence have shown the expected REM-related penile tumescence (Karacan et al., 1978).

PSYCHOENDOCRINOLOGY It is now well established that such hormones as cortisol, thyroxine, growth hormone, prolactin, estrogen, progesterone, and testosterone are regulated by the CNS via the regulatory neurochemical agents of the hypothalamic-anterior pituitary. Because of its broad influence on major bodily functions, the neuroendocrine system holds special interest for psychosomatic researchers. They believe that investigating these hormones during defined psychological conditions will ultimately lead to an understanding of the hitherto mysterious link between mind and body in health and disease. Selye's (1976) work on adrenocortical response to noxious physical and psychological stimuli eventually led to his theory of stress influencing disease. Selye defined *stress* as the nonspecific response of the body to any demand. His definition of *stressor* as an agent that produces stress at any time is an unfortunate tautology.

While no one has offered a truly satisfactory definition of stress and authors have used the term variously to refer to environmental events, individual responses, or both, psychoendocrinologists are devoted to the notion of noxious influences on endocrine activity. Theoretically, the endocrine stress responses should cause functional and structural changes in the body and then cause disease (Henry, 1982). The observation of an increase in urinary or plasma 17-hydroxycorticosteroids in subjects engaged in a variety of stressful situations (competitive boat racing, aircraft flight, anticipation of examinations or surgery, military combat, hospital admission, and so forth) provides evidence of pituitary-adrenocortical response to emotional disturbance (Mason, 1975a; 1975b). Similarly, other endocrine systems, such as growth hormone, testosterone, prolactin, thyroid hormone, insulin, aldosterone, β-endorphin, and (possibly) Substance P, respond to psychological stress. While cortisol, growth hormone, and prolactin levels increase following exposure to stressful stimuli, plasma testosterone levels decrease (Rose, in press). All these observations are consistent with the importance of the brain in mediating endocrine responses to psychosocial stimuli.

The various endocrine responses to stressful events are not always uniform. For example, rhesus monkeys exposed to a prolonged conditioned emotional disturbance exhibited a stereotypical pattern of multiple-hormone response. Some hormones rose initially (e.g., corticosteroids, catecholamines, thyroxine, and growth hormone). Others fell (e.g., insulin, androgens, and estrogens) and then, following termination of the disturbance, rebounded above the baseline (Mason, 1968). Furthermore, endocrine responses to emotional stress are not always persistent or consistent. Experiments have shown that animals do not continue to show adrenocortical hormone response to repeated shocks (Mason, 1968; Pollard et al., 1976), and clinical studies have shown an absence in some individuals of hormone responses associated with stress. Such reduced hormonal responsivity is found in people whose coping styles protect them from being unduly distressed or aroused, though these styles are not necessarily psychologically adaptive (Rose, in press). For example, among women awaiting breast tumor biopsy, those who showed psychological defenses such as denial and isolation of affect had low cortisol secretion. Those who were visibly anxious and distressed, on the other hand, had higher cortisol secretion (Katz et al., 1970).

The evidence that endocrine responses to stress invariably cause disease in man is not definitive. For example, retrospective psychiatric studies suggest that certain personality characteristics, emotional conflicts, or defenses predispose to Graves' disease (Weiner, 1977). Theoretically, major or prolonged psychological distress would induce thyroid overactivity via the hypothalamic-hypophyseal-thyroid axis. Yet while some experiments on animals and man have shown that thyroid-stimulating hormone (TSH) increases with psychological stress, other studies have reported the opposite effect (McKenzie, 1979) or no effect. Severe anxiety induced by treating phobic subjects with the behavioral technique of "flooding" is not associated with any consistent or specific change in TSH response (Nesse et al., 1982). Animal experiments have not shown that stressful circumstances produce hyperthyroidism. Furthermore, changes in the immune system are considered to be important in the pathogenesis of Graves' disease, but no experimental evidence to date indicates that emotional distress plays a role in the formation of the long-acting thyroid stimulator, or immunoglobin G, which is related to that disease (McKenzie, 1979).

Whereas the "stress" research on hormones as causal agents in disease has not been very profitable, research on the contribution of their circadian rhythms to the clinical features of illness has been encouraging. For example, women with anorexia nervosa show a regulatory dysfunction of thyroid, growth, and arginine vasopressin hormones, as well as altered circadian rhythms of serum gonadotropins. A state of starvation is associated with reduced levels of serum triiodothyronine (T_3), an increase in inactive reverse form of T_3, and elevated levels of resting growth hormone (Garfinkel and Garner, 1982). With considerable weight loss, anorectic women show circadian patterns of luteinizing hormone (LH) that are typical of prepubertal or pubertal girls: they have low day and low night or low day and high night LH secretion (Boyar et al., 1974). With restoration of weight and menses, the LH secretory pattern matures to higher levels during both day and night. In a subgroup of bulimic women at near normal body weight, the LH pattern remains immature (Boyar and Katz, 1977).

Future studies of the influences of the newly discovered neuropeptides on metabolism and behavior will help to elucidate the mediating psychobiological mechanisms. Cholecystokinin is found not only in the central and peripheral nervous systems, but also in the gut, and it may play an important role in regulating satiety in man (Rehfeld, 1981). The endogenous opioid peptides, the enkephalins, β-endorphins, and dymorphins, are involved in a signaling system that seems to relate to pain perception, mood regulation, and aspects of learning (Koob and Bloom, 1983).

PSYCHOIMMUNOLOGY (BEHAVIORAL IMMUNOLOGY) The immunological system has specialized adaptive humoral- and cell-mediated functions. The rapid responding, humoral-mediated, hypersensitivity response depends on antigenic sensitization of B-lymphocytes. The slower, or delayed, cell-mediated immunity is controlled by T-lymphocytes. These immune operations protect against foreign substances such as bacteria, viruses, and exogenous tissues (grafts or organ transplants). The immune system is believed to be vital in the pathogenesis of autoimmune and neoplastic diseases. Much attention has been directed to deciphering the complex structural code of antigen-antibody activities. Not until recently have researchers seriously investigated the respective roles of the brain and psychological phenomena in immune responses (Rogers et al., 1979; Ader, 1981).

The research suggests that the CNS, neurotransmitter, and endocrine processes are important in mediating hypothalamic influences on the immune system (Stein et al., 1981; Fauman, 1982). Such neuropharmacologic agents as histamine agonists and antagonists, atropine, and adrenergic drugs affect allergic symptoms, e.g., bronchial hyperreactivity in asthma (Boushey, 1981).

The immune system appears to be responsive to emotional stress. Bereaved persons (Bartrop et al., 1977) and students prior to oral examinations (Dorian et al., 1982) have shown reduced T-lymphocyte response to mitogens. Following 48 hours of sleep deprivation, normal subjects have reduced reaction to phytohemagglutinin. The immune reactions return to baseline levels after five days (Palmblad et al., 1979). Immunoglobulin A was elevated in women who suppressed their anger prior to breast biopsy (Pettingale et al., 1977b). In a follow-up study, immunoglobulins correlated with the extent of metastatic breast disease, but they did not discriminate between benign and cancer groups (Pettingale et al., 1977a).

Behaviorally conditioned immunological suppression has been demonstrated in animal studies (Ader and Cohen, 1981). When a neutral conditioning stimulus (saccharin) is paired with a noxious immunosuppressive pharmacologic agent (cyclophosphamide), the neutral stimulus subsequently exerts a suppressive effect on the immune response to an exogenous antigen (sheep red blood cells). The antibody response of the conditioned animals is small and transient, but the consistency of the response, especially in mice showing low spontaneous activity in an open field (Gorczynski et al., 1983), suggests that the immune system mediates individual behavioral differences in regard to disease activity.

Personality features, mood, and attitude are all related to immune features of disease. For example, those rheumatoid arthritis patients who do not have rheumatoid factor in their sera differ psychologically from those patients who do. Seronegative patients are more aggressive (Rimon, 1973) and show more anxiety and psychological distress (Crown et al., 1975; Gardiner, 1980; Vollhardt et al., 1982) than seropositive patients. Alteration of the psychological state of an allergic individual affects tissue reactivity to the specific antigen. Following the suggestion under hypnosis not to react to the skin test (Black et al., 1963) or holding the expectation of no skin response (Smith and McDaniel, 1983), tuberculin-positive subjects showed an inhibited, delayed-type hypersensitivity reaction to skin tuberculin injection. Similarly, suggestion has affected airway reactivity in asthmatic subjects (Luparello et al., 1968).

DEVELOPMENTAL PSYCHOBIOLOGY The contribution of faulty childhood emotional experience to later medical illness has interested psychosomatic investigators. Recent animal research casts new light on the importance of infant psychobiological influences for subsequent distress. Noxious stimuli, such as electric shocks delivered to an infant rat, or removal of a rat pup from the nest and holding it for a few minutes, predispose the animal to various gastric lesions, infections, and neoplastic disease. The results are not simple or uniform (Ader, 1977). Animals with different infantile experiences appear to react differently to the same pathogenic stimulus. For example, rats housed in social groups rather than individually show reduced susceptibility and resistance to gastric erosions. The group-housed rodents also vary in their susceptibility to other diseases. They may be more suspectible to whole body x-irradiation, alloxan diabetes, trichinosis, malaria, immobilization-induced gastric erosions, anaphylactic shock, and adjuvant-induced arthritis. They appear to be more resistant than individually housed animals to mammary tumors, ruminal ulceration, encephalomyocarditis virus, E. coli, and spontaneous convulsions (Ader, 1981).

Animal research demonstrates that maternal separation at a specific time in infantile maturation increases susceptibility to later pathology. Rat pups which are prematurely weaned at around the age of 15 days show an 80 to 90 percent incidence of gastric erosions when physically restrained on postnatal day 30 and a marked reduction in erosions by day 200. Gastric erosions rarely occur in rats restrained prior to day 21. Factors involved in this animal model include premature loss of maternal milk and hypothermia during food deprivation and physical restraint (Ackerman, 1981). Premature weaning of mice, together with social isolation, results in later marked elevation of blood pressure and high mortality (Henry et al., 1967). The early separation of the animal from its mother appears to disrupt a variety of psychobiological regulatory processes that govern the mother-infant relationship. These maternally derived regulatory processes include neurochemical and neuroendocrine growth processes, sleep-wake organization, emotional behavior (Hofer, 1982), and immune reactivity (Keller et al., 1983).

Some evidence suggests that these animal models are in fact applicable to human behavior and illness. A young adult who had had a gastric fistula as an infant showed maternal behavior reminiscent of her early feeding experiences (Engel, G.L. et al., 1974). The so-called deprivation dwarfism of childhood that stems from distorted parent-child relationships results not only in growth retardation with bizarre eating behavior, disturbed sleep, retarded speech, and social withdrawal, but also in deficiencies of adrenocorticotrophic and growth hormones (Powell et al., 1967a; 1967b; Imura et al., 1971). When these children are removed from the stressful situation, they grow at a remarkable rate, and their hormonal abnormalities disappear.

Psychosocial Studies

FAMILY CONSTELLATIONS Family relationships can influence childhood psychosomatic disorders. Children with anorexia nervosa, unstable diabetes mellitus, and intractable asthma have been studied using systems analysis in the context of family psychotherapy (Minuchin et al., 1975). Specific features in the families' organization and functioning suggest the concept of the "psychosomatogenic family." Such a family supports or predisposes to the child's expression of somatic symptoms which are thought to reflect emotional distress. The affected child not only expresses the family's problems but also relieves its difficulties (Rosman et al., 1977). Five characteristics of faulty family functioning have been proposed: enmeshment (overinvolvement in one another's lives), overprotectiveness, rigidity, lack of conflict resolution, and involvement of the affected child in the parental conflict in order to detour, avoid, or suppress it.*

A systems analysis of family functioning along these lines does not imply specific etiology of illnesses. The observations of the Philadelphia group (Minuchin et al., 1975) on the families of anorectic patients, for example, differ from the findings of other authors. The observed overall rate of parental psychopathology ranges from 33 percent (Dally, 1969) to 54 percent (Morgan and Russell, 1975). While some authors suggest that marital discord and unfavorable parent-child relationships are related to an unfavorable outcome (Crisp et al., 1974; Hsu et al., 1979), others have not found this association (Theander, 1970; Pierloot et al., 1975). The discrepant observations suggest that a variety of family relationships may contribute to anorexia nervosa (Garfinkel and Garner, 1982).

*Editor's note: Part III of Psychiatry Update: Volume II deals more extensively with family systems. Particularly relevant here are the chapters by Dr. Donald A. Bloch on family dynamics and individual patients (pages 203–215) and Dr. Charles A. Malone on the child in the context of family interaction patterns (pages 228–241).

ENVIRONMENTAL AND SOCIAL INFLUENCES The study of human disease has also focused on the influence of the social environment. Illness is believed to result from various social-environmental or personal life-change stressors. Mediating variables between disease and these psychosocial stressors include (1) the qualities of the stressor, i.e., its intensity, duration, predictability, and novelty; (2) personality characteristics; and (3) social status and supports (Rabkin and Struening, 1976). Epidemiologic studies on the connection between life events, stressors, mediating factors, and disease onset or frequency offer some evidence that psychosocial factors affect health. The frequency of a person's recent life changes has been measured by the Schedule of Recent Experience and the amount of adjustment required by the Social Readjustment Rating Questionnaire (Holmes and Rahe, 1967; Masuda and Holmes, 1978). The studies showed that the greater the social stress requiring change in the life situation, the greater the risk that the person will become ill and that the illness will be serious. Those life events that demand intense or prolonged readjustment (e.g., death of a spouse) are more likely to be followed by the development of physical or psychiatric illness.*

Recent reviews of this research suggest caution in drawing definite conclusions about life events as related to illness. Many factors, including age, marital status, sex, socioeconomic status, ethnicity, level of education, and culture, influence the perception of life events and reports of their frequency (Masuda and Holmes, 1978). Young people accumulate more life events than old people; single individuals tend to have more of them than those who are married, widowed, separated, or divorced. Furthermore, methodological problems surround the interpretation of statistics involving studies of large populations. Correlation coefficients relating the number and nature of life events to subsequent illness episodes are statistically significant but small (typically below .30), indicating that life events account for only a small percentage of the variance in illness. Thus, for practical purposes, life events may not be reliable predictors of future illness (Rabkin and Struening, 1976).

THERAPEUTIC STUDIES

Theoretically, the methods for treating psychosomatic disorders should originate from an understanding of the psychological and biological processes which contribute to the disease. The early use of psychoanalytic theory for understanding personality disturbances and emotional conflicts led to the use of insight-oriented psychotherapy with the psychosomatic disorders. When psychoanalysis did not prove particularly expedient or effective, psychoanalysts withdrew from the psychosomatic arena (Wittkower, 1977). Psychoanalysis failed in part because psychoanalysts failed to appreciate the importance of genetic and acquired biological influences in disease. Moreover, they claimed that psychosomatic patients were poor candidates for psychotherapy because of their inherently impoverished fantasy life. The psychosomatic patients seemed dull, lifeless, colorless, and boring, and they did not respond to the psychoanalytic interventions used with psychoneurotic

*Editor's note: Dr. Robert M.A. Hirschfeld and Christine K. Cross offer a review of the research on life events and depressive disorders in Part V of *Psychiatry Update: Volume II* (pages 394–404).

patients (Nemiah and Sifneos, 1970). These views about an entire class of patients and a whole set of interventions are not universally held, however. Indeed, the apparently alexithymic characteristics of psychosomatic patients may result from poor doctor-patient relationships in which aggression plays a leading role (Musaph, 1977).

The observations of behavioral psychology about the importance of cognition and learning have recently permitted a shift away from psychodynamic explanations and treatments to the application of behavioral methods in the treatment of medical disorders. The new field of research and therapy called behavioral medicine has been defined as "an interdisciplinary field concerned with the development and integration of behavioral and biomedical science, knowledge and techniques relevant to health and illness and the application of this knowledge and these techniques to prevention, diagnosis, treatment and rehabilitation." (Schwartz and Weiss, 1978, 250). The objectives of behavioral medicine differ little from those of psychosomatic medicine, and their differences may be more historical and political than substantive. Behavioral medicine's roots lie in behaviorism and psychology, while psychosomatic medicine's origins are in psychoanalysis and medicine. Each emphasizes specific psychological approaches derived from its particular theories. As with psychoanalytic therapy, behavioral treatments have proven unnecessarily biased theoretically and neglectful of biological processes. The treatment methods of behavioral medicine include psychophysiological techniques such as biofeedback and psychological methods such as operant conditioning and cognitive-behavioral intervention.

Psychophysiological Techniques

BIOFEEDBACK Biofeedback is an instrumental procedure that senses, records, and provides the subject with information about those physiological functions in relation to which there is usually no awareness or voluntary control. The motivated subject learns to regulate the physiological activity by monitoring information that he or she perceives or receives through feedback. Measurement procedures yield information about bodily functions influenced by the autonomic nervous system (e.g., heart rate, blood pressure, skin temperature, gastrointestinal activity) or about certain aspects of musculoskeletal and CNS electrophysiology.

The theoretical basis for this technique stems from animal and human experimental research. In animals, operant conditioning appeared in early studies to modify autonomic bodily functions through its system of aversive or rewarding stimuli. For example, rats were trained to slow the heart rate or to increase blood flow in one ear while decreasing flow to the other ear. The animals were curarized in order to eliminate the contaminating influence of motor activity (Miller, 1969). Later researchers could not replicate the early findings (Orne et al., 1980).

Although the scientific foundation for biofeedback is rather shaky, clinical research suggests that unconscious physiological functions can be altered by psychological means. Biofeedback has been used successfully in man to explore the regulation in normal subjects of blood pressure, heart rate, peripheral vasomotor tone, EEG, electromyographic (EMG), and various other physiological responses (e.g., gastric acidity and penile tumescence) (Shapiro and Surwit, 1979). EMG activity, even as small as single motor units, can be trained. Some EEG frequencies, e.g., α (8 to 13 Hz) may be brought under operant control. However, the initial reports relating increased α-frequency production to subjective calm were not uniformly substantiated in later studies (Orne et al., 1980). Increases in blood pressure and heart rate and decreases in skin temperature have been demonstrated consistently, but the converse functions have been demonstrated less successfully (Shapiro and Surwit, 1979).

A major question in much of this research is whether the response is specific to the biofeedback technique. Similar alterations in physiological functions can be produced by various relaxation or meditative procedures. This lack of specificity raises doubts about the actual utility of biofeedback procedures for specific medical disorders. EMG biofeedback training for tension headache is better than no treatment in reducing chronic headache (Orne et al., 1980; Neuchterlein and Holroyd, 1980; Stoyva, 1982). However, relaxation training also provides relief from headache. There is controversy about whether a decrease in frontalis EMG activity is essential for improved pain relief, as well as whether biofeedback training is any better than relaxation (Beatty and Haynes, 1979). Similarly, increasing the finger temperature through biofeedback appears to be an effective treatment for migraine and Raynaud's disease. For migraine, though, the therapeutic response may not depend on the ability to warm one's hands. Relaxation training is reportedly just as effective for migraine symptoms (Orne et al., 1980), Raynaud's disease, and hypertension (Shapiro and Surwit, 1979). Finally, although operant conditioning to increase the amount of 12-to-15 Hz activity seems promising for some patients with intractable epileptic seizures, the specificity of this EEG frequency for seizure reduction remains open to question (Callaway, 1980).

Measurable benefits of biofeedback are reported in selected medical disorders. Training in external anal sphincter contraction synchronous with the relaxation of the internal sphincter helps to control severe fecal incontinence (Engel, B.T. et al., 1974; Cervulli et al., 1976). EMG biofeedback is useful in rehabilitating patients with a variety of neuromotor disorders (Inglis et al., 1976). Further research must determine the practical benefits of biofeedback versus relaxation and/or drugs in the management of tension headache, migraine cardiac arrhythmias, essential hypertension, and Raynaud's disease.

Psychological Techniques

OPERANT CONDITIONING   Operant conditioning techniques have been used to eliminate or modify faulty behavior believed to contribute to psychosomatic disorders. The initial phase of the method entails careful observation and detailed measurements of environmental cues and the patient's faulty response patterns. The second phase attempts to modify the illness by extinguishing undesirable behavior and by shaping and strengthening desirable behavior through such reinforcers as praise or material reward. The therapist monitors and evaluates the patient's progress, and may introduce modifications during the course of treatment.

This behavioral approach has been applied in the treatment of chronic pain and eating disorders such as anorexia nervosa and obesity. While the operant conditioning or so-called multidimensional pain management methods have proven helpful in the short-term management of chronic pain (Fordyce et al., 1973; Swanson et al., 1979; Kerns et al., 1983), the benefits have not continued on follow-up. Long-term, controlled follow-up studies are required.

The early enthusiastic reports of success in patients with eating disorders have been tempered by the results of controlled follow-up studies. Operant conditioning techniques were reported no better in facilitating weight gain in anorectic patients than conventional treatments such as psychotherapy, drugs, or milieu therapy (Garfinkel et al., 1977b; Eckert et al., 1979). At one-year follow-up, patients who received behavioral modification were no more successful in sustaining weight loss than those who received traditional dietary manipulation (Stunkard and Penick, 1979).

COGNITIVE-BEHAVIORAL METHODS   Cognitive behavioral methods and cognitive-social learning theory have recently been applied to the treatment of chronic pain syndromes and the reduction of postoperative anxiety and pain (Kerns et al., 1983; MacDonald and Kuiper, 1983). The method begins with an analysis of how the patient's thoughts and feelings influence his or her perception of pain. Patients learn cognitive coping skills, such as relaxation training, imagery, and distraction, and they consolidate their coping skills through practice. For helping patients tolerate chronic pain and alleviating their anxiety, these methods are allegedly superior to relaxation therapy alone or group supportive treatment. The cognitive-behavioral therapy and social support may also help patients to cope with postoperative anxiety and pain, reduce their need for analgesics, and facilitate their recovery from surgery. Further research should determine whether this behavioral method actually alleviates pain or whether it merely teaches patients not to complain.

Psychosocial Therapies

A number of studies have suggested that social supports lower the risk and severity of illness in persons involved in stressful experiences (Caplan, 1981). Complications of pregnancy, for example, are increased in women who are both under high emotional stress and without social supports (Nuckolls et al., 1972). Men who develop rheumatoid arthritis after losing their jobs have more articular complaints if they lack social supports (Cobb, 1976). Emotionally disturbed asthmatic patients who have little support require more steroids than those with much support (De Aravjo et al., 1973). Clearly, such observations argue for providing patients with social support. For example, asthmatic patients who frequently visited the hospital emergency department improved after the introduction of an outpatient program of group education and support (Green, 1974). Studies of individual support measures with patients who have had myocardial infarction show modest psychological and possible physiological gains. Group support intervention also benefits these patients psychologically, and there are some indications of reduced mortality and morbidity (Razin, 1982).

CONCLUSIONS

Investigations of chronic medical disease based on psychoanalytic and behavioristic theories of mental functioning have led to an excessive emphasis on specific psychological etiologies and treatments and to an insufficient regard for scientific advances in pathology and normal biology. Understanding the role of psychological and social influences in disease will result not from the psychological abstractions of theory, but rather from the traditional pragmatism of science. The major advances in understanding psychosomatic disease will come from applying sophisticated methods, careful research designs, and statistical analyses to the exploration of associations in biological and psychological processes.

The pragmatic scientific approach has demonstrated that disordered psychological and social operations may play nonspecific roles in illness. As with Type A behavior and coronary heart disease, aspects of psychosocial functioning may participate as risk factors for disease. Individual dysphoric states, such as bereavement or depression, disturbed family relationships, or distressing life events, are inconsistently associated with the onset or course of medical diseases. Disorders in cognitive operations, such as a faulty visual self-image and faulty responses to eating cues, are often found in patients with anorexia nervosa or obesity.

Technological advances and biological discoveries have led to specialized disciplines in psychobiological inquiry. The scientific methods and observations of psychoimmunology (behavioral immunology) and developmental psychobiology promise to uncover specific predispositions to disease resistance and vulnerability. Research on the psychological correlates of neurohormone, neuropeptide, and neurotransmitter metabolism over the temporal course of sleep-wake rhythms may advance our understanding of the interactions of mind, brain, and body functions in health and disease. Recent observations suggest that the psychobiological pathways to selected diseases are multifactorial and varied.

Methods of treatment can also profit more from scientific pragmatism than from preconceived theoretical notions derived from psychoanalysis or psychological behaviorism. For example, psychoanalytic therapy alone has not proved expedient or effective with psychosomatic disorders. Biofeedback has not been shown to be a specific therapeutic technique for chronic headache, migraine, Raynaud's disease, or hypertension, but it does appear beneficial for disorders normally under volitional control, such as certain varieties of fecal incontinence and neuromotor disorders. Another behavioral technique, operant conditioning, is no better than other conventional treatments for eating disorders. While operant conditioning offers short-term benefits for patients with chronic intractable pain, the long-term benefits are uncertain. Cognitive-behavioral therapies that instruct patients in acquiring coping skills show promise in the overall management of postoperative pain and anxiety. Absence of social support measures appears harmful for disease prognosis. Some selected efforts to provide support have helped patients with intractable asthma and patients following myocardial infarction. Finally, some cost-benefit studies should examine and compare the practical application of these psychological, psychophysiological, and psychosocial techniques and of drug treatments for medical disorders.

Chapter 15

Psychiatry and Geriatric Medicine
by Charles V. Ford, M.D.

Consultation-liaison psychiatry has increasingly involved the concurrent practice of geropsychiatry. Recent statistics indicate that elderly people make up a large proportion of hospitalized medical patients, and a continuing increase both in their percentage of the total population and in total numbers is predicted (McFarland, 1978). The psychiatrist based in the general hospital must therefore develop particular skills in order to serve these older patients. Fortunately, the basic principles of consultation-liaison psychiatry are fully compatible with those of geriatric psychiatry. Both emphasize the multifactorial approach to clinical practice (Ford, 1981). Lipowski (1983) has stressed the overlap between the activities of consultation-liaison psychiatrists and geropsychiatrists, and he has recommended establishing combined training programs which would further link these two subspecialities.

PATTERNS OF CONSULTATION

Reports from various psychiatric consultation services have indicated that between 14 and 31 percent of all referred patients are 60 years of age or older (Anstee, 1972; Bustamente and Ford, 1981; Kornfeld and Feldman, 1965; Shevitz et al., 1976). Although this percentage is high, it is lower than the overall percentage of general hospital patients who are 60 or older (Bustamente and Ford, 1981; Folks and Ford, 1983). Elsewhere the author has suggested that attitudes reflecting ageism and therapeutic nihilism may be contributing to an underutilization of psychiatric consultation services for older patients (Ford, 1981).

A recent study of 1,000 consecutive psychiatric consultations in a general hospital found that approximately one in five consultation requests was for a patient 60 years of age or older (Folks and Ford, 1983). Psychiatric diagnoses assigned by the psychiatric consultant included organic mental disorders (51.4 percent), depressive disorders (35.9 percent), somatoform disorder (6.2 percent), and miscellaneous categories (16.4 percent). Referring physicians had failed to recognize organic mental disorder in over 60 percent of the cases, but they missed depressive disorder in only 14 percent of the cases. These findings are comparable with those of Shevitz et al. (1976) who also found that organic brain syndromes and depression were the most frequent psychiatric diagnoses of elderly patients seen in psychiatric consultation.

PSYCHIATRIC DIAGNOSIS

Frequently, psychiatric consultation is requested because of ward management difficulties, uncooperative behavior, or dispositional problems (Karasu et al., 1977; Papastamou, 1970). The consultation-liaison psychiatrist must first establish a diagnosis for the patient and may then assist the medical care team by making practical recommendations for management. In this regard, the consultation can also involve liaison activity and have benefits extending beyond the individual patient.

Consideration of all the psychiatric disorders which might face the consultant would fill a textbook of geriatric psychiatry. The following discussion must be limited to the more common diagnostic issues relevant to elderly patients who are hospitalized with medical or surgical ailments. Busse and his colleagues reviewed the major psychiatric syndromes affecting elderly people in the previous volume of *Psychiatry Update* (Grinspoon, 1983).

Organic Brain Syndromes

The incidence and prevalence of brain disease increase with advancing age. An elderly patient must therefore be carefully evaluated for the possibility of an organic mental disorder. Most such disorders involve the syndromes of delirium, dementia, and organic affective syndrome. Each of these syndromes is discussed separately in regard to the problems it poses to the consultation-liaison psychiatrist.

DELIRIUM   Delirium is common among hospitalized elderly patients. One study reported the incidence of "confusional" episodes (delirium) among elderly medical patients to be 56 percent (Chisholm et al., 1982). Despite its high prevalence and incidence, delirium is frequently unrecognized, and the psychiatric consultation may be requested because of "agitation," "uncooperative behavior," or suicidal ideation (Folks and Ford, 1983). In their recent comprehensive reviews of delirium in elderly patients, Lipowski (1980a) and Liston (1982) noted that nearly every disease and therapeutic intervention which has systemic effects can produce delirium. The etiology of delirium is frequently multifactorial and represents the cumulative effects of a variety of physiological insults and psychological stressors.

The tasks of the consultation psychiatrist are to determine the factor or factors that are responsible for the delirium and to propose proper therapeutic intervention. Cardiopulmonary, renal, and hepatic diseases and electrolyte imbalance are among the commonest causes of delirium in elderly patients. Infections which primarily or secondarily affect the brain, such as pneumococcal pneumonia or viral encephalitis, may also lead to delirium. The syndrome may be induced in an elderly person by inadequate sensory input, such as after cataract surgery (Weisman and Hackett, 1958), or by intensive care experiences (Kornfeld et al., 1965), or even as a result of hospitalization itself (Lipowski, 1980a).

One of the most common causes of delirium in elderly patients is an adverse reaction to medication, and numerous medications have been implicated (Levenson, 1979; Lipowski, 1980a; Shader, 1972). Drugs which have been especially associated with delirium in elderly patients include cimetidine, the cardioglycosides, and the anticholinergic agents.

Cimetidine, used primarily for the treatment of peptic ulcer, has become one of the most frequently prescribed drugs in the world. A number of clinical centers have reported delirium associated with cimetidine, and almost one-half of these reports have involved patients who were 60 years of age or older (Weddington et al., 1982). In most cases, the delirium has resulted from inadvertently overdosing the patient (Strauss, 1982). Overdosing is most likely to occur with impairment of renal and/or hepatic function, since approximately 50 percent of the oral dosage is cleared by the kidney in a metabolically unchanged state (Walkenstein et al., 1978). Cimetidine delirium usually begins within 24 to 48 hours of beginning treatment, and its symptoms include auditory and visual hallucinations, agitation, paranoia, lethargy, stupor, and coma (Weddington et al., 1982). It tends to clear up within 24 hours after discontinuing the cimetidine or decreasing the dosage. In addition to delirium, cimetidine has also been reported to induce depression (Jefferson, 1979; Crowder and Pate, 1980; Billings et al., 1981).

With digitalis toxicity, neuropsychiatric symptoms may appear as an early or as the sole finding (Portnoi, 1979), and the symptoms may include lethargy, depression, delirium, confabulation, restlessness, emotional instability, hyperventilation, vertigo, and visual hallucinations (Portnoi, 1979; Gregory, 1980; Volpe and Soave, 1979). Headache may be a sign of early toxicity, and anorexia may develop insidiously. Other gastrointestinal symptoms seen are nausea, vomiting, and diarrhea. Disorders of vision, when present, are a diagnostic clue and can involve scotomas and alterations of color vision. Blue-yellow vision is characteristic of toxicity due to digitalis preparations, while disturbance of green perception is frequently seen with the synthetic glycosides (Anderson, 1980). Although serum levels of cardioglycosides can yield useful ancillary information, they must be interpreted cautiously and used in conjunction with clinical findings and the electrocardiogram. There is a high degree of individual variability and a narrow therapeutic-toxic ratio (Anderson, 1980). Treatment of digitalis delirium involves withholding the drug until serum levels return to normal and the sensorium clears. Normal mental status may not return for a number of days.

Anticholinergic agents are among the most common causes of delirium in elderly patients. Not only do elderly people use a large number of prescribed and over-the-counter drugs which have anticholinergic activity, but they also have increased physiological sensitivity to these agents. Brain acetylcholinesterase decreases with age and shows dramatic decreases with Alzheimer's disease (Bartus et al., 1982). As a consequence, the central nervous system has an increased susceptibility to anticholinergic side effects.

The psychological symptoms of anticholinergic delirium are often dramatic. Patients are agitated, confused, and disoriented, and they demonstrate marked memory impairment. Vivid visual and auditory hallucinations are frequently a part of the clinical picture, and one may observe the patient grasping imaginary objects or picking at the bedclothes (Greenblatt and Shader, 1973; Shader, 1972). Physical findings of dilated pupils, increased heart rate, ataxia and myoclonic twitching, and dry mucous membranes contribute to making the diagnosis of anticholinergic toxicity.

Numerous medications have anticholinergic activity, and the potential for delirium is additive when the patient takes more than one such medication. Anticholinergic drugs frequently used by elderly patients include belladonna derivatives, tricyclic antidepressants, and antihistaminic agents (Shader, 1972). When the offending medications are discontinued, anticholinergic delirium usually clears rapidly. Many patients can be managed by reassurance only (Greenblatt and Shader, 1973).

If a more rapid response is required, both the peripheral and central effects of anticholinergic activity can be reversed by the intramuscular administration of physostigmine. However, physostigmine is not risk free, and it is contraindicated in such conditions as diabetes, heart block, coronary artery disease, cardiac arrhythmias, and bronchitis (Hall et al.,

1981). Because these disorders are common in elderly patients, physostigmine has a limited use in this age group, and conservative supportive management is preferable. Some of the phenothiazines (particularly thioridazine) have a high level of anticholinergic activity, so that using these drugs to treat delirium may have the paradoxical effect of increasing its severity. The treatment of the delirious patient should be directed primarily at correcting the underlying cause of the delirium. General supportive measures must also be applied (Lipowski, 1980a). If the patient is severely agitated, haloperidol may be employed to ensure sedation.

DEMENTIA   Dementia is defined as a loss of intellectual abilities that is of sufficient severity to affect social or occupational functioning. It features impairment of abstract thinking, memory, and judgment. Unlike delirium, dementia does not entail clouded consciousness.

The most common cause of dementia in late life is termed Primary Degenerative Dementia in DSM-III (American Psychiatric Association, 1980), a disorder which is synonymous with Alzheimer's disease (Reisberg and Ferris, 1982). Although therapeutic endeavors can make these patients and their families more comfortable (Rabins, 1981), the disease process is irreversible. A major responsibility of the psychiatric consultant, therefore, is to ensure a full exploration of the possibility that the dementia might be due to some treatable disorder. Potentially reversible dementias have been termed pseudosenility (Libow, 1973) or pseudodementia (Wells, 1979; Janowsky, 1982). These terms have been criticized as misleading (Folstein and McHugh, 1978; Reifler, 1982), though; since patients who have a reversible dementia do exhibit clear-cut cognitive dysfunction, the dementia itself is not really "pseudo." One exception is a specific subtype of depression in which the patient repetitively complains of a failing memory and other symptoms of dementia, but is actually cognitively intact (Wells, 1979). However, many patients with severe depression and psychomotor retardation exhibit dementia-like symptoms which cannot be distinguished clinically from primary degenerative dementia even with the aid of neuropsychological testing. The problem is further complicated by the fact that early dementia is often associated with depression and that treatment of the depression will improve the level of cognitive functioning. Thus, dementia and pseudodementia may not be as distinct and separate from each other as some authors have asserted (Folstein and McHugh, 1978; Wells, 1982).

Other causes of reversible dementia include endocrinopathies (e.g., hypothyroidism), normal pressure hydrocephalus, chronic drug intoxication, pernicious anemia, syphilis, and other infections, toxic, or metabolic disorders. To rule out treatable forms of dementia, a diagnostic workup is essential, and this should include a careful history, physical, neurological, and mental status examinations, and the following laboratory studies: urinalysis, complete blood count, serum folate and B_{12} levels, computerized tomography of the head, chest X ray, a metabolic screening test (SMAC), a serological test for syphilis, and thyroid function tests. Note that the finding of cortical atrophy on computerized tomography is *not* diagnostic of dementia; such atrophy occurs normally with aging (Ford and Winter, 1981). Rather, a congruence of information obtained from all sources, including the history, will underlie the diagnosis (Wells and Duncan, 1977). Highlighting the difficulty in diagnosing dementia accurately, a study by Ron et al. (1979) demonstrated that 31 percent of patients who had been diagnosed as having presenile dementia were subsequently shown not to be demented.

ORGANIC AFFECTIVE SYNDROME Organic Affective Syndrome is a disorder of mood caused by a physical illness or an exogenous agent such as a medication. Examples of diseases and disorders associated with depression include hypercalcemia, hypothyroidism, Parkinson's disease, stroke, and carcinoma of the pancreas (Blumenthal, 1980; Ouslander, 1982; Salzman and Shader, 1978a). Often it is unclear whether the mood disturbance is caused directly by the disease or represents a psychological response to the knowledge that one has a serious disease.

A number of the medications used frequently with elderly patients have been observed to precipitate depression or mania (Hall et al., 1980; Levenson, 1979; Perl et al., 1980; Salzman and Shader, 1978b). Among the medications which can cause depression, the most notorious are the antihypertensive agents (resperine, α-methyldopa, propranolol, and clonidine). Drugs implicated in mania include the antidepressant medications, L-dopa, and baclofen.

The diagnosis of Organic Affective Syndrome requires a high index of suspicion. At times, the mood disturbance will remit with treatment of the underlying medical illness or with discontinuation of the offending medication. This is not always the case, however, and it may be necessary to treat depression or mania as if the disorder were primary (Lipowski, 1980b).

Affective Disorders

Depressive mood is so highly prevalent both in the elderly population (Blazer, 1982) and in hospitalized medically ill patients (Dovenmuehle and Verwoerdt, 1962; Moffic and Paykel, 1975; Schuckit et al., 1975) that some people draw the unwarranted conclusion that depression is "normal" for these groups. Such an attitude impedes the initiation of psychiatric consultation and the implementation of effective treatment for the depressed medically ill elderly patient.

Depressive symptoms are common in medically ill elderly people for several reasons. Old age has been described as a "season of loss," and loss of health is one of the losses for which one may grieve. In addition, many diseases, and medications used to treat them, have a high association with depression, either because they induce an organic affective syndrome or because they precipitate depression in susceptible persons. Finally, elderly people may be more prone to endogenous depression, as suggested by the finding that brain monoamine oxidase increases with age (Robinson, 1975).

The consulting psychiatrist should avoid ascribing depressive symptoms to grief too readily. One study has shown that elderly people actually handle bereavement better than younger people (Clayton, 1974). The symptoms of acute grief, including physiological changes, are similar to those of depression, but their persistence beyond a few weeks to months suggests a diagnosis of a depressive disorder rather than grief (Clayton, 1980).

The assessment of a mood disorder in an elderly patient requires a careful evaluation which takes into account the possibilities that the symptoms may be due to an underlying disease process, may be secondary to a prescribed medication, or may signify the presence of a major depression. One pitfall in the differential diagnosis of both depression and mania in elderly patients is that the symptoms may be mistakenly attributed to dementia. A depressed patient with psychomotor retardation may exhibit the symptoms of cognitive impairment and regressed behavior such as incontinence, which suggest dementia. Similarly, the elderly manic patient who is excited, grandiose, or delusional or who displays impaired judgment may appear to be demented. The patient may be a poor historian, and the history must be obtained from other sources (Spar et al., 1979). The dexamethasone suppression test has been suggested for distinguishing dementia from depression (McAllister et al., 1982), but many demented patients fail to suppress cortisol levels in response to the dexamethasone (Spar and Gerner, 1982). On tests such as cerebral blood flow measurements, several depressed patients have shown findings similar to findings with demented patients (Mathew et al., 1980). Differentiation between dementia and depression is further complicated by the fact that many demented patients have depressive symptoms early in the course of their disease (Liston, 1977; Reifler et al., 1982). With treatment of the depression, some demented patients may show an improvement in cognitive function even though some degree of dementia remains (McAllister and Price, 1982). Ultimately, differential diagnosis between dementia and depression may depend upon the results of a therapeutic trial with antidepressants. In one study, the majority of patients who were later proven to have "pseudodementia" due to depression had a previous psychiatric history (McAllister, 1983).

Many depressed older patients present with what appear to be somatoform disorders such as hypochondriasis or psychogenic pain disorder. Somatoform disorders do occur in elderly patients, simply because patients with primary hypochondriasis and Briquet's syndrome (somatization disorder) do grow old (Ford, 1983). However, the available data (Denney et al., 1965) suggest that the elderly people as a group are no more hypochondriacal than younger patients, and the emergence in late life of hypochondriacal symptoms therefore strongly suggests either an adjustment disorder (Goldstein and Birnbom, 1976) or major depression (Blumenthal, 1980). The diagnosis of depression may be confirmed if further inquiry reveals vegetative symptoms, a mood change, or a favorable response to a therapeutic trial of antidepressant medication.

Depression and mania in elderly people are eminently treatable, and patients often demonstrate a favorable response in a fairly short period of time (Jarvik et al., 1982; Rothblum et al., 1982). One should not discontinue treatment too early, however, or lose the patient to follow-up, because relapses are common (Murphy, 1983; Sadavoy and Reiman-Sheldon, 1983).

ROLES OF THE CONSULTATION-LIAISON PSYCHIATRIST

The liaison psychiatrist usually gains entry into the medical care delivery system in the role of a consultant. Consultation techniques for the elderly patient do not differ basically from those applicable to younger persons, but some special points deserve emphasis.

It is preferable to see an elderly patient for several short interviews than to spend the same amount of time in a single long interview. The first reason for this is that such an approach facilitates discovery of a fluctuating sensorium. Furthermore, older patients who are medically ill often tire easily and find the shorter interviews more comfortable. Finally, the multiple visits show the patient an ongoing interest and help to establish rapport. Every patient must be evaluated from several perspectives. Too narrow a theoretical orientation would limit the consultant's effectiveness with a great many of the elderly patients encountered in medical settings. The patient's distress may be due to a single factor or a combination of factors related to intrapsychic conflicts, interpersonal relationships, economic problems, and physiological dysfunctions. The psychiatric consultant must retain his or her identity as a physician and carefully review the patient's medical history, the information in the medical record, and any results of laboratory tests. At times, the psychiatric consultant may need to conduct a physical or a neurological examination or both to obtain more clinical data. Often it will be mandatory for the consultant to interview other people to obtain a more complete history. At most times a spouse or children are available for such interviews, but at other times a distant relative, or even someone such as an apartment manager, can provide the vital information.

With elderly patients, no less than with those who are younger, the psychiatric consultant must complete a skillful mental status examination. This must include an evaluation of attention, memory, abstract thinking, language, and constructional-spatial capabilities (functions of the nondominant hemisphere) (McEvoy, 1981). Failure to complete such a thorough evaluation may result in misdiagnosis; for example, a "thought disorder" may later prove to be dysphasia secondary to a small stroke. Using a standardized and scorable mental status examination, the consultant can objectively follow cognitive function through the course of illness (Folstein et al., 1975).

The psychiatric consultant must appreciate that psychopharmacologic intervention with elderly medically ill patients involves special care (Salzman, 1982; Salzman et al., 1976). Not only does age markedly change the pharmacokinetics of many agents prescribed for older patients, but concurrent disease may affect a given drug's metabolism or excretion (Hicks et al., 1981). Adverse drug reactions, such as orthostatic hypotension, may be potentiated by physical illness, while potential side effects may contraindicate the use of a given drug in certain disease states (for example, tricyclic antidepressants are relatively contraindicated in patients with cardiac conduction defects). The elderly medically ill patient is frequently receiving multiple medications (Salzman et al., 1976), and the probability of adverse drug interactions expands exponentially with the number of drugs prescribed. Any recommendation to use a psychotropic drug must take into account other medications that the patient is concurrently receiving (Gaultieri and Powell, 1978). Advice on the use of psychotropic medications for older patients must be precise in regard to both the type of medication and the specific dosage recommended. An explanation of the logic underlying the choice of a medication and its dosage is helpful. For example, if the consultant recommends a markedly reduced dose of lithium for an elderly manic patient, he or she should explain that the patient has reduced renal clearance and that older patients generally tend to develop toxicity with lower serum levels of lithium (Foster et al., 1977).

Psychiatric treatment of the geriatric patient is not limited to psychopharmacology. The consulting psychiatrist must bear in mind that many clinical problems are responsive to psychotherapy, both individual and family, and that psychotherapy does not carry with it the risk of potentially life-threatening complications that pharmacotherapy may have (Steuer, 1982). At times, electroconvulsive therapy may be useful. Not only is ECT highly effective in treating depressed elderly patients, but it is often safer than antidepressant medications (Weiner, 1982).

The consultant should employ teaching skills as well, so that as the patient receives clinical service, the consultee receives some education. This may not be easy, since the referring physician may only be interested in a disposition for the aged patient. Ignorance about effective psychopharmacology with elderly patients or pervasive nihilistic attitudes toward them sometimes constitute formidable obstacles to the consultant's efforts. Communications with consultees must therefore offer precise descriptions of clinical details, and recommendations must be specific.

Liaison opportunities are plentiful in geriatric medicine. Multiproblem patients lend themselves to multidisciplinary therapeutic approaches (Blumenfield et al., 1982), and liaison psychiatrists are generally skilled in leading and cooperating with multidisciplinary treatment teams. Furthermore, Levitan and Kornfeld (1981) have shown that liaison psychiatry can improve cost-effectiveness: psychiatric liaison service to elderly women with hip fractures led to shorter hospitalizations. Further studies of this type are urgently needed.

CONCLUSION

To be effective in the evaluation and treatment of elderly medically ill patients, the psychiatrist must possess medical diagnostic skills. The psychiatrist cannot serve these patients well without being knowledgeable about their physiological status, about the psychological effects of disease, and about the psychiatric complications of various treatment modalities. Psychological and organic issues are inseparably bound together.

Consultation-liaison psychiatrists have always been geriatric psychiatrists, too; they just may not have known it. Their work has included a significant amount of care for elderly patients, and the future holds a large increase in the proportion of elderly patients requiring consultation-liaison services. Consultation-liaison psychiatrists must acquire skills in geriatric psychiatry, and consultation-liaison services should teach geriatric psychiatry to medical students and house officers (Lipowski, 1983).

Chapter 16

Psychiatry and Oncology
by Mary Jane Massie, M.D. and Jimmie C. Holland, M.D.

In the past decade, interest in psychiatric, psychological, and social issues in cancer has burgeoned. The impetus for this phenomeon has arisen from several sources. First, psychiatry has markedly increased its interest in the psychological problems of medically ill patients, and particularly in the problems of patients with cancer. We have begun defining cancer patients' emotional problems and psychiatric disorders and have begun to understand the difficulties of their families and the staff who care for them (Holland, 1982). Second, the social climate in the United States has changed such that most patients demand more knowledge of their diagnosis and more participation in decisions about their treatment. Third, the speciality of oncology has developed rapidly from the time thirty years ago when little was known about causes or cures of cancer; today, research in cancer is providing exciting new insights into basic patterns of both abnormal and normal cell growth.*

RISK FACTORS AND MANAGEMENT ISSUES IN CANCER

Risk Factors

The fact has long been known that certain behaviors and personal habits increase the risk of cancer through exposure to environmental carcinogens (Higginson and Muir, 1979). The first cancer related to an environmental exposure was identified in 1775 when Percival Potts observed that scrotal cancer occurred frequently among the chimney sweeps of London. The association of cigarette smoking and the epidemic of lung cancer in the United States was recognized in 1956; it represents the single most important finding of a personal habit related to cancer. In both instances, 200 years apart, encouraging individuals to alter their behavior to reduce risk proved to be a formidable task, and the challenge to social scientists remains today. In addition, the potential contribution to cancer risk of "life-style," which includes diet and personal habits, has yet to be studied systematically. The international cancer epidemiologists Higginson and Muir (1979) have estimated that life-style currently represents the major inadequately studied area in cancer cause and prevention.

In a paradigm described by Weiner (1977), the increased risk of cancer which results from behavior is considered the "external loop." (See Figure 1.) This is an indirect route whereby personality, through behavior, alters risk by controlling exposure to a carcinogen. Once cancer has developed, behavior also affects survival, through patients' compliance and adherence to cancer treatment. Many of the chemotherapeutic regimens for cancer, while arduous, are curative if given in full amount, but they result in less chance of cure if the patient cannot or will not take

*Preceptor's note: The reader will find no discussion of the important area of mastectomy and related procedures in this chapter. Rather, Milano and Kornfeld have prepared a review of this topic for their chapter on psychiatry and surgery.

Two Routes:

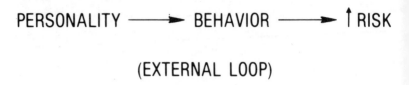

PERSONALITY ——————▶ BEHAVIOR ——————▶ ↑ RISK

(EXTERNAL LOOP)

PERSONALITY ——————▶ CELLULAR ——————▶ ↑ RISK
OR
HUMORAL RESPONSE

(INTERNAL LOOP)

Figure 1. Psychological and social risk factors in cancer

the full treatment. Problems with noncompliance are particularly common in young men with testicular neoplasms and generally in teenagers, who have difficulty tolerating short-term discomforts to obtain long-term gain.

Of considerable interest to psychiatrists has been the "internal loop," a possible direct route whereby personality, through some cellular or humoral mechanism, could alter both premorbid risk and length of survival. Since these issues are beyond the scope of this review, the reader is referred to the excellent overviews by Fox (1979; 1981), who combines skillfully the thoroughness and skepticism of a psychologist and an epidemiologist.

Survival Rates and Management Issues

Figure 2 shows data from the National Cancer Institute on cancer mortality and population trends in the United States since 1954. In persons under 30, cancer deaths have been dropping sharply since 1966, due largely to dramatically improved survival among patients with Wilms's tumor, acute lymphocytic leukemia, osteogenic sarcoma, testicular neoplasms, and Hodgkin's disease. Patients under 45 have a clear but less impressive reduction in cancer mortality. Those under 60 show a plateau which began in 1968. The development of therapies which combine surgery, radiation, and increasingly effective chemotherapy account for these changes. As these facts have become more widely known, optimism about cancer has increased. Physicians themselves, recognizing better chances for survival, have become more insistent about patients' accepting and adhering to treatment.

Greater attention has turned to the emotional, physical, and behavioral consequences of rigorous treatment regimens, especially in young

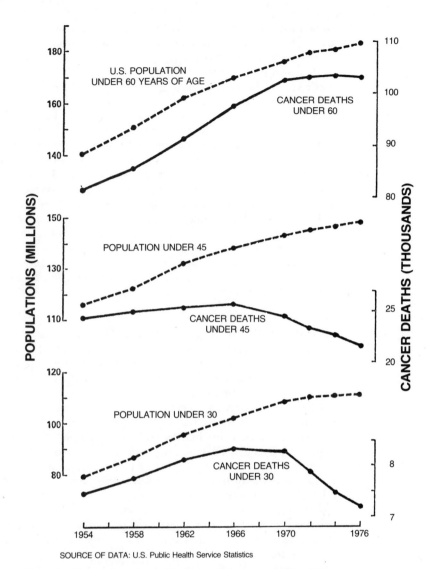

Figure 2. Cancer mortality and U.S. population trends: 1954–1976

SOURCE OF DATA: U.S. Public Health Service Statistics

people. Quality of life and delayed treatment effects in long survivors and cured patients have become important issues. Patients no longer accept the statement, "You should be grateful just to be alive." Their concerns about the long-term sequelae of treatment on psychological and physical function, particularly sexual, are discussed below.

Quality of life is equally important for the patient whose treatment is palliative only. When patients have advanced illness and cure is no longer possible, the oncologist must carefully weigh the likely benefits of a given treatment versus toxicity. These issues fall into bold relief when conventional treatments have failed and the physician, patient, and family must decide between supportive care with maximum comfort and participation in a clinical investigation of new, unapproved anticancer agents.

The ethical issues surrounding this important decision constitute a new area of medical ethics and are of interest to psychiatrists working with patients who have cancer.

Measuring the quality of life is difficult, but it has become an important issue in the clinical trials of new agents. The national cooperative group, Cancer and Leukemia Group B (CALGB), has been carefully measuring the toxicity and side effects of new drugs over the past twenty years, but the group had not until recently measured patients' subjective perception and the "psychological toxicity" of the treatments. Since 1976, when the CALGB psychiatric research component was instituted, quality of life (e.g., function in physical, social, work, and family areas) has been measured in ten protocol studies. For instance, Silberfarb et al. (1983) studied two chemotherapy regimens for palliative treatment of lung cancer. They found that although survival rates were identical, patients who received the treatment which contained vincristine (Oncovin), known to have significant neurotoxic side effects, were significantly more depressed. Studies of this kind are important since they also provide new clinical insights and research direction for studying the neurochemical parameters of depression.

PHYSICIAN-PATIENT INTERACTIONS The nature of the physician-patient interaction has changed markedly over the past 25 years. In large part, this reflects changes in telling or not telling the diagnosis of cancer, which was once the primary (and highly emotional) issue that engaged psychiatrists in cancer.

Changes in the management of children with acute leukemia and their parents exemplify the trends. CALGB has carried out increasingly more successful protocols in children with acute lymphocytic leukemia. (See Figure 3.) Using the best-known treatment in 1956, all children died within 14 months. Physicians at that time understandably tried to shield family and patient from the dreaded words leukemia and cancer. Psychological intervention focused on helping the patient and family manage the certain and rapidly fatal outcome. Then, as each new protocol produced cures and longer survivals, particularly in the last ten years, it became easier for doctors to discuss the diagnosis and treatment. Today, children know their diagnosis and are encouraged to be part of all discussions about treatment plans.

The marked changes in patient-physician interactions thus result from two factors: the patient's demands to know about treatment options and to participate in the treatment decisions and the physician's acceptance of a less authoritarian and paternalistic role. Treatment options, especially in regard to investigational therapy, must be reviewed with patients and strict guidelines adhered to for the protection of human rights. Truly informed consent is difficult to obtain, however. Patients are anxious, are given more information than they can comprehend at one sitting, and tend to hear the positive, while failing to hear the negative. Physicians, though trying to give appropriate information, are still hesitant to distress the patient unduly. The Psychosocial Collaborative Oncology Group (PSYCOG) (Penman et al., 1980) demonstrated that even when the consent forms stated that no benefit could be expected from an investigational new treatment, 80 percent of patients believed that their disease would be helped by the treatment. Improving the quality

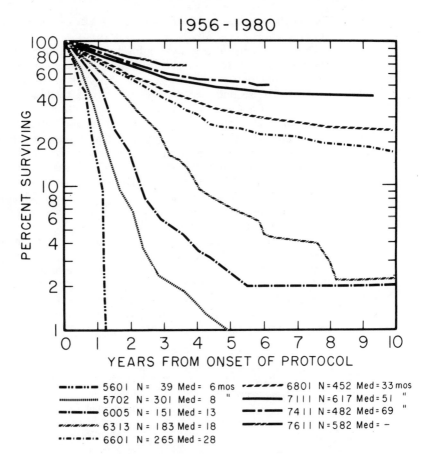

1956-1980

PERCENT SURVIVING

YEARS FROM ONSET OF PROTOCOL

▬▪▬▪▪▬	5601 N = 39 Med = 6 mos	▬▬▬▬ 6801 N = 452 Med = 33 mos
▬▬▬▬▬	5702 N = 301 Med = 8 "	▬▬▬▬ 7111 N = 617 Med = 51 "
▬▪▬▪▬	6005 N = 151 Med = 13	▬▪▬▪▬ 7411 N = 482 Med = 69 "
▬▬▬▬	6313 N = 183 Med = 18	▬▬▬▬ 7611 N = 582 Med = −
▪▬▪▬▪▬	6601 N = 265 Med = 28	

Figure 3. Acute lymphocytic leukemia survival in children under 20 (Cancer and Leukemia Group B)
Source: Adapted from Holland JF: Cancer Medicine, 2nd ed. Philadelphia, Lea and Febiger, 1982. Used with permission.

of informed consent and the information given to patients is a fruitful area for research at the interface of psychiatry and oncology.*

The range and intensity of the psychological and social needs of cancer patients and their families have led medical and pediatric oncologists to make use of multidisciplinary teams. The oncologist often becomes the primary care physician for the cancer patient, and the health care team also includes strong roles for the oncology nurse, social workers, clergy, and supportive participants from rehabilitation. To be effective, the team approach requires a high level of communication among team members and with the patient.

Roles of the Consultation-Liaison Psychiatrist

Psychiatric consultations for cancer patients have caused greater attention to be directed to the psychological stresses imposed by cancer and its treatment on the patient, the family, and the staff who care for them.

*Preceptor's note: In their chapter, Milano and Kornfeld discuss the topics of consent and refusal in greater detail and review some of the relevant research regarding patient recall.

The problems of the health care setting as a social system have also come under study.

The psychiatrist in a cancer setting has several important functions. The central one is to serve as consultant, providing expertise in the recognition, diagnosis, and management of psychiatric disorders in cancer patients. The second role involves outlining a treatment plan and assuring that it is carried out. In the oncology setting, three major therapeutic modalities are used: (1) psychotherapeutic (which includes individual and group psychotherapy and which may be carried out by professional or self-help groups); (2) psychopharmacologic (which includes the use of antianxiety agents, antidepressants, analgesics, and antipsychotics); and (3) behavioral interventions (which are increasingly being used to control pain, anxiety, and both the anticipatory and the treatment-induced nausea and vomiting that are associated with many chemotherapeutic agents). (See Table 1.)

An eclectic philosophy has evolved in most cancer centers today so that a combination of these three approaches is used, either concurrently or sequentially, depending on the nature of the symptoms and their response. Since the most common psychiatric disorders require a range of therapeutic approaches, each approach is discussed below where its role in management is most appropriate. Table 2 outlines the primary indications for each modality.

Table 1. Principal Therapeutic Approaches in Cancer

Psychotherapeutic	Individual
	Professional
	Counseling and advice
	Support/crisis intervention
	Psychotherapy
	Nonprofessional
	Veteran and fellow
	Group
	Professional
	Education
	Support
	Psychotherapy
	Nonprofessional
	Self-help
	(Make Today Count, Cansurmount)
Psychopharmacologic	Antianxiety
	Antidepressant
	Analgesic
	Antipsychotic
	(emesis and psychiatric indications)
Behavioral	Relaxation
	Biofeedback
	Systematic desensitization
	Hypnosis
	Guided imagery
Combined Approaches	

Table 2. Primary Indications for Each Therapeutic Approach

Psychotherapeutic	Professional
	Crisis intervention at times of maximal stress
	At time of diagnosis
	Prior to a new treatment
	At relapse
	At treatment failure
	Ongoing psychotherapy
	For preexisting psychiatric disorders
	Nonprofessional
	Provision of "practical" advice at times of crisis
	Ongoing support
Psychopharmacologic	Some Adjustment Disorders
	Anxiety Disorders
	Major Depression
	Delirium/dementia
	Schizophrenic Disorders
	Bipolar Disorders
	Pain
	Nausea and vomiting
	Insomnia
Behavioral	Anxiety and discomfort with procedures
	(bone marrow aspiration, lumbar puncture)
	Pain (adjunct to analgesics)
	Nausea and vomiting (anticipatory, treatment-related)
	Eating disorders

    The psychiatrist who establishes credibility as a valuable consultant in patient care has no difficulty in carrying out the liaison function. The liaison role evolves naturally when a single psychiatrist routinely makes rounds with the oncology staff and sees all the patients who require consultation. The consultant can then encourage staff members to discuss their reactions to the stresses of the treatment environment and to patients who arouse painful emotions.

    Dealing daily with critically ill patients and with the ethical issues involved in their care can be draining and may lead to the syndrome called staff burnout. When the oncologist, nurse, or house officer experiences transient personal difficulties or has preexisting personality problems, he or she may feel overwhelmed by the combined personal and work stresses. Psychiatrists have developed both intra- and interdisciplinary meetings to address these staff needs. The meetings have been particularly valuable with physicians (Artiss and Levine, 1973), nurses (Vachon et al., 1978), and medical students (Massie et al., 1982).

PSYCHIATRIC DISORDERS IN CANCER PATIENTS

Prevalence

The diagnosis of cancer clearly causes an individual to experience stress related both to the actual symptoms of the disease and to the psychological meaning attached to cancer. A given patient's ability to manage these stresses depends on his or her prior level of emotional adjustment, the threat the cancer poses to his or her age-appropriate goals (career, family, and so forth), the presence of emotionally supportive persons in the environment, and variables determined by the disease (disabling symptoms, site, treatments required, prognosis). When the cancer patient's emotional distress exceeds what would seem expectable or normal, the psychiatric symptoms must be evaluated.

There has been an increasing need for information regarding the actual prevalence of significant psychiatric disorders among cancer patients. PSYCOG recently reported on a study of 215 randomly selected hospitalized and ambulatory patients at three major cancer centers (Johns Hopkins, Rochester, and Memorial Hospital) (Derogatis et al., 1983). Clinical interviews which permitted a DSM-III diagnosis revealed that 47 percent met criteria for a psychiatric disorder and 53 percent did not. Of the 47 percent who had a recognizable psychiatric disorder, 68 percent had an Adjustment Disorder with Depressed, Anxious, or Mixed Mood, 13 percent had a Major Depression, 8 percent had an Organic Mental Disorder, 7 percent had a Personality Disorder, and 4 percent had an Anxiety Disorder. The spectrum of depressive disorders encompassing Adjustment Disorder with Depressed Mood and Major Depression, accounted for the most common problems. (See Table 3.)

Table 3. Rates of DSM-III Disorders

	N (Percent in Diagnostic Class)	Percent of Total Sample
Adjustment Disorders	69 (68)	32
Major Affective Disorders	13 (13)	6
Organic Mental Disorders	8 (8)	4
Personality Disorders	7 (7)	3
Anxiety Disorders	4 (4)	2
Total DSM-III Disorders	101 (100)	47
Total No DSM-III Disorder	114 (0)	53
TOTAL	215 (47)	100

Source: Adapted from Derogatis LR, et al: The prevalence of psychiatric disorders among cancer patients. JAMA 249:751–757, 1983. American Medical Association, copyright 1983.

In another study, Bukberg et al. (1983) explored the prevalence of depression in hospitalized cancer patients at Memorial Hospital. They found that 24 percent were severely depressed, 18 percent were moderately depressed, and 14 percent had depressive symptoms of sadness. The remaining 44 percent showed no depression at all, despite their cancer illness. The factor most significantly related to the presence of severe depression was the level of impaired physical function; 77 percent of those who were most depressed were also the most physically impaired. Separation of cancer symptoms from vegetative signs of depression is almost impossible in the very ill, making interpretation of such studies difficult. However, the finding of 24 percent with severe depression is similar to that of Plumb and Holland (1977). This study found that approximately 23 percent of cancer patients were significantly depressed. Two studies of patients on a general medical floor found a similar prevalence of depression, suggesting that cancer patients are no more or less depressed than equally physically ill patients with other diseases (Schwab et al., 1967; Moffic and Paykel, 1975).

Up to a quarter of all cancer patients may thus be experiencing significant emotional distress, most often of a depressive nature. However, in two studies of psychiatric consultations, one at Memorial Hospital (Massie et al., 1979) and the other at Dartmouth (Levine et al., 1978), patients who were referred for consultation and found to be depressed constituted less than 3 percent of the patient population hospitalized for cancer. A PSYCOG survey of psychotropic drugs ordered by physicians for cancer patients in five centers over an eight-month period found that only 1 percent of the prescriptions were for antidepressant medication (Derogatis et al., 1979). Taken together, the studies of prevalence of depression and the studies of psychiatric consultations in cancer patients suggest that while 20 to 25 percent of cancer patients are depressed, a large number of the depressions go unrecognized and untreated.

Causes and Management of Primary Psychiatric Disorders

The most common psychiatric disorders encountered in cancer patients are reactions to crises in cancer, major depressive disorder, delirium and dementia, and anxiety disorders.

REACTIONS TO CRISES The ubiquitous human responses documented in other situations of threatened or actual loss (Hamburg et al., 1953; Lindemann, 1944; Lifton, 1967) are seen with similar symptoms in cancer patients at times of crisis. When individuals are told about their diagnosis of cancer, they are transiently distressed, and reactions vary from minimal to major disruptions of emotions and activities. The psychological symptoms are initial shock and disbelief, followed by anxiety symptoms, depressive symptoms, anger, and a disruption of appetite and sleep. The ability to concentrate and to carry out the normal daily patterns of work and home life may be impaired, and intrusive thoughts about the diagnosis and fears for the future may be uncontrollable. The acute response is ordinarily resolved in seven to ten days. Using DSM-III terminology, these patients would receive a diagnosis of Adjustment Disorder with Depressed or Anxious Mood, or a combination of both, in which the stressor is news of threat to life. DSM-III is poorly suited to making a more refined diagnosis of secondary and reactive responses to medical illness.

Psychiatric consultation should be requested when the acute symptoms of distress last longer than a week, when they worsen rather than improve, or when they interfere with the patient's ability to cooperate with the planned treatment. Short-term supportive psychotherapy, based on a crisis intervention model with four to six sessions, is usually sufficient to reduce symptoms to a tolerable level. The sessions deal with the here and now of adaptation to the diagnosis and treatment.*

*Editor's note: In Part I of this volume, Bellak offers a detailed discussion of the technique of brief, crisis-oriented psychotherapy.

MAJOR DEPRESSIVE DISORDER Differentiating between a severe adjustment disorder with depressed mood and major depression is difficult in the cancer setting. In the authors' experience, these two diagnoses encompass a continuum according to the severity of depressive symptoms. Choice of treatment is based on severity of symptoms, and the major depression seen in cancer is rarely related to an underlying bipolar illness. The depression seen in cancer patients is almost always secondary to the physical illness.

While the diagnosis of depression in physically healthy patients depends heavily on the somatic symptoms of anorexia, fatigue, and weight loss, these indicators are of little value with a cancer patient, since they are common to both cancer and depression. Diagnosis must therefore rest upon psychological, not somatic, symptoms: presence of dysphoric mood, feelings of helplessness or hopelessness, loss of self-esteem, and feelings of worthlessness or guilt. Psychotic depressions are exceedingly rare. Cancer patients who are at higher risk for depression are those with poorer physical state, those with inadequately controlled pain, and those with advanced stages of illness, particularly pancreatic cancer (Holland et al., 1983).

In addition to supportive psychotherapy, tricyclic antidepressants are used for the depressed cancer patient who has symptoms severe enough to interfere with function. Imipramine, amitriptyline, doxepin, and nortriptyline are most commonly prescribed. For reasons which are unclear, cancer patients appear to respond to antidepressants in shorter time and at lower doses (10 to 25 mg). One hypothesis is that tumors alter the activity of the hepatic enzymes involved in the metabolism of antidepressants.

Treatment should start at a low dose, especially in debilitated patients, beginning with 10 mg of amitriptyline twice a day and increasing as tolerated up to 75 to 150 mg per day. When insomnia is a dominant symptom and sedation is desired, amitriptyline is the drug of choice, starting with 25 mg at bedtime. When given intramuscularly, a more rapid effect is obtained. Amitriptyline is particularly useful in the cancer setting because it combines analgesic, sedative, and antidepressant actions. Nortriptyline is available in liquid form for patients who cannot take a tablet. Parenteral imipramine or amitriptyline can be used with patients who cannot take medication by mouth.

Anticholinergic side effects are troublesome with cancer patients who have gastrointestinal or genitourinary cancer, who have had gastrointestinal surgery, or who have stomatitis secondary to chemotherapy or radiation. Antidepressants with the weakest anticholinergic effects, such as doxepin, trazodone, or maprotiline, are indicated for these patients. Tricyclic antidepressants are contraindicated with only one chemotherapeutic agent: procarbazine (Matulane), a monoamine oxidase (MAO) inhibitor.

Another anticholinergic side effect, delirium, occasionally develops in older patients and in those receiving other anticholinergic drugs: atropine, scopolamine, or antipsychotics. Agranulocytosis can result from the use of tricyclics, and they should therefore be used cautiously with neutropenic patients.

Amitriptyline is widely used in the management of cancer patients' pain. A suggested dose is 25 mg at bedtime. The initial assumption was that the analgesic effect resulted indirectly from the tricyclics' effect upon depression. While it is now clear that the tricyclics have a separate analgesic action that is not mediated through endorphins, the mechanism of action is unclear (Spiegel et al., 1983).

The other psychopharmacologic treatments for depression are lithium, MAO inhibitors, and psychostimulants. Patients who have been receiving lithium prior to their cancer illness should be maintained on it throughout treatment, and they should be monitored closely during the pre- and postoperative periods when fluids and salt may be restricted. Lithium should be used most cautiously with patients who are receiving cis-platinum (cisplatin, DDP) since both lithium and cis-platinum are both potentially nephrotoxic. Lithium has been used in several cancer centers in an attempt to stimulate granulocyte production in neutropenic patients or to prevent leukopenia during chemotherapy. The stimulation effect appeared transient, and no mood changes were noted in the patients.

If a patient has responded well to a MAO inhibitor for depression prior to treatment for cancer, its continued use is warranted. However, most psychiatrists in oncology settings do not prescribe MAO inhibitors, since cancer patients often have other extensive dietary restrictions.

The psychostimulants, dextroamphetamine or methylphenidate, are sometimes used with cancer patients who are depressed or in the terminal phases of illness. Dextroamphetamine may improve appetite and promote an increased sense of well-being, starting at 2.5 mg twice a day and increasing as tolerance develops. Amphetamines can also be used to potentiate the analgesic effect of opiates.

Cancer patients rarely abuse psychotropic or narcotic medications. In contrast, they often reduce or stop taking them on their own as the need seems to diminish, thus requiring that the psychiatrist encourage them to take enough.

DELIRIUM AND DEMENTIA: CAUSES Delirium, the second most common psychiatric diagnosis among cancer patients, is due both to the direct effects of cancer on the CNS and the indirect CNS complications of the disease and treatment. CNS complications affect 15 percent of all cancer patients (Posner, 1971). Recognition of delirium is important since the underlying cause may be a treatable complication of cancer. Any patient who shows impaired cognitive function, altered attention span, or a fluctuating level of consciousness should be evaluated for presence of delirium.

CNS complications in cancer patients occur directly through a structural change effect caused by a primary brain tumor or intracranial metastases, or indirectly and more commonly through nonmetastatic CNS complications (Posner, 1971). Primary brain tumors account for only 4 percent of all cancer; intracranial metastases, particularly from lung, breast, and kidney, are much more common. Patients may present with a profoundly altered personality related to a solitary metastasis, or they may have multiple metastases and minimally impaired personality or mental function. The reasons for this are not understood. Few neuropsychological studies have been done on patients with primary or metastatic brain lesions. Patients may become depressed, even suicidal, when they recognize the threatened loss of their highly valued intellectual function.

The indirect CNS complications of cancer usually present with symptoms of delirium. Indirect CNS complications are in most cases due to metabolic factors and side effects of chemotherapy or radiation. Rarely are they due to the remote effects of cancer most often seen as multifocal leukoencephalopathy.

Delirium is usually due to one or more of seven causes (Lipowski, 1980): medications, electrolyte imbalance, failure of a vital organ or system, nutritional state, infections, vascular complications, and/or hormone-producing tumors.

Cancer patients are often placed simultaneously on multiple *medications* which can produce delirium. Analgesics (levorphanol or meperidine), steroids (dexamethasone or prednisone), hypnotics, and chemotherapeutic agents are notorious offenders.

Electrolyte imbalance, such as hypercalcemia, occurs in patients with cancers which frequently metastasize to bone, breast, prostate, lung, kidney, multiple myeloma, and lymphoma. Patients with elevated calcium may show mild confusion which can progress to frank delirium.

Encephalopathy occurs with failure of a *vital organ:* liver, kidney, lung, adrenals, and thyroid. Hepatic encephalopathy, uremia, and hypoxia associated with impaired lung function are the most common sources of cerebral dysfunction in patients with disseminated or metastatic disease.

Poor nutritional state, resulting in hypoalbuminemia and vitamin deficiencies, particularly B_1, may contribute to impaired mental function in debilitated cancer patients.

Infections producing generalized sepsis are common in neutropenic or immunologically impaired cancer patients. Delirium in this situation is usually transient. Opportunistic infections of the CNS are more common in immunosuppressed patients. Delirium in patients with acquired immunodeficiency syndrome (AIDS) often appears to be due to cytomegalovirus (CMV) encephalitis (Gapen, 1982).

Vascular complications are uncommon, but they occur with some tumors, particularly those of the lung. Disseminated intravascular coagulation (DIC) presents with a coagulation defect, producing cerebral embolism and microinfarcts, which sometimes result in delirium.

Certain tumors produce *hormones* which affect mental function, cognition, and mood. These tumors include the "APUDomas" (tumors of dispersed neuroendocrine cell systems with the capacity for *a*mine *p*recursor *u*ptake and *d*ecarboxylation), medullary thyroid carcinoma, carcinoid tumors, tumors of the adrenal medulla, parathyroid tumors, and small cell cancer of the lung. Altered mental states range from mood disturbance to delirium and psychosis (Delellis and Wolfe, 1982).

Among the sixty or more chemotherapeutic agents now available for cancer, neurotoxicity is not generally a prominent feature. Nevertheless, neurological side effects are significant and limiting with some agents. Table 4, adapted from Young's excellent 1982 review, lists the CNS symptoms of the commonly used chemotherapeutic agents.

Methotrexate, used in the treatment of leukemia, leukemic meningitis, breast carcinoma, lymphoma, and osteogenic sarcoma, has few neurotoxic effects when used in standard systemic doses. However, when

Table 4. CNS Symptoms and Toxicity of Major Chemotherapeutic Agents Used for Cancer

	Delirium	Lethargy	Hallucinations	Dementia	Depression	Personality Change	Mania	Psychosis	Extrapyramidal Symptoms
Methotrexate	+			+		+			
Fluorouracil	+								+
Vincristine/ Vinblastine	+	+			+				
Bleomycin	+								
BCNU	+			+					
Cis-platinum	+								
Dacarbazine				+					
Hydroxyurea			+						
Asparaginase	+	+	+						
Procarbazine	+	+	+		+		+		
Prednisone	+	+	+		+	+	+	+	

Source: Adapted from Young (1982).

a high-dose intravenous or intrathecal route is used, methotrexate can cause delirium. Dementia has been reported in a small number of cases (Allen et al., 1980). Whole brain radiation, combined with intrathecal methotrexate, enhances the development of encephalopathy (Price and Jamieson, 1975). Rowland et al. (1982) retrospectively studied children with acute lymphocytic leukemia who were treated with intrathecal methotrexate and cranial radiation as prophylaxis against CNS recurrence. They found that children who received both radiation and intrathecal methotrexate had a mean 10-point-lower IQ than children who received only intrathecal methotrexate. Abnormalities in growth hormone and soft neurological signs were also evident.

Radiation causes a transient syndrome in children known as the radiation somnolence syndrome. It usually occurs several weeks after radiation and is caused by radiation-induced demyelinization. Doses of radiation required to treat brain tumors at times result in cognitive impairment and occasionally in progressive dementia, which cannot be avoided. Lower doses used for prophylaxis in adults with lung cancer and leukemias are still being assessed for side effects.

Fluorouracil (5-FU), used in the treatment of colorectal and breast carcinoma, occasionally produces cerebellar ataxia and Parkinson-like syndromes (Young, 1982). High-dose infusions cause encephalopathy in up to 40 percent of patients (Bagley, 1975; Greenwald, 1976).

Vincristine and vinblastine (Velban), chemotherapeutic agents derived from periwinkle plants, are used in the treatment of leukemia and solid tumors. In addition to peripheral neuropathy, which can be severe, lethargy, hallucinations, and depression have been described with the use of these drugs (Holland, J.F. et al., 1973).

Bleomycin, (Blenoxane), combined with methotrexate, cyclophosphamide (Cytoxan), and fluorouracil, is used in the treatment of several solid tumors and lymphomas. Delirium has been reported (Fazio et al., 1976).

Carmustine (BCNU) is a nitrosourea used to treat lung cancer, Hodgkin's disease, leukemia, and multiple myeloma. In the treatment of malignant glioma, BCNU acts synergistically with cranial radiation, occasionally producing dementia and cerebral atrophy (Young and Posner, 1980). Intracarotid injection of BCNU for treatment of primary and metastatic brain tumor has resulted in encephalopathy (Yamada et al., 1979).

Cis-platinum, the first heavy metal compound to be used as an antineoplastic agent, has been highly successful in the treatment of testicular and ovarian cancer. It can produce an acute reversible encephalopathy (Young, 1982).

Dacarbazine (DTIC), used in the treatment of malignant melanoma, glioma, refractory Hodgkin's disease, and certain soft tissue sarcomas, can cause dementia (Sawicka et al., 1977).

Hydroxyurea (Hydrea), used to treat both acute and chronic phases of chronic myelogenous leukemia and carcinoma of the prostate, causes headache, drowsiness, and hallucinations (Young, 1982).

Asparaginase (Elspar), useful in acute lymphoblastic leukemia, can have significant CNS toxicity at commonly used doses. Subtle memory and personality change may precede lethargy and confusion. Marked symptoms of depression, delirium, and impaired recent memory have been reported (Young, 1982).

Procarbazine is an agent which crosses the blood-brain barrier and acts as a MAO inhibitor. Used to treat Hodgkin's disease and lymphoma, it produces few neurological side effects at the usual dose. At higher levels, however, up to 30 percent of patients develop CNS toxicity, with somnolence, lethargy, depression, mania, or delirium (Mann and Hutchinson, 1967; DeConti, 1971). Procarbazine, as a MAO inhibitor, potentiates the effects of alcohol, barbiturates, narcotics, and tricyclic antidepressants.

Glucocorticosteroids are widely used in cancer. Prednisone is a critical component of the treatment for Hodgkin's disease, acute leukemia, and lymphoma. Dexamethasone is used to diminish cerebral edema with brain and spinal cord tumors. All the steroid compounds may cause psychiatric disturbances ranging from minor mood disturbances to a frank steroid psychosis (Hall et al., 1979; Lipowski, 1980). Disturbances may include affective changes (emotional lability, depressed mood), anxiety, fears, or paranoid interpretation of events and suspiciousness of others, with illusions, delusions, and hallucinations. Symptoms often develop four to five days after beginning high-dose steroids or when the dose is rapidly tapered, but psychiatric symptoms can also develop while patients are on maintenance dose. No relationship has been shown between the development of steroid psychosis and premorbid personality or psychiatric history.

DELIRIUM AND DEMENTIA: MANAGEMENT Frequently, the cause of delirium in a patient with cancer cannot be traced to a single cause, since the potential contributing factors are so numerous. When the patient is confused, disruptive, and unable to cooperate with diagnostic tests, sedation may be necessary to enable doing the workup. Furthermore, when the etiology is organ failure or some irreversible complication, it is often impossible to correct the cause. In a study of terminally ill cancer patients, the authors and Glass (1983) found that over three-quarters of them developed a delirium and that the etiology was most often due to more than one cause (e.g., a combination of analgesics, infection, encephalopathy, or hemorrhage).

Haloperidol is the most effective drug for prompt control of agitated, disruptive behavior. Intramuscular injection of 0.5 to 2.0 mg reduces agitation without causing sedation or hypotension. It can be administered intravenously at 1 mg per minute if necessary. Doses which can be repeated at thirty- to sixty-minute intervals are titrated against behavior. The patient should be changed to an oral dose of three-fourths the parenteral dose as soon as possible. For lesser degrees of disturbed behavior, 1 to 2 mg of trifluoperazine or 10 to 25 mg of thioridazine may be given orally twice a day.

SCHIZOPHRENIC DISORDERS The possibly lower incidence of cancer in chronically hospitalized schizophrenic patients was once thought to be due to a protective effect either of the mental illness or of phenothiazines. However, it now appears likely that this could be explained by the mildly protective effects of environment in the long-term hospital patient. Despite the fact that reserpine and phenothiazines cause elevations of prolactin, there is no evidence in human beings that taking these drugs alters the risk of developing breast cancer or that they might promote tumor growth. Women with breast cancer can safely be prescribed these drugs.

ANXIETY DISORDERS　Cancer patients have peaks of reactive anxiety at times of crisis. These reactions may occur when a symptom of cancer is discovered, during the diagnostic workup, on being told the diagnosis, and when a new treatment is started. Patients with generalized anxiety disorder or panic disorder antedating the diagnosis of cancer may experience a severe exacerbation of their psychological symptoms, requiring aggressive psychopharmacologic management. It is sometimes difficult to differentiate symptoms of anxiety from those of underlying cancer. A common consultation request in a cancer hospital is that the psychiatrist evaluate anxiety (accompanied by hyperventilation) in a lung cancer patient who is complaining of shortness of breath. Concern about compromising the respiratory function should not preclude a judicious trial of an antianxiety drug, since the patient's shortness of breath may be remarkably improved when the secondary anxiety is reduced. Benzodiazepines are the treatment of choice for anxiety states. Dose is titrated to control symptoms. Sedation and somnolence, the common side effects of the benzodiazepines, occur more frequently in older patients and in those with impaired liver function.

NAUSEA AND VOMITING
Control of both pre- and posttreatment nausea and vomiting is important toward improving compliance wth anticancer chemotherapy, and many of the chemotherapeutic agents produce immediate nausea and vomiting. They act on the chemoreceptor trigger zone in the floor of the fourth ventricle, thereby stimulating the vomiting center in the lateral reticular formation. Cis-platinum and doxorubicin hydrochloride (Adriamycin) are prime offenders. Prochlorperazine (Compazine) has been the traditional antiemetic used, but more recently other agents have proved more effective. Metoclopramide (Reglan) given intravenously is the most effective agent for nausea and vomiting (Gralla et al., 1981). Marijuana smoking is often helpful, but its utility is tightly connected to set and setting. Tetrahydrocannabinol, the active agent in marijuana, has an antiemetic effect, but the level required produces significant dysphoria, particularly in older patients. About 30 percent of patients who receive weekly cycles of chemotherapy which produces significant nausea and vomiting have been noted after four or five cycles to develop anticipatory nausea and vomiting in response to cues such as smells or sights. This appears to be a classical conditioning paradigm. Desensitization has been used successfully by Morrow and Morrell (1982) to reduce the development of anticipatory nausea and vomiting.

PSYCHOLOGICAL SEQUELAE IN CURED AND LONG-SURVIVING PATIENTS
The psychological problems of long-term survivors constitute a new area of psychiatric concern (Holland and Rowland, 1982). Common psychological problems include fears associated with termination of treatment, fears of recurrence or second malignancy, adaptation to "unanticipated" late effects (infertility, CNS dysfunction, organ failure), chronic

stress on patient and family, development of "survivor syndrome" (guilt), and adaptation to negative social responses (job, friends).

The authors' observations of patients finishing radiotherapy treatments revealed an unexpected and significant increase in psychological distress at the *end* of treatment (Holland et al., 1979). This distress seemed to be related to fear that the tumor might recur when treatment was stopped. Loss of daily supportive contact with staff and of the security provided by close physical monitoring caused heightened distress. The even more difficult question of when maintenance therapy should end, particularly in leukemia, is a source of fear. Patients continue years later to experience anxiety when they develop minor symptoms which earlier they would have ignored.

The patient's quality of life can also be directly affected by his or her adaptation to the delayed side effects of treatment. Neurotoxicity, damage to renal and cardiovascular systems, and infertility caused by radiation and/or chemotherapeutic agents do alter normal functioning and thus cause emotional distress (Holland and Rowland, 1982).

Ovarian failure related to chemotherapy regimes accounts for sexual dysfunction and diminished libido in a high percentage of young women who have had the MOPP regimen for Hodgkin's disease (Mustargen, Oncovin, procarbazine, prednisone) and adjuvant chemotherapy for breast cancer (Chapman et al., 1979; Schilsky et al., 1980). Frequently, women have not been prepared for this treatment-related early menopause, and an explanation of hormonal replacement therapy can be helpful.

Men also experience a high frequency of sterility with the MOPP regimen for Hodgkin's disease. Men who receive unshielded pelvic radiation become aspermic after three or four treatments and remain sterile. While retroperitoneal node dissection for testicular neoplasms causes no loss in sexual performance, ejaculation is impaired, and sterility may result due to interruption of the sympathetic chain (von Eschenbach, 1980). Sperm banking should be an integral part of management.

The following guidelines are recommended to minimize psychological sequelae in long-term survival:

1. *Honesty about the diagnosis and clear communication* between the physician, patient, and family about diagnosis and treatment
2. *Honesty about possible long-term adverse side effects*
3. *Support* for patients as active treatment terminates
4. *Continuity of the treating physician and staff* (The complexity of cancer treatment requires that many consultants and specialists be involved in a patient's care. However, continuity of one physician adds greatly to the security of patient and family.)
5. *Monitoring* the effects of cancer and treatment on the patient's ability to attain age-appropriate developmental tasks with early referral for rehabilitation as needed (This may entail neurological, endocrinological, and psychological evaluation to arrive at a diagnosis and to introduce remediation.)
6. *Psychological intervention* for significant anxiety and depression
7. *Evaluation* of family interaction for possible impact of the stress on other family members

8. *"Veteran" patient support* (The psychological gains from discussion with others who have had the same neoplasm and have experienced similar treatment is invaluable.)

SUMMARY

The nature and prevalence of the common psychiatric disorders in cancer patients are now known. Diagnosis and management of these disorders are the major tasks of the psychiatrist in an oncology unit, and interventions are psychotherapeutic, psychopharmacologic, and behavioral. Longer survival and cure of patients with cancer have led to a new emphasis on the long-term psychiatric sequelae and guidelines for their management.

Chapter 17 # Psychiatry and Surgery
by Michael R. Milano, M.D. and Donald S. Kornfeld, M.D.

The psychiatrist consulting with a surgical patient confronts a welter of possible influences on the patient's course. As well as considering the effects of the underlying disease and the patient's style of coping, the psychiatrist must consider the effects of anesthesia, surgery, possible mutilation, and numerous postoperative possibilities. The newer surgical procedures such as organ transplantation and gastric or jejunoileal bypass for obesity have given rise to special psychological adaptation issues. Similarly, the availability of new surgical techniques for mastectomy and breast reconstruction may alter the typical patient's postoperative course and thus influence psychological adaptation.

This chapter reviews new developments in understanding the surgical patient in the preoperative, perioperative, and postoperative phases and considers the effects of intervention in each phase. Next, the chapter explores the special effects of new surgical procedures and of psychosocial intervention, focusing on those areas of surgery that are most typical or instructive. Finally, attention is given to progress in liaison work with surgery services.

THE PREOPERATIVE PHASE

Anxiety

Most studies of surgical patients presume that anxiety peaks at the time of the operative event. They therefore infer that the purpose of intervention is to reduce immediate and delayed postoperative psychological, and perhaps physical, sequelae. However, Silberfarb et al. (1980) and Jamison et al. (1978) have reported that mastectomy patients are most anxious well before surgery, at the time illness is discovered and surgery is recommended, and after surgery, while postoperative results are pending and when illness recurs. The immediate preoperative period was a time of lessened anxiety. Johnston (1980) studied orthopedic and elective gynecology patients and found that only 12 percent of these patients reached a peak of anxiety on the day of surgery. The highest levels of anxiety occurred before admission and five to six days postoperatively.

The same results have been obtained in studies based on illnesses which are life threatening and lead to mutilative surgery and studies based on illnesses which are not life threatening and lead to surgery that improves functioning. In neither case is the operative event the apparent cause of peak anxiety. In the authors' experience, the nature of the underlying illness, the degree of success of surgery, and the intensity of postoperative pain and complications are the major determinants of when anxiety occurs during the surgical experience. Although the recent findings do challenge prior thinking about the psychological stress of surgery, more detailed studies are needed so that we can properly evaluate the role of denial and isolation of affect. Only then can we draw accurate prognostic inferences for the postoperative course.

Quantification of preoperative anxiety has led to arbitrary assignments of patients to high-, medium-, and low-anxiety groups. Janis (1959), Andrew (1970), and Cohen and Lazarus (1973) have developed typologies of preoperative anxiety which combine degree of anxiety with patient coping style and which attempt to predict the nature and quantity of postoperative anxiety. Patients with low degrees of anxiety have been characterized as repressors, avoiders, or deniers and typically have an external locus of control. These patients see themselves as passive participants in their treatment and often show little interest in understanding either the nature of their illness or the treatment outlined. There may, in fact, be two groups of low-anxiety patients, those who deny anxiety in a counterphobic way and who have the poor postoperative course described by Janis (1959), and a much larger group who accept the authority and ministrations of medical personnel. Such optimistic, unwary, and unquestioning patients warm the hearts of most surgeons and liaison psychiatrists.

Patients with contrasting coping styles have been characterized as sensitizers (Andrew, 1970) or vigilant (Cohen and Lazarus, 1973) and have an internal locus of control. Such patients are keenly aware of their own sensations and monitor the interventions of medical staff. Their vigilance seems to accompany heightened anticipatory anxiety, and they ask many more questions of medical staff. They may be more aggressive in dealing with their doctors, demand more medication, report more pain, and have longer stays after minor surgical procedures (Cohen and Lazarus, 1973). While there is no necessary correlation between coping style and degree of anxiety, most highly anxious patients will be found in the group of vigilant copers. Perhaps vigilance is inappropriate to the helplessness and dependency of the postoperative state and therefore leads to more anxiety. An alternate causal explanation would be that excessive anxiety leads to sensitization and vigilance. From a systems standpoint, however, they reinforce each other. Consequently, the preoperative patient is hereafter discussed only in terms of degree of anxiety.

Does the level of preoperative anxiety affect postoperative recovery? This most important question unfortunately has been answered in conflicting fashion by recent papers. Highly anxious preoperative patients have reported more postoperative fear, helplessness, and negative affect in all studies (Janis, 1959; Andrew, 1970; Cohen and Lazarus, 1973;

Johnson et al., 1971; Wolfer and Davis, 1970; Sime, 1976; Egbert et al., 1964). While all researchers have found a correlation with subjective symptoms, only Sime (1976) and Egbert et al. (1964) reported that high preoperative anxiety correlated positively with increased pain medication and prolonged hospital stay. However, George et al. (1980) described delayed wound healing in high- versus low- and medium-anxiety patients who had had molars extracted. Gonzdilov et al. (1977) described double the rate of major postoperative complications in high- versus low- and medium-anxiety patients undergoing abdominoperineal resection. They related this finding to observed elevations in urinary catecholamines and serum hydroxycorticosteroids. Johnston and Carpenter (1980) have agreed with most of the authors cited above that the low-anxiety patient, in contrast, has no increased postoperative physical or psychic morbidity and that low-anxiety patients are not at increased risk for subjective or objective complications.

Some of the conflict noted among these studies may result from failure to discriminate between groups of patients experiencing major versus minor surgery. Certainly the effects of high preoperative anxiety may be obscured by a complication-ridden postoperative course. The later section on cardiac surgery sheds further light on the relationship between preoperative anxiety and the postoperative course.

Preoperative Preparation

Even if the only effect of heightened preoperative anxiety was to increase subjective psychological pain, it would be worthwhile and instructive to consider the effects of intervention. Much of the research on preoperative intervention has been done in the past ten years, and it has recently been summarized by Wilson (1981) and Mumford et al. (1982). Neither the repressing, denying patients nor the sensitizing, vigilant patients with extreme preoperative anxiety have been affected much by a simple enhanced preparation that merely recounts the imminent surgical events. Information and support alone are insufficient to deal with the neurotic bases of anxiety in these patients. Psychiatric consultation is indicated, and the sooner the better. The surgeon's fear that a quiet, low-anxiety patient will be damaged by too much preoperative preparation is also groundless. While low-anxiety patients who are given additional preoperative preparation may complain more frequently in the postoperative period, they ultimately express heightened satisfaction with their treatment (Mumford et al., 1982).

In all studies of systematic preparation, lessened postoperative anxiety and distress have been reported by both patient and independent observer. Decreased hospital stay, lessened analgesic need, and increased patient satisfaction are common. A decrease in minor complications such as urinary retention and paralytic ileus has been reported and may reflect lessened anxiety and increased patient activity (Wilson, 1981). The absence of any study reporting negative effects is striking. Similar findings apply to surgery with children (Gabriel and Danilowicz, 1978; Visintainer and Wolfer, 1975).

The recent literature on patient preparation includes a dazzling variety of techniques. Hypnosis, relaxation tapes, talking with investigators or other medical personnel, postoperative exercises, and interventions including family and other patients have all produced positive results.

Extensive psychiatric training of the preparer may be unnecessary, for it is impossible to discern differences in the relative effectiveness of psychiatrists, surgeons, nurses, and sensitive nonmedical personnel who establish contact in the preoperative period and continue to work with the patient postoperatively.

A general distinction can be drawn between active and passive modes of preparation. Langer et al. (1975) found that patients who were given a preoperative coping strategy which focused on active coping had far less postoperative anxiety than patients who were merely given information and reassurance without encouragement toward increased activity and participation in recovery. While minimizing passivity may be the best currently identified technique for helping the preoperative patient, it is not possible to define ideal ratios of activity versus passivity, nor is it clear which specific techniques are superior.

Thus far, preparation has been studied primarily with respect to the initial surgical procedure. The need for postoperative preparation is continuous, however, where the surgical course is fraught with complications and additional procedures are necessary. Little attention has been paid to this issue or to the development of refined or standardized interventions for high-risk, extremely anxious or depressed patients.

Consent and Refusal*

The area of informed consent is of concern to patients, to their physicians and attorneys, and to liaison psychiatrists. It has been demonstrated that patients undergoing minor surgery have excellent postoperative recall of carefully elicited informed consent (88 percent) and that they appreciate the careful approach (Reading, 1981). Patients undergoing major cardiac surgery have a lower rate of recall (29 percent) (Robinson, 1976), but this may reflect an intervening organic brain syndrome or the role of inattention and denial in the anxious preoperative period. Rockwell and Pepitone-Rockwell (1979) have published an excellent recent review of the legal issues, timing, technique, and value of eliciting informed consent and treat the subject comprehensively. They urged that physicians view informed consent as a variant of preoperative information giving, rather than as a legal interference with medical practice.

Frequently, advances in surgical treatment complicate informed consent issues. Auchincloss (1981), for example, has commented on the difficulty currently faced by surgeon and patient in selecting the best treatment for breast cancer where options range from lumpectomy and/or radiation to modified radical mastectomy. While statistics on long-range survival are unclear or controversial, patients must still decide on the relative merits of a more or less mutilating procedure. The liaison psychiatrist may be able to play an important role in helping some patients to resolve these conflicts.

The paucity of recent and past literature on refusal of surgery reflects both incidental and substantial issues. Most surgery is elective and by

*Editor's note: For a broader legal treatment of the consent and refusal issue, the reader may want to refer to Part IV of *Psychiatry 1982 (Psychiatry Update: Volume I)*. In particular, Dr. Loren H. Roth discusses the legal issues surrounding competency to consent to or refuse treatment (pages 350–360), and Dr. Thomas G. Gutheil examines some of the difficulties involved in the legal and judicial concepts of the right to refuse treatment (pages 379–384).

definition not refused. Nonelective procedures are most commonly assented to prior to hospitalization, so that those who might refuse are not seen by a consulting psychiatrist in the hospital. The cases of refusal of surgery are scattered through consultation surgery literature (Hackett and Weisman, 1960b), melded with the literature about signing out against medical advice (Albert and Kornfeld, 1973) and treatment refusal (Applebaum and Roth, 1983). These cases suggest that fear of the surgical procedure itself is rarely the prime issue in refusal of surgery. Rather, the predominant issues are hopelessness and the wish to die, general failure of coping defenses, and fears of the consequences of surgery (e.g., impotence after abdominoperineal resection). Problems in communication with the physician are also contributing factors, which may account for the higher incidence of treatment refusal in ward patients (Applebaum and Roth, 1983). This corroborates the authors' initial observation that operative anxiety may not be the major problem in the surgical process. It also underlines the complexity of the issues that face physicians consulting with preoperative patients whose distress often arises more from fear of the underlying illness or postoperative sequelae than from the operative event.

THE PERIOPERATIVE PHASE

Anesthesia

The fear of anesthesia has been recognized as a preoperative phenomenon since Deutsch's (1942) paper on the psychological aspects of surgery. Typically, this fear has been related to concerns about respiration among patients with asthma or emphysema and to commonplace fears of death. Unconscious concerns about loss of control or about forbidden wishes emerging under states of suspended consciousness may also color the fear of anesthesia. Williams and Jones (1969) demonstrated that excessive anxiety prolonged induction time and increased thiopental tolerance in operative patients. In later papers they demonstrated that preoperative benzodiazepines (Williams et al., 1975a) and supportive instruction (Williams et al., 1975b) were both capable of reversing these trends for highly anxious patients.

Approximately 1 percent of surgical patients accurately recall operative events (Hilgenberg, 1981), usually in cardiac and obstetrical cases where anesthesia levels are lighter. The proportion of recall can be heightened with postoperative hypnosis (Cheek, 1959). While most recall is unthreatening, cases of classical traumatic neurosis have been described for cardiac surgery patients awake during surgery (Guerra, 1980). Patients experienced postoperative nightmares about the surgery or about being attacked, and they manifested marked anxiety and fears of death for days after surgery. Guerra (1980) found these patients to be less distressed about the recall, which was incomplete and blunted by anesthesia, than they were by difficulties in communicating their postoperative psychic distress to the surgical team. These patients are best helped by applying the principles for treating traumatic neurosis, i.e., explanation and reassurance, repeated abreaction, and minor tranquilizers or hypnotics.

The nature of the anesthesia used may also shape the patient's postoperative curve of anxiety. Winkelstein et al. (1965) found that patients who had spinal anesthesia and were awake during surgery showed immediate signs of anxiety, irritability, and tearfulness in the recovery room, while patients who had general anesthesia showed peak anxiety several days later, when concerns about diagnosis, recovery, and pain were preeminent. Pre- and postoperative assessment should therefore include an inquiry regarding a patient's prior anesthetic history.

Intervention in the Surgical Environment

The operating room, recovery room, and surgical ICUs have in recent years become focal points for the attention of liaison psychiatrists. While patients spend relatively brief periods of time in these environments, moments of the highest human drama occur. Douduin and Katz (1980) discovered that awake herniorraphy patients showed a marked increase in anxiety (measured by GSR) whenever operating personnel discussed the ongoing surgery or the patients' medical care. They urged surgeons and anesthesiologists to pay special care to operating room talk about the patient.

It is in the recovery room that some patients, discovering that a mutilating procedure has been done, realize that they have a malignancy. Important observations about the patients' further postoperative course may also be made here, for failure of coping mechanisms in the recovery room frequently presages later problems. Menger et al. (1951) found a correlation between childlike, tearful, demanding, or uncooperative behavior in the recovery room and poor long-range coping with the effect of hysterectomy. One of the authors (Kornfeld, 1969) has described the atmosphere of the surgical ICU, with its critically ill patients, noisy mechanistic environment, pain, sleep deprivation, enforced dependency and restriction of movement, and recurrent emergencies. He and Nadelson (1976) have outlined methods for dealing with the effects of these special stresses.

Recent evidence of the efficacy of intervention has come from the study of special surgical environments. Preoperative visits by operating room nurses to acquaint patients with the sights and sounds of the operating room, along with occasional tours when requested, decreased postoperative anxiety for minor, though not major, surgery cases (Lindemann and Stetzer, 1973). A medically unsophisticated patient advocate accompanying patients while they awaited entrance to the operating room was warmly received and credited with relieving preoperative anxiety, especially where delays in surgery occurred (MacDonald, 1981). For the patient in a special environment, the counteraction of isolation and loneliness by any medical personnel seems helpful.

The range of helpful interventions may be further expanded in light of two studies of postoperative delirium, or "interval psychosis," occurring in surgical ICUs.(The multicausal nature of delirium is considered elsewhere in this Part.)* Delirium is the primary psychological disturbance seen in the surgical ICU. Lazarus and Hagens (1968) lowered the incidence of postcardiotomy delirium in the ICU from 33 to 14 percent through psychosocial intervention. Liaison nurses developed preopera-

*Preceptor's note: See especially Ford's discussion of organic brain syndromes in elderly patients and Massie and Holland's review of the many factors which can cause delirium and dementia in cancer patients.

tive relationships with patients and maintained brief but frequent contact throughout the patients' stays in the ICU. The nurses' interventions were simple and standardized: they offered frequent verbal contact and reassurance, assured better sleep, and consistently oriented the patients. Similar interventions by briefly trained family members were also effective in diminishing postcardiotomy delirium (Chatham, 1978).

THE POSTOPERATIVE PHASE

The fundamental techniques of consultative intervention for postoperative surgical patients were elaborated in 1960 by Hackett and Weisman (1960a; 1960b). This aspect of the psychiatric effects of surgery has received little recent attention for a number of reasons. Once past the unique impact of the surgical event, the patient begins to assume psychological tasks that differ little from those of medical patients, so the literature on the postoperative phase is less distinctive. What is special about the postoperative course tends to be linked to specific illnesses and operations and is considered later in this chapter.

It has been difficult to outline the frequency of prolonged psychological sequelae for general surgery. Barker (1968) found that cholecystectomy patients had no higher rate of referral versus comparable nonoperative cases. In contrast, the careful prospective study by Titchener et al. (1957) revealed that 15 percent of 200 surgical patients had improved surgically but worsened psychiatrically one year after surgery. They inferred that the surgery itself was the noxious agent. Rates of psychiatric morbidity vary so widely in retrospective studies that it is best to consider postoperative sequelae only in relationship to specific illnesses and procedures.

Postoperative delirium remains the commonest postoperative psychosis. Its incidence has been reported to vary from 15 to 70 percent (Titchener et al., 1956; Skoug, 1968; Morse and Litin, 1968; Kornfeld et al., 1965), depending on the nature of the study (retrospective versus prospective) and the procedure (general surgery versus cardiac valve replacement). More elaborate exploration of the causes, symptoms, and treatment in cardiac surgery is undertaken below. Psychosocial intervention, as described above, can have ameliorative effects.

PSYCHIATRIC ASPECTS OF
SPECIFIC PROCEDURES AND FIELDS

Cardiac Surgery

An association between cardiac surgery and psychiatric difficulties has been noted since the 1950s when high psychiatric morbidity in the immediate postoperative period was reported after mitral commissurotomy (Fox et al., 1954; Bliss et al., 1955). Proposed explanations were organic factors (Zaks, 1958) and psychological factors ((Fox et al., 1954; Bliss et al., 1955; Meyer et al., 1961). By the early 1960s, the problem had diminished significantly, and this was attributed to improved techniques.

As surgeons shifted to open-heart techniques in the 1960s, independent observers reported a high incidence of a transient syndrome dubbed postcardiotomy delirium (Kornfeld et al., 1965; Blachly, 1964; Edgerton and Kay, 1964). Typically, the patient experienced a three- to four-day lucid interval, followed by perceptual distortions, visual and auditory hallucinations, disorientation, and paranoid ideation. Not all patients experienced the entire syndrome. The incidence varied from 38 to 70 percent of all adults, with the highest incidence in those series of patients who had daily psychiatric examinations. The delirium was rare in children (Kornfeld et al., 1965). An early organic brain syndrome was also described, in which the patients did not experience a lucid interval after surgery (Heller et al., 1970). Some of the reports in the literature suffered from a failure to separate postcardiotomy delirium from early organic brain syndrome.

A variety of preoperative, operative, and postoperative factors have been associated with postcardiotomy delirium. Preoperative factors cited include the symbolism of the heart (Abram, 1965; Kennedy and Bakst, 1966), increasing age and the severity of the illness (Kornfeld et al., 1965; Blachly, 1964; Heller et al., 1970), evidence of organicity (Layne and Yudofsky, 1970), unexpressed anxiety (Layne and Yudofsky, 1970; Kornfeld et al., 1974), and an active dominant personality (Kornfeld et al., 1974). Operative factors mentioned include the length of time on cardiac bypass (Edgerton and Kay, 1964; Fox et al., 1954; Kennedy and Bakst, 1966), and intraoperative hypotensive episodes (Tufo and Ostfeld, 1968). Postoperative factors include a shift in biogenic amines (Blachly, 1967), the severity of the illness, and the stresses of the open-heart recovery room, specifically sleep deprivation, sensory monotony, and anxiety (Kornfeld et al., 1965; Edgerton and Kay, 1964; Heller et al., 1970; Sveinsson, 1975; Orr and Stahl, 1977). Heller et al. (1979) found that a decline in postoperative cardiac index (a measure of cardiac output) after aortic valve surgery or a failure to increase on the index after mitral valve surgery was associated with delirium. That finding confirmed the findings of Blachly and Koster (1966). The delirium most likely results from an interaction of these multiple factors, with the relative importance of any one factor varying from patient to patient. The preoperative and operative factors probably contribute to subclinical cerebral dysfunction, which makes the patient vulnerable to the subsequent stresses of the open-heart recovery room.

Observations on the stressful nature of open-heart recovery room experiences have led to specific recommendations for modifications in intensive care settings (Kornfeld et al., 1965). Recommendations include providing more separation between patients, reorganizing nursing procedures to allow for more uninterrupted sleep, reducing sensory monotony by changes in the placement of monitoring equipment, and encouraging more mobility. Such modifications, along with preoperative preparation of the patient by an open-heart recovery room nurse, have reportedly led to significant reduction in the incidence of delirium (Lazarus and Hagens, 1968).

With open-heart surgery, as with closed-heart surgery, there has now been a reduction in the incidence and severity of delirium. The authors' group at Columbia reported the incidence to be about 25 percent in a sample of coronary bypass cases (Frank et al., 1972; Kornfeld et al., 1978). Sveinsson (1975) reported a 13 percent incidence in a mixed patient population from a Cleveland clinic. That low incidence was associated with very short bypass times, and decreased time on the cardiopulmonary bypass seems to have been a primary factor in reducing the incidence of delirium. However, better preoperative preparation, reduced anxiety in staff and patients regarding the procedures, and modifications in the environment of the recovery room may also have contributed to the decline.

The patient's preoperative psychological state may also be a predictor of surgical morbidity and mortality, with depression being a correlate of poor outcome (Meyer et al., 1961; Kornfeld et al., 1978). This association may be related to biochemical changes associated with depression or to the inability of the severely disturbed or depressed patient to cooperate adequately in his or her own care.

Such a high incidence of delirium following cardiac surgery has raised the question of possible persistent organic deficits. A follow-up study of patients six months after surgery found that intellectual functioning was preserved, with no adverse effects in those patients who had experienced postcardiotomy delirium (Frank et al., 1972). However, no follow-up data were available on those patients who had experienced early organic brain syndrome, the group most likely to experience neurological deficit. A Swedish study did report a small percentage of patients with residual evidence of intellectual impairment two months postoperatively (Aberg, 1974). A subsample who had an arterial micropore filter showed no detectable deficits. Open-heart surgery techniques have now developed to the point that uncomplicated surgery is unlikely to produce detectable intellectual impairment in those centers with very low operative and postoperative mortality and morbidity.

In the 1960s and early 1970s, cardiac surgery was performed primarily for the repair of valves damaged by childhood rheumatic fever. Many of these patients had experienced years of life with serious impairment of function and a relatively dependent existence. Most surprisingly, some of these patients received their "cure" ambivalently. For example, Heller et al. (1974) reported on a sample followed prospectively for one year. Although more than 90 percent showed improvement in their physical conditions, about one-third had declined in general and psychological adjustment, posing significant psychological hindrances to recovery. On the average, poorly adapted patients tended to become passive and had impaired sexual and marital functioning. The patients at high risk for relatively poor postoperative outcome were those with generally poor psychological adjustment characterized by disorganization, high levels of anxiety, and paranoid tendencies. Patients who tended to deal with life in an aggressive, unreflective manner also did not do well; they may have had difficulty submitting to surgery and convalescent regimens. Depression and reluctance to have surgery were also predictors of poor outcome.

Coronary artery bypass graft surgery is now the most common cardiac surgery procedure. It has been found to reduce angina and prolong life in some subsets of patients (National Institute of Health Consensus Development Conference Statement, 1981). Studies of the postoperative quality of life have been done to evaluate the cost-benefit ratio of this expensive procedure.

The earliest studies focused on return to work as a quantifiable variable. Lamendola and Pelligrini (1979) found that while 60 percent of their sample were working prior to surgery, only 40 percent had returned to work six months after surgery. However, 79 percent of those who wanted to work were working. One of the authors and his colleagues (Kornfeld et al., 1982) found that 77 percent of their patients were working just prior to surgery and 78 percent at nine months postoperatively. Other studies also suggest that the best predictor of work postoperatively is working status at the time of surgery. While it is possible that the patients out of work preoperatively might have been sicker at the time of surgery, it is more likely that psychological or social factors determined whether they returned to work. For some, the stress of working may have been perceived as contributing to coronary heart disease; for others, disability or retirement income may have been enough to justify giving up a less than satisfactory job. It is therefore important that we learn to distinguish between patients who freely choose not to resume work and those who are prevented from doing so by a fear of working or by employers' policies or attitudes.

In the second study (Kornfeld et al., 1982), most patients reported overall satisfaction with the results of the surgery, with marked reduction in angina, increased general pleasure, and reduction in anxiety and depression. However, they had less improvement in sexual functioning, with some patients tending to decrease sexual activity despite an apparent improvement in their physical status. Physicians may need to discuss postoperative sexual activity with their patients routinely to relieve misconceptions and inhibitions. Patients who undergo cardiac valve surgery tend to have personalities marked by pre- and postoperative passivity. In contrast, a high percentage of patients who have coronary artery bypass surgery manifest very active Type A coronary-prone behavior patterns. Follow-up assessment found a persistence of the Type A behavior (Kornfeld et al., 1982), and prospective studies are needed to determine whether the Type A pattern is associated with more rapid arteriosclerosis in the grafted vessels.

Organ Transplantation

The latest medical procedure to challenge human adaptability is organ transplantation. The advent of immunosuppressive techniques in the middle 1960s triggered organ transplantation programs around the country. The kidney has been the most commonly transplanted organ. In the early 1970s, there was a worldwide flurry of interest in heart transplantation. Although very few heart transplantation programs are currently operating in the United States, improved immunosuppressive drugs may bring about additional interest. Psychiatric studies have led to a better understanding of the psychology of coping and have highlighted the potential problem area. Most individuals who have organ transplantations manage to adapt reasonably well (Eisendrath, 1976). However, there have been psychiatric difficulties, and, in such critical situations, these complications can have dire consequences.

KIDNEY The kidney donor, the recipient, and the families have all been the subjects of reports. For the recipient, a patient with end-stage renal disease, a new kidney represents freedom from total dependence on a dialysis machine. Kaplan-DeNour (1976) has comprehensively reviewed the serious psychological issues involved in chronic dialysis.

In the early years of limited access to dialysis and transplants, psychiatrists were usually included in the committees that determined who should be accepted into the programs (Abram and Wadlington, 1963). With the greater availability of dialysis machines and cadaver kidneys, the psychiatrist's role now is to determine whether there are psychiatric contraindications to the transplantation procedure. The two questions at issue are (1) Does the patient have the ability to tolerate the procedure and to cooperate adequately in the relatively complex programs required to prevent rejection? (2) Will the patient become psychiatrically disabled by his or her reaction to the procedure? The answers are necessarily based on subjective clinical judgments.

Beard (1969) suggested several psychological criteria: the absence of disabling psychiatric disease, the presence of sufficient emotional stability to enable the patient to react in a predictable fashion, sufficient maturity to comprehend the nature of the illness and the complexity of the treatment, and consistent and sufficient motivation for recovery. Eisendrath (1976), however, suggested that in most cases psychiatric status ought not to be a criterion for transplantation. He believed that it would be too difficult to predict posttransplantation behavior and that with psychiatric treatment disturbed patients could be helped to cooperate and to adapt to the procedure. Crammond (1971) also opted for giving every possible patient a trial of medical and surgical therapy with the full support of the psychiatric staff. He believed that intractable chronic schizophrenic psychosis and severe degrees of intellectual retardation would be the only psychiatric contraindications to transplantations.

The donor and the process by which he or she is selected have been the subjects of some study. Obviously, a good tissue match is more likely with close family members than with nonrelatives. A 1979 series reported the three-year survival rates for different donor types as 69 percent from a relative and 45 percent from a cadaver (Krakauer et al., 1983). With recent advances in matching and immunosuppressive techniques, cadaver donations are becoming increasingly common. However, living donors are still used, and both research and consultation must continue to focus on minimizing the psychological and physical harm to all involved.

Simmons et al. (1971) emphasized the stresses of the decision-making process on the family unit. Nondonors often experienced great feelings of ambivalence and long periods of indecision. Complex family dynamics were often the determinants of the final decision. While Hayes and Gunnels (1969) noted that donors had usually reserved their decisions until they had examined the problem carefully and discussed it with others, Fellner and Marshall (1970) reported that the decision-making process seemed to be an instantaneous and irrational response that was later justified by a number of defensive mechanisms. Kemph et al. (1969) reported that consciously altruistic donors harbored considerable unconscious resentment toward the recipients and toward those who had requested and encouraged the transplant. Resentment was more common in sibling donors than in maternal donors.

Eisendrath (1969) suggested three criteria for donor selection: the donor must understand the risks and the possibility of failure for him- or herself and the recipient; the donor must be free from undue external coercion; and the donor must be free of any previous history of significant mental or emotional instability. He believed that any understanding physician could make those determinations and that a psychiatrist would be needed only where the medical team had doubts. Crammond (1971) disagreed and recommended routine psychiatric evaluation of all donors to deal with the complexities of the donation process.

Kemph et al. (1969) found that shortly after surgery donors experienced a period of depression of varying duration. While in the preoperative period the donors are showered with praise for their sacrifice, in the postoperative phase the attention shifts to the recipient and the fate of the donated kidney. The postsurgical depression required brief supportive psychotherapy in every case. Eisendrath (1969) concurred that more attention should be shown to the donors after surgery. In contrast, Fellner and Marshall (1970) did not find much evidence for a postoperative depressive phenomenon. They were more impressed with reports from donors that the act of donation had turned out to be the most meaningful experience of their lives. Kemph et al. (1969) also reported that the procedure can be perceived as rebirth by the patient and as a chance for the donor to alter his or her identity.

The data are inadequate concerning long-range effects on the donor. Eisendrath (1969) did report on a retrospective questionnaire survey of 57 donors. Almost all said they would do it again and had derived a sense of worthwhile accomplishment. However, 21 reported having had physical or emotional difficulties, with a greater incidence of complaints from people involved in unsuccessful transplantations. No control group was provided, however, and it was not possible to determine to what extent the difficulties reported were related to the kidney donations. More comprehensive prospective long-term studies are required in this important area.

The candidate for kidney transplantation arrives at that point beset with multiple stresses. Progressive kidney failure impairs cerebral function. Chronic invalidism causes dependency conflicts and threatens self-esteem. Despite the prospect of transplantation, the candidate must also face the prospect of early death. Nonetheless, most patients make a workable adjustment. Anxiety and unhappiness are understandable; psychosis, depression, and panic are much less common. With kidney transplantation patients, there is no clear-cut pattern of postoperative psychiatric disturbances as there is with cardiac surgery.

In a series of 292 patients, Penn et al. (1971) found significant psychopathology in 32 percent (94 patients). Thirty-six of the 94 patients had psychiatric symptoms before the transplantation. Anxiety and depression were the most common diagnoses (55 patients). Personality disorders were present in 7 patients. Organic mental disorder was diagnosed in 30 patients and functional psychoses in 2 patients. Mild depression in reaction to some physical problem was transiently present in almost all of the other patients.

The only other study with a sizable sample was Eisendrath's (1969) study of 200 patients. He reported only a 5 percent rate of problems serious enough to warrant psychiatric consultation. However, he indicated that many other patients displayed anxiety, depression, or impulsive behavior which the transplantation staff were able to manage effectively. The psychiatrist was often most useful in helping the staff understand the patient's unspoken fears.

Kemph (1969), in his intensive work with a smaller sample, found that both donors and recipients had fantasies regarding possible damage to their sexual organs. Like Beard (1969), he emphasized the need to help the patients verbalize their fears of death, which he felt were a frequent cause of recurring depression. A number of analysts have dealt with the intriguing question of the intrapsychic processes by which the recipient deals with the unique experience of receiving an organ from another person (Kemph, 1969; Muslin, 1971; Castelnuovo-Tedesco, 1973). Viederman (1974) suggested that the patient's affective response is related to the degree to which the donor's representation is imbued with the qualities of either a benevolent or a hostile introject.

Some have suggested that unconscious factors can play a role in the rejection of a kidney transplant. Eisendrath (1969) reported that 8 of 11 patients who died after renal transplantation were either abandoned during their illness by a significant figure or manifested more anxiety than survivors. All had experienced more panic and more extensive pessimism about the outcome than had the patients who survived. Eisendrath suggested that this observation was compatable with the theoretical formulations of Engel and Schmale (1976), who stated that hopelessness and helplessness can produce pathophysiological changes that can in turn adversely affect the physical well-being of the patient. Viederman (1975) also reported on the rejection of a kidney by a young man after the death of a father surrogate. The patient was believed to be psychologically vulnerable because he had experienced the death of his own father in adolescence.

HEART In view of the relatively limited surgical experience with heart transplantation, psychiatric studies with large samples are not available, but one would certainly expect the procedure to have considerable psychological impact. In his description of the early experience at Stanford, Lunde (1969) pointed out that the heart is viewed not only as an organ absolutely essential for life, but also as the center of love, loyalty, and other strong feelings. There are therefore significant differences between heart and kidney donations. Removal of a kidney from a cadaver does not carry the same emotional charge as the removal of a heart from a living person. The cessation of cardiac function has traditionally been thought to be the criterion for death. Consequently, with heart transplants, all parties involved, including staff and families, must be comfortable with the concept of brain death.

In one report, a number of different factors seemed to motivate a family to make a heart donation: a family history of heart disease, academic or medical sophistication, the deceased person having previously expressed the desire to be a donor, and the family's desire to give some meaning to the death of the donor by helping others to continue life (Christopherson and Lunde, 1971a). The family's intense interest in the recipient seemed to subside about four to six weeks after the donation, and this seemed to coincide with the course of their own acute grief responses. In none of the instances where a secondary grief response followed the later death of the recipient did the families express regret about their original decision.

The Stanford team stated that the only nonmedical criteria for rejection of a potential recipient should be mental deficiency or active psychosis that would make cooperation with the procedure difficult, but they were also concerned about serious depression because of its prognostic significance (Christopherson and Lunde, 1971b; Kraft, 1971). Three preoperative factors seemed to play a role in predicting good postoperative adjustment: (1) the presence of extended family support for the procedure, (2) the patient's ability to discuss the possibility of his or her own death, and (3) the expression of specific uses for the additional lifetime that the procedure might give to him or her. A group of twenty patients from Houston described by Kraft (1971) showed a high incidence of preoperative cerebral organic impairment that was related to the effects of chronic heart disease or associated cerebral arteriosclerosis. In the early postoperative period, organic impairment was present in the majority of the patients.

Both research groups were concerned with the question of what the relationship should be between the donor family, the recipient, and the recipient's family (Kraft, 1971; Christopherson and Lunde, 1971a). Kraft (1971) found that the family of the recipient often felt that a relationship with the donor family was an emotional drain, since special demands were made on them. They were forced to share the donor family's grief over their lost member, while they themselves, with the recipient, needed to think of the heart as just a pump. The donor family, on the other hand, needed to think of themselves as having made a noble humanitarian gesture and felt their sense of sacrifice diminished by mechanistic references to the organ. Some donor families also indicated that they believed their own dead loved one lived on symbolically in the recipient, and this placed an additional burden on the recipient and his or her family. The Stanford group believed that personal contact between the donor and the recipient family would not be productive, except in special situations in which there was a mutual desire for one such meeting (Christopherson and Lunde, 1971a).

Christopherson and Lunde (1971b) found that most recipients showed only limited personality changes postoperatively and that those changes were primarily accentuations of characteristics that were present preoperatively. Of course, the patients did need to integrate the new role of transplant survivor into their self-images. The maintenance prednisone also produced some difficulties in concentration, emotional lability, and irritability, but no psychoses. Kraft (1971) noted marked improvement in mood associated with postoperative pain relief and increased alertness. A variety of psychodynamic mechanisms were called into play in the postoperative period. Both reports commented on the use of denial, especially when patients became aware of the death of another transplant patient (Christopherson and Lunde, 1971b; Kraft, 1971). Kraft (1971) noted that some male patients associated the receipt of a new heart from a young donor with increased virility and that some expressed concern about receiving a heart from a female donor. For the patient who had been chronically ill, the need to adapt to a new, more independent status posed serious problems. Most patients had to compromise high expectations with the real emotional and physical burdens of life after a transplantation.

Mastectomy

The study of the psychological consequences of mastectomy has generated over 200 research papers in the past fifteen years and is a paradigm for the study of postsurgical psychological complications in general. Early papers anecdotally delineated the dynamics of loss of sexual self-esteem and shame about deformity. Some authors emphasized marital dynamics (Ervin, 1973), while others focused on the defensive structure of patients (Bard and Sutherland, 1955) or on the specific patterns which created risk for psychosocial morbidity (Renneker and Cutler, 1952).

The next phase of research used preoperative and postoperative interviews to delineate the incidence of various psychological disorders in the postoperative year. Studies had somewhat variable results, but those of Maguire et al. (1978) are typical. Their 200 patients experienced peaks of psychological distress at the time of first diagnosis and while awaiting the results of biopsies from axillary nodes. Four months after mastectomy, 32 percent of the patients were depressed, 30 percent were anxious, 46 percent described sexual difficulties, and 61 percent had not resumed regular work. One year postoperatively, the respective figures were somewhat lower: 20 percent were depressed, 10 percent were anxious, 38 percent described sexual difficulties, and 44 percent had not resumed work. Based on several studies, the overall incidence of psychological complications appears to vary around 20 percent, a figure lower than predicted by earlier authors.

Recent research has begun to question the specificity of the "postmastectomy syndrome" and may point the way for a redefinition of areas for future study. Silberfarb et al. (1980) found that adjuvant chemotherapy produced far more distress than loss of the breast, and they also determined that breast cancer patients on chemotherapy were no more distressed than other cancer patients undergoing similar treatment. Concomitant studies of patients (Jamison et al., 1978) and their spouses (Wellisch et al., 1978) showed that patients and their spouses had the same frequency and types of psychological distress in the first postoperative year. This suggests that issues of death and separation may predominate or that the psychic trauma of losing the breast is borne equally by the patient and the marital partner. Using preoperative and postoperative interviews and psychological tests, Worden and Weisman (1977) found incidence rates of 20 percent postoperative psychological difficulty for mastectomy patients and 18 percent incidence for patients with other cancers treated surgically. No pathognomonic differences in the type of psychopathology were described, and the breast cancer patients minimized the impact of losing the breast. These authors concluded that the so-called postmastectomy syndrome is a nonspecific response to cancer surgery and that issues of body image and damage to sexual self-esteem are of secondary importance, while the dynamics of illness, operation, and possible death seem to dominate. Confirmation of these conclusions as they pertain to organ loss, including the loss of a breast, will have important implications for consultation-liaison psychiatry.

The study of postmastectomy psychological phenomena is complicated by recent changes in surgical approaches to breast cancer. Since the early 1970s, various new procedures have emerged, including two-stage surgery, routine adjuvant chemotherapy, modification of the radical mastectomy to include lumpectomy and a variety of procedures designed to spare some or all of the pectoral muscle, and the advent of reconstructive breast surgery. Surgical treatment has become individualized in response both to new medical data and to the intense pressure of patients to make their own choices of surgical procedures. Assessing the effects of two-stage mastectomies, modified procedures, and reconstructive surgery is limited by the self-selected nature of the procedures. Furthermore, with the development of new techniques, the results of earlier studies based upon modified radical mastectomy may be invalid.

Results to date show that advances in surgical technique are contributing greatly to minimizing problems of damaged sexual self-esteem and body image. Modification of surgical procedure by lumpectomy improves immediate postoperative self-image but does not change overall psychosocial morbidity (Sanger and Reznikoff, 1981). Noone et al. (1982) showed that early reconstruction was well accepted by mastectomy patients, and Stevens et al. (1983) showed that reconstruction at the time of mastectomy produced more benefit in self-image than delayed reconstruction also decreased the incidence of depression.

Finally, the study of mastectomy offers us the broadest view of various strategies of intervention. Reach to Recovery and inpatient counseling are well received by almost all patients (Winick and Robbins, 1977). In one of the few detailed prospective studies of routine postsurgical interventions, Maguire et al. (1980) screened 75 mastectomy patients and referred them for psychiatric treatment when indicated. After one year, 12 percent of the sample showed significant psychopathology, compared with 39 percent, a high figure, for an unscreened mastectomy control group. Closer examination of these results revealed that most of the benefit came from improved case finding and referral of at-risk patients and that random brief counseling for all patients had insufficient preventive impact. Future models for intervention in consultation-liaison psychiatry should involve both screening and subsequent in-depth treatment for patients showing evidence of adaptive failure.

Total Parenteral Nutrition

Respect for patients' adaptability is further enhanced by recent studies of total parenteral nutrition (TPN), a technique involving an indwelling intravenous catheter. Loss of the entire small bowel through volvulus, vascular occlusion, or enteritis is no longer fatal since TPN can give adequate nutritional support. Important modifications of psychiatric intervention strategies have developed from work with TPN patients.

Permanent loss of eating activity initially produces feelings of shock, and an immediate grief response ensues (MacRitchie, 1978). After one year of successful TPN, however, patients seem well adapted to living without ingesting any food. In fact, most psychological complications have their greatest intensity in the immediate postoperative period and resemble the psychological problems seen in renal dialysis patients. Like dialysis, TPN requires protracted connection to a feeding apparatus and the management of numerous medical and surgical complications. Twenty percent of patients experience serious psychological effects, primarily delirium, in the first year, and the rate of residual psychopathology is 5 percent thereafter (Malcolm et al., 1980). In the early stages of adaptation, crying spells, feelings of hopelessness, and body image distortions are common (Hall et al., 1980; Perl et al., 1981). The most effective psychiatric interventions closely follow the unfolding medical symptoms as they interact with underlying characterological patterns.

When permanent TPN is carried out at home, major strains are placed on both patient and family, and new issues for intervention arise. Gulledge et al. (1980) found that the psychiatrist continued to encounter many questions related to drugs and medical issues. Close coordination with medical personnel was crucial. However, the most effective interventions challenged patient demoralization and provided support for family members. Loss of the small bowel and permanent TPN require ongoing surgical management with continuous outpatient and home treatment, a different role for many surgeons. Psychiatric interventions are accordingly guided by the different medical and social issues of the later stages of treatment.

Amputation and Phantom Pain

The study of limb amputation illustrates par excellence the degree to which psychological sequelae of surgery are shaped by the underlying disease process. The young man with a limb amputation secondary to an accident suffers an immediate traumatic neurosis with a clearly defined grief reaction and a nearly universal phantom sensation (Frank, 1973). Persistent phantom pain and lasting psychological disability are uncommon, however, in the absence of unresolved mourning, secondary gain, or preexisting psychopathology (Ewatt et al., 1947; Frazier and Kolb, 1970). The young patient with a below-the-knee amputation of a chronically osteomyelitic leg, in contrast, experiences relief of pain and the opportunity for a prosthesis which allows improved locomotion. The issue of amputation in children has only recently received attention (Turgay, 1983; Eule, 1979). Psychological response is highly dependent on the age of the child and family responses, but denial followed by grief and mourning is usual.

A very different course is seen for the vascular amputee. The surgical event may remove a chronically painful, dysfunctional extremity and allow the patient to move from a protracted, unsuccessful period of conservative management and failed femoral-popliteal bypass to the stage of active rehabilitation. A common course is that described by Parkes and Napier (1975). Peaks of depression occur one week after surgery and when the patient returns home. Functional disability is severe. A third of Parkes and Napier's 46 patients returned to work, and a third remained disabled by psychological difficulties beyond what one would expect from the surgical deficits. In addition, progression of vascular disease may dominate the patient's recovery.

Parkes (1973) also found that severe, persistent phantom pain in vascular amputees reflected a blend of physical and psychodynamic factors. Immediate or persistent postoperative stump pain and a prior history of more than a year of limb pain predicted persisting phantom pain, as did marked denial, perfectionism, rigid self-reliance, and unemployment after one year. Phantom sensations, it should be noted, are protean phenomena, and they may represent many organs or even body sensations such as micturition. Patients with persistent breast phantoms may in fact bear some psychological resemblance to amputees with lasting limb phantoms (Jamison et al., 1979).

Clearly, the surgeon and the liaison psychiatrist face not one but many tasks in assessing and counseling a person who undergoes an amputation. Friedmann (1978) has outlined an extremely flexible approach attuned to the different types of amputation and to the various stages experienced by each type of amputee. Muiltidisciplinary supportive approaches are recommended (Kindon and Pearce, 1982), and there is a growing literature on group intervention for vascular amputees (Keistein, 1980).

Ostomies

Defining the psychological impact of an ostomy begins with a consideration of the underlying illness. Druss et al. (1968) found that 41 patients with ulcerative colitis and permanent ileostomies felt shame and embarrassment about problems of odor and spillage, but they vastly preferred their ileostomies to active ulcerative colitis. Their postoperative psychological adjustment was improved. Thirty-six patients undergoing abdominoperineal resection for rectal cancer, despite better-functioning colostomies, had far more shame, phobic response, and depression, as well as frequent organic impotence due to interruption of sacral efferents (Druss et al., 1969). Seventy-two percent reported deteriorated personal relationships. Wirschung et al. (1975) found considerable psychosocial morbidity after both abdominoperineal resection with a permanent colostomy and anterior resection with primary anastomosis. Only impotence had a higher incidence for the first group, suggesting further that disruption of the sacral plexus rather than colostomy itself was the major cause of the impotence.

The grim postoperative psychology of the colostomy patient, initially described by Sutherland et al. in 1952, has been modified by many factors. New appliances and the widespread use of a continent colostomy have nearly eliminated problems of spillage and odor. Surgeons and society have become more aware of the psychological effects of colostomy. Self-help groups are available, and nursing literature exists on helping colostomy patients (Freyberger, 1979; Bille, 1979). Ostomy nurses now specialize in helping patients cope with problems of adapting to colostomies. These developments parallel those seen in mastectomy and point to the variety of interventions capable of ameliorating the psychosocial sequelae of surgery.

Pelvic Exenteration and Hysterectomy

Recent developments contrasting the psychological consequences of pelvic exenteration and hysterectomy permit further commentary on a question for consultation psychiatry. To what degree does postoperative psychiatric morbidity come from the illness, the procedure, or antecedent psychopathology? Of the two operations, the inherently more devastating is pelvic exenteration, with removal of rectum, urinary bladder, and/or internal and external sexual organs. Both Knorr (1967) and Dempsey et al. (1975) have described a transient postoperative depression. Psychological recovery began to occur after four months, however, and at three-year follow-up both Dempsey et al. (1975) and Brown et al. (1972) found a remarkably well-adapted group of patients. Only 2 of 31 patients showed severe and enduring postoperative psychopathology, and both of these patients had antecedent psychiatric illness. Six patients remained sexually active, and expressions of shame were rare. For these patients, cure of their cancer proved to be a powerful adaptive stimulus. Family support was critical in overcoming early demoralization.

In contrast, early retrospective studies of hysterectomy, summarized by Turpin and Heath (1979), reported an incidence of depression of about 30 percent and a psychiatric referral rate of 7 percent in the year after surgery. The term posthysterectomy syndrome was coined. Recent literature, however, has contradicted the seemingly higher incidence of psychopathology following this lesser surgical procedure. In a prospective study, Meikle et al. (1977) found no greater postoperative mood disturbances in hysterectomy than cholecystectomy patients. Gath and Cooper (1981) found a 29 percent incidence of psychopathology in the year after hysterectomy for benign conditions. For 58 percent of these cases, they found preoperative psychopathology, and in the others, they found intervening medical illness. In both of these studies, salpingectomy, oophorectomy, and choice of operation (abdominal versus vaginal) or surgeon were insubstantial variables.

Recent prospective studies by Roeske (1978) and Coppen et al. (1981) confirm the common experience for much elective surgery. Their patients reported fewer symptoms, better well-being, and less psychopathology after hysterectomy for benign but troublesome gynecological conditions. Rather than continuing to describe a posthysterectomy syndrome, recent studies have refined our understanding of groups at high risk for psychopathology after surgery. These include patients whose surgery is in response to somatic complaints reflecting psychopathology, patients with preexisting psychopathology or subsequent medical illness, young women desirous of childbirth (Kaltreiden et al., 1979), and unsophisticated rural patients whose sociocultural expectations lead them to anticipate damage (Iacovides et al., 1981).

Brief postoperative counseling by nurses was found to have little effect on postoperative sexual functioning (Krueger et al., 1979). This confirmed the finding by Maguire et al. (1980) that the major value of brief postoperative counseling was good case finding. If patients who manifest overt symptomatology are referred for effective treatment, the overall morbidity is decreased. However, when Capone and Good (1980) offered more extensive postoperative counseling on an unselected basis, they were able to reduce the incidence of postoperative sexual dysfunction in patients undergoing hysterectomy for cancer from 50 percent to 25 percent. They also noted improvement in other areas of psychological functioning.

Advances in Other Surgical Fields

ORTHOPEDIC SURGERY In recent years, psychiatrists have begun to produce a substantial literature outlining the psychological factors that influence functional results for orthopedic patients. Findings accepted in the assessment of lumbar disc patients (Wiltse, 1975) have been extended to new procedures. Wise et al. (1979) assessed patients prior to knee repair or replacement, and Wiltse and Rochio (1975) studied patients undergoing chemonucleolysis for herniated discs. In both studies, elevated hysteria or hypochondriasis scales on the MMPI were better than surgical assessment in predicting a poor functional result. Perhaps passivity impedes the vigorous rehabilitative program such patients need, but only more detailed clinical studies and intervention trials can confirm this possibility.

Studies of the psychiatric sequelae of orthopedic procedures for pectus excavatum (Holcomb, 1977), scoliosis (Clayson and Levine, 1976), and spina bifida (Gerber, 1973) have demonstrated that the predominant trauma is the underlying deformity rather than the surgery itself. These studies emphasize the individual variability in responses to deformities present in childhood. Similar conclusions arise from the study of two new orthopedic procedures. Rogers et al. (1982) found a 6 percent rate of psychiatric referrals after total joint replacement. Major factors in precipitating the referrals included faulty expectations that were rarely related to an inadequate surgical process, decreased cognitive functioning due to organic brain dysfunction, loss of the sick role, and phobias focusing on activity but largely unrelated to surgery. A series of thirty patients undergoing replantation surgery had a 60 percent incidence of traumatic neurosis and a 20 percent incidence of prior chronic substance abuse (Schweitzer and Rosenbaum, 1982). Their 33 percent incident of preaccident psychopathology and the traumatic impact of the accident were important issues in postoperative management. This again emphasizes how liaison psychiatrists need to understand each procedure and the preoperative psychiatric and social background of each patient.

The elderly patient with a fracture of the femoral neck is a candidate for a variety of postoperative psychiatric difficulties. Kupfer et al. (1971) found that 10 of 25 patients with femoral neck fractures showed marked worsening of cognitive functioning one year after surgery. Levitan and one of the authors worked in the immediate postoperative period with a wide range of problems, including delirium, anxiety, depression, and family pathology, and demonstrated that such psychiatric complications of hospitalization and surgery can be treated successfully and cost-effectively (Levitan and Kornfeld, 1981).

UROLOGY　The psychiatric literature on urology has in the past been unaccountably sparse, but a new procedure will be attracting attention in the future. The treatment of organic and functional impotence through insertion of rigid or inflatable prostheses opens a new area for psychological research (Gregory, 1981). Thus far, results have been measured primarily by patient and partner ratings of subjective satisfaction, reported by Besser et al. (1982) to be 81 percent for patients and 83 percent for partners where impotence was secondary to diabetes. Buikholder and Bewell (1979) described the successful use of prostheses to ameliorate psychological distress due to partial penile amputation. The psychiatrist consulting with patients facing possible or probable impotence from abdominoperineal resection or radical prostatectomy should be familiar with these procedures.

PLASTIC SURGERY　No other area of liaison psychiatry with surgery has produced as steady and consistent a growth in theoretical and clinical understanding as that seen in plastic and reconstructive surgery. Space limitations prevent more than a brief mention here of the areas of consensus.

For selective cosmetic surgery, psychological evaluation techniques and criteria governing acceptance and rejection for surgery are now established. Techniques and criteria vary for the different procedures and for different groups of applicants. Patient profiles have been developed for rhinoplasty, face lift, abdominoplasty, body sculpturing, augmentation and reduction mammoplasty, and breast reconstruction after mastectomy. These profiles form the basis for informed consultation with the cosmetic surgery patient before and after surgery. Psychiatrists may be predisposed to minimize the psychological benefits of cosmetic surgery, or they may be unfamiliar with the problems posed in evaluating the contemplated surgery. An excellent survey of these issues, *Changing the Body: Psychological Effects of Plastic Surgery* (Goin and Goin, 1981), reviews the past and recent literature and offers an introduction to this field.

Patients who experience disfiguring surgery for cancer in the head and neck seem to adapt remarkably well to their altered appearance. West (1977) surveyed 152 disfigured patients and found that 93 percent had adapted well socially, with minimal alteration in their patterns of work, pleasure, and so forth. For these patients, the cure was a major ameliorative force. This is striking in view of the considerable preoperative psychopathology, especially alcoholism, described for this group by David and Bairitt (1977). Reconstructive orthognathic surgery also has a high rate of acceptance (93 percent) (Ouellette, 1978).

PSYCHIATRIC LIAISON WITH SURGERY

Teaching surgeons the psychological aspects of patient care has thus far been the subject of only one paper (Baudry and Wiener, 1969), suggesting that liaison psychiatrists have been more comfortable with surgical patients than with surgeons. The early papers of Deutsch (1942) and Meerloo (1956) did show a decided skepticism about the motivations of surgeons and their results. Recent papers have been less judgmental, focusing on the distinctive features of surgery as a professional activity. Surgeons still hold a special position in the medical community. They may be feared or held in awe and may be treated with scorn or respect. Surgeons describe themselves as different in favoring the most active pursuit of rewards for the patient. Finding the definitive answer to a problem and solving it by direct, technical intervention remains their ultimate professional gratification. For them, communication is a handmaiden to operating. Operating itself is time-consuming, an impersonal but intense experience that promotes a sense of detachment and a suspended awareness of the patient as a person. Meyer (1967) speculated that emotional detachment in the surgeon may be a necessary prerequisite to operating effectively. We do not know whether the practice molds the physician or vice versa.

In a study of 56 plastic surgeons and their patients, Wright (1980; 1981) confirmed some stereotypical notions about surgeons. Both doctor and patient saw the doctor as possessing the character traits of intelligence, ambition, an intense need for both internal and external control, independence, and self-sufficiency. In addition, surgeons revealed themselves as cautious, essentially conservative, and somewhat lacking in individuality and spontaneity. Such a description contrasts nicely with the liaison psychiatrist's familiarity with ambiguity, lack of clarity, and openendedness. This may help to explain the sense of discomfort that psychiatrists express with surgeons, and the sense of dismay that surgeons experience when they try to "pin down" the psychiatric consultant to a specific plan of action. Optimal teaching of the surgeon requires that the liaison psychiatrist be aware of these differences.

Baudry and Wiener's (1969) paper focused on teaching psychologically oriented patient care to surgeons. They included a didactic curriculum easily suited to the surgeon but also conducted joint interviewing sessions with patient, surgeon, and liaison psychiatrist. This method allowed for a gradual expansion of the surgeon's interviewing skills and for consideration of countertransference issues. On the other hand, the method is time-consuming and labor intensive, and no documentation of its effectiveness has been published. Surgeons, and especially house staff, are frequently preoccupied with mastering technical procedures and are not aware that they must also understand psychic processes and acquire interviewing techniques.

While some didactic emphasis seems essential, much of the psychological teaching must occur close to the surgeon's working situation, on ward rounds, and in routine admission, preoperative, and postoperative interviews. Under these circumstances, ongoing patient interactions are the basis for teaching structured modes of intervention. Mere exhortations to be more attentive to psychological needs are most often guilt inducing and counterproductive. Although surgeons' conservatism frequently leads them to avoid using patient interviews as experiments in relatedness, their fear of harming the patient can be allayed by using simulated interviews where no patient is at risk, and by having the liaison psychiatrist at hand during the interviews. In the future, liaison psychiatrists can help surgeons to deepen their interview skills with videotape observation and with instructional videotapes that are specially designed for teaching surgeons.

References for Part III

References for the Introduction

Lipowski ZJ: Holistic-medical foundations of American psychiatry: A bicentennial. Am J Psychiatry 138:888–895, 1981

Lipowski ZJ: What does the word "psychosomatic" really mean? A historical and semantic inquiry. Psychosom Med, in press

References for Chapter 12

History, Definition, and Scope of Consultation-Liaison Psychiatry

Barsky AJ, Klerman GL: Overview: Hypochondriasis, bodily complaints and somatic styles. Am J Psychiatry 140:273–283, 1983

Beigler JS, Robbins FP, Lane EW, Miller AA, Samelson C: Report on liaison psychiatry at Michael Reese Hospital, 1950–1958. AMA Arch Neurol Psychiatry 81:733–746, 1959

Beresford TP: Alcoholism consultation and general hospital psychiatry. Gen Hosp Psychiatry 1:293–300, 1979

Bernstein S, Kaufman RM: The psychiatrist in a general hospital. J Mount Sinai Hosp 29:385–394, 1962

Billings EG: Liaison psychiatry and intern instruction. J Assoc Med Coll 14:375–385, 1939

Billings EG: Value of psychiatry to the general hospital. Hospitals 15:305–310, 1941

Brown HN, Zinberg NE: Difficulties in the integration of psychological and medical practices. Am J Psychiatry 139:1576–1580, 1982

Cassem EH: Teaching liaison psychiatry as medicine at Massachusetts General Hospital. Presented at the Annual Meeting of the American Psychiatric Association, New York, May 4, 1983

Dunbar FH, Wolfe TP, Rioch JM: Psychiatric aspects of medical problems. Am J Psychiatry 93:649–679, 1936

Eaton JS, Goldberg R, Rosinski E, Allerton WS: The educational challenge of consultation-liaison psychiatry. Am J Psychiatry Suppl 134:20–23, 1977

Ebaugh FG, Rymer CA: Psychiatry in Medical Education. New York, Commonwealth Fund, 1942

Engel GL, Greene WA, Reichsman F, Schmale A, Ashenburg N: A graduate and undergraduate teaching program on the psychological aspects of medicine. J Med Educ 32:859–870, 1957

Faguet RA, Fawzy FI, Wellisch DK, Pasnau RO, (eds): Contemporary Models in Liaison Psychiatry. New York, SP Medical & Scientific Books, 1978

Ford CV: The Somatizing Disorders. New York, Elsevier Biomedical, 1983

Glazer WM, Astrachan BM: A social systems approach to consultation-liaison psychiatry. Int J Psychiatry Med 9:33–47, 1978–79

Glickman LS: Psychiatric Consultation in the General Hospital. New York, Marcel Dekker, 1980

Goldiamond I: Behavioral approaches and liaison psychiatry. Psychiatr Clin N Am 2:379–401, 1979

Greenberg IM: Approaches to psychiatric consultation in a research hospital setting. Arch Gen Psychiatry 3:691–697, 1960

Greenhill MH: The development of liaison programs, in Psychiatric Medicine. Edited by Usdin G. New York, Brunner/Mazel, 1977

Hall RCW (ed): Psychiatric Presentations of Medical Illness. New York, SP Medical & Scientific Books, 1980

Henry GW: Some modern aspects of psychiatry in general hospital practice. Am J Psychiatry 86:481–499, 1929–30

Kahana RJ, Bibring GL: Personality types in medical management, in Psychiatry and Medical Practice in a General Hospital. Edited by Zinberg NE. New York, International Universities Press, 1964

Kaufman RM: The role of the psychiatrist in a general hospital. Psychiatr Q 27:367–381, 1953

Levitan SJ, Kornfeld DS: Clinical and cost benefits of liaison psychiatry. Am J Psychiatr 138:790–793, 1981

Lipowski ZJ: Review of consultation psychiatry and psychosomatic medicine. I. General principles. Psychosom Med 29:153–171, 1967a

Lipowski ZJ: Review of consultation psychiatry and psychosomatic medicine. II. Clinical aspects. Psychosom Med 29:201–224, 1967b

Lipowski ZJ: Consultation-liaison psychiatry: An overview. Am J Psychiatry 131:623–630, 1974

Lipowski ZJ: Psychiatry of somatic diseases: Epidemiology, pathogenesis, classification. Compr Psychiatry 16:105–124, 1975

Lipowski ZJ: Consultation-liaison psychiatry: Past failures and new opportunities. Gen Hosp Psychiatry 1:3–10, 1979

Lipowski ZJ: Holistic-medical foundations of American psychiatry: A bicentennial. Am J Psychiatry 138:888–895, 1981a

Lipowski ZJ: Liaison psychiatry, liaison nursing, and behavioral medicine. Compr Psychiatry 22:554–561, 1981b

Lipowski ZJ: Current trends in consultation-liaison psychiatry. Can J Psychiatry 28:329–338, 1983a

Lipowski ZJ: The need to integrate liaison psychiatry and geropsychiatry. Am J Psychiatry 140:1003–1005, 1983b

Lipowski ZJ: Psychosocial reactions to physical illness. Can Med Assoc J 128:1069–1072, 1983c

Lipowski ZJ, Wolston EJ: Liaison psychiatry: Referral patterns and their stability over time. Am J Psychiatry 138:1608–1611, 1981

Lipsitt IR, Lipsitt MP: The family in consultation-liaison psychiatry. Gen Hosp Psychiatry 3:231–236, 1981

McKegney FP, Beckhardt RM: Evaluative research in consultation-liaison psychiatry. Review of literature, 1970–1981. Gen Hosp Psychiatry 4:197–218, 1982

Meyer E, Mendelson M: Psychiatric consultations with patients on medical and surgical wards: Patterns and processes. Psychiatry 24:197–220, 1961

Mohl PC: The liaison psychiatrist: Social role and status. Psychosomatics 20:19–23, 1979

Pasnau RO (ed): Consultation-Liaison Psychiatry. New York, Grune & Stratton, 1975

Perl M, Shelp EE: Psychiatric consultation masking moral dilemmas in medicine. New Engl J Med 307:618–621, 1982

Ripley HS: Psychiatric consultation service in a medical inpatient department. Am J Med Sci 199:261–268, 1940

Sandt JJ, Leifer R: The psychiatric consultation. Compr Psychiatry 5:409–418, 1964

Schiff SK, Pilot ML: An approach to psychiatric consultation in the general hospital. AMA Arch Gen Psychiatry 1:349–357, 1959

Schubert DSP, McKegney FP: Psychiatric consultation education—1976. Arch Gen Psychiatry 33:1271–1273, 1976

Schwab JJ: Handbook of Psychiatric Consultation. New York, Appleton-Century-Crofts, 1968

Shader RI (ed): Psychiatric Complications of Medical Drugs. New York, Raven Press, 1972

Solow C: Psychotropic drugs in somatic disorders. Int J Psychiatry Med 6:267–282, 1975

Starkman MN, Youngs DD: Psychiatric consultation with patients who refuse medical care. Int J Psychiatry Med 5:115–123, 1974

Strain JJ, Grossman S: Psychological Care of the Medically Ill. New York, Appleton-Century-Crofts, 1975

Sweeney GH: Pioneering general hospital psychiatry. Psychiatr Q (Suppl) 36:209–268, 1962

Tarnow JD, Guttstein SE: Systemic consultation in a general hospital. Int J Psychiatry Med 12:161–186, 1982–83

Wain HJ: Hypnosis on a consultation-liaison service. Psychosomatics 20:678–689, 1979

Weisman AD, Hackett TP: Organization and function of a psychiatric consultation service. Int Rec Med 173:306–311, 1960

Wise TN, Berlin RM: Burnout: Stresses in consultation-liaison psychiatry. Psychosomatics 22:744–751, 1981

Wise TN, Goldberg RL: Group dynamics in liaison psychiatry. J Psychiatr Treat Eval 3:501–505, 1981

References for Chapter 13

Prevalence of Psychiatric Morbidity in Medical Populations

Cavanaugh S: The prevalence of emotional and cognitive dysfunction in a general medical population: Using the MMSE, GHQ, and BDI. Gen Hosp Psychiatry 5:15–24, 1983

Cheah KC, Baldridge JA, Beard OW: Geriatric evaluation unit of a medical service: Role of a geropsychiatrist. J Gerontol 34:41–45, 1979

Clayton PJ, Halikas JA, Maurice WL: The depression of widowhood. Br J Psychiatry 120:71–78, 1972

Cohen F: Stress and bodily illness. Psychiatr Clin North Am 4:269–286, 1981

Culpan MB, Davies B: Psychiatric illness at a medical and a surgical outpatient clinic. Compr Psychiatry 1:228–235, 1960

Culpan MB, Davies B, Oppenheim, AN: Incidence of psychiatric illness among hospital outpatients. Br Med J 1:855–857, 1960

Denney D, Quass RM, Rich DC: Psychiatric patients on medical wards. Arch Gen Psychiatry 14:530–535, 1966

Derogatis LR, Morrow GR, Fetting J, Penman D, Piasetsky S, Schmale AM, Henrichs M, Carniche CLM: The prevalence of psychiatric disorders among cancer patients. JAMA 249:751–757, 1983

Dhadphale M, Ellison RH, Griffin L: The frequency of psychiatric disorders among patients attending semi-urban and rural general out-patient clinics in Kenya. Br J Psychiatry 142:379–383, 1983

Eastwood MR: The Relation Between Physical and Mental Illness. Toronto, University of Toronto Press, 1975

Farley J, Woodruff RA, Guze SB: The prevalence of hysteria and conversion symptoms. Br J Psychiatry 114:1121–1125, 1968

Fava GA, Pilowsky I, Pierfederici A, Bernardi M, Pathak D: Depressive symptoms and abnormal illness behavior in general hospital patients. Gen Hosp Psychiatry 4:171–178, 1982

Finlay-Jones RA, Burvill PW: The prevalence of minor psychiatric morbidity in the community. Psychol Med 7:475–489, 1977

Finn R, Huston PE: Emotional and mental symptoms in private medical practice. Iowa Med Soc 56(2):138–143, 1966

Gardner EA: Emotional disorders in medical practice. Ann Intern Med 73:651–653, 1970

Glass RM, Allan AT, Uhlenhuth EH, Kimball CP, Borinstein DI: Psychiatric screening in a medical clinic: An evaluation of a self-report inventory. Arch Gen Psychiatry 35:1189–1195, 1978

Goldberg DP: The Detection of Psychiatric Illness by Questionnaire. London, Oxford University Press, 1972

Goldberg DP, Blackwell B: Psychiatric illness in general practice. Br Med J 2:439–443, 1970

Goldberg DP, Cooper B, Eastwood MR, Kedward HB, Shepherd M: A standardized psychiatric interview for use in community surveys. Br J Prev Soc Med 24:18–23, 1970

Graduate Medical Education National Advisory Committee, Report of Graduate Medical Education National Advisory Committee. U.S. Department of Health and Human Services (HRA) 7:81–657, 1981

Hankin JR, Locke BZ: Extent of depressive symptomatology among patients seeking care in a prepaid group practice. Psychol Med 13:121–129, 1983

Hankin JR, Oktay JS: Mental Disorder and Primary Medical Care: An Analytical Review of the Literature. National Institute of Mental Health: U.S. Department of Health, Education, and Welfare, 1979

Hankin JR, Steinwachs DM, Regier DA, Burns BJ, Goldberg ID, Hoeper EW: Use of general medical care services by persons with mental disorders. Arch Gen Psychiatry 39:225–231, 1982

Harding TW, De Arango MV, Baltazar J, Climent CE, Ibrahim HHA, Ladrido-Ignacio L, Srinivasa Murhy R, Wig NN: Mental disorders in primary health care: A study of their frequency and diagnosis in four developing countries. Psychol Med 10:213–241, 1980

Hilkevitch A: Psychiatric disturbances in outpatients of a general medical outpatient clinic. Int J Neuropsych 1:371–375, 1965

Hoeper EW, Nycz GR, Cleary PD, Regier DA, Goldberg ID: Estimated prevalence of RDC mental disorder in primary medical care. Int J Mental Health 8:6–15, 1979

Johns MW: Symptoms of neurotic illness in general hospital patients: Use of the Cornell Medical Index. Med J Aust 2:41–44, 1972

Johnstone A, Goldberg D: Psychiatric screening in general practice. Lancet 1:605–608, 1976

Jones KR, Vischi TR: Impact of alcohol, drug abuse and mental health treatment on medical care utilization: A review of the research literature. Med Care 17 (Suppl 2):1–82, 1979

Kathol RG, Petty F: Relationship of depression to medical illness. J Affective Disord 3:111–121, 1981

Kaufman MR, Lehrman S, Franzblau AN, Tabbat S, Weinroth L, Friedman S: Psychiatric findings in admissions to a medical service in a general hospital. J Mt Sinai Hosp NY 26:160–170, 1959

Kessel WIN: Psychiatric morbidity in a London general practice. Br J Prev Soc Med 14:16–22, 1960

Kessler LG, Tessler RC, Nycz GR: Co-occurrence of psychiatric and medical morbidity in primary care. J Fam Pract 16:319–324, 1983

Kimball CP: Psychological responses to the experience of open heart surgery: I. Am J Psychiatry 126:96–107, 1969

Klerman GL: Depression in the medically ill. Psychiatr Clin North Am 4:301–317, 1981

Kurland HD, Hammer M: Emotional evaluation of medical patients. Arch Gen Psychiatry 19:72–78, 1968

Lewis WC, Berman M: Studies of conversion hysteria. Arch Gen Psychiatry 13:275–282, 1965

Linn LS, Yager J: The effect of screening, sensitization, and feedback on notation of depression. J Med Educ 55:942–949, 1980

Lipowski ZJ: Psychiatry of somatic diseases: Epidemiology, pathogenesis, classification. Compr Psychiatry 16:105–123, 1975

Lipowski ZJ: Physical illness and psychiatric disorder: A neglected relationship. Psychiatria Fennica (Suppl) 32–57, 1979.

Lloyd GG, Cawley RH: Psychiatric morbidity after myocardial infarction. Q J Med 201:33–42, 1982

Locke BZ, Gardner EA: Psychiatric disorders among the patients of general practitioners and internists. Public Health Rep 84:167–173, 1969

Lucente FE, Fleck S: A study of hospitalization anxiety in 408 medical and surgical patients. Psychosom Med 34:304–312, 1972

McIntosh ID: Alcohol-related disabilities in general hospital patients: A critical assessment of the evidence. Int J Addict 17:609–639, 1982

Maguire GP, Julier DL, Hawton KE, Bancroft JHJ: Psychiatric morbidity and referral on two general medical wards. Br Med J 1:268–270, 1974

Majerus PW, Guze SB, Delong WB, Robins E: Psychologic factors and psychiatric disease in hyperemesis gravidarum: A follow-up study of 69 vomiters and 66 controls. Am J Psychiatry 117:421–428, 1960

Marks JN, Goldberg DP, Hillier VF: Determinants of the ability of general practitioners to detect psychiatric illness. Psychol Med 9:337–353, 1979

Meyer E, Derogatis LR, Miller MJ, Park LC, Whitmarsh GA: Medical clinic patients with emotional disorders. Psychosom 19:611–619, 1978

Moffic HS, Paykel ES: Depression in medical in-patients. Br J Psychiatry 126:346–353, 1975

Mumford E, Schlesinger HJ, Glass GV: The effects of psychological intervention on recovery from surgery and heart attacks: An analysis of the literature. Am J Public Health 72:141–151, 1982

Murphy GE, Robins E, Kuhn NO, Christensen RF: Stress, sickness and psychiatric disorder in a "normal" population: A study of 101 young women. J Nerv Ment Dis 134:228–236, 1962

Nielsen AC, Williams TA: Depression in ambulatory medical patients. Arch Gen Psychiatry 37:999–1004, 1980

Ostfeld AM, Stein M, Clayton P: Seminar: Bereavement: Psychosocial, endocrine, and immunological aspects. Annual Meeting of the American Psychosomatic Society, New York, March 25–27, 1983

Payson HE, Davis JM: The psychosocial adjustment of

medical inpatients after discharge: A follow-up study. Am J Psychiatry 123:1220–1225, 1967

Pincus HA, Strain JJ, Haupt JL, Gise LH: Models of mental health training in primary care. JAMA 249:3065–3068, 1983

Purtell JJ, Robins E, Cohen ME: Observations on clinical aspects of hysteria: A quantitative study of 50 hysteria patients and 156 control subjects. JAMA 146:902–909, 1951

Querido A: Forecast and follow-up: An investigation into the clinical, social, and mental factors determining the results of hospital treatment. Br J Prev Soc Med 13:33–49, 1959

Rahe RH, Arthur RJ: Life change and illness studies: Past history and future directions. J Human Stress 4:3–15, 1978

Regier DA, Goldberg ID, Taube CA: The de facto US mental health service system. Arch Gen Psychiatry 35:685–693, 1978

Roberts BH, Norton NM: The prevalence of psychiatric illness in a medical outpatient clinic. N Eng J Med 246:82–86, 1952

Rosen BM, Locke BZ, Goldberg ID, Babigian HM: Identification of emotional disturbance in patients seen in general medical clinics. Hosp Community Psychiatry 23:364–370, 1972

Salkind MR: Beck Depression Inventory in general practice. J R Coll Gen Pract 18:267–271, 1969

Schleifer SJ, Keller SE, Camerino M, Thornton JC, Stein M: Suppression of lymphocyte stimulation following bereavement. JAMA 250:374–377, 1983

Schlesinger HJ, Mumford E, Glass GV, Patrick C, Sharfstein S: Mental health treatment and medical care utilization in a fee-for-service system: Outpatient mental health treatment following the onset of a chronic disease. Am J Public Health 73:422–429, 1983

Schwab JJ, Bialow M, Brown JM, Holzer CE: Diagnosing depression in medical inpatients. Ann Intern Med 67:695–707, 1967a

Schwab JJ, Bialow M, Holzer CE, Brown JM, Stevenson BE: Sociocultural aspects of depression in medical inpatients. Arch Gen Psychiatry 17:533–538, 1967b.

Seller RH, Blascovich J, Lenkei E: Influence of stereotypes in the diagnosis of depression by family practice residents. J Fam Pract 12:849–854, 1981

Shepherd M, Cooper B, Brown AC, Kalton G: Psychiatric Illness in General Practice. London, Oxford University Press, 1966

Sime AM: Relationship of preoperative fear, type of coping, and information received about surgery to recovery from surgery. J Pers Soc Psychol 34:716–724, 1976

Stern MJ, Pascale L, Ackerman A: Life adjustments postmyocardial infarction. Arch Intern Med 137:1680–1685, 1977

Strain JJ: The uses and abuses of screening devices. Presented at the Annual Psychosomatic Meeting, 1979

Strain JJ: Diagnostic considerations in the medical setting. Psychiatr Clin North Am 4:287–300, 1981

Taylor MA, Abrams R: The prevalence of schizophrenia: A reassessment using modern diagnostic criteria. Am J Psychiatry 135:945–948, 1978

Weissman MM, Boyd JH: The epidemiology of affective disorders: Rates and risk factors, in Psychiatry Update: The American Psychiatric Association Annual Review, Vol II. Edited by Grinspoon L. Washington DC, American Psychiatric Press, 1983

Widmer RB, Cadoret RJ: Depression in primary care: Changes in pattern of patient visits and complaints during a developing depression. J Fam Pract 7:293–302, 1978

Woodruff RA: Hysteria: An evaluation of objective diagnostic criteria by the study of women with chronic medical illness. Br J Psychiatry 114:1115–1119, 1967

Woodruff RA, Clayton PJ, Guze SB: Hysteria: Studies of diagnosis, outcome, and prevalence. JAMA 215:425–428, 1971

World Health Organization: Psychiatry and Primary Medical Care. Report on a Working Group Convened by the Regional Office for Europe of the World Health Organization, Lysebu, Oslo. April 10–13, 1973

Wright JH, Bell RA, Kuhn CC, Rush EA, Tatel N, Redmon JE: Depression in family practice patients. South Med J 73:1031–1034, 1980

Zung WWK, Magill M, Moore JT, George DT: Recognition and treatment of depression in a family medicine practice. J Clin Psychiatry 44:3–6, 1983

References for Chapter 14

Clinical Research at the Interface of Medicine and Psychiatry

Ackerman SH: Premature weaning, thermoregulation and the occurrence of gastric pathology, in Brain, Behavior and Bodily Disease, vol 59. Research Publications: Association for Research in Nervous and Mental Disease. Edited by Weiner H, Hofer MA, Stunkard AJ. New York, Raven Press, 1981

Adamson JD, Schmale AH: Object loss, giving up and the onset of psychiatric disease. Psychosom Med 27:557–576, 1965

Ader R: The role of developmental factors in susceptibility to disease, in Psychosomatic Medicine, Current Trends and Clinical Applications. Edited by Lipowski ZJ, Lipsitt DR, Whybrow PC. New York, Oxford University Press, 1977

Ader R: Animal models in the study of brain, behavior and bodily disease, in Brain, Behavior and Bodily Disease, vol 59. Research Publications: Association for Research in Nervous and Mental Disease. Edited by Weiner H, Hofer MA, Stunkard AJ. New York, Raven Press, 1981

Ader R (ed): Psychoneuroimmunology. New York: Academic Press, 1981

Ader R, Cohen N: Conditioned immunopharmacologic responses, in Psychoneuroimmunology. Edited by Ader R. New York, Academic Press, 1981

Ader R, Schmale AH: George Libman Engel: On the occasion of his retirement. Psychosom Med 42:79–101, 1980

Alexander F, French TM, Pollock GH: Psychosomatic Specificity. Chicago, University of Chicago Press, 1968

Anderson, CD: Expression of affect and physiological response in psychosomatic patients. J Psychosom Res 25:143–149, 1981

Apfel RJ, Sifneos PE: Alexithymia: Concept and measurement. Psychother Psychosom 32:180–190, 1979

Bartrop RW, Luckhurst E, Lazarus L, Kiloh LG, Penny R: Depressed lymphocyte function with bereavement. Lancet 1:834–836, 1977

Beatty ET, Haynes SN: Behavioral intervention with muscle–contraction headache: A review. Psychosom Med 41:165–180, 1979

Black S, Humphrey JH, Niven JS: Inhibition of Mantoux reaction by direct suggestion under hypnosis. Br Med J 1:1649–1652, 1963

Blumenthal JA, Williams RB, Kong D, Schanberg SM, Thompson LW: Type A behavior pattern and coronary atherosclerosis. Circulation 58:634–639, 1978

Boushey HA: Neural mechanisms in asthma, in Brain, Behavior and Bodily Disease, vol 59. Research Publications: Association for Research in Nervous and Mental Disease. Edited by Weiner H, Hofer MA, Stunkard AJ. New York, Raven Press, 1981

Boyar RM, Katz J: Twenty-four-hour gonadotropin secretory patterns in anorexia nervosa, in Anorexia Nervosa. Edited by Vigersky R. New York, Raven Press, 1977

Boyar RM, Katz J, Finkelstein JW, Kapen S, Weiner H, Weitzman ED, Hellman L: Anorexia nervosa: Immaturity of the 24-hour luteinizing hormone secretory pattern. N Engl J Med 291:861–865, 1974

Bruch H: Eating Disorders: Obesity, Anorexia Nervosa and the Person Within. New York, Basic Books, 1973

Callaway E: Biofeedback of Brain Electrical Activity, in Biofeedback, Task Force Report 19. Edited by Orne MT, Weiss T, Callaway E, Struebel C. Washington DC, American Psychiatric Association, 1980

Cannon WB: Bodily Changes in Pain, Hunger, Fear and Rage, 2nd ed. New York, D Appleton, 1920

Caplan G: Mastery of stress: Psychosocial aspects. Am J Psychiatry 138:413–420, 1981

Casper RC, Halmi KA, Goldberg SC, Eckert ED, Davis JM: Disturbances in body image estimation as related to other characteristics and outcome in anorexia nervosa. Br J Psychiatry 134:60–66, 1979

Cervulli M, Nikoomanesh P, Schuster MM: Progress in biofeedback treatment in fecal incontinence (abstract). Gastroenterology 70:869, 1976

Clayton PJ: Mortality and morbidity in the first year of widowhood. Arch Gen Psychiatry 30:747–750, 1974

Clayton PJ: The sequelae and nonsequelae of conjugal bereavement. Am J Psychiatry 136:1530–1534, 1979

Cobb S: Social support as a moderator of stress. Psychosom Med 38:300–314, 1976

Coll M, Meyer A, Stunkard AJ: Obesity and food choices in public places. Arch Gen Psychiatry 36:795–797, 1979

Corse CD, Manuck SB, Cantwell JD, Giordoni B, Mathews KA: Coronary-prone behavior pattern and cardiovascular response in persons with and without coronary heart disease. Psychosom Med 44:449–459, 1982

Crisp AH, Kalucy RS: Aspects of the perceptual disorder in anorexia nervosa. Br J Med Psychol 47:349–361, 1974

Crisp AH, Harding B, McGuiness B: Anorexia Nervosa: Psychoneurotic characteristics of parents: Relationship to prognosis. A quantitative study. J Psychosom Res 18:167–173, 1974

Crown S, Crown JM, Fleming A: Aspects of the psychology and epidemiology of rheumatoid disease. Psychol Med 5:291–299, 1975

Dally P: Anorexia Nervosa. New York, Grune & Stratton, 1969

De Aravjo G, van Arsdel PP, Holmes TH: Life change, coping ability and chronic intrinsic asthma. J Psychosom Res 17:359–363, 1973

Dembrowski TM, MacDougall JM, Shields JL, Petitto J, Lushene R: Components of the Type A coronary-prone behavior pattern and cardiovascular responses to psychomotor performance challenge. J Behav Med 1:159–176, 1978

Dexter JD, Weitzman ED: The relationship of nocturnal headaches to sleep stage patterns. Neurology 10:513–518, 1970

Dimsdale JE, Hackett TP, Hutter AM, Block PC: The risk of Type A-mediated coronary artery disease in different populations. Psychosom Med 42:55–62, 1980

Dorian B, Garfinkel P, Brown G, Shore A, Gladman D, Keystone E: Aberrations in lymphocyte subpopulations and function during psychological stress. Clin Exp Immunol 50:132–138, 1982

Dunbar HF: Psychosomatic Diagnosis. New York, Hoeber, 1943

Eastwood MR, Stiasny S, Meier RMH, Woogh CM: Mental illness and mortality. Psychiatry 23:377–385, 1982

Eckert ED, Goldberg SC, Halmi KA, Casper RC, Davis JM: Behavior therapy in anorexia nervosa. Br J Psychiatry 134:55–59, 1979

Engel BT: Stimulus-response and individual-response specificity. Arch Gen Psychiatry 2:305–313, 1960

Engel BT, Nikoomanesh P, Schuster MM: Operant conditioning of rectosphincter responses in the treatment of fecal incontinence. N Engl J Med 290:646–649, 1974

Engel GL: A psychological setting of somatic disease: The "giving up–given up" complex. Proc R Soc Med 60:553–555, 1967

Engel GL: The need for a new medical model: A challenge for biomedicine. Science 196:129–136, 1977

Engel GL, Reichsman F, Segal HL: A study of an infant with a gastric fistula: I. Behavior and the rate of total hydrochloric acid secretion. Psychosom Med 18:374–398, 1956

Engel GL, Reichsman F, Harway V, Hess DW: Follow up of an infant with gastric fistula and depression: VI. Infant feeding behavior as a mother 19 years later. Psychosom Med 36:459, 1974

Evans NJR, Baldwin JA, Gath D: The incidence of cancer among patients with affective disorders. Br J Psychiatry 124:518–525, 1974

Fauman MA: The central nervous system and the immune system. Biol Psychiatry 17:1459–1482, 1982

Fordyce WE, Fowler RS, Lehman JF, De Lateur BJ, Sand PL, Trieschmann RB: Operant conditioning in the treatment of chronic pain. Arch Phys Med Rehabil 54:399–408, 1973

Frank KA, Heller SS, Kornfeld DS, Sporn AA, Weiss MB: Type A behavior pattern and coronary angiographic findings. JAMA 240:761–762, 1978

Friedman M, Rosenman RH: Association of specific overt behavior pattern with blood-cardiovascular findings. JAMA 169:1286–1296, 1959

Friedman M, Rosenman RH, Straus R, Wurm M, Kositchek R: The relationship of behavior pattern A to the state of the coronary vasculature: A study of fifty-one autopsy subjects. Am J Med 44:525–537, 1968

Gardiner BM: Psychological aspects of rheumatoid arthritis. Psychol Med 10:159–163, 1980

Garfinkel PE, Garner DM: Perceptual and conceptual disturbances, in Anorexia Nervosa, A Multidimensional Pespective. New York, Brunner Mazel, 1982

Garfinkel PE, Moldofsky H, Garner DM: The outcome of anorexia nervosa: Significance of clinical features, body image, and behavior modification, in Anorexia Nervosa. Edited by Vigersky RA. New York, Raven Press, 1977a

Garfinkel PE, Moldofsky H, Garner DM: Prognosis in anorexia nervosa as influenced by clinical features, treatment and self-perception. Can Med Assoc J 117:1041–1045, 1977b

Garfinkel PE, Moldofsky H, Garner DM: The stability of

perceptual disturbances in anorexia nervosa. Psychol Med 9:703–708, 1979

Garner DM, Garfinkel PE: Body image in anorexia nervosa: Measurement, theory and clinical implications. Int J Psychiatry Med 11:263–284, 1981

Garner DM, Garfinkel PE, Stancer HC, Moldofsky H: Body image disturbances in anorexia nervosa and obesity. Psychosom Med 38:227–336, 1976

Glass DC, Krakoff LR, Contrada R, Hilton WF, Kehoe K, Mannucci EG, Collins C, Snow B, Elting E: Effect of harassment and competition upon cardiovascular and catecholamine responses in Type A and Type B individuals. Psychophysiology 17:453–463, 1980

Goldberg SC, Halmi KA, Casper R, Eckert E, Davis JM: Pretreatment predictors of weight change in anorexia nervosa, in Anorexia Nervosa. Edited by Vigersky R. New York, Raven Press, 1977

Goldhand S: Stimulus specificity of physiological response to stress and the Type A coronary-prone behavior pattern. J Pers Soc Psychol 39:670–679, 1980

Gorczynski RM, MacRae S, Kennedy M: Factors involved in the classical conditioning of antibody responses in mice. Proceedings of Workshop on Psychoneuroimmunology. Edited by Ballieux R, Ader R. Commission of the European Communities, 1983

Green LW: Towards cost-benefit evaluations of health education. Some concepts, methods, and examples. Health Education Monographs, vol 2 (Suppl 1):34–36, 1974

Greene SM, O'Mahony PD, Rungasamy P: Levels of measured hopelessness in physically ill patients. J Psychosom Res 26:591–593, 1982

Greer S, Morris T, Pettingale KW: Psychological response to breast cancer: Effect on outcome. Lancet 2:785–787, 1979

Guilleminault C, van den Hoed J, Mitler M: Clinical overview of the sleep apnea syndromes, in Sleep Apnea Syndromes. Edited by Guilleminault C, Dement WC. New York, Liss, 1978

Halmi KA, Mason E, Falk JR, Stunkard A: Appetitive behavior after gastric bypass for obesity. Int J Obes 5:457–464, 1981

Henry JP: The relation of social to biological processes in disease. Soc Sci Med 16:359–380, 1982

Henry JP, Stevens PM, Meehan JP: The use of psychosocial stimuli to induce prolonged hypertension in mice. Psychosom Med 29:408–443, 1967

Herman CP: Restrained eating. Psychiatr Clin North Am 1:593–607, 1978

Hofer MA: Some thoughts on "The transduction of experience" from a developmental perspective. Psychosom Med 44:19–28, 1982

Holmes TH, Rahe RH: The Social Readjustment Rating Scale. J Psychosom Res 11:213–218, 1967

Hsu LKG, Crisp AH, Harding B: Outcome of anorexia nervosa. Lancet 1:61–65, 1979

Hsu LKG, Crisp AH, Kalucy RS, Koval J, Chen CN, Caruthers M, Zilka KJ: Early morning migraine nocturnal plasma levels of catecholamines tryptophan, glucose and free fatty acids and sleep encephalogram. Lancet 1:447–450, 1977

Imura H, Yoshimi T, Ikekubo K: Growth hormone secretion in a patient with deprivation dwarfism. Endocrinol Jpn 18:301–304, 1971

Inglis J, Campbell D, Donald DW: Electromyographic biofeedback and neuromuscular rehabilitation. Can J Behav Sci 8:299–323, 1976

Jenkins CD, Rosenman RH, Zyzanski SJ: Prediction of clinical coronary heart disease by a test for the coronary-prone behavior pattern. N Engl J Med 290:1271, 1974

Kahn JP, Kornfeld DS, Blood DK, Lynn RB, Heller SS, Frank KA: Type A behavior and the thallium stress test. Psychosom Med 44:431–436, 1982

Karacan I, Salis PJ, Williams RL: The role of the sleep laboratory in diagnosis and treatment of impotence, in Sleep Disorders, Diagnosis and Treatment. Edited by Williams RL, Karacan I. New York, John Wiley & Sons, 1978

Katz JL, Weiner H, Gallagher TF, Hellman L: Stress, distress and ego defenses. Arch Gen Psychiatry 23:131–142, 1970

Kayed K, Godtlibsen OB, Sjaastad O: Chronic paroxysmal hemicrania IV: "REM sleep locked" nocturnal headache attacks. Sleep 1:91–95, 1978

Keller SE, Ackerman SH, Schleifer SJ, Shindledecker RD, Camerino MS, Hofer MA, Weiner H, Stein M: Effect of premature weaning on lymphocyte stimulation in the rat (abstract). Psychosom Med 45:75, 1983

Kerns RD, Turk DC, Holzman AD: Psychological treatment for chronic pain: A selective review. Clinical Psychol Review 3:15–26, 1983

Kerr RA, Shapira K, Roth M: The relationship between premature death and affective disorders. Br J Psychiatry 115:1277–1282, 1969

Kinsman RA, Dirks JF, Jones NF, Dahlem NW: Anxiety reduction in asthma: Four catches to general application. Psychosom Med 43:397–405, 1980

Knapp PH, Mathe AA, Vachon L: Psychosomatic aspects of bronchial asthma, in Bronchial Asthma: Mechanism and Therapeutics. Edited by Weiss EG, Segal MS. Boston, Little Brown & Co, 1976

Koob GE, Bloom FE: Behavioural effects of opioid peptides. Br Med Bull 39:89–94, 1983

Lader M: Psychophysiological research and psychosomatic medicine, in Physiology, Emotion and Psychosomatic Illness; Ciba Foundation Symposium 8 (new series). Amsterdam, Elsevier/Excerpta Medica/North Holland/Associated Scientific Publishers, 1972

Leigh H, Reiser MF: The Patient: Biological, Psychological and Social Dimensions of Medical Practice. New York, Plenum Medical Book Co, 1980

Lesser IM: A review of the alexithymia concept. Psychosom Med 43:531–543, 1981

Luparello T, Lyons HA, Bleecker ER, McFadden ER: Influences of suggestion on airway reactivity in asthmatic subjects. Psychosom Med 30:819–825, 1968

MacDonald MR, Kuiper NA: Cognitive-behavioral preparations for surgery: Some theoretical and methodological concerns. Clinical Psychol Review 3:27–39, 1983

McKenzie JM: Stress and thyroid function, in Clinical Neuroendocrinology: A Pathophysiological Approach. Edited by Tolis G, Martin J, Labrie F, Natolin F. New York, Raven Press, 1979

Manuck SB, Garland FN: Coronary-prone behavior pattern, task incentive and cardiovascular response. Psychophysiol 16:136–142, 1979

Marty P, de M'Uzan M: La "pensée opératoire". Rev Franc Psychanal 27(Suppl):1345, 1963

Mason JW: Organization of the multiple endocrine responses to avoidance in the monkey. Psychosom. Med. 30:774–790, 1968

Mason JW: A historical view of the stress field: Part one. J Human Stress 1:6–12, 1975a

Mason JW: Clinical psychophysiology, psychoendocrine mechanisms, in American Handbook of Psychiatry, vol 6. Edited by Arieti S. New York, Basic Books, 1975b

Masuda M, Holmes TH: Life events: Perceptions and frequencies. Psychosom Med 40:236–261, 1978

Mellstrom D, Nilsson A, Oden A, Ake R, Svanborg A: Mortality among the widowed in Sweden. Scand J Soc Med 10:33–41, 1982

Miller NE: Learning of visceral and glandular responses. Science 163:434–445, 1969

Minuchin S, Baker L, Rosman B, Liebman R, Milman L, Todd T: A conceptual model of psychosomatic illness in children. Arch Gen Psychiatry 32:1031–1038, 1975

Moldofsky H: Sleep and psychosomatic illness, in The Biology of Anxiety. Edited by Mathew R. New York, Brunner/Mazel, 1982

Moldofsky H, Chester WJ: Pain and mood patterns in patients with rheumatoid arthritis. Psychosom Med 32:309–318, 1970

Moldofsky H, Scarisbrick P: Induction of neurasthenic musculoskeletal pain syndrome by selective sleep stage deprivation. Psychosom Med 38:35–44, 1976

Moldofsky H, Lue FA, Smythe HA: Alpha EEG sleep and morning symptoms in rheumatoid arthritis. J Rheumatol 10:373–379, 1983

Moldofsky H, Scarisbrick P, England R, Smythe HA: Musculoskeletal symptoms and Non-REM sleep disturbance in patients with "Fibrositis Syndrome" and in healthy subjects. Psychosom Med 37:341–351, 1975

Moldofsky H, Tullis C, Lue FA, Quance G, Davidson J: Sleep-related myoclonus in rheumatic pain modulation disorder (Fibrositis Syndrome) and in excessive daytime somnolence. Psychosom Med, in press.

Morgan HG, Russell GFM: Value of family background in clinical features as predictors of long-term outcome in anorexia nervosa: Four-year follow-up study of 41 patients. Psychol Med 5:355–371, 1975

Musaph H: The role of aggression in somatic symptom formation, in Psychosomatic Medicine, Current Trends and Clinical Applications. Edited by Lipowski ZJ, Lipsitt DR, Whybrow PC. New York, Oxford University Press, 1977

Neill JR, Marshal JR, Yale CE: Marital changes after intestinal bypass surgery. JAMA 240:447–450, 1978

Nemiah JC, Sifneos PE: Affect and fantasy in patients with psychosomatic disorders, in Modern Trends in Psychosomatic Medicine. Edited by Hill OW. London, Butterworth, 1970

Nesse RM, Curtis GC, Brown GM: Phobic anxiety does not affect plasma levels of thyroid stimulating hormone in man. Psychoneuroendocrinology 7:69–74, 1982

Neuchterlein KH, Holroyd JC: Biofeedback in the treatment of tension headache. Arch Gen Psychiatry 37:866–873, 1980

Niemi T, Jaaskelainen J: Cancer morbidity in depressive persons. J Psychosom Res 22:117–120, 1978

Nuckolls KB, Cassel J, Kaplan BH: Psychosocial assets, life crisis, and the prognosis of pregnancy. Am J Epidemiol 95:431–441, 1972

Orne MT, Weiss T, Callaway E, Stroebel CF: Biofeedback. Task Force Report 19. Washington DC, American Psychiatric Association, 1980

Palmblad J, Petrini B, Wasserman J, and Akerstedt T: Lymphocyte and granulocyte reactions during sleep deprivation. Psychosom Med 41:273–278, 1979

Parkes CM, Brown RJ: Health after bereavement: A controlled study of young Boston widows and widowers. Psychosom Med 34:449–469, 1972

Parkes CM, Benjamin B, Fitzgerald R: Broken heart: A statistical study of increased mortality among widowers. Br Med J 1:740, 1969

Pettingale KW, Merrett TG, Tee DEH: Prognostic value of serum levels of immunoglobulins (IgG, IgA, IgM, and IgE) in breast cancer: A preliminary study. Br J Cancer 36:550–557, 1977a

Pettingale KW, Greer S, Tee DEH: Serum IgA and emotional expression in breast cancer patients. J Psychosom Res 21:395–399, 1977b

Pierloot RA, Houben ME: Estimation of body dimensions in anorexia nervosa. Psychol Med 8:317–324, 1978

Pierloot RA, Wellens W, Houben ME: Elements of resistance to a combined medical and psychotherapeutic program in anorexia nervosa. Psychother Psychosom 26:10–117, 1975

Pittner MS, Houston BK: Response to stress, cognitive coping strategies and the Type A behavior pattern. J Pers Soc Psychol 39:147–157, 1980

Pollard T, Bassett, JR, Cairnscross KD: Plasma glucocorticoid elevation and ultrastructural changes in the adenohypophysis in the male rat following prolonged exposure to stress. Neuroendocrinol 21:312–330, 1976

Powell GF, Brasel JA, Blizzard RM: Emotional deprivation and growth retardation simulating idiopathic hypopituitarism. Clinical evaluation of the syndrome. N Engl J Med 276:1271–1278, 1967a

Powell GF, Brasel JA, Raiti S, Blizzard RM: Emotional deprivation and growth retardation simulating idiopathic hypopituitarism. Endocrinologic evaluation of the syndrome. N Engl J Med 276:1279–1283, 1967b

Rabkin JG, Struening EL: Social change, stress, and illness: A selective literature review. Psychoanalysis and Contemporary Science, vol 5. New York, International Universities Press, 1976

Razin AM: Psychosocial intervention in coronary artery disease: A review. Psychosom Med 44:363–387, 1982

Rees WD, Lutkins SG: Mortality of bereavement. Br Med J 4:13–16, 1967

Rehfeld JF: Cholecystokinin as a satiety signal. Int J Obes 5:465–469, 1981

Review Panel on Coronary-Prone Behavior and Coronary Heart Disease: Coronary-prone behavior and coronary heart disease: A critical review. Circulation 63:1199–1255, 1981

Rimon RA: Rheumatoid factor and aggression dynamics in female patients with rheumatoid arthritis. Scand J Rheumatol 2:119–122, 1973

Rodin J: The role of perception of internal and external signals on the regulation of feeding in overweight and nonobese individuals, in Appetite and Food Intake, Life Science Report 2. Edited by Silverstone T. Berlin, Dahlem Konferenz, 1976

Roessler R, Engel BT: The current status of the concepts of physiological response specificity and activation, in Psychosomatic Medicine, Current Trends and Clinical Applications. Edited by Lipowski ZJ, Lipsitt DR, Whybrow PC. New York, Oxford University Press, 1977

Rogers MP, Dubey D, Reich P: The influence of the psyche and the brain on immunity and disease susceptibility: A critical review. Psychosom Med 41:147–164, 1979

Rose RM: Overview of endocrinology of stress, in Neuroendocrinology and Psychiatric Disorders. Edited by Brown GM, Koslow SH, Reichlin S. New York, Raven Press, in press

Rosman BL, Minuchin S, Baker L, Liebman R: A family approach to anorexia nervosa: Study, treatment and outcome, in Anorexia Nervosa. Edited by Vigersky RA. New York, Raven Press, 1977

Schachter S: Emotion, Obesity and Crime. New York, Academic Press, 1971

Scherwitz L, Berton K, Leventhal H: Type A assessment and interaction in the behavior pattern interview. Psychosom Med 39:229–240, 1977

Schiebel D, Castelnuovo-Tedesco P: Studies of superobesity III. Body image changes after jejuno-ileal bypass surgery. Int J Psychiatry Med 8:117–123, 1978

Schmale AH: Relationship of separation and depression to disease. Psychosom Med 20:259–277, 1958

Schmale AH, Engel GL: The giving up–given up complex illustrated on film. Arch Gen Psychiatry 17:135–145, 1967

Schmale AH, Meyerowitz S, Tinling DC: Current concepts of psychosomatic medicine, in Modern Trends in Psychosomatic Medicine, 2nd ed. Edited by Hill OW. London, Butterworth & Co, 1970

Schucker B, Jacobs DR: Assessment of behavioral risk for coronary disease by voice characteristics. Psychosom Med 39:219–228, 1977

Schwartz GE, Weiss SM: Behavioral medicine revisited. An amended definition. J Behav Med 1:249–251, 1978

Sclafani A: Appetitive behavior after jejunoileal bypass. Int J Obes 5:449–455, 1981

Selye H: Forty years of stress research. Can Med Assoc J 115:53–59, 1976

Shapiro D, Surwit RS: Biofeedback, in Behavioral Medicine: Theory and Practice. Edited by Pomerleau OF, Brady JP. Baltimore, Williams & Wilkins, 1979

Sifneos PE: The prevalence of "alexithymic" characteristics in psychosomatic patients. Psychother Psychosom 22:255–262, 1973

Slade PD, Russell GFM: Experimental investigations of bodily perception in anorexia nervosa and obesity. Psychother Psychosom 22:259–263, 1973

Smith GR, McDaniel SM: Psychologically mediated effect on the delayed hypersensitivity reaction to tuberculin in humans. Psychosom Med 45:65–69, 1983

Stein M: Biopsychosocial factors in asthma, in Critical Issues in Behavioral Medicine. Edited by West LJ, Stein M. Philadelphia, JB Lippincott Co, 1982

Stein M, Keller S, Schleifer S: The hypothalamus and the immune response, in Brain, Behavior and Bodily Disease, vol 59. Research Publications: Association for Research in Nervous and Mental Disease. Edited by Weiner H, Hofer MA, Stunkard AJ. New York, Raven Press, 1981

Steptoe A: Psychologic Factors in Cardiovascular Disorders. New York, Academic Press, 1981

Stoyva J: Biofeedback and relaxation in stress management. Modern Med Can 37:1661–1668, 1982

Stunkard A, Koch C: The interpretation of gastric motility: I. Apparent bias in the reports of hunger by obese persons. Arch Gen Psychiatry 11:74–82, 1964

Stunkard AJ, Penick SB: Behavior modification in the treatment of obesity: The problems of maintaining weight loss. Arch Gen Psychiatry 36:801–804, 1979

Suess WM, Alexander AB, Smith DD, Sweeney HW, Marion RJ: The effects of psychological stress on respiration: A preliminary study of anxiety and hyperventilation. Psychophysiology 17:535–540, 1980

Swanson DW, Maruta T, Swenson WM: Results of behavioral modification in the treatment of chronic pain. Psychosom Med 41:55–61, 1979

Theander S: Anorexia nervosa: A psychiatric investigation of 44 female cases. Acta Psychiatr Scand (Suppl) 214:1–194, 1970

Van Egeren LF: Social interactions, communications and the coronary prone behavior pattern. A psychophysiological study. Psychosom Med 41:2–28, 1979

Verrier RL, Lown B: Autonomic nervous system and malignant cardiac arrhythmias, in Brain, Behavior, and Bodily Disease, vol. 59. Research Publications: Association for Research in Nervous and Mental Disease. Edited by Weiner H, Hofer MA, Stunkard, AJ. New York, Raven Press, 1981

Vollhardt BR, Ackerman SH, Grayzel AI, Barland P: Psychologically distinguishable groups of rheumatoid arthritis patients: A controlled single blind study. Psychosom Med 44:353–362, 1982

Ward AWM: Mortality of bereavement. Br Med J 1:700–702, 1976

Weiner, H: The heterogeneity of psychosomatic disease. Psychosom Med 37:371–372, 1976

Weiner H: Psychobiology and Human Disease. New York, Elsevier/North Holland, 1977

Weiner H: Psychobiology of Essential Hypertension, vol 1. New York, Elsevier/North Holland, 1979

Weiner H: The prospects for psychosomatic medicine: Selected topics. Psychosom Med 44:491–518, 1982

Whitlock FA, Siskind M: Depression and cancer: A follow-up study. Psychol Med 9:747–752, 1979

Wise TN, Rosenthal JB: Depression, illness beliefs and severity of illness. J Psychosom Res 26:247–253, 1982

Wittkower ED: Historical perspective of contemporary psychosomatic medicine, in Psychosomatic Medicine, Current Trends and Clinical Application. Edited by Lipowski ZJ, Lipsitt DR, Whybrow PC. New York, Oxford University Press, 1977

Wolf S, Wolff HG: Human Gastric Function: An Experimental Study of a Man and His Stomach. New York, Oxford University Press, 1947

Young M, Benjamin B, Wallis C: The mortality of widowers. Lancet 2: 454–456, 1963

Zyzanski SJ, Jenkins CD, Ryan TJ: Psychologic correlates of coronary angiographic findings. Arch Int Med 136:1234–1237, 1978

References for Chapter 15

Psychiatry and Geriatric Medicine

American Psychiatric Association: Diagnostic and Statistical Manual of Mental Disorders, Third Edition. Washington DC, American Psychiatric Association, 1980

Anderson GJ: Clinical clues to digitalis toxicity. Geriatrics 35:57–65, 1980

Anstee BA: The pattern of psychiatric referrals in a general hospital. Br J Psychiatry 120:631–634, 1972

Bartus RT, Dean RL, Beer B, Lippa AS: The cholinergic hypothesis of geriatric memory dysfunction. Science 217:408–417, 1982

Billings RF, Tang SW, Rakoff VM: Depression associated with cimetidine. Can J Psychiatry 26:260–261, 1981

Blazer D: The epidemiology of late life depression. J Am Geriatr Soc 30:587–592, 1982

Blumenfield S, Morris J, Sherman FT: The geriatric team in the acute care hospital: An educational and consultation modality. J Am Geriatr Soc 30:660–664, 1982

Blumenthal MD: Depressive illness in old age: Getting behind the mask. Geriatrics 35:34–43, 1980

Bustamante JP, Ford CV: Characteristics of general hospital patients referred for psychiatric consultation. J Clin Psychiatry 42:338–341, 1981

Chisholm SE, Deniston OL, Igrisan RM, Barbus AJ: Prevalence of confusion in elderly hospitalized patients. J Gerontol Nurs 8:87–96, 1982

Clayton PJ: Mortality and morbidity in the first year of widowhood. Arch Gen Psychiatry 30:747–750, 1974

Clayton PJ: Clinical insights into normal grief. RI Med J 63:107–109, 1980

Crowder MK, Pate JK: A case report of cimetidine-induced depressive syndrome. Am J Psychiatry 137:1451, 1980

Denney D, Kole DM, Matarazzo RG: The relationship between age and the number of symptoms reported by patients. J Gerontol 20:50–53, 1965

Dovenmuehle RH, Verwoerdt A: Physical illness and depressive symptomatology. I. Incidence of depressive symptoms in hospitalized cardiac patients. J Am Geriatr Soc O:932–947, 1962

Folks DG, Ford CV: Psychiatric consultation for the geriatric medical/surgical patient. Unpublished paper. Submitted for publication, 1983

Folstein MF, McHugh PR: Dementia syndrome of depression, in Alzheimer's Disease: Senile Dementia and Related Disorders. Edited by Katzman R, Terry RD, Bick KL. New York, Raven Press, 1978

Folstein MF, Folstein SE, McHugh PR: "Mini-mental state" a practical method for grading the cognitive state of patients for the clinician. J Psychiatr Res 12:189–198, 1975

Ford CV: Psychiatrists and elderly patients. Psychosomatics 22:190–192, 1981

Ford CV: The Somatizing Disorders: Illness as a Way of Life. New York, Elsevier Biomedical, 1983

Ford CV, Winter J: Computerized axial tomograms and dementia in elderly patients. J Gerontol 36:164–169, 1981

Foster JR, Gershell WJ, Goldfarb AI: Lithium treatment in the elderly. J Gerontol 32:299–302, 1977

Gaultieri CT, Powell SF: Psychoactive drug interactions. J Clin Psychiatry 39:720–729, 1978

Goldstein SE, Birnbom F: Hypochondriasis and the elderly. J Am Geriatr Soc 24:150–154, 1976

Greenblatt DJ, Shader RI: Anticholinergics. N Engl J Med 288:1215–1219, 1973

Gregory DW: Digitalis delirium: A reminder. South Med J 73:371–372, 1980

Grinspoon L (ed): Psychiatry Update: The American Psychiatric Association Annual Review. Vol. II. Washington DC, American Psychiatric Press, Inc, 1983

Hall RCW, Feinsilver DL, Holt RE: Anticholinergic psychosis: Differential diagnosis and management. Psychosomatics 22:581–587, 1981

Hall RCW, Stickney SK, Gardner ER: Behavioral toxicity of nonpsychiatric drugs, in Psychiatric Presentations of Medical Illness. Edited by Hall RCW. New York, Spectrum Publications, 1980

Hicks R, Dysken MW, Davis JM, Lesser J, Ripeckyj A, Lazarus L: The pharmacokinetics of psychotropic medication in the elderly: A review. J Clin Psychiatry 42:374–385, 1981

Janowsky DS: Pseudodementia in the elderly: Differential diagnosis and treatment. J Clin Psychiatry 43:(9-Section 2) 19–25, 1982

Jarvik LF, Mintz J, Steuer J, Gerner R: Treating geriatric depression: A 26-week interim analysis. J Am Geriatr Soc 30:713–717, 1982

Jefferson JW: Central nervous system toxicity of cimetidine: A case of depression. Am J Psychiatry 136:346, 1979

Karasu TB, Plutchik R, Steinmuller RI, Conte H, Siegel B: Patterns of psychiatric consultation in a general hospital. Hosp Community Psychiatry 28:291–294, 1977

Kornfeld DS, Feldman M: The psychiatric service in the general hospital. NY State J Med 65:1332–1336, 1965

Kornfeld DS, Zimberg S, Malm JR: Psychiatric complications of open heart surgery. N Engl J Med 273:287–292, 1965

Levenson AJ: Neuropsychiatric side-effects of drugs in the elderly, In Aging, vol 9. Edited by Levenson AJ. New York, Raven Press, 1979

Levitan SJ, Kornfeld DS: Clinical and cost benefits of liaison psychiatry. Am J Psychiatry 138:790–793, 1981

Libow LS: Pseudo-senility: Acute and reversible organic brain syndromes. J Am Geriatr Soc 21:112–120, 1973

Lipowski ZJ: Delirium: Acute Brain Failure in Man. Springfield Ill, Charles C Thomas, 1980a

Lipowski ZJ: Organic mental disorders: Introduction and review of syndromes, in Comprehensive Textbook of Psychiatry/III, vol 2. Edited by Kaplan HI, Freedman AM, Sadock BJ. Baltimore, Williams & Wilkins, 1980b

Lipowski ZJ: The need to integrate liaison psychiatry and geropsychiatry. Am J Psychiatry, 140:1003–1005, 1983

Liston EH: Occult presenile dementia. J Nerv Ment Dis 164:263–267, 1977

Liston EH: Delirium in the aged. Psychiatr Clin North Am 49:66, 1982

McAllister TW: Overview: Pseudodementia. Am J Psychiatry 140:528–533, 1983

McAllister TW, Price TRP: Severe depressive pseudodementia with and without dementia. Am J Psychiatry 139:626–629, 1982

McAllister TW, Ferrell RB, Price TRP: The dexamethasone suppression test in two patients with severe depressive pseudodementia. Am J Psychiatry 139:479–481, 1982

McEvoy JP: Organic brain syndromes. Ann Intern Med 95:212–220, 1981

McFarland DD: The aged in the 21st century: A demographic view, in Aging Into the 21st Century. Edited by Jarvik LF. New York, Gardner Press, 1978

Mathew RJ, Meyer JS, Francis DJ, Semchuk KM, Mortel K, Claghorn JL: Cerebral blood flow in depression. Am J Psychiatry 137:1449–1450, 1980

Moffic HS, Paykel ES: Depression in medical in-patients. Br J Psychiatry 126:346–353, 1975

Murphy E: The prognosis of depression in old age. Br J Psychiatry 142:111–119, 1983

Ouslander JG: Physical illness and depression in the elderly. J Am Geriatr Soc 30:593–599, 1982

Papastamou PA: Psychiatric consultations in a general hospital. Psychosomatics 11:57–62, 1970

Perl M, Hall RCW, Gardner ER: Behavioral toxicity of psychiatric drugs, in Psychiatric Presentations of Medical Illness. Edited by Hall RCW. New York, Spectrum Publications, 1980

Portnoi VA: Digitalis delirium in elderly patients. J Clin Pharmacol 19:747–750, 1979

Rabins PV: Management of irreversible dementia. Psychosomatics 22:591–597, 1981

Reifler BV: Arguments for abandoning the term pseudodementia. J Am Geriatr Soc 30:665–668, 1982

Reifler BV, Larson E, Hanley R: Coexistence of cognitive impairment and depression in geriatric outpatients. Am J Psychiatry 139:623–626, 1982

Reisberg B, Ferris SH: Diagnosis and assessment of the older patient. Hosp Community Psychiatry 33:104–110, 1982

Robinson DS: Changes in monoamine oxidase and monoamines with human development and aging. Fed Proc 34:103–107, 1975

Ron MA, Toone BK, Garralda ME, Lishman WA: Diagnostic accuracy in presenile dementia. Br J Psychiatry 134:161–168, 1979

Rothblum ED, Sholomskas AJ, Berry C, Prusoff BA: Issues in clinical trials with the depressed elderly. J Am Geriatr Soc 30:694–699, 1982

Sadavoy J, Reiman-Sheldon E: General hospital geriatric psychiatric treatment: A follow-up study. J Am Geriatr Soc 31:200–205, 1983

Salzman C: A primer on geriatric psychopharmacology. Am J Psychiatry 139:67–74, 1982

Salzman C, Shader RI: Depression in the elderly. I. Relationship between depression, psychologic defense mechanisms and physical illness. J Am Geriatr Soc 26:253–260, 1978a

Salzman C, Shader RI: Depression in the elderly. II. Possible drug etiologies; differential diagnostic criteria. J Am Geriatr Soc 27:303–308, 1978b

Salzman C, Shader RI, van der Kolk BA: Clinical psychopharmacology and the elderly patient. NY State J Med 76:71–77, 1976

Schuckit MA, Miller PL, Hahlbohm D: Unrecognized psychiatric illness in elderly medical/surgical patients. J Gerontol 30:655–660, 1975

Shader RI: Psychiatric Complications of Medical Drugs. New York, Raven Press, 1972

Shevitz SA, Silberfarb PM, Lipowski ZJ: Psychiatric consultation in a general hospital: A report on 1000 referrals. Dis Nerv Syst 37:295–300, 1976

Spar JE, Gerner R: Does the dexamethasone suppression test distinguish dementia from depression? Am J Psychiatry 139:238–240, 1982

Spar JE, Ford CV, Liston EH: Bipolar affective disorder in aged patients. J Clin Psychiatry 40:504–507, 1979

Steuer J: Psychotherapy with the elderly. Psychiatr Clin North Am 5:199–213, 1982

Strauss A: Cimetidine and delirium: Assessment and management. Psychosomatics 23:57–62, 1982

Volpe BT, Soave R: Formed visual hallucinations as digitalis toxicity. Ann Intern Med 91:865–866, 1979

Walkenstein SS, Dubb JW, Randolph WC, Westlake WJ, Stote RM, Intoccia AP: Bioavailability of cimetidine in man. Gastroenterology 74:360–365, 1978

Weddington WW, Muelling AE, Moosa HH: Adverse neuropsychiatric reactions to cimetidine. Psychosomatics 23:49–53, 1982

Weiner RD: The role of electroconvulsive therapy in the treatment of depression in the elderly. J Am Geriatr Soc 30:710–712, 1982

Weisman AD, Hackett TP: Psychosis after eye surgery. N Engl J Med 258:1284–1289, 1958

Wells CE: Pseudodementia. Am J Psychiatry 136:895–900, 1979

Wells CE: Refinements in the diagnosis of dementia. Am J Psychiatry 139:621–622, 1982

Wells CE, Duncan GW: Dangers of overreliance on computerized axial tomography. Am J Psychiatry 134:811–813, 1977

References for Chapter 16

Psychiatry and Oncology

Allen JC, Rosen G, Mehta BM, Horten B: Leukoencephalopathy following high-dose IV methotrexate chemotherapy with leucovorin rescue. Cancer Treat Rep 64:1261–1273, 1980

Artiss LK, Levine AS: Doctor-patient relation in severe illness: A seminar for oncology fellows. N Engl J Med 288:1210–1214, 1973

Bagley CM: Single IV doses of 5-fluorouracil—a phase I study (abstract). Proc Amer Association Cancer Res 16:12, 1975

Bukberg J, Penman D, Holland J: Depression in hospitalized cancer patients. Psychosom Med, in press

Chapman RM, Sutcliffe SB, Malpas JS: Cytotoxic-induced ovarian failure in women with Hodgkin's disease. I. Hormone function. JAMA 242:1877–1880, 1979

DeConti RC: Procarbazine in the management of late Hodgkin's disease. JAMA 215:927–930, 1971

Delellis R, Wolfe HJ: Multiple endocrine adenomatosis syndrome, in Cancer Medicine. Edited by Holland JF, Frei E. Philadelphia, Lea & Febiger, 1982

Derogatis LR, Feldstein M, Morrow GR, Schmale A, Schmitt M, Gates C, Murawski B, Holland J, Penman D, Melisaratos N, Enelow AJ, Adler LM: A survey of psychotropic drug prescriptions in an oncology population. Cancer 44:1919–1929, 1979

Derogatis LR, Morrow GR, Fetting J, Penman D, Piasetsky S, Schmale AM, Henrichs M, Carnicke CM: The prevalence of psychiatric disorders among cancer patients. JAMA 249:751–757, 1983

D'Angio GJ: Complications of treatment encountered in lymphoma leukemia long-term survivors. Cancer 42:1015–1025, 1978

Fazio M, Cavallero P, Minetto E, Rattalino PG, Sartoris S: Polichemotherapy of advanced head and neck malignancies. Tumori 62:599–608, 1976

Fox BH: Psychosocial factors and the immune system in human cancer, in Psychoneuroimmunology. Edited by Ader R. New York, Academic Press, 1981

Fox BH: Behavioral issues in cancer, in Perspectives in Behavioral Medicine. Edited by Weiss SM, Herd JA, Fox BH. New York, Academic Press, 1979

Gapen P: Neurological complications now characterizing many AIDS victims. JAMA 248:2941–2942, 1982

Gralla R, Itri L, Pisko S, Squillante AE, Kelsen DP, Braun DW, Bordin LA, Braun TJ, Young CW: Antiemetic efficacy of high-dose metaclopramide: Randomized trials with placebo and prochlorperazine in patients with chemotherapy-induced nausea and vomiting. N Engl J Med 305:905–909, 1981

Greenwald ES: Organic mental changes with fluorouracil therapy (ltr to ed). JAMA 235:248–249, 1976

Hall RCW, Popkin MK, Stickney SK, Gardner ER: Presentation of the steroid psychoses. J Nerv Ment Dis 167:229–236, 1979

Hamburg D, Hamburg B, de Goza S: Adaptive problems and mechanisms in severely burned patients. Psychiatry 16:1–20, 1953

Higginson J, Muir CS: Environmental carcinogenesis: Misconceptions and limitations to cancer control. J Nat Cancer Inst 63:1291–1298, 1979

Holland JC: Psychosocial aspects of cancer, in Cancer Medicine, 2nd ed. Edited by Holland JF, Frei E. Philadelphia, Lea & Febiger, 1982

Holland J, Rowland J: Emotional effects of cancer and cancer therapy. Proc XIII International Cancer Congress. Abstract No. 2069:363, 1982

Holland JC, Rowland J, Lebovits A, Rusalem R: Reactions to cancer treatment: Assessment of emotional response to adjuvant radiotherapy as a guide to planned intervention. Psychiatr Clin North Am 2:347–357, 1979

Holland JC, Hughes A, Silberfarb P, Feldman M, Perry M, Comis R, Oster M: Patients with depression in pancreatic and gastric cancer (abstract). Proc Am Soc Clin Oncol 2:127, 1983

Holland JF (ed): Cancer Medicine, 2nd ed. Philadelphia, Lea & Febiger, 1982

Holland JF, Scharlau C, Gailani S, Krant MJ, Olson KB, Horton J, Shnider BI, Lunch JJ, Owens A, Carbone PP, Colsky J, Grob D, Miller SP, Hall TC: Vincristine treatment of advanced cancer: A cooperative study of 392 cases. Cancer Res 33:1258–1264, 1973

Levine PM, Silberfarb PM, Lipowski ZJ: Mental disorders in cancer patients: A study of 100 psychiatric referrals. Cancer 42:1385–1391, 1978

Lifton RJ: Death in Life: Survivors of Hiroshima. New York, Random House, 1967

Lindemann E: Symptomatology and management of acute grief. Am J Psychiatry 101:141–148, 1944

Lipowski ZJ: Delirium: Acute Brain Failure in Man. Springfield, Ill, Charles C Thomas, 1980

Mann AM, Hutchinson JL: Manic reaction associated with procarbazine hydrochloride therapy of Hodgkin's disease. Can Med Assoc J 97:1350–1353, 1967

Massie MJ, Holland JC, Glass E: Delirium in terminally ill cancer patients. Am J Psychiatry 140:1048–1050, 1983

Massie MJ, Holland JC, Myers WPL: Psychosocial teaching of third year medical/surgical clerks in a cancer research hospital (abstract No 42). American Association for Cancer Education, 1982

Massie MJ, Gorzynski G, Mastrovito R, Theis D, Holland J: The diagnosis of depression in hospitalized patients with cancer (abstract). Proc Amer Assoc for Cancer Res and Amer Soc for Clin Oncol 20:432, 1979

Moffic HS, Paykel ES: Depression in medical inpatients. Br J Psychiatry 126:346–353, 1975

Morrow GR, Morrell C: Behavioral treatment for the anticipatory nausea and vomiting induced by cancer chemotherapy. N Engl J Med 307:1476–1480, 1982

Penman D, Gahna G, Holland JC, Morrow G, Morse I, Schmale A, Derogatis L: Patients' perception of giving informed consent for investigational chemotherapy (abstract). Proc Amer Assoc for Cancer Res and Amer Soc for Clin Oncol 21:188, 1980

Plumb MM, Holland JC: Comparative studies of psychological function in patients with advanced cancer. I. Self-reported depression symptoms. Psychosom Med 39:264–276, 1977

Posner JB: Neurological complications of systemic cancer. Med Clin North Am 55:625–646, 1971

Price RA, Jamieson PA: The central nervous system in childhood leukemia. II. Subacute leukoencephalopathy. Cancer 35:306–318, 1975

Rowland J, Glidewell O, Sibley R, Holland JC, Brecher M, Tull B, Berman A, Glicksman A, Forman E, Harris M, McSweeney J, Jones B, Black M, Cohen M, Freeman A: Effect of cranial radiation (CRT) on neurologic function in children with acute lymphocyte leukemia (ALL) (abstract). Proc Amer Soc for Clin Oncol 1:123, 1982

Sawicka J, Dawson DM, Blum R: Neurologic aspects of the treatment of cancer, in Current Neurology, vol 1. Edited by Tyler HR. Boston, Houghton Mifflin, 1977

Schilsky RL, Lewis BJ, Sherins RJ, Young RC: Gonadal dysfunction in patients receiving chemotherapy for cancer. Ann Intern Med 93:109–114, 1980

Schwab JJ, Bialow M, Brown JM, Holzer CE: Diagnosing depression in medical inpatients. Ann Intern Med 67:695–707, 1967

Silberfarb P, Holland J, Anbar D, Gahna G, Maurer H, Chahinian A, Comis R: Psychological response of patients receiving two drug regimens for lung cancer. Am J Psychiatry 140:110–111, 1983

Spiegel K, Kalb R, Pasternak GW: Analgesic activity of tricyclic antidepressants. Ann Neurol 13:462–465, 1983

Vachon MLS, Lyall WAL, Freeman SJJ: Measurement and management of stress in health professionals working with advanced cancer patients. Death Education 1:365–375, 1978

von Eschenbach AC: Sexual dysfunction following therapy for cancer of the prostate, testis and penis. Front Radiat Ther Oncol 14:42–47, 1980

Weiner H: Psychobiology and Human Disease. New York, Elsevier, 1977

Yamada K, Bremer AM, West CR, Ghoorah J, Park H, Takita A: Intra-arterial BCNU therapy in the treatment of metastatic brain tumor from lung carcinoma. Cancer 44:2000–2007, 1979

Young DF: Neurological complications of cancer chemotherapy, in Neurological Complications of Therapy: Selected Topics. Edited by Silverstein A. New York, Futura Publishing Co, 1982

Young DF, Posner JB: Nervous system toxicity of the chemotherapeutic agents, in Handbook of Clinical Neurology, vol 39. Edited by Viken PJ, Bruyn GW. Amsterdam, North-Holland Publishing Co, 1980

Zubrod CG: The clinical toxicities of L-asparaginase: In treatment of leukemia and lymphoma. Pediatrics 45:555–559, 1970

References for Chapter 17

Psychiatry and Surgery

Aberg T: Effects of open-heart surgery on intellectual functioning. Scand J Thorac Cardiovasc Surg 8(suppl)15:1–63, 1974

Abram HS: Adaptation to open-heart surgery: A psychiatric study of response to the threat of death. Am J Psychiatry 122:659–668, 1965

Abram HS, Wadlington W: Selection of patients for artificial and transplanted organs. Ann Intern Med 69:615–620, 1963

Albert H, Kornfeld DS: The threat to sign out against medical advice. Annals of Internal Medicine, 79:888–891, 1973

Andrew JM: Recovery from surgery, with and without preparatory instruction, for three coping styles. J Pers Soc Psychol 15:223–226, 1970

Appelbaum PS, Roth L: Why medical patients refuse treatment. APA Annual Meeting, New York, 1983

Auchincloss H: A surgeon views the patient's options for the treatment of carcinoma of the breast. Surg Gynecol Obstet 153:247–249, 1981

Bard M, Sutherland AM: Psychological impact of cancer and its treatment: Adaptation to radical mastectomy. Cancer 8:656–679, 1955

Barker MG: Psychiatric illness after hysterectomy. Br Med J 2:91–92, 1968

Baudry F, Wiener AD: Initiation of a psychiatric teaching program for surgeons. Am J Psychiatry 125:1192–1197, 1969

Beard BH: Fear of death and fear of life. Arch Gen Psychiatry 21:373–380, 1969

Besser RS, Van der Hock C, Jacobson AM, Flood TM, Desautels RE: Experience with penile prostheses in the treatment of impotence in diabetic men. JAMA 248:943–948, 1982

Bille DA: Teaching the patient to adapt to colorectal surgery. QRB 5:29–31, 1979

Blachly PH: Post-cardiotomy delirium. Am J Psychiatry 121:371–375, 1964

Blachly PH: Open-heart surgery: Physiological variables and mental functioning, in Psychological Aspects of Surgery. Edited by Abrams HS. Boston, Little, Brown & Co, 1967

Blachly PH, Koster F: Relation of cardiac output to postcardiotomy delirium. J Thorac Cardiovasc Surg 52:422–427, 1966

Bliss EL, Rumel WR, Branch DHH: Psychiatric complications of mitral surgery. Arch Neurol Psychiatry 74:249–252, 1955

Brown RS, Haddox V, Posada A, Rubio A: Social and psychological adjustment following pelvic exenteration. Am J Obstet Gynecol 114:162–171, 1972

Bruckburg JB, Straker N: Psychiatric consultation with the ambivalent cancer surgery candidate. Psychosomatics 23:1043–1051, 1982

Buikholder GU, Bewell ME: Amelioration of problems of partial penile amputation. J Urol 122:562–563, 1979

Capone MA, Good RS: Sex counselling for cancer patients. Contemp OB/GYN 15:131–140, 1980

Castelnuovo-Tedesco P: Organ transplant, body image, psychosis. Psychoanal Q 42:349–363, 1973

Chatham MA: The effect of family involvement on patients' manifestations of postcardiotomy psychosis. Heart Lung 7:995–999, 1978

Cheek DS: Unconscious perception of meaningful sounds during surgical anesthesia as revealed under hypnosis. Am J Clin Hypn 1:101–113, 1959

Christopherson LK, Lunde DT: Heart transplant donors and their families, in Psychiatric aspects of Organ Transplantation. Edited by Castelnuovo-Tedesco P. New York, Grune & Stratton, 1971a

Christopherson LK, Lunde DT: Selection of cardiac transplant recipients and their subsequent psycho-social adjustment. Seminars in Psychiatry 3:36–45, 1971b

Clayson D, Levine DB: Adolescent scoliosis patients. Personality patterns and effects of corrective surgery. Clin Orthop 116:99–102, 1976

Cohen F, Lazarus RS: Active coping processes, coping

dispositions, and recovery from surgery. Psychosom Med 356:375–389, 1973

Coppen A, Bishop M, Beard R, Barnard GL, Collens WP: Hysterectomy, hormones and behavior. A prospective study. Lancet 17:126–128, 1981

Crammond WA: Renal transplantation experience with recipients-donors, in Psychiatric Aspects of Organ Transplantation. Edited by Castelnuovo-Tedesco P. New York, Grune & Stratton, 1971

David DJ, Bairitt JA: Psychosocial aspects of head and neck cancer surgery. Aust NZ J Surg 47:584–589, 1977

Dempsey GM, Buchsbaum HJ, Morrison J: Psychosocial adjustment to pelvic exenteration. Gynecol Oncol 3:325–334, 1975

Deutsch H: Some psychoanalytic observations in surgery. Psychosom Med 4:105–115, 1942

Douduin T, Katz A: Emotional reactions during lumbar extradural anaesthesia. Anaesthesia 35:822–824, 1980

Druss RG, O'Connor JF, Prudden JF, Stein LO: Psychologic response to colostomy. Arch Gen Psychiatry 18:53–58, 1968

Druss RG, O'Connor JF, Stein LO: Psychologic response to colectomy. 1. Adjustment to a permanent colostomy. Arch Gen Psychiatry 20:419–424, 1969

Egbert LD, Battit GE, Welch CE, Bartlett MK: Reduction of postoperative pain by encouragement and instruction of patients. N Engl J Med 270:827–837, 1964

Edgerton MT, Kay JH: Psychological disturbances associated with open-heart surgery. Br J Psychiatry 110:433–439, 1964

Eisendrath RM: The role of grief-fear in kidney transplant rejection. Am J Psychiatry 129:381–387, 1969

Eisendrath RM: Adaptation to transplantation, in Modern Perspectives in the Psychiatric Aspects of Surgery. Edited by Howells JG: New York, Brunner/Mazel, 1976

Engel GL, Schmale AH: Psychoanalytic theory of somatic disorder. J Am Psychoanal Assoc 15:344–366, 1976

Ervin CW: Psychologic adjustment to mastectomy. Med Aspects Hum Sex 11:42–51, 1973

Eule EM: The psychological effects of mutilating surgery in children and adolescents. Psychoanal Study Child 34:527–546, 1979

Ewatt JR, Randall GC, Morris H: The phantom limb. Psychosom Med 9:118–130, 1947

Fellner CH, Marshall JR: Kidney donors: The myth of informed consent. Am J Psychiatry 126:1245–1251, 1970

Fox HM, Rizzo ND, Gifford S: Psychological observations of patients undergoing mitral surgery. Psychosom Med 16:186–208, 1954

Frank JL: The amputee war casualty in a military hospital: Observations on psychiatric management. Int J Psychiatry Med 4:1–13, 1973

Frank KA, Heller SS, Kornfeld DS, Malm JR: Long term effects of open-heart surgery on intellectual functioning. J Thorac Cardiovasc Surg 64:811–815, 1972

Frazier SH, Kolb LC: Psychiatric aspects of pain in the phantom limb. Orthop Clin North Am 1:481–495, 1970

Freyberger H: Psychosomatic aspects in self-help groups made up of medical patients. The example of the ostomy groups. Psychother Psychosom 31:114–120, 1979

Friedmann LW: The Psychological Rehabilitation of the Amputee. Springfield Ill, Charles C Thomas, 1978

Gabriel HP, Danilowicz D: Postoperative responses in the "prepared" child after cardiac surgery. Br Heart J 40:1046–1051, 1978

Gath D, Cooper P: Psychosomatic aspects of gynecological conditions: Psychiatric disorder after hysterectomy. J Psychosom Res 25:347–356, 1981

George JM, Scott DS, Turner SP, Gregg JM: The effects of psychological factors and physical trauma on recovery from oral surgery. J Behav Med 3:291–310, 1980

Gerber LA: Issues in the psychotherapy of patients with previous successful spina bifida surgery. Psychiatr Q 47:117–123, 1973

Goin JM, Goin MK: Changing the Body: Psychological Effects of Plastic Surgery. Baltimore, Williams & Wilkins Co. 1981

Gonzdilov AV, Alexandrin GP, Simono NN, Entzebrun AI, Babrovu F: The role of stress factors in the postoperative course of patients with rectal cancer. J Surg Oncol 9:517–523, 1977

Gregory JG: Impotence: The surgical approach. Surg Clin North Am 62:981–998, 1981

Gulledge AD, Gipson WT, Steiger E, Hooley R, Srp F: Home parenteral nutrition for the short bowel syndrome: Psychological issues. Gen Hosp Psychiatry 2:271–281, 1980

Guerra F: Awareness during anesthesia (ltr to ed). Can Anaesth Soc J 27:178, 1980

Hackett TP, Weisman AD: Psychiatric management of operative syndrome: 1. The therapeutic consultation and effect of noninterpretive intervention. Psychosom Med 22:267–278, 1960a

Hackett TP, Weisman AD: Psychiatric management of operative syndromes: 2. Psychodynamic factors in formulation and management. Psychosom Med 22:356–368, 1960b

Hall RGW, Stickney SK, Gardner ER, Popkin MK: Psychiatric reactions to long term intravenous hyperalimentation. Psychosomatics 22:428–443, 1981

Hayes CP, Gunnels JC: Selection of recipients and donors for renal transplantation. Arch Intern Med 123:521–530, 1969

Heller SS, Frank KA, Malm J: Psychiatric complications of open-heart surgery: A re-examination. N Engl J Med 283:1015–1020, 1970

Heller SS, Frank KA, Kornfeld DS: Psychological outcome following open-heart surgery. Arch Intern Med 134:908–914, 1974

Heller SS, Frank K, Kornfeld DS: Post-cardiotomy delirium and cardiac output. Am J Psychiatry 136:337–339, 1979

Hilgenberg JC: Intraoperative awareness during high-dose fentanyl-oxygen anesthesia. Anesthesiology 54:341–343, 1981

Holcomb GW, Jr: Surgical correction of pectus excavatum. J Pediatr Surg 12:295–302, 1977

Iacovides A, Ierodiabonou C, Bikos C, Kantarakias S: Prevention of psychiatric gynaecologic operations. Bibl Psychiatr 160:84–91, 1981

Jamison KR, Wellisch DK, Pasnau RO: Psychosocial aspects of mastectomy: 1. The woman's perspective. Am J Psychiatry 135:432–442, 1978

Jamison K, Wellisch DK, Katz RL, Pasnau RO: Phantom breast syndrome. Arch Surg 114:93–95, 1979

Janis IL: Psychological Stress: Psychoanalytic and Behavioral Studies of Surgical Patients. New York, John Wiley & Sons, 1959

Johnson JE, Leventhal H, Dobbs JM: Contributions of emotional and instrumental response processes in adaptation to surgery. J Pers Soc Psychol 20:550–64, 1971

Johnston M: Anxiety in surgical patients. Psychol Med 10:145–152, 1980

Johnston M, Carpenter L: Relationship between pre-operative anxiety and postoperative states. Psychol Med 10:361–367, 1980

Kaltreiden NB, Wallace A, Horowitz MJ: A field study of the stress response syndrome. Young women after hysterectomy. JAMA 242:1499–1503, 1979

Kaplan-DeNour A: Psychiatric aspects of renal hemodialysis, in Modern Perspectives in the Psychiatric Aspects of Surgery. Edited by Howells JG. New York, Brunner/Mazel, 1976

Keistein MD: Group rehabilitation for the vascular disease amputee. J Am Geriatr Soc 28:40–41, 1980

Kemph JP: Psychotherapy with patients receiving kidney transplant. Am J Psychiatry 124:77–83, 1969

Kemph JP, Bermann EA, Coppolillo HR: Kidney transplants and shifts in family dynamics. Am J Psychiatry 125:1485–1490, 1969

Kennedy J, Bakst J: The psychological parameter in cardiac surgery. Bull NY Acad Med 42:811–845, 1966

Kimball CP: Psychological response to the experience of open-heart surgery, I. Am J Psychiatry 126:348–359, 1969

Kindon D, Pearce T: Psychological assessment and management of the amputee, in Rehabilitation Management of Amputees. Edited by Banejie SN. Baltimore, Williams & Wilkins Co, 1982

Knorr NJ: A depressive syndrome following pelvic exenteration and colostomy. Arch Surg 94:258–260, 1967

Kornfeld DS: Psychiatric agents of patient care in the operating suite and special areas. Anesthesiology 31:106–171, 1969

Kornfeld DS, Zimberg S, Malm J: Psychiatric complications of open-heart surgery. N Engl J Med 273:287–297, 1965

Kornfeld DS, Heller SS, Frank KA, Moskowitz R: Personality and psychological factors in post-cardiotomy delirium. Arch Gen Psychiatry 31:249–253, 1974

Kornfeld DS, Heller SS, Frank KA: Delirium after coronary artery bypass surgery. J Thorac Cardiovasc Surg 76:93–96, 1978

Kornfeld DS, Heller SS, Frank KA, Wilson SN, Malm J: Psychological and behavioral responses after coronary artery bypass surgery. Circulation 66 (Suppl 3):24–28, 1982

Kraft IA: Psychiatric complications of cardiac transplantation, in Psychiatric Aspects of Organ Transplantation. Edited by Castelnuovo-Tedesco P. New York, Grune & Stratton, 1971

Krakauer H, Grauman JS, McMullan MR, and Creede CC: The recent U.S. experience in the treatment of end stage renal disease by dialysis and transplantation. N Engl J Med 308:1558–1563, 1963

Krueger JC, Hassel J, Gaggins DB, Ishimatsu T, Pablico MR, Tuttle EJ: Relationship between nurse counselling and sexual adjustment after hysterectomy. Nurs Res 28:145–150, 1979

Kupfer DJ, Detre TP, Swigar ME, Southwick WD: Adjustment of patients after hip surgery. J Am Geriatr Soc. 19:709–720, 1971

Lamendola NF, Pelligrini RV: Quality of life and coronary artery bypass surgery patients: Soc Sci Med 134:457–462, 1979

Langer EJ, Janis IL, Wolfer JA: Reduction of psychological stress in surgical patients. J Exp Soc Psychol 2:155–165, 1975

Layne OZ, Yudofsky SC: Postoperative psychosis in cardiotomy: The role of organic and psychiatric factors. N Engl J Med 283:518–520, 1970

Lazarus HR, Hagens JH: Prevention of psychosis following open-heart surgery. Am J Psychiatry 124:1190–1195, 1968

Levitan SJ, Kornfeld DS: Clinical and cost benefits of liaison psychiatry. Am J Psychiatry 138:790–793, 1981

Lindemann CA, Stetzer SL: Effects of preoperative visits by operating room nurses. Nurs Res 22:4–16, 1973

Lunde DT: Psychiatric complications of heart transplants. Am J Psychiatry 126:369–373, 1969

MacDonald NE: Patient representatives come to the operating room. AORN J 34:332–340, 1981

MacRitchie KL: Life without eating or drinking. Total parenteral nutrition outside hospital. Can Psychiatr Assoc J 23:373–379, 1978

Maguire GP, Lee EG, Bevington DJ, Kuehmann, GS: Psychiatric problems in the first year after mastectomy. Br Med J 1:963–965, 1978.

Maguire P, Tait A, Brooke M, Thomas C, Sellwood R: Effect of counselling on the psychiatric morbidity associated with mastectomy. Br Med J 281:1454–1456, 1980

Malcolm RM, Robson JR, Vanderveen TW, O'Neil, PM: Psychosocial aspects of total parenteral nutrition. Psychosomatics 21:115–125, 1980

Meerloo JAM: The fate of one's face. Psychiatr Q 30:31–43, 1956

Meikle S, Brody H, Pysh F: An investigation into the psychological effects of hysterectomy. J Nerv Ment Dis 164:36–41, 1977

Menger D, Movis T, Gates P, Sabbath J, Robey H, Plaut T, Sturgis SH: Patterns of emotional recovery after hysterectomy. Psychosom Med 19:379–387, 1951

Meyer BC: Some Considerations in the Doctor-Patient Relationship in the Practice of Surgery. Boston, Little, Brown & Co, 1967

Meyer BC, Blacher RS, Brown F: A clinical study of psychiatric and psychological aspects of mitral surgery. Psychosom Med 23:194–218, 1961

Morse RM, Litin EM: Postoperative delirium: A study of etiologic factors. Am J Psychiatry 126:388–496, 1968

Mumford E, Schlesinger HJ, Glass GU: The effects of psychological intervention on recovery from surgery and heart attack: An analysis of the literature. Am J Public Health 72:141–151, 1982

Muslin HC: On acquiring a kidney. Am J Psychiatry 127:1185–1188, 1971

Nadelson T: The psychiatrist in the surgical intensive care unit: 1. Postoperative delirium. Arch Surg 3:113–117, 1976

National Institutes of Health Consensus Development Conference Statement: Coronary artery bypass surgery: Scientific and clinical aspects. N Engl J Med 304:680–684, 1981

Noone RB, Fraxier TG, Hayward CZ, Skiles MS: Patient acceptance of immediate reconstruction following mastectomy. Plast Reconstr Surg 69:632–638, 1982

Orr WC, Stahl ML: Sleep disturbances after open-heart surgery. Am J Cardiol 39:196–201, 1977

Ouellette DL: Psychological ramifications of facial change in relation to orthodontic treatment and orthognathic surgery. J Oral Surg 36:787–790, 1978

Parkes CM: Factors determining the persistence of phantom pain in the amputee. J Psychosom Res 17:97–108, 1973

Parkes CM, Napier GG: Psychiatric sequelae of amputation. Br J Psychiatry Special Publication No. 9, 440–446, 1975.

Penn I, Bunch D, Olenik D, Abouna G: Psychiatric experience with patients receiving renal and hepatic transplants, in Psychiatric Aspects of Organ Transplantation. Edited by Castelnuovo-Tedesco P. New York, Grune & Stratton, 1971

Perl M, Peterson LG, Dutrick SL, Benson, DM: Psychiatric effects of long term hyperalimentation. Psychosomatics 22:1047–1063, 1981

Reading AE: Psychological preparation for surgery: Patient recall of information. J Psychosom Res 25:57–63, 1981

Renneker R, Cutler M: Psychological problems of adjustment to cancer of the breast. JAMA 148:833–838, 1952

Robinson J: Patient consent given but forgotten. Med World News 17:26–28, 1976

Rockwell DA, Pepitone-Rockwell F: The emotional impact of surgery and the value of informed consent. Med Clin North Am 63:1341–1351, 1979

Roeske NA: The emotional response to hysterectomy. Psychiatr Opin 15:11–20, 1978

Rogers MP, Liang MIT, Poss R, Cullen K: Adverse psychological sequelae associated with total joint replacement surgery. Gen Hosp Psychiatry 4:155–158, 1982

Sanger CK, Reznikoff M: A comparison of the psychological effects of breast-saving procedures with the modified radical mastectomy. Cancer 48:2341–2346, 1981

Schweitzer I, Rosenbaum M: Psychiatric aspects of replantation surgery. Gen Hosp Psychiatry 4:271–281, 1982

Silberfarb PM, Maurer LH, Crouthamel CS: Psychosocial aspects of neoplastic disease: 1. Functional status of breast cancer patients during different treatment regimens. Am J Psychiatry 137:450–456, 1980

Sime M: Relationship of pre-operative fear, type of coping, and information received about surgery to recovery from surgery. J Pers Soc Psychol 34:716–724, 1976

Simmons RG, Hickey K, Kjellstrand CM, Simmons Rl: Family tension in the search for kidney donors. JAMA 215:909–912, 1971

Skoug G: The course of acute confusional states. Acta Psychiatr Scand (Suppl) 203:29–32, 1968

Stevens LA, McGrath MH, Druss RG, Kister SJ, Gump PE, Forde KD: The psychological impact of immediate breast reconstruction for women with early breast cancer. Paper presented at the Annual Meeting of the American Society for Aesthetic Plastic Surgery, April 1983

Sutherland AM, Orbach CE, Dyk RB, Bard M: The psychological impact of cancer surgery: 1. Adaptation to dry colostomy. Preliminary report and summary findings. Cancer 5:857–877, 1952

Sveinsson IS: Postoperative psychosis after surgery. J Thorac Cardiovasc Surg 70:717–726, 1975

Titchener JL, Zwerling I, Gottschalk LA, Levine M, Culbertson W, Cohen S, Silver H: Psychosis in surgical patients. Surg Gynecol Obstet 102:59–67, 1956

Titchener JL, Zwerling I, Gottschalk LA, Levine M, Silber H, Gowett A, Cohen S, Culberson W: Consequences of surgical illness and treatment. Arch Neurol Psychiatry 77:623–637, 1957

Tufo HM, Ostfeld AM: A prospective study of open-heart surgery. Psychosom Med 30:552–553, 1968

Turgay A: Emotional aspects of arm or leg amputations in children. American Psychiatric Association Annual Meeting, 1983

Turpin TJ, Heath DS: The link between hysterectomy and depression. Am J Psychiatry 24:247–252, 1979

Viederman M: The search for meaning in renal transplant rejection. Psychiatry 37:283–290, 1974

Viederman M: Psychogenic factors in kidney transplant rejection: A case study. Am J Psychiatry 132:957–959, 1975

Visintainer MA, Wolfer JA: Psychological preparation for surgery with pediatric patients: The effects on childrens' and parents' stress responses and adjustment. Pediatrics 56:187–202, 1975

Wellisch DK, Jamison KR, Pasnau RO: Psychosocial aspects of mastectomy. 2. The man's perspective. Am J. Psychiatry 135:543–546, 1978

West DW: Social adaptation patterns among cancer patients with facial disfigurements resulting from surgery. Arch Phys Med Rehabil 58:673–679, 1977

Williams JGL, Jones JR: Psychophysiological responses to anesthesia and operation. JAMA 203:415–420, 1969

Williams JGL, Jones JR, Williams B: The chemical control of preoperative anxiety. Psychophysiology 12:46–49, 1975a

Williams JGL, Jones JR, Workhave MN, Williams B: The psychological control of preoperative anxiety. Psychophysiology 12:50–54, 1975b

Wilson JF: Behavioral preparation for surgery: Benefit or harm. J Behav Med 4:79–102, 1981

Wiltse LL: Psychological testing in predicting the success of low back surgery. Orthop Clin North Am 6:317–318, 1975

Wiltse L, Rochio P: Preoperative tests as predictors of success of chemonucleolysis. J Bone Joint Surg 57A:478–483, 1975

Winick L, Robbins GF: Physical and psychologic readjustment after mastectomy: An evaluation of Memorial Hospital's PMRG program. Cancer 39:478–486, 1977

Winkelstein C, Blacker RS, Weger B: Psychiatric observations on surgical patients in the recovery room. NY State J Med 65:865–870, 1965

Wirschung M, Druner HU, Hermann G: Results of psychosocial adjustment to long term colostomy. Psychother Psychosom 26:245–256, 1975

Wise A, Jackson DW, Rochio P: Preoperative psychologic testing as a predictor of success in knee surgery. A preliminary report. Am J Sports Med 7:287–292, 1979

Wolfer JA, Davis CE: Assessment of surgical patient's preoperative emotional condition and postoperative recovery. Nurs Res 19:402–414, 1970

Worden JW, Weisman AD: The fallacy in postmastectomy depression. Am J Med Sci 273:169–175, 1977

Wright MR: Self-perception of the elective surgeon and some patient perception correlates. Arch Otolaryngol 106:460–465, 1980

Wright MR: The elective surgeon's personality and role confusion. Otolaryngol Head Neck Surg 89:776–779, 1981

Zaks MS: Disturbances in psychological functions and neuropsychiatric complications in heart surgery, in Cardiology: An Encyclopedia of the Cardiovascular System, vol 3. Edited by Luisada AA. New York, McGraw-Hill, 1958.

IV

Alcohol Abuse and Dependence

Alcohol Abuse and Dependence

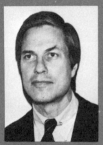

George E. Vaillant, M.D.,
Preceptor

Raymond Sobel Professor
   of Psychiatry
Dartmouth Medical School

Authors for Part IV

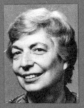

Lee N. Robins, Ph.D.
Professor of Sociology
   and Psychiatry
Washington University
   of Saint Louis

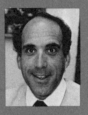

Marc A. Schuckit, M.D.
Professor of Psychiatry
University of California
   at San Diego
Medical School
Director of Alcohol
   Treatment Program
Veterans Administration
   Medical Center

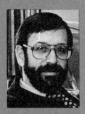

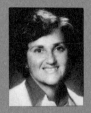

Peter E. Nathan, Ph.D.

Henry and Anna Starr
   Professor of Psychology
Director, Center of Alcohol Studies
Rutgers, the State University

Sheila B. Blume, M.D.

Medical Director
National Council on Alcoholism

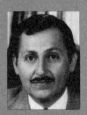

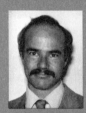

Ernest P. Noble, Ph.D., M.D.

Pike Professor of Alcohol Studies
Director, Alcohol Research Center
University of California
   at Los Angeles

Dean Gerstein, Ph.D.

Study Director
Committee on Substance Abuse
   and Habitual Behavior
National Research Council
National Academy of Sciences

	Page
Introduction to Part Four *George E. Vaillant, M.D.*	*299*
Chapter 18 The Diagnosis of Alcoholism After DSM-III *Lee N. Robins, Ph.D.*	*301*
Overview of DSM-III Alcohol-Related Diagnoses	301
Diagnostic Scheme for Alcohol Abuse and Alcohol Dependence	302
Criteria for Alcohol Abuse and Alcohol Dependence	303
The Construction and Current Status of the Criteria	307
Chapter 19 The Course of Alcoholism and Lessons for Treatment *George E. Vaillant, M.D.*	*311*
Introduction	311
Illusions About Etiology	311
Illusions About Incurability	313
Is Alcoholism a Progressive Disease?	314
Treatment Goals	317
Natural Healing Processes	318
Chapter 20 Genetic and Biochemical Factors in the Etiology of Alcoholism *Marc A. Schuckit, M.D.*	*320*
Introduction	320
Methodological Considerations	321
Possible Biological Markers	323
Conclusions	327
Chapter 21 Contributions of Learning Theory to the Diagnosis and Treatment of Alcoholism *Peter E. Nathan, Ph.D.*	*328*
Historical Perspectives	328
Behavioral Assessment of Alcoholism	329
Behavioral Treatment of Alcoholism	331
Future Trends	337

Chapter 22   338
Psychotherapy in the Treatment of Alcoholism
    Sheila B. Blume, M.D.
Introduction   338
Conceptual Framework for Psychotherapy
    with Alcoholic Patients   339
Psychotherapeutic Technique   343
Conclusion   346

Chapter 23   346
Pharmacotherapy in the Detoxification
    and Treatment of Alcoholism
    Ernest P. Noble, Ph.D., M.D.
Introduction   346
Amethystic Agents   347
The Pharmacotherapy of the
    Alcohol Withdrawal Reaction   351
Drugs in the Long-Term Treatment
    of Alcoholism   356

Chapter 24   359
Alcohol Policy: Preventive Options
    Dean Gerstein, Ph.D.
Governing Ideas About Alcohol   359
Types of Prevention Policies   362
Conclusion   370

References for Part Four   371

Introduction
by George E. Vaillant, M.D.

Psychiatrists need to know a great deal more about alcoholism and its treatment than they do. In recent years, many forces have discouraged psychiatrists from taking great interest in alcoholism. These forces have compounded the denial of the illness, a tendency that afflicts the medical profession as a whole. On the one hand, psychiatrists have been told that there is nothing to be done. Psychotherapy by itself does not cure alcoholism; tranquilizers are contraindicated; and hospitalization for alcoholism is no more effective than brief outpatient counseling (Orford and Edwards, 1977) or just letting the natural history of the disorder run its course (Vaillant, 1983). On the other hand, psychiatrists have been told that much can be done to help alcoholics, but that they as a profession need not be concerned. They are told that the illness is really best seen as a medical disorder and that detoxification should occur on medical, not psychological, units. Alternatively, psychiatrists are advised that the disease is best treated by self-help groups like Alcoholics Anonymous (AA) or by paraprofessionals (Armor et al., 1978). Finally, in the last decade, work by the Sobells (1976) and others has suggested that alcoholism, like enuresis and simple phobias, should best be turned over to behavioral psychologists.

Such denial serves neither alcoholics nor psychiatrists well. In psychiatry, alcoholism is simply too pervasive for us to sit on our hands. A recent unpublished survey from the outpatient department of an active community mental health center revealed that 40 percent of the patients abused alcohol, but only 2 percent carried a diagnosis of alcoholism. A similar survey of a child guidance clinic revealed that 50 percent of the children referred to the clinic had an alcohol-abusing parent (M. Bennett, personal communication, 1983). A study of so-called borderline patients, surely a major focus of psychiatric effort, revealed that up to 85 percent of such patients have abused drugs or alcohol (Perry, 1983). Thus, providing psychiatrists with an update on the treatment of alcoholism is not an idle exercise.

But if psychiatry cannot ignore alcoholism, what is the basic knowledge that psychiatrists need in order to help? It is in the spirit of responding to this question that this Part has been designed. Treatment is the emphasis. Therefore, recent research on etiology, epidemiology, and pathology is subordinated to advances in diagnosis and prognosis and the treatment modalities with which every psychiatrist should be familiar.

First, Dr. Lee N. Robins provides the history and the rationale behind the DSM-III diagnostic system for alcoholism, with an emphasis on Alcohol Abuse and Alcohol Dependence. There is increasing evidence (Vaillant et al., 1982) that the DSM-III criteria for alcoholism may be about as good as we are likely to receive.

Second, the Preceptor presents the findings of recent prospective studies regarding prognosis. The chapter shows how prospective study can dispel illusions and elucidate the responses to some fundamental questions. What variables are important? What variables affect outcome? What might appropriate treatment choices be?

Third, Dr. Marc A. Schuckit reviews the evidence for the risk of alcoholism being seriously influenced by genetic factors. In part, effective treatment response rests upon psychiatrists having a realistic model of causation. Despite the dramatic familial nature of alcoholism, its etiology rests less on a model of identification with the aggressor and of distorted intrafamilial dynamics than previously thought. Instead, since alcoholism probably runs in families for predominantly genetic reasons, then family therapy in alcoholism should take the form that it would in diabetes or Huntington's chorea. Family therapy should aim to mitigate the ravages of the disease on family dynamics rather than to hold family dynamics responsible for the ravages of the disease.

Fourth, Dr. Peter E. Nathan helps psychiatrists appreciate the psychological underpinnings of alcohol abuse and its treatment. If psychopathology does not cause alcoholism and if psychotherapy alone does not cure it, which etiologic psychological factors should psychiatry address? To what extent is behavioral modification the answer? Should we believe the Sobells or Mary Pendery?

In the fifth and sixth chapters, Drs. Sheila B. Blume and Ernest P. Noble examine what psychiatrists can do directly. Dr. Blume reviews the place of psychotherapy in the overall treatment of alcoholism and offers practical guidance on technique. Dr. Noble discusses the pharmacotherapy of alcoholism, including those agents which may be helpful in sobering, in managing withdrawal reactions, in treating psychological symptoms, and in long-term treatment.

The final chapter, by Dr. Dean Gerstein, puts into realistic perspective the economic, political, and social risk factors that we might manipulate in order to achieve primary prevention. For example, Dr. Gerstein points out the catch-22 dilemma of American society. We forbid children in late adolescence to drink because they lack the judgment to do it wisely, and then we allow them to drink in unlimited fashion at age 20 without ever having given them cultural instruction. Obviously, many Mediterranean countries, which have no minimum drinking ages, handle the instruction of children in intelligent drinking decisions with more wisdom and with less morbidity.

Some readers may wonder why this Part on treatment has no chapter on AA and its companion organization for family members, Al-Anon. In the first place, the knowledge that these organizations are important for the treatment of alcoholism is not new, so there is no need to review them in an update. Second, in the Preceptor's experience, one can *tell* neither physicians nor patients about AA. They must be *shown*. Thus, it is the Preceptor's sincere hope that any clinician reading this update who has not personally attended AA and Al-Anon meetings will rectify that educational deficiency as soon as possible. As with foreign travel, only experience, not guidebooks, will dispel prejudice and bias toward alternative ways of life. The conflicting ideologies of AA and dynamic psychiatry can only be bridged by each one "walking a mile in the other's moccasins."

Finally, the reader is reminded that alcoholism in the United States costs the nation more money than all cancers and all respiratory illnesses combined (Institute of Medicine, 1980). Alcoholism certainly causes more depression, more familial misery, and more psychosocial invalidism than any other single psychiatric disorder, including schizophrenia and bipolar affective disorder. Psychiatrists need to become better educated about alcoholism than they are at the present time.

Chapter 18

The Diagnosis of Alcoholism After DSM-III[+]
by Lee N. Robins, Ph.D.

OVERVIEW OF DSM-III ALCOHOL-RELATED DIAGNOSES

Diagnoses related to alcohol use or abuse appear in two sections of the third edition of the *Diagnostic and Statistical Manual of Mental Disorders* (DSM-III), Organic Mental Disorders and Substance Use Disorders (American Psychiatric Association, 1980). Under Organic Mental Disorders, as Table 1 shows, are seven diagnoses attributed to the use of alcohol: Alcohol Intoxication, Alcohol Idiosyncratic Intoxication, Alcohol Withdrawal, Alcohol Withdrawal Delirium, Alcohol Hallucinosis, Alcohol Amnestic Disorder, and Dementia Associated with Alcoholism. The first two diagnoses do not imply either chronic or prolonged alcohol intake. The other five, however, occur only after excessive alcohol consumption over some period of time. The diagnoses under Substance Use
· Disorders are Alcohol Abuse and Alcohol Dependence. This terminology was used instead of using the terms probable alcoholism and definite alcoholism in order to emphasize that alcohol is a drug and in order

Table 1. Diagnoses Related to Alcohol in DSM-III

Alcohol Organic Mental Disorders
   303.00 Alcohol Intoxication
   291.40 Alcohol Idiosyncratic Intoxication
   291.80 Alcohol Withdrawal
   291.00 Alcohol Withdrawal Delirium
   291.30 Alcohol Hallucinosis
   291.10 Alcohol Amnestic Disorder
   291.2x Dementia Associated with Alcoholism

Substance Use Disorders
   305.0x Alcohol Abuse
   303.9x Alcohol Dependence

Source: American Psychiatric Association (1980).

[+]This work is supported by Grants No. DA 00013, No. AA 03852, and MH 33883 from the United States Public Health Service. The chapter is adapted from: Robins LN: The diagnosis of alcoholism after DSM-III, in Research Monographs #5, Evaluation of the Alcoholic: Implications for Research, Theory and Treatment. Edited by Meyer RE and Babor TF. Washington DC, Government Printing Office, 20402, 1981.

to describe the disorders associated with its excessive use in terms similar to those used for disorders associated with other drugs. Alcohol Dependence corresponds to what used to be called alcoholism, and Alcohol Abuse corresponds to what used to be called probable alcoholism.

This chapter concentrates on the diagnoses classified under Substance Use Disorders. It explains how to make a diagnosis according to DSM-III, how the DSM-III criteria were developed, and what problems remain in the diagnosis of alcohol abuse and dependence. Finally, the chapter examines the accuracy and consistency of alcohol diagnoses compared with other psychiatric diagnoses.

DIAGNOSTIC SCHEME FOR ALCOHOL ABUSE AND ALCOHOL DEPENDENCE

The DSM-III descriptions of alcohol abuse and dependence follow the manual's general pattern for other diagnoses. First, each diagnosis is assigned a number corresponding to the number of the syndrome in ICD-9, so that the two documents will be compatible. Next, each diagnosis is assigned to Axis I or Axis II. Alcohol Abuse and Alcohol Dependence fall on Axis I. Although some diagnostic combinations are not allowed on Axis I, no other diagnoses on Axis I preclude the diagnosis of Alcohol Abuse or Alcohol Dependence.

The DSM-III text for Substance Use Disorders first describes symptoms, subclassifications, associated features, age of onset, complications, predisposing factors, prevalence, sex ratio, and differential diagnosis of Substance Use Disorders as a whole. Then the text for the alcohol disorders describes the course, family patterns, and diagnostic criteria specific to Alcohol Dependence and Alcohol Abuse. This chapter focuses on the specific criteria.

Throughout DSM-III, diagnostic criteria are listed as groups of symptoms, and each group is designated by a capital letter. To receive a positive diagnosis, an individual must present at least one symptom from each lettered group. Table 2 shows the titles under which alcohol symptoms are grouped. For Alcohol Abuse, group A includes symptoms of a pattern of pathological alcohol use, B includes symptoms of impairment in social or occupational functioning due to alcohol use, and C contains the single criterion of duration for at least one month. (The C criterion thus distinguishes Alcohol Abuse from Alcohol Intoxication, which can arise from a single drinking bout, but which can also impair social and occupational function.)

Table 2.   DSM-III Criteria for the Diagnoses of Alcohol Abuse and Alcohol Dependence

---

Alcohol Abuse
   A. Pattern of pathological alcohol use . . .
   B. Impairment in social or occupational functioning due to alcohol use . . .
   C. Duration of disturbance at least 1 month

Alcohol Dependence
   A. Either a pattern of pathological use or impairment in social or occupational functioning due to alcohol use . . .
   B. Either tolerance or withdrawal . . .

Source: American Psychiatric Association (1980).

For Alcohol Dependence, group A combines the criteria from groups A and B for Alcohol Abuse, and group B here is either tolerance or withdrawal. Thus, for Alcohol Dependence, one must have either tolerance or withdrawal and in addition have *either* a pattern of pathological alcohol use *or* impairment of social or occupational function. To be considered dependent, one need not have both a pathological pattern of use and social or occupational impairment.

CRITERIA FOR ALCOHOL ABUSE AND ALCOHOL DEPENDENCE

Origins

The DSM-III diagnostic system grew out of the RDC (Spitzer et al., 1975), which in turn grew out of the Feighner criteria (Feighner et al., 1972). The RDC were originally developed for the ongoing Collaborative Depression Study of the National Institute of Mental Health (NIMH). During the study's planning years, Eli Robins and Robert Spitzer were members of the discussion group. Dr. Spitzer had for a long time been interested in systematic diagnostic methods and while he was participating in the United States–United Kingdom study of depression and schizophrenia, he had developed a systematic interview known as the Psychiatric Status Schedule (Spitzer et al., 1970). As the discussion group considered what instruments to use in the collaborative study, Dr. Spitzer became enthusiastic about the Feighner criteria. He, Jean Endicott, and Eli Robins then worked together to modify the Feighner criteria, and their revision was called the Research Diagnostic Criteria, or RDC (1975).

A number of years ago, Dr. Spitzer was asked to lead the task force to create DSM-III. His work with the RDC inspired him to try to give DSM-III the same kind of rigor as RDC, so that diagnoses across medical centers would be more comparable than they had previously been. Not surprisingly, he sought help from some of the Washington University group who had been responsible for the Feighner criteria. The author served on the substance abuse panel, which had as one of its jobs writing the section on alcohol. Other members of that group were Drs. Henry Rosett, Robert Morse, Sheldon Zimberg, and Milton Gross, who had in 1975 worked with a World Health Organization (WHO) steering group on alcoholism led by Griffith Edwards.

Tables 3 through 6 show the extent to which DSM-III evolved from the RDC and the Feighner criteria. From left to right, the tables display the DSM-III criteria, the comparable criteria as they appeared in the RDC, and the same items in the Feighner criteria. A number of new symptoms appear in DSM-III, representing input from many people.

Criteria by Symptom Groups

PATHOLOGICAL PATTERNS OF USE One symptom unique in the DSM-III criteria for a pathological pattern of use is the daily need for alcohol in order to function adequately (see Table 3). This particular item has been the subject of considerable discussion because of the vagueness of the term *adequate functioning.* Some researchers have been concerned that such a vague term might lead to including individuals who have functioned perfectly well all day without alcohol and who will function well the next day, but who are upset if they cannot have their

Table 3. Symptoms of a Pattern of Pathological Use

DSM-III	RDC	Feighner
Need for daily use for adequate functioning	———	———
Inability to cut down or stop	Admits often can't stop	Not able to stop
———	*Says he or she drinks too much*	*Thinks he or she drinks too much*
Repeated efforts to control by "going on the wagon" or restriction to certain times of day	———	Allowing self to drink . . . only after 5 P.M., only on weekends, *only with others*
Binges (at least two days) Drinks more than one fifth per day	*Three* occasions of *three* days drinking more than one fifth per day	Binges—two days *with default of obligations*
Blackouts	*Frequent* blackouts	Blackouts
Drinking exacerbates serious physical disorder	———	———
Drinks nonbeverage alcohol	———	Nonbeverage alcohol

Notes: Italicized phrases within the table are not specifically covered in DSM-III.
A dash (———) means a symptom in another system is not included in the one under which the dash is shown.

daily drink before dinner. The difficulty here is in distinguishing between signs of pathology and an individual's desire to preserve pleasant habits.

All three systems refer to a person's inability to control or stop drinking. DSM-III, however, omits the person's own opinion that he or she drinks too much, which in fact is the most common symptom found among alcoholics. Only DSM-III includes a person's efforts to control drinking by "going on the wagon." Restricting drinking to certain times of day or week is found in both DSM-III and the Feighner criteria; Feighner also includes a person's efforts to control drinking by having rules against drinking alone.

Binge drinking appears in all three systems, although the binge must be of somewhat longer duration in RDC than in the other two. The RDC requirement that the binge drinker consume more than one fifth a day guarantees that the individual will be intoxicated during these binges. DSM-III also uses drinking more than a fifth a day as an indicator of pathological drinking, but the quantity consumed need not be associated with a binge. Thus, DSM-III does not exclude people who drink a great deal every day and whose consumption varies little from day to day. Blackouts are accepted in all three systems as a sign of pathological drinking.

DSM-III also includes drinking that exacerbates a serious physical disorder. This criterion was added to include persons whose drinking would not be pathological if they were healthy, but who should not drink at all because of their physical state. Their drinking is pathological for them, even though their consumption patterns are well within the social norms of the group in which they live. The difficulty here is in defining the

Table 4. Symptoms of Impairment in Social or Occupational Functioning

DSM-III	RDC	Feighner
Violence while intoxicated	Physical violence	Fighting
Absence from work	Missed work, *impaired job performance, unable to take care of household responsibilities*	*Trouble at* work
Loss of job	Job loss	———
Arrest for intoxicated behavior	Picked up by police due to behavior	Arrests for drinking
Traffic accidents while intoxicated	Traffic difficulties due to drinking, *reckless driving*, accidents, *speeding*	Traffic *difficulties*
Arguments or difficulties with family or friends	Others complain	Others object
	Frequent difficulties with family members, friends, or *associates*	Family objects Lost friends
	Divorce or separation where drinking is primary reason	

Notes: Italicized phrases within the table are not specifically covered in DSM-III.
A dash (———) means a DSM-III criterion does not appear in RDC or Feighner.

severity of the physical illness. Clearly, many people still drink who would like to lose weight, even though alcohol gives them excess calories. Weight problems, however, are generally not classified as serious medical disorders and would not cause individuals to be included here.

IMPAIRMENT OF SOCIAL OR OCCUPATIONAL FUNCTIONING Table 4 shows the indicators of impaired social and occupational functioning. Alcohol-related violence appears in all three systems, although it is more broadly defined in the RDC and DSM-III than in the Feighner criteria. Job loss and absence from work because of drinking are the only occupational impairments listed in DSM-III; RDC and Feighner define work troubles more generally. Arrests for intoxication are also listed in all three systems, as are traffic accidents while intoxicated; again, both RDC and Feighner include broader definitions of traffic difficulties. Interpersonal difficulties are mentioned in all three systems. DSM-III globally describes these as difficulties with family and friends, while RDC generally includes more detail. Only Feighner includes losing friends because of drinking. Losing friends is actually a rare occurrence, because people tend to choose friends with drinking patterns similar to their own.

TOLERANCE AND WITHDRAWAL Table 5 shows the indicators of tolerance and withdrawal. Tolerance does not appear in the RDC or the Feighner criteria at all, but was added to Alcohol Dependence in DSM-III so that alcohol problems could be measured comparably to problems with other drugs.

Table 5. Symptoms of Withdrawal or Tolerance to Alcohol

DSM-III	RDC	Feighner
Tolerance		
Need for increased amounts to achieve desired effect or diminished effect with same amount	_____	_____
Withdrawal		
Morning "shakes" and malaise after cessation or reduction (relieved by drinking)	Tremors Drinking before breakfast	Tremulousness Drinking before breakfast

Determining personal tolerance to alcohol is something of a problem. Even inexperienced drinkers vary enormously in the amounts they can drink. Clearly, people do develop tolerance to alcohol (alcoholics regularly drink amounts no inexperienced drinker can), but it is hard to obtain evidence of their tolerance. You can ask alcoholics whether they have had to increase their intake to get a desired effect or whether they have experienced a diminished effect from the same intake. But by the time alcoholics see a physician to discuss drinking, most have been tolerant at about the same level for many years. They may not remember how much less they used to drink to achieve the same effect.

DSM-III restricts evidence of withdrawal to shakes and malaise re-

Table 6. Medical Complications of Dependence as Criteria

DSM-III	RDC	Feighner
NOT USED AS CRITERIA	USED AS CRITERIA	USED AS CRITERIA
Hepatitis, cirrhosis	Cirrhosis	Cirrhosis
Peripheral neuropathy	Polyneuropathy	Polyneuropathy
Gastritis	_____	Gastritis
Alcohol Withdrawal Delirium	DTs	Delirium
Alcohol Hallucinosis	Hallucinations	Hallucinations
Alcohol Amnestic Syndrome	Korsakoff's psychosis	Korsakoff's psychosis
Dementia Associated with Alcoholism	_____	_____
Other Disorders		
Neurological	Withdrawal seizures	Convulsions
_____	_____	*Myopathy*
_____	_____	Pancreatitis

lieved by drinking. These also appear in the RDC and the Feighner criteria as tremors or tremulousness and drinking before breakfast.

MEDICAL COMPLICATIONS   Medical complications of dependence are used as criteria in the RDC and Feighner systems, but not in DSM-III (see Table 6). In DSM-III they are discussed in the text preceding the diagnostic criteria. They are omitted as diagnostic criteria for Alcohol Dependence or Abuse no doubt because of their separate enumeration under Organic Mental Disorders and Brain Syndromes, and because they could be classified in Axis III.

Pancreatitis and myopathy appear in the Feighner criteria, but not in DSM-III or the RDC. The author's experience suggests that this omission is wise. The records of medical and surgical patients with diagnoses of pancreatitis in one hospital study showed no elevated rate of problem drinking in their histories. Myopathy was too rare a disease to be subjected to this kind of analysis.

THE CONSTRUCTION AND CURRENT STATUS OF THE CRITERIA

History

The history of the DSM-III criteria may explain some of the differences between DSM-III and the systems from which it originated. The first draft of the DSM-III section on alcohol abuse and dependence was written in 1975. There was little criticism of the specific criteria then, but reviewers did argue over the natural history of the disorder.

Some reviewers said that alcoholics tend to have early onset and a history of antisocial behavior. Some treated only private patients and thought that alcoholism tended to be of much later onset and to occur frequently in people of middle-class origins. These reviewers did not believe that alcoholism was associated with antisocial personality. Data from the literature were produced to convince them that their patients were somewhat atypical.

In 1976, Dr. Frank Seixas reviewed the proposed criteria. He asked that the National Council on Alcoholism definition be used instead of the one in the draft and objected to DSM-III's dropping the word alcoholism. The term alcoholism now does appear, but only in the statement, "Alcohol dependence has also been called alcoholism," and in the title of one of the alcohol-related Organic Mental Disorders, Dementia Associated with Alcoholism. Seixas particularly wanted to see psychological criteria omitted from the criteria for Alcohol Dependence and to have them discussed only under Alcohol Abuse. Psychological dependence, disguised by the terminology, pathological use, is still part of the group A criteria for Alcohol Dependence, however.

The DSM-III task force resisted adopting the NCA definition in part because it implied that any drinking at all after the occurrence of alcohol problems is associated with progression of the disorder. The task force felt that the NCA statement would be better if limited to *heavy* drinking. NCA's viewpoint on the factors contributing to progression of the disorder has figured into its battle against the Rand study findings (Armor et al., 1978). The DSM-III panel decided not to include prognosis in the criteria. In the first place, the criteria for a diagnosis should be applicable early in the course of an illness, before the prognosis is known. Second, there is considerable evidence that at least a few persons who have been dependent on alcohol eventually drink moderately without problems, although the number who can do so is still very much in dispute. Finally, if one were to include prognosis in the criteria for a diagnosis, the criteria would have to be changed as improvement in treatment brought about changes in prognosis.

In 1976, the criterion of one month's duration was adopted. Initially, it referred to one month's continuous or episodic use, because those working on early drafts of DSM-III were still considering using the same criteria for licit and illicit drugs. Use of a drug for a least one month was intended to eliminate the person who was only an experimenter. But this criterion did not prove very useful when related to alcohol use. Almost everyone who drinks at all has used alcohol episodically for more than one month. Thus, the criterion was changed to make the month's duration refer to "duration of disturbance."

At the same time that DSM-III was being developed, the author's research group was devising an interview schedule for making DSM-III diagnoses in the general population (Robins et al., 1979). While writing computer programs to go with the draft DSM-III criteria, the group noticed that while the criteria for Alcohol Dependence required tolerance or withdrawal and social complications, they did not initially mention pathological drinking. Therefore, if someone were tolerant, had withdrawal symptoms, and *said* that drinking could not be controlled, that person would still not have qualified as dependent on alcohol. The panel considered changing the criteria by dropping social complications as a requirement. Then, however, a person could have been scored as positive for dependence if the only symptom was tolerance. Since tolerance is probably an invariable consequence of considerable experience with alcohol, a large proportion of the population would have been diagnosable as dependent, making the diagnosis trivial. Finally, the panel decided on the current criteria for Alcohol Dependence. Tolerance alone is not enough; there must be at least some evidence of either pathological drinking or social problems. This vignette illustrates the difficulty of writing criteria. One has to consider both the maximum case that could be missed and the minimum case that could be included and then strike some compromise between the two.

Remaining Problems

The DSM-III criteria for Alcohol Dependence and Alcohol Abuse represent the input of a great many people trying to produce a system that reasonably reflects both research and clinical experience. But many problems remain in the diagnosis of alcohol-related disorders. One that frequently comes up stems from the WHO idea that an alcohol disorder represents a way of drinking that is not acceptable in one's own subculture. The problem arises here in trying to define exactly what the norms are for a subculture. Another issue is whether the norms of a subculture are necessarily compatible with good functioning. In the subcultures of some fraternity houses or some Indian reservations, for example, the drinking norms are incompatible with optimal functioning.

Another difficulty, and one that pertains to all drug disorders, is how to decide when the intake of a drug is responsible for the behavioral problems. Arrests, traffic accidents, suicide, or death for unexplained reasons may or may not be the result of drug consumption. People who tend to have high arrest rates, high suicide rates, and high rates of impulsive behavior also tend to use drugs and alcohol heavily. Thus, the drug or alcohol use and the event may both be caused by some preexisting factors.

Reliability and Scalability

Although problems remain in diagnosing alcohol abuse and dependence, it would be a mistake to be pessimistic about the potential research and clinical value of the DSM-III criteria. While the DSM-III criteria themselves are too new to have had their efficacy fully examined, the RDC and the Feighner criteria from which they grew have been studied extensively.

The author's research group performed a test-retest study of the reliability of all the Feighner diagnoses in 99 inpatients (Helzer et al., 1981). All patients had the same interview on two successive days, with two psychiatrists, with two lay interviewers, or with one psychiatrist and one lay interviewer. Alcoholism, as it was called in the Feighner diagnosis, had the highest reliability of any diagnosis tested (with a kappa of .77 out of a possible 1.00). In comparison, depression had a value of .58, phobia a value of .53, and mania a value of .52. These results show that psychiatrists agree with each other when they diagnose alcoholism and that lay interviewers can make the same diagnosis with considerable accuracy if they use the kinds of criteria listed in DSM-III. These findings were corroborated in a test of DSM-III criteria as operationalized by the NIMH Diagnostic Interview Schedule (DIS). When a largely clinical sample with diverse diagnoses was independently given this structured interview by lay interviewers and psychiatrists, the kappa for alcohol abuse or dependence was .86, sensitivity was 86 percent, and specificity was 98 percent (Robins et al., 1981). These results again compared very favorably with those for other diagnoses. Kappas for the DSM-III alcohol diagnoses were very similar to those for Feighner and RDC (both .85); sensitivity of the DSM-III diagnosis by the DIS was not quite as good (Feighner and RDC were 90 percent), while its specificity was slightly better (Feighner and RDC were both 95 percent). Thus, the DSM-III diagnosis of alcoholism appears to share the high reliability of its parent systems.

Regarding scalability, in another study the author's group found that the symptoms typically used to diagnose alcoholism tend to form a Guttman-type scale in which the rarer symptoms are those that require the longest period of drinking (Robins et al., 1977). The results shown in Table 7 come from a study of white and black men aged 45 to 64, who were patients in a St. Louis public hospital and members of the Teamsters Union. The study focused on those who admitted to having been heavy drinkers (having had at least seven drinks on one occasion at least once a week for some period). Heavy drinkers were asked which alcohol symptoms they had had and over how many years they had been heavy drinkers. The more frequent the alcohol symptoms in this sample, the shorter the average history of heavy drinking; the rarer the

Table 7. Symptoms and Duration of Heavy Drinking in Men Aged 45 to 64

Symptom	Percentage with this Symptom	Median Years of Heavy Drinking with this Symptom
DTs	7	30
Hospitalization for drinking problem	15	27
Job loss because of drinking	16	26
Drinking led to arrest	19	26
Trouble on job from drinking	21	25
Benders (more than two days without sobering up)	25	22
Trouble with wife over drinking	28	22
Family objected to drinking	38	21
Felt guilty about drinking	41	20
Concerned about drinking too much	53	17

symptoms, the longer the average history. Men with delirium tremens, the rarest symptom, averaged 30 years of heavy drinking, while men concerned about drinking too much, which was the most common symptom, had been heavy drinkers for an average of only 17 years.

Generally, alcohol symptoms have a similar pattern of frequency to the pattern observed in the St. Louis study. The most common symptoms are those of personal and family concern; the rarest are loss of employment, hospitalization, and delirium tremens. A study of alcoholics in the Veterans Administration showed exactly this pattern (Gomberg, 1975). Symptoms of other psychiatric disorders are not known to occur in such a regular pattern nor to be so well predicted by the duration of the illness. Thus, the diagnosis of alcoholism or alcohol dependence may be more reliable and valid than other common psychiatric diagnoses.

Conclusion

The story of developing the DSM-III alcohol-related diagnoses reveals the logical complexities involved in describing the mixture of physical, social, and psychological correlates of alcohol use. Some of these correlates are clearly the effects of alcohol intake, while others, particularly the antisocial acts seen in heavy drinkers, may often be what DSM-III calls associated features. As such, they may indicate personality types predisposed to heavy drinking rather than the consequences of drinking. Some of these correlates, such as auto accidents, can occur in response to a single ingestion of large amounts, while others, like DTs and cirrhosis, require years of exposure.

Given these logical difficulties, the assembly of symptoms from grossly different conceptual realms, and the reported unreliability of alcoholics as historians, it is remarkable that the diagnosis of alcoholism by symptom self-report is found repeatedly to be among the most valid and reliable psychiatric diagnoses. There seems little doubt that, crude as our methods remain, we are tapping a sturdy entity as we research the social, medical, and psychological problems associated with alcohol abuse and dependence.

Chapter 19

The Course of Alcoholism and Lessons for Treatment

by George E. Vaillant, M.D.

Alcoholism is cunning, baffling, powerful . . . and patient.
—(Alcoholics Anonymous saying)

INTRODUCTION

Understanding the course of alcoholism is essential to an update on its treatment. If we fail to understand the course of alcoholism, we risk retaining dangerous illusions about it. Just as water refracts the passage of light and thus produces visual illusions, so do lives passing through time bend memory and understanding and thus produce cognitive illusions. Prospective study is needed to dispel the illusions produced by memory and time. This chapter addresses five areas that prospective study of the lives of alcoholics helps to clarify.

First, prospective study can dispel the illusion that alcoholism is but a symptom of unhappy childhood, familial discord, and personality disorder. Second, prospective study of community samples can dispel enduring mythologies that are maintained by selection bias. Such a bias has resulted in hopelessness toward treating the chronically relapsing alcoholics who attend clinics. Third, prospective studies not only validate diagnosis but lend coherence to an evolving symptom picture. For as Lee Robins's chapter suggests, it requires decades of follow-up to understand that alcoholism is often a progressive disorder. Fourth, in the case of highly correlated symptoms, prospective study can elucidate "cart-and-horse" relationships. In other words, prospective study clarifies treatment goals. (In a depressed alcoholic, should we treat the depression or the alcohol abuse?) Finally, only a prospective design can elucidate natural healing processes.

ILLUSIONS ABOUT ETIOLOGY

In 1941 Paul Schilder wrote, "The chronic alcoholic person is one who from his earliest childhood has lived in a state of insecurity" (290). Since the illness of alcoholism profoundly distorts the individual's own recollection of relevant childhood variables, the only study design suited to test Schilder's generalization is a prospective one.

The author and a colleague (Vaillant and Milofsky, 1982a) undertook a reexamination of the junior-high-school boys whom the Gluecks (1950) had described as a control group in their monograph *Unraveling Juvenile Delinquency*. In this reexamination, few significant differences were observed in the childhoods of alcoholics and nonalcoholics. Although as adults many more alcoholics than nonalcoholics were in social class V, no such differences had been observed in the social class of their parents. Nor did the alcoholics and nonalcoholics show any differences in IQ. Although as adults many more alcoholics than nonalcoholics were diagnosed as mentally ill, as children the alcoholics had not been rated more emotionally disturbed, nor had they come more often from multiproblem families. As adults, alcoholics were much less likely to have had stable employment than nonalcoholics, but in childhood they had shown no differences in their capacity for schoolwork or part-time employment. No differences appeared between the groups' relationships with their mothers, in terms of either maternal affection or maternal supervision. The implication is that alcoholics may exaggerate childhood difficulties after the fact to explain difficulties engendered by alcoholism.

While many alcoholics do come from chaotic families, the effect of broken homes upon adult alcoholism vanishes when one controls for parental alcoholism, a potent cause of chaotic home life. For example, of the 51 men who had *few* childhood environmental weaknesses but who did have an alcoholic parent, 27 percent became alcohol dependent as adults; in contrast, of the 56 men with *many* environmental weaknesses but no alcoholic parent, only 5 percent became alcohol dependent. (In his chapter, Schuckit reviews the persuasive evidence that the etiologic effect of familial alcoholism is more genetic than environmental.)

By prospective study, the McCords were also able to refute several hypotheses regarding the childhood etiology of alcoholism, refutations that have been upheld in subsequent prospective studies (Vaillant, 1983). The McCords undertook an imaginative follow-up of the 325 treated members of the Cambridge-Somerville Study (Powers and Witmer, 1959). Each boy in the original study had been seen at least weekly by a counselor who kept extensive progress notes, and a family investigation had been undertaken to assess delinquency risks. Using these records, the McCords were able to make extensive judgments about the premorbid characteristics of the boys and their families (McCord and McCord, 1960). Fifteen years later, when the "boys" were between 30 and 35, raters who were blind to any earlier judgments obtained evidence for alcoholism from public records, clinics, probation officers, and social agencies.

The McCords observed, contrary to prior impressions, that children with nutritional disorders, glandular disorders, "strong inferiority feelings," phobias, and "more feminine feelings" were *not* more likely to develop alcoholism. More important, boys with "strong encouragement of dependency" from their mothers and manifest oral tendencies (thumb sucking, playing with their mouths, early heavy smoking, and compulsive eating) were actually less likely to develop alcoholism. Contrary to popular belief, prealcoholics were outwardly more self-confident, less disturbed by normal fears, more aggressive and active, and more heterosexual.

Reactive depression is so frequently associated with alcoholism that psychiatric texts have consistently suggested that depression is a major cause of alcoholism. However, the prospective studies by Kammeier et al. (1973) suggest that this, too, may be an illusion. These authors contrasted the MMPIs of 38 men in college with their MMPIs many years later when they were admitted to an alcohol clinic. Only the later of the MMPIs showed an elevated depression scale. The composite MMPI of the subjects, once alcoholic, revealed the pathological profile of a self-centered, immature, dependent, resentful, and irresponsible person who was unable to face reality. For example, once they had developed alcoholism, the men were far more likely ($p<.01$) to answer "false" to "I am happy almost all the time" and "true" to "I shrink from facing a crisis," "I am high-strung," and "I am certainly lacking in self-confidence." At the Carrier Clinic, Pettinatti et al. (1982) made the same observations, in reverse sequence. At time of admission for alcoholism treatment, alcoholics manifested pathological elevations on the MMPI depression scale. After four years of abstinence, their mean values on the MMPI depression scale had returned to normal.

A retrospective study by Ullman (1953), as well as the testimonials of AA speakers, suggests that alcohol abuse and craving can begin after an alcoholic's first drink. If true, this would support the possibility of a metabolic predisposition to alcoholism. However, as with tobacco dependence, prospective study suggests that progression from asymptomatic social drinking to frank alcohol abuse to frank alcohol dependence occurs gradually over a span of three to thirty years. Before any real difficulties in the control of alcohol could be discerned, many of the alcohol abusers in a prospective study of college men had been drinking asymptomatically for as long as twenty years (Vaillant, 1983).

Admittedly, there is enormous individual variation in the evolution of alcoholism: in the rapidity of onset of abuse, in the "progression" of symptoms, and in the eventual severity of alcohol dependence. Compared with alcoholism in the well-socialized, upper-middle-class college sample, alcoholism in the most sociopathic members of the Gluecks' (1950) inner-city sample was far more extreme and manifested a far more rapid onset (Vaillant, 1983). However, rather than postulate, as did Goodwin (1979), a genetic difference between sociopathic alcoholics and those with a less rapid onset, the author suggests an environmental hypothesis. Among antisocial adolescent personalities, alcohol intake, like many other mood-altering behaviors, is used from the beginning to alter consciousness, to obliterate conscience, and to defy social canons. Such use of a potentially addictive substance can only hasten the onset of dependence.

ILLUSIONS ABOUT INCURABILITY

A second broad set of illusions that can be dispelled by prospective study are those regarding the hopelessness of treatment. These failures in reasoning arise from many sources. One source is the tendency to regard the individuals who attend clinics as representative of all individuals who have a given disease. But clinical populations are biased in several ways. First, individuals who frequent clinics—whether for heart disease, tuberculosis, alcoholism, or any other chronic illness—tend to be more dependent, more physically ill, and more psychologically vulnerable than those who do not attend clinics. Thus, personality-disordered individuals are oversampled. Second, clinical samples tend to exclude those who spontaneously recover and who have alternative social supports. Prospective follow-up of an entire cohort avoids these pitfalls by beginning with a normal population sample and then following it until those at risk have developed the disease.

As a result of sampling bias, alcoholics are usually presumed to be personality disordered. Three premorbid personality types have been repeatedly postulated to play an etiologic role in alcoholism: the emotionally insecure, anxious, and dependent (Simmel, 1948; Blane, 1968), the chronically depressed (Winokur et al., 1969), and the sociopathic (Robins, 1966). However, long-term studies suggest that such personality patterns are often the cart and not the horse to alcoholism.

Several examples will illustrate how longitudinal study can expose sampling bias. Because of the observed association of alcohol abuse with bipolar affective disorder, some investigators have suggested that alcoholism might be a variant of major depressive disorder (Winokur et al., 1969). However, in an impressive thirty-year follow-up study of the life course of over 1,700 Scandinavian alcoholics, Sundby (1967) determined that the prevalence of psychotic depression (0.35 percent) was, if anything, less than the lifetime prevalence observed in the general population. Sundby's finding, which suggests that major depressive disorder and alcoholism are quite independent disorders, has received recent confirmation from a variety of sources (Morrison, 1974; Schlesser et al., 1980). In other words, if alcoholism is often observed in affectively disordered patients, it is because such patients are particularly likely to elicit psychiatric attention rather than because alcoholism is caused by affective disorders.

In a prospective study of alcoholics with late onset (Vaillant, 1980), the author was able to study the effect of adult psychopathology upon alcoholism. In this sample, bleak childhoods and psychological instability in college had predicted, and presumably played a causal role, in the young adults' development of personality disorder and "oral" traits (pessimism, passivity, self-doubt, and heightened dependency). The men who in later life developed alcohol abuse did not come disproportionately from this subgroup, but rather appeared similar to those men who continued to drink asymptomatically until age 60. Once they began to abuse alcohol, however, oral-dependent traits and personality disorder were very common.

Many believe that it is futile to treat alcoholics, especially those who come to public clinics and emergency rooms. This myth, too, results from selection bias and from cross-sectional designs which tend to count relapses rather than remissions. An unpublished review of admissions to the Springfield, Massachusetts, freestanding detoxification center illustrates this point (Carlson, 1980). During a 78-month interval, roughly 5,000 clients received over 19,000 detoxifications. One-eighth of these 19,000 admissions encompassed the 2,500 easily forgotten clients who never returned. Another one-eighth, however, were visits from the 25 indelibly remembered clients who returned sixty times or more. Thus, the most intractable 0.5 percent were admitted as often and became far more deeply etched in clinicians' consciousness than did the 50 percent who never came back and who must have included the best outcomes.

IS ALCOHOLISM A PROGRESSIVE DISEASE?

Prospective study lends coherence to an evolving symptom picture. One reason why our understanding of alcoholism is so confused is that investigators who scrutinize the behavior of alcoholics for short periods of time come to doubt that alcoholism is a stable or progressive disorder. Indeed, some believe that there are as many alcoholisms as there are problem drinkers. Certainly, the elderly retired stockbroker who first comes to medical attention due to cirrhosis and polyneuritis appears to have a different disorder from that of the young motorcyclist who comes to police attention due to drunken episodes of belligerence and community complaints. They come to the attention of different people, but is their illness different?

In a middle-aged sample, when the correlation of *symptoms ever present* was substituted for the correlation of *symptoms currently present*, there did not appear to be many different alcoholisms (Vaillant et al., 1982). The lifetime prevalence of the five items that define the hypothetical stockbroker's alcohol dependence from the vantage point of the medical model (morning drinking, alcohol-related medical problems, going on the wagon, clinical diagnosis of alcoholism, and self-admission of loss of control) were correlated with five items that identify the motorcyclist's problem drinking from the vantage point of the social deviance model (alcohol-related arrests, occupational problems, social problems, marital problems, and fights). For 110 47-year-old alcohol abusers, the correlations (r) between the five individual symptoms drawn from the medical model with those drawn from the sociological model ranged from .40 to .60. When the 3-point DSM-III scale of no abuse, abuse, and physiological dependence was correlated with the 11-point Cahalan scale of socially deviant drinking behaviors, the correlation was .87. In other words, given a long enough period of observation, the clinician's "disease" and the sociologist's "continuum of drinking behaviors" merge. Given enough time, the stockbroker may be arrested for drunken driving, and the motorcyclist may damage his liver.

To address the problem of different alcoholisms, Jellinek (1960) devised a five-group typology of alcohol abuse: alpha (symptoms and psychological, but not physical, dependence), beta (medical symptoms but no physical dependence), gamma (symptoms *and* physical dependence), delta (physical dependence but few or no symptoms), and epsilon (binge drinking). Jellinek viewed the gamma and delta groups as reflecting the "disease" of alcoholism and suggested that the disease might be progressive.

Viewed over the short term, however, all alcoholism appears extemely unstable and in no sense progressive. For example, in their month-by-month study of 100 alcoholics, Orford and Edwards (1977) questioned the validity of any black-and-white definition of the disorder. Every month they interviewed their alcoholic subjects and their wives. On the average, the wives believed that their husbands—a majority of whom met the criteria for gamma alcoholism—engaged in drinking in only 31 of the 52 weeks under study; for only 23 of those 31 weeks did they regard their husband's drinking as unacceptable. Thus, during the year, the average alcoholic was abstinent for 21 weeks and engaged in perfectly acceptable "social" drinking for 8 weeks more. The standard deviations were small. In other words, on a day-by-day basis many alcoholics do not have trouble with their drinking. What is equally important, however, is that in contrast to nonalcoholics, alcoholics do have difficulty on a year-by-year basis. At the year's end, 20 of Orford and Edwards's alcoholics appeared in clear clinical remission, and 55 more men could be unambiguously classified as problem drinkers. The status of only 25 remained ambiguous.

In the past decade, a compelling and coherent body of empirical work has appeared contradicting the idea that alcoholism has an orderly evolution (Knupfer, 1972; Cahalan and Room, 1974; Clark, 1976; Clark and Cahalan, 1976; Roizen et al., 1978). Summarizing this work, Clark and Cahalan (1976) wrote: "The common conception of alcoholism as a disease fails to cover a large part of the domain of alcohol problems and a more useful model would be to place further emphasis on the development and correlates of particular problems related to drinking, rather than assuming that alcoholism as an underlying and unitary progressive disease is a source of most alcohol problems" (Clark and Cahalan, 1976, 258). At first glance, this evidence, like that of Orford and Edwards, would seem to contradict Jellinek's (1952) concept of a natural progression of the symptoms underlying the "disease" of gamma alcoholism. Whom are we to believe, Jellinek or Clark and Cahalan?

Aamark (1951) and Keller (1975) have each elucidated the distinction between the unstable *problem drinker* studied by Clark and Cahalan and the *progressive alcoholic* described by Jellinek and Alcoholics Anonymous. The critical distinction between these categories is where individuals are in their alcoholic careers. The modal problem drinker is 25 to 35, married, and working and has never been treated for alcoholism. His or her use of alcohol is markedly responsive to environmental factors and can, over time, become either more or less symptomatic. In such individuals, symptoms of alcohol abuse are likely to be "disjunctive." A symptom is disjunctive in that its presence will not significantly predict the presence of other symptoms that might, according to Jellinek's sequence of progression, theoretically precede the index symptom.

In contrast, the modal chronic alcoholic is seen less commonly, but his or her alcohol abuse has evolved and become far less plastic. He or she is 10 years older, aged 35 to 45, and exhibits unstable marital and employment status. Such individuals may have sought treatment for alcoholism and exhibit a pattern of alcohol abuse that is relatively insensitive to environmental variables. They often become stably abstinent but rarely evolve into patterns of asymptomatic drinking. In such individuals, the appearance of a given symptom will be statistically associated with the preexistence of earlier symptoms in the chain of progression outlined by Robins in the preceding chapter. Obviously, to elucidate such a relationship, a prospective view is imperative.

Illuminating the reversibility of the 25- to 35-year-old problem drinker, the eight-year follow-up by Goodwin et al. (1971) is noteworthy. They reported the lowest death rate and the highest rate of return to asymptomatic drinking in the long-term follow-up literature. The felons who made up their sample were very young (average age 27), and, unlike the men in most other longitudinal samples, they had not sought treatment for alcohol dependence. Rather, when the felons in the Goodwin et al. sample were interviewed in prison, they had merely reported a past history of alcohol-related problems. This study is heuristically important because it underscores a fundamental principle involved in the reversibility of alcohol abuse. By inadvertently selecting alcoholics who had abused alcohol for only a short time and with little physical dependence, Goodwin and his coworkers were able to identify problem drinkers, a large proportion of whom were to return to asymptomatic drinking.

Illuminating the progression of the 35- to 45-year-old individual with alcohol dependence, the study by Ojesjo (1981) is useful. Ojesjo began with a representative community cohort drawn from the district of Lundby in Sweden (Essen-Möller, 1956). The average age of the 96 male alcohol abusers identified in the Lundby study was 47. Half of the 96 would have met the DSM-III criteria for alcohol dependence. The sample was followed up after 15 years. In 1957 and in 1972, each subject's problem drinking had been classified as alcohol abuse, alcohol dependence, or chronic alcoholism (dependence with serious medical sequelae). At first glance, these categories seemed most unstable over time. Of 49 men categorized as alcohol abusers in 1957, only 4 were still categorized as alcohol abusers in 1972. Of 29 men classified as alcohol dependent in 1957, only 8 were still classified as alcohol dependent in 1972. Nonetheless, concealed in this apparent instability was clear support for Jellinek's concept of progression. Among the 49 men who were counted as alcohol abusers in 1957, 17 men were no longer classified as alcohol abusers in 1972 because their alcoholism had progressed either to death or to chronic alcoholism. Another 25 had achieved stable remission. Of the 29 alcohol-dependent men, 13 had progressed to death or chronic alcoholism, 4 had achieved stable remission, and, as noted above, 8 remained alcohol dependent. Thus, after 15 years, only 4 alcohol dependent men contradicted Jellinek's concept of a progressive disease and were reclassified as alcohol abusers.

To summarize, in conceptualizing the clinical course of alcoholism, methodological considerations are crucial. On the one hand, the course of a chronic relapsing disease may appear very unstable if many mild cases are included, if data are gathered by questionnaires, if deaths are excluded, if periods of observation are short, if syndromes are broken down into individual symptoms, and if integrated individual case histories are ignored. On the other hand, the course of a chronic disease may appear stable and progressive if only severe cases are included, if data are gathered by skilled clinical interviews, if all deaths are reported, if symptoms, however individually unstable, are treated as clusters, if long periods of observation are used, and if individual lives rather than statistical analyses are scrutinized.

TREATMENT GOALS

A fourth advantage of prospective study is that it can help us determine appropriate treatment goals. For example, does abstinence cure the alcoholic? Gerard et al. (1962) thought not. These authors, however, ignored the fact that their clinic population was drawn from a public city hospital and that their abstinent alcoholics, in fact, fared far better than those who continued to drink. By studying a community sample prospectively, the author and a colleague (Vaillant and Milofsky, 1982b) observed that 21 former alcoholics who had achieved the most stable abstinence (mean duration of ten years) did not significantly differ in psychosocial adjustment from men who had never abused alcohol. In other words, their abstinence was associated with full recovery. In contrast, the psychosocial adjustment of alcoholics who had only recently become abstinent (less than three years) did not seem very different from that of active alcoholics. The three groups did not differ, however, in terms of childhood predictors associated with midlife psychosocial adjustment. The implication from these and other data (Vaillant, 1983) is that abstinence is the treatment goal of choice for most severe alcoholics, but that recovery from alcoholism requires prolonged convalescence.

Long-term follow-up also addresses the question, Can alcoholics be taught to return to social drinking? Recently, the Sobells (1976), in a comparatively well-controlled study, suggested that a major etiologic factor in alcoholism was a failure to self-monitor blood alcohol levels. The Sobells' effort to teach alcoholics to drink socially provided the illusion that increasing alcoholics' awareness of such internal cues would facilitate their return to asymptomatic drinking. Their findings at two years were impressive and influential. However, if one examines their two-year data carefully, one discovers that the reason that patients trained in controlled drinking had the fewest "problem days" was that they had even more abstinent days than the patients who received abstinence training. A ten-year reevaluation of the Sobells' patients by Pendery et al. (1982) confirmed that the Sobells' original deduction was incorrect. The 6 patients who recovered did so by achieving stable abstinence, and 13 of the 14 remaining patients died or repeatedly relapsed to alcohol dependence. Alcoholism is often a progressive disease.

NATURAL HEALING PROCESSES

The fifth value of prospective study is that it helps us understand effective prognosis and treatment. Over the short term, the law of initial values blurs the frequently progressive nature of alcoholism and magnifies the effect of treatment. The law of initial values reflects the tendency of extreme physiological or psychological values to regress toward the mean over time. Alcoholics tend to present themselves for medical attention at their clinical nadir and at the time when their symptoms are most exacerbated. Thus, if follow-up has a brief or rigid time frame, most alcoholic patients will appear to improve regardless of the treatment offered. Eighteen months after admission, 67 percent of the Rand study patients were reported to have fewer alcohol-related problems than they had during the one month prior to admission (Armor et al., 1978). However, when the Rand investigators extended their follow-up to four years and substituted a six-month observation period for a one-month period, much of the improvement that they had originally noted appeared evanescent (Polich et al., 1981).

Students of alcoholism have long been impressed by the value of multimodality treatment. The more eclectic and enthusiastic the inpatient treatment, the better the reported results. However, Costello (1980) observed that although multimodality inpatient treatment and subsequent attendance at alcohol outpatient clinics were associated with good outcome, prospective study rendered the apparent causal association illusory. Two premorbid variables, marriage and stable employment, strongly predicted that an alcoholic would receive multimodality treatment, attend clinics conscientiously, and enjoy remission from alcoholism. When premorbid social stability was controlled, however, the treatment components (e.g., group therapy, disulfiram [Antabuse] treatment, and outpatient clinic attendance) explained little further independent variance in outcome.

Is the apparent effectiveness of AA based on a similar illusion? In a prospective eight-year study of clinic alcoholics (Vaillant et al., 1983), 100 alcoholics were studied in terms of premorbid variables known to affect prognosis. These patients were then followed every 18 months for eight years (1972–1980). The authors examined the relationship between AA attendance, premorbid variables and outcome. At the end of the eight years, of the 29 patients with stable remissions of three years or more, 15 patients had made 300 or more visits to AA. This was true of only 1 of the 37 still active alcoholics. As expected, social stability on admission predicted stable abstinence eight years later for the group as a whole, but social instability on admission predicted AA attendance over the subsequent eight years. Thus, 32 patients attended AA meetings 100 or more times (mean 600 visits) between 1972 and 1980; of these individuals, the number with stable employment and living arrangements went from 2 in 1972 to 15 in 1980. Put differently, the alcoholics who were socially stable premorbidly tended to become abstinent without AA; but if the socially unstable alcoholics were to recover, frequent AA attendance appeared to be an important intervening variable.

Finally, if controlling the effect of premorbid variables shows that formal treatment modalities may add relatively little to treatment outcome (Costello, 1980), how do we explain the fact that over time alcoholics enjoy a 50 percent recovery rate? What natural treatment variables are working to help alcoholics to recover?

Following an entire cohort of 120 inner-city alcohol abusers from adolescence until the age of 47, the author and a colleague (Vaillant and Milofsky, 1982b) identified 49 men who had achieved a year or more of abstinence. Only one-third of the 49 had sought professional help during the first year of their abstinence, but over half had found an external superego or some form of natural behavior modification that altered the consequences of their alcohol use. The external superego could include disulfiram, probation, or a medical affliction that made heavy drinking aversive. Over half found a substitute dependency such as gambling, meditation, smoking or eating, or compulsive overinvolvement in a job or hobby. Parenthetically, one reason why by itself disulfiram therapy is rarely the answer is that it renders one habit impossible but fails to provide a substitute. Over half became very involved in AA or some other quasi-religious organization that in Jerome Frank's terms raised their morale and helped to provide hope and enhanced self-esteem.* Finally, a third of the men found a new love object during their first year of abstinence, someone whom they had not injured in the past.

To conclude, there are many lessons to be learned from the prospective study of alcoholism. One is that long-term follow-up shatters our retrospective illusions. A second lesson to be learned is therapeutic humility. Instead of only studying the effects of our favorite therapeutic interventions ever more closely, we must learn from those who have recovered from alcoholism without our help. Still a third lesson is hope. If alcoholism is both a baffling and a patient disorder, unlike most chronic diseases alcoholism enjoys a high rate of stable remission. If we do not always understand natural healing processes, we can still learn to harness them.

*Editor's note: In Part V of this volume, Frank discusses his morale concept with particular reference to patients with anxiety disorders and shows how the various schools of psychotherapy work to raise patients' hopes and feelings of self-efficacy.

Chapter 20

Genetic and Biochemical Factors in the Etiology of Alcoholism[†]

by Marc A. Schuckit, M.D.

INTRODUCTION

The nature-versus-nurture controversy over the etiology of alcoholism has been replaced by the recognition that both sets of factors are important. This chapter reviews the data supporting the concept that genetically mediated biological influences contribute to the development of alcoholism, which is seen as a multifactorial, polygenic disorder (Schuckit and von Wartburg, in press; Cloninger and Reich, 1981). While environmental factors are important and must be incorporated into any theory, they are not the focus of this chapter.[*]

This review has a number of inherent biases. First, whenever possible the author emphasizes information gathered over the last five to ten years. The field is relatively new, and the tentative conclusions reached in the last five years interdigitate closely with prior findings. Second, the author's approach is that of a clinically oriented researcher, a bias which dictates the use of objectively stated diagnostic criteria which outline as homogeneous a diagnostic group as possible and which relate diagnosis to prognosis and probable treatment (Goodwin and Guze, 1979).

The work reviewed has built on the four types of studies which have supported a genetic influence in alcoholism. These include, first, the studies of the familial nature of alcoholism and the manner in which it tends to run in families (Cotton, 1979); second, the animal studies which support the importance of inherited factors in the organism's decision to drink and in the quantity consumed (Meisch, 1982); and, third, the twin studies which demonstrate a two-times-greater risk or more for alcoholism in an identical twin of an alcoholic than in a fraternal twin (Schuckit, 1981c). The fourth and most compelling source of evidence is the adoption studies done in the United States and Scandinavia. They have revealed a fourfold or higher elevated alcoholism risk for the sons and daughters of alcoholics adopted at birth and raised without knowledge of their biological parent's problem when compared with children of nonalcoholics adopted at birth (Schuckit et al., 1972; Goodwin et al., 1974; Bohman et al., 1981). Indeed, once one controls for the possible effects of alcoholism in a biological parent, being raised by an alcoholic adoptive parent or experiencing a broken home early in life adds nothing to the alcoholism risk. Recognizing the strong data which support the importance of genetics in the development of alcoholism, as well as the importance of environmental factors, researchers have begun to search for genetically mediated biological factors which could contribute to the

†This work was supported by the Medical Research Service of the Veterans Administration and by National Institutes of Alcohol Abuse and Alcoholism Grant No. AA 04353.

*Preceptor's note: Environmental influences are covered in the Preceptor's discussion of etiology and course and in Nathan's review of learned behavior and behavioral interventions that focus on environmental contingencies. In his chapter, Gerstein discusses the various ways in which primary prevention policies attempt to alter environmental factors.

alcoholism risk. Before reviewing this research, though, some methodological considerations must be addressed briefly.

METHODOLOGICAL CONSIDERATIONS

Studies of genetic factors in alcoholism recognize the probable influence of multiple genes, which interact with a variety of unknown environmental factors to establish a final risk for alcoholism (Schuckit and von Wartburg, in press). Any methodology which decreases the heterogeneity in study samples will therefore help to elucidate the combination of most relevant factors.

The first methodological issue arises in choosing a definition of alcoholism. Most of the adoption studies have used relatively severe alcoholic cases. Samples have included those who qualify for the diagnosis based on the occurrence of any one of the major life problems related to alcohol, marital separation or divorce, multiple arrests related to alcohol, job loss or layoff, or physical evidence that alcohol had harmed health (withdrawal, alcoholic cirrhosis, and so forth) (Schuckit, 1979). The next definitive step in the investigation is to select alcoholics who have no major preexisting psychiatric disorder so that the study focuses on primary alcoholics. When severe alcohol-related life problems occur in the context of a manic episode, an antisocial personality, or schizophrenia, for example, the genetic influences in the psychiatric disorder could obscure the genetic factors relating to the alcoholism (Schuckit, 1982b; 1983c).

A next commonsense but important step is to establish the behavioral focus of the genetic research. Possible choices include the acquisition of drinking, the decision to continue to drink once alcohol has been tasted, the development of temporary alcohol-related problems, which are seen in up to 40 percent of men in the United States by the age of 40 (Cahalan, 1970), or the transition from usual drinking with some minor problems to the persistent, severe alcohol-related difficulties that characterize alcoholism (Schuckit and von Wartburg, in press; Schuckit, 1980d). The studies to be reviewed examine how genetic factors might influence the transition from more normal drinking to severe and persistent alcohol-related problems in individuals who have no preexisting major psychiatric disorders.

Once these parameters have been established, the next step is to select from among the possible genetically influenced risk factors those that will be studied (Schuckit, 1980b; 1982c). Possible genetically influenced pathways for enhancing the risk of alcoholism include:

1. Unusual metabolism of ethanol and/or acetaldehyde
2. Personality attributes
3. Enhanced ethanol-related risk for organ damage
4. Enhanced development of tolerance or physical dependence
5. Altered acute reaction to ethanol
6. Risk mediated through other psychiatric disorders

In a heavy-drinking society the risk for alcoholism might increase when an unusual metabolism of alcohol has affected the rate of ethanol disappearance or acetaldehyde accumulation. An unusual acute reaction to alcohol (i.e, either more reinforcement or less warning that intoxication is developing) is another possible factor. Personality characteristics may also indirectly increase the risk for alcohol-related problems. An increased risk of organ damage when drinking may result in higher chances of being identified as an alcoholic with such symptoms as cirrhosis or brain damage. Another factor could be an unusual predisposition to the development of tolerance or physical dependence. Any of these or other states might be reached through multiple genetic mechanisms, which might affect the risk differently in different families (Schuckit and von Wartburg, in press). Thus, in studying possible factors increasing the predisposition to alcoholism, an investigator might focus on measuring some final common pathway, such as a distinctive metabolism, which might be controlled by different genetic factors in different families.

Finally, the mechanism of investigation must be chosen. Some scientists have compared alcoholics versus controls, but the differences observed between two such groups could result from many years of heavy drinking and not have been contributors to the original elevated alcoholism risk. Others have observed linkage by studying close relatives in a limited number of families of alcoholics (Watt, 1982). While this method does allow for determining the genetic distribution within families, the focus on a limited number of individuals and a small number of families may be misleading if different factors are operating in different families. To be most effective, it might be best to have a high index of suspicion about which specific biological factors should be observed. Furthermore, in a multifactorial disorder, relatives may be carrying the biological predisposition but not actually demonstrate the disorder, a problem which can be exceptionally important in studies of a limited number of individuals.

The method used by the author and his colleagues is to identify nonalcoholic close relatives of alcoholics, limiting the study to men who are young enough not to have entered the major age of risk for alcoholism. In such high-risk studies, many relatives of a large number of alcoholics are identified and compared with controls. The assets of this method include an almost inexhaustible number of potential subjects, the large number of different families investigated permitting different factors to be studied, and the investigators' ability to observe individuals at high risk before alcoholism actually develops. Potential subjects are male students and nonacademic staff aged 21 to 25 who have responded to a questionnaire. Individuals are excluded if they already have serious alcohol or drug-related life problems or if they have a past or current major medical or psychiatric disorder. Then, those drinking but nonalcoholic young men who report an alcoholic parent or sibling are placed in the high-risk group and matched on demography and drinking history with similar men who report no close alcoholic relative. Members of these family-history-positive (FHP) and family-history-negative (FHN) matched pairs then come to the laboratory, and raters blind to their family history measure personality attributes, alcohol metabolism, physical reactions to ethanol, neurological functioning using event-related potentials, and cognitive as well as psychomotor performance. After baseline procedures have been completed, the subjects are administered 0.75 ml/kg of pure ethanol as a 20 percent solution in a sugar-free carbonated beverage, and performance measures as well as biochemical markers are followed for five hours. (Results of these high-risk studies are briefly reviewed in the next section.)

POSSIBLE BIOLOGICAL MARKERS

The studies reviewed are based on the premise, established through other investigations, that alcoholism appears to be a genetically influenced disorder. The goal is to identify possible genetically influenced biological factors which, interacting with environmental events, might increase the risk for alcoholism. As a result of these studies, data are now available in five main areas: (1) possible differences in metabolism, (2) personality factors which might influence the development of alcoholism, (3) a possible mediation by the risk for other psychiatric disorders, (4) a difference in the response to acute ethanol intoxication, and (5) electrophysiological differences.

Metabolic Factors

Using orally administered ethanol, studies by the author's group have consistently shown no difference by family history on the time to peak blood alcohol concentration (BAC), the magnitude of that peak, or the rate of disappearance of ethanol (Schuckit, 1981b). However, there are possible differences between the FHP and FHN matched pairs on the drinking-related accumulation in the blood of the first breakdown product of ethanol, acetaldehyde (Schuckit and Rayses, 1979; Zeiner, 1982). These results are admittedly compromised by the lack of agreement on the best method of establishing acetaldehyde in blood (Schuckit, 1980a; Lindros, 1982). Nonetheless, they are consistent with the slightly higher levels found in alcoholics after drinking compared with controls (Korsten et al., 1975; Lindros et al., 1980), and they raise speculations about the possible biological meanings of higher acetaldehyde.

A mild elevation could counteract some of the brain depressant effects of ethanol and might decrease the sedation at modest BACs (Schuckit and von Wartburg, in press). Increases in this toxic substance could also increase the risk for organ damage, since acetaldehyde appears to be toxic to striated muscle (including the heart) as well as to liver, brain, and so forth. Of course, while small increases in acetaldehyde could increase the alcoholism risk, very large increases could produce an effect like that of disulfiram, with a resulting lowered risk (Schuckit and Duby, 1982).

Acetaldehyde is also capable of combining with brain transmitters to form neuronally active compounds with some morphinelike properties (Myers et al., 1982; Bloom, 1982). The problem is that these catecholamine-derived products (tetrahydroisoquinolines, or TIQs) and serotonin-derived products (β-carbolines) are exceptionally difficult to measure in biological samples. Methodological problems arise from the possibility of spurious production during sample processing, as can also happen with acetaldehyde. While no solid conclusions can be drawn about the importance of these substances in vivo, artificially produced TIQs administered intraventricularly in rats have been reported to produce long-term modest increases in voluntary oral ethanol intake, which in turn may be attenuated with naloxone (Myers and Critcher, 1982). The β-carboline salsolinol has been reported to be self-administered in rodents (Bloom, 1982). Even though these studies have not been widely replicated and their findings might not be produced in biologically active amounts in vivo (Weiner, 1982), some interesting leads remain regarding possible mechanisms of biologically related factors which might increase alcoholism risk. An alteration in the acute reaction to alcohol, an increased risk for alcohol-related body damage, and effects on the development of tolerance or physical dependence may yet be shown to have some connection with TIQ levels and production.

Finally, the genetically influenced risks for alcoholism may be connected to some genetic control over the enzyme responsible for most of the destruction of ethanol and production of acetaldehyde, alcohol dehydrogenase (ADH), and the enzyme responsible for the destruction of acetaldehyde, aldehyde dehydrogenase (ALDH) (Li, 1977; Lieber, 1977). A variation in either of these enzymes could result in a more rapid metabolism of ethanol or a slower destruction of acetaldehyde.

Investigators have given extensive attention to the genetic factors responsible for the 15 isoenzyme forms of ADH (von Wartburg, 1980; Bosron and Li, 1981). Each form has been shown to have a potential different optimum ethanol concentration, optimum acid base balance, and rate of ethanol destruction. ADH isoenzyme patterns are different in different ethnic subgroups. A slower, more "atypical" form appears in 20 percent of the Swiss, 5 to 10 percent of North Americans, and 90 percent of Orientals (Harada et al., 1980; Li and Magnes, 1975). However, the differing patterns of ADH have not yet been actively associated with the alcoholism risk. Of potentially greater importance to the genetics of alcoholism are the minimum of two to four isoenzymes of ALDH known to exist in human liver (Greenfield and Pietruszko, 1977; Goedde et al., 1979a), although some disagree about which isoenzyme forms are the most clinically important (Jenkins and Peters, 1980). It is agreed, however, that the Japanese, who reportedly have lower rates of alcoholism, show a different pattern of ALDH with a subsequent different pattern of accumulation of acetaldehyde from the pattern seen in Occidentals. Fifty percent of the Japanese are missing the form of ALDH which is more active at lower acetaldehyde levels, with the result that when they drink they feel great discomfort, including obvious facial flushing (Harada et al., 1980; Goedde et al., 1979b). This in turn may relate to the risk for drinking and the subsequent risk for alcoholism (Harada et al., 1982).

In summary, one possible genetically influenced biological mechanism affecting the risk for alcoholism could be the manner of ethanol metabolism. Consistent with the modestly higher levels of acetaldehyde observed in alcoholics after drinking, the offspring of alcoholics may also demonstrate this pattern even before alcoholism develops. If so, this could increase the risk for alcoholism via increased organ damage or a different type of intoxication at modest blood alcohol levels. Modest levels of acetaldehyde could also be responsible for producing some biologically active substances which might increase the chances of developing alcoholism. Very high levels of acetaldehyde, on the other hand, could decrease the alcoholism risk by bringing on a discomfort like that caused by disulfiram. All of these factors are of heuristic value at present. They are increasing our knowledge about genetic controls in ethanol metabolism and about the biological factors which could mediate the drinking experience.

Personality Factors

Along with the evidence that personality factors can be genetically in-fluenced (Schuckit and Haglund, 1982), studies also have demonstrated that alcoholics have particular personality patterns. They tend to show a unique pattern on the MMPI, and they have higher levels of extro-version, demonstrate higher levels of anxiety, and tend to feel that their lives are controlled by external factors and not by themselves. When the author and his colleagues administered personality tests to the sons of alcoholics and controls before the subjects imbibed ethanol, however, they found no clinically significant personality differences between the groups. No differences appeared on the Eysenck Personality Inventory measures of extroversion and neuroticism, on the MMPI subtests usu-ally noted to differ in alcoholics versus controls (with the possible but weak exception of the McAndrew Score), on the Shipley Trait Anxiety Scale, or on the locus-of-control measure (Saunders and Schuckit, 1981; Schuckit, 1983a; Morrison and Schuckit, 1983; Schuckit, 1982a). Thus, the high-risk studies reveal few differences on personality variables be-tween the sons of alcoholics and matched controls.

Mediation by Risk for Other Psychiatric Disorders

Genetic influences are believed to contribute to the development of ma-jor psychiatric disorders, including schizophrenia, the major affective disorders, the antisocial personality, and so forth.* A genetic predispo-sition to these disorders could possibly masquerade as primary alcohol-ism under certain biological or environmental conditions.

This speculation received indirect investigation in studies showing decreased monoamine oxidase (MAO) activity in alcoholics (Sullivan et al., 1979), since lower MAO values have been related to behavioral traits including psychiatric disorders (Coursey et al., 1979). Although such decreases have been noted for alcoholism, with abstinence the level of MAO activity may return to normal (Brown, 1977). To test this possi-bility in the FHP-FHN pairs, the author's group determined MAO lev-els before ethanol administration. They found only a nonsignificant trend for lower MAO activity in the higher-risk FHP men: 5.06 ± 1.26 for FHP men versus 5.60 ± 1.00 for FHN men (n mol/mg protein/hr) (Schuckit et al., 1982).

The author's group followed a similar line of reasoning with dopa-mine β-hydroxylase (DBH), which is believed to be an indirect measure of noradrenergic activity. Abnormal levels of DBH are reportedly asso-ciated with major psychiatric disorders, and DBH levels may be low in the spinal fluid of alcoholics, which could in turn be associated with a decreased response to modest levels of ethanol (Schuckit et al., 1981a). The author's group found no significant DBH differences between their matched pairs, although there was a trend for the higher-risk group to

Part IV

Psychiatry
Update:
Volume III

325

*Editor's note: In Part II of Volume I of *Psychiatry Update* (*Psychiatry 1982*), Dr. Robert Cancro reviews and evaluates the evidence for genetic factors in the etiology of the schizophrenic dis-orders (pages 92–97). Genetic factors in the major affective disorders are the subject of Dr. Elliot S. Gershon's chapter in Part V of *Psychiatry Update: Volume II* (pages 434–457). Readers may also want to refer to Dr. Larry J. Siever's chapter on genetic factors in borderline personality disor-ders (Volume I, pages 437–456).

show lower levels: 38.2±5.6 for FHP men versus 45.6±9.7 for FHN men (IU/l).

Some investigators have reported an increased risk for affective disorder in the families of alcoholics. However, this may relate in part to diagnostic confusion over primary alcoholic relatives who develop symptoms of depression during heavy drinking (Schuckit, 1979; 1983b; 1983c). Alcohol alone can cause serious mood disturbances in alcoholics or normal subjects during experimental intoxication, but even suicidal depressions associated with heavy drinking are likely to clear within days of abstinence (Schuckit, 1982b; 1983c). The studies conducted by the author's group have failed to show any significant correlation between the occurrence of depressions in primary alcoholics and a family history of affective disorder (Schuckit 1982b; 1983b).

No compelling evidence to date links the genetic factors increasing the risk for primary alcoholism with genetic factors mediating any other major psychiatric disorder. Part of the confusion in the literature may come from the studies having used relatively loose definitions of disorders and not limiting themselves to primary alcoholics. Thus, the studies have often included antisocial personality subjects who have alcohol-related problems (and may be carrying a genetic predisposition toward their primary antisocial personality) and individuals who demonstrate alcohol-related problems in the midst of schizophrenic and major affective disorders (Schuckit, 1983c).

Response to Acute Ethanol Intoxication

The risk for developing serious and persistent alcohol-related problems could increase if an individual were less able to moderate drinking because of an impaired ability to estimate intoxication at a given BAC (Nathan and Lisman, 1976). Some evidence suggests that alcoholics are less able than others to estimate their blood alcohol levels after drinking. To test the possibility that a less intense reaction to modest doses of alcohol might relate to the future alcoholism risk, the author's group administered a series of subjective, cognitive, and psychomotor tests to higher-risk and lower-risk young men and monitored the effects of 0.75 ml/kg of ethanol. Despite identical mean BACs, the higher-risk FHP men reported less subjective intoxication when compared with controls. They also demonstrated less impairment than controls on some cognitive tests (the Trails Test) and some motor tests (body sway) (Schuckit, 1980c; 1981b; 1982c). Similarly, two hours after drinking, the FHP men demonstrated lower levels of prolactin, which is believed to be released from the anterior pituitary in response to ethanol, and they showed lower levels of cortisol (Schuckit et al., in press). These studies suggest that one mechanism for increasing the alcoholism risk could be a lessened response to the acute effects of modest ethanol doses, which might in turn impair the high-risk drinker's ability to tell when it is time to stop.

Electrophysiological Differences

If alcohol affects the nervous tissue of higher-risk individuals and controls differently, this might mediate the quality or intensity of the intoxication. A number of studies address this possibility.

Propping's group has demonstrated a deficiency in EEG α-rhythm activity in alcoholics compared with controls (Propping, 1977). Similar findings have been reported for the relatives of alcoholics, as has a tendency of alcohol itself to increase the α-rhythms (Pollock et al., in press). If an α-rhythm pattern is associated with relaxation and comfortable feelings, then one motive behind an increased risk for alcoholism could be that alcohol gives a greater reinforcing effect to individuals who have "deficiencies" in α-rhythms.

A second finding of interest has been the possible differential effect of ethanol on muscle tension. The higher-risk FHP men tested in the author's laboratory demonstrated significantly greater levels of muscle relaxation at rest than controls when given ethanol (Schuckit et al., 1981b). This could be yet another way that ethanol is differentially reinforcing, suggesting another source of alcohol risk mediation in some families.

A more complex alcohol-sensitive measure of brain activity is found with brain-stem auditory event-related potentials. Computer-averaged brain waves are measured by exposing subjects to a train of stimuli (e.g., clicks or flashes of light), and they are asked to discriminate a randomly occurring unusual stimulus. When the anticipated unusual event occurs (e.g., a tone much shorter or of a different frequency than the others), a positive brain wave will appear between 300 and 500 milliseconds following the stimulus. The amplitude and latency of this brain wave are related to the importance of the task, how unpredictable or infrequent the event is, and the subject's motivation (Porjesz and Begleiter, 1982). Since acute administration of ethanol increases the latency and decreases the P300 amplitude, the P300 amplitude has been used as one possible marker of neurological differences between higher- and lower-risk groups before ethanol and their response to the drug. While the results to date are tentative, the high-risk sons of alcoholics may demonstrate a decreased P300 amplitude even without ethanol or when receiving placebo (Elmasian et al., 1982; Begleiter and Porjesz, 1983), or alcohol may produce an enhanced increase in latency (Schuckit and Stockard, 1983). Although these studies have methodological drawbacks in the comparability of high- and low-risk samples and in their small sample sizes, the results still have heuristic importance. They suggest that young men with a higher future risk for alcoholism may be unwilling or unable to pay attention to their surroundings when they are becoming intoxicated. This in turn might support the possibility that they feel less intoxicated because they pay less attention to how they are feeling or responding to their environment.

CONCLUSIONS

The data to date supply some interesting leads for future research. Any interpretations must of course recognize that the findings may only represent some final common pathways, which may themselves involve a number of different genetic mechanisms in different families (Schuckit and von Wartburg, in press). The findings reviewed here may be succinctly summarized. First, men at higher and lower risk for alcoholism may differ in their accumulation of acetaldehyde after drinking. Evidence of this possibility has stimulated further research into the effects of acetaldehyde on body functioning, its possible role in mediating intoxication, and the biologically active compounds which might be produced through the interaction of acetaldehyde and brain monoamines. Second, no evidence to date supports the role of measurable personality factors in contributing to the risk for alcoholism. Third, little evidence to date supports the hypothesis that the genetic factors which increase the risk for alcoholism are the same as those which mediate other major psychiatric disorders. Of course, the evidence in this area depends upon a careful definition of primary alcoholism. Fourth, consistent but preliminary data show that decreased sensitivity to acute ethanol effects may occur in young men at higher alcoholism risk, and this may impair their ability to discern when they are becoming intoxicated and should stop drinking. Fifth and finally, high- and low-risk groups may have differences in inherent α-rhythms, the effect of ethanol on muscle tension, and EEG correlates of the level of vigilance during a task. These differences in turn might either cause high-risk subjects to experience more reward from ethanol or help explain the differences between higher- and lower-risk groups on the acute effects of the drug.

Investigation into the possible biological mediators of a genetic predisposition to alcoholism is a recent development. Investigation is difficult because important but unknown environmental factors may mediate the effects of genetic influences, because there are difficulties in establishing homogeneous study groups, and because specific problems surround the accuracy of the measurements involved. Nonetheless, enough evidence has accumulated to warrant future investigation into the possible importance of genetic factors in alcoholism.

Chapter 21

Contributions of Learning Theory to the Diagnosis and Treatment of Alcoholism

by Peter E. Nathan, Ph.D.

HISTORICAL PERSPECTIVES

Over fifty years ago, the Soviet physician, N.V. Kantorovich, had apparent success when he used electrical aversion to treat a group of chronic alcoholics. Not until the 1960s, however, did behavioral treatment procedures begin to find widespread application with a range of behavioral disorders. The only continuing use of behavioral methods with alcoholics during the thirty years separating Kantorovich's demonstration and the 1960s was at the Shadel Sanatorium in Seattle (Lemere and Voegtlin, 1950). Chemical aversion was employed there with apparent success to induce conditioned aversion to alcohol.

Intensive clinical application of behavioral methods began in the early 1960s. The range of methods expanded to include systematic desensitization and covert sensitization, as well as chemical aversion and electrical aversion. Applications extended well beyond alcoholism to virtually the full range of psychopathology: from normal children in classroom settings, to individuals and families with no more than the usual "problems in living," to psychotic, demented, criminal, and retarded individuals. During the same time, more and more persons began to focus their efforts on alcoholism. At first, these efforts began where Kantorovich left off, with vain attempts to induce conditioned aversion to alcohol by electrical aversion and other unidimensional methods. Gradually, however, more comprehensive and sophisticated behavioral treatment programs came to the fore. These latter programs are the focus of this chapter's summary review.

The unidimensional behavioral treatment methods, epitomized by electrical aversion, reflected a comparatively uncomplicated view of etiology. Early learning theorists believed that alcoholics drink abusively because they have learned that alcohol is an effective means of reducing conditioned anxiety. Empirical support for this view derived from the animal laboratory (Conger, 1951; 1956); clinical support came from the observation that alcohol seems to ease prevailing high levels of anxiety in alcoholics. Behavioral research with humans suggesting just the opposite, however, weakened support for this unidimensional view of alcoholism's etiology (Mello, 1972; Nathan and O'Brien, 1971; Okulitch and Marlatt, 1972). In its place, multidimensional theories of etiology were proposed.

Etiologic theories of alcoholism from the behavioral perspective have since grown both more numerous and more sophisticated and have been more closely tied to research findings. As with social learning theory generally, behavioral views on alcoholism have added cognitive elements as mediating variables to the learning factors considered responsible for the development of abusive drinking. Marlatt, active in the development of the cognitive, social learning conceptualizations of alcoholism, has portrayed this contemporary view of alcoholism: "Problem drinking is viewed as a multiply determined, learned behavioral disorder. It can be understood best through the empirically derived principles of social learning, cognitive psychology, and behavior therapies . . . Particular attention is paid to the determinants of drinking behavior . . . An equal emphasis is placed on the consequences of drinking, which serve to maintain the behavior" (Marlatt and Donovan, 1982, 561).

Acceptance of contemporary social learning views of alcoholism does not require rejection of other etiologic factors, either the sociocultural (Cahalan and Room, 1974; Vaillant and Milofsky, 1982) or the genetic and physiological ones (Goodwin and Guze, 1974). The behavioral position, instead, presumes that while learning may play a prepotent role in the alcoholism of some individuals, it does not necessarily do so in the absence of other important etiologic factors.

BEHAVIORAL ASSESSMENT OF ALCOHOLISM

The behavioral view of assessment assumes that much maladaptive (and adaptive) behavior is learned and, hence, subject to continual alteration and modification by past and present environmental circumstance. Many who assess psychopathology from the behavioral perspective focus on the five crucial assessment elements first outlined by Tharp and Wetzel (1969).

1. The target behavior itself—the frequency, intensity, and pattern of psychopathological behavior
2. Antecedent events—the "setting events" for the individual's maladaptive behavior

3. Maintaining stimuli—the environmental factors which reinforce the target behaviors
4. Reinforcement hierarchy—the range of factors in the environment which reinforce both target and nontarget behaviors
5. Potentials for remediation in the environment

Limitations of space preclude a detailed review of each of these assessment elements as applied to alcoholism. Target behaviors and antecedent events in alcoholism have been assessed in the laboratory (e.g., Mello and Mendelson, 1965; 1966; Nathan et al., 1970; Nathan and O'Brien, 1971; Bigelow et al., 1974; Tracey et al., 1976; Marlatt et al., 1975; Higgins and Marlatt, 1973; 1975; Caudill and Marlatt, 1975) and in natural settings (Marlatt, 1976; 1981; Selzer, 1971; Oates and McCoy, 1973; Cahalan et al., 1969). With regard to reinforcement hierarchies and environmental potentials, Cohen, Bigelow, Griffiths, Liebson, and their colleagues at the Baltimore City Hospitals have been almost alone in their systematic exploration of environmental reinforcers capable of modifying maladaptive drinking (e.g., Bigelow et al., 1972; Bigelow et al., 1981). This review focuses on the third element, maintaining stimuli, primarily because of the availability of recent findings in this area.

In an earlier review of research on the assessment of maintaining stimuli, the author and Lisman discussed three determinants of drinking which behavioral researchers had studied most extensively to that time (Nathan and Lisman, 1976). First, social interaction was clearly seen as facilitating alcohol consumption for most alcoholics but had little or no effect on others, and the reciprocal reinforcement between alcohol and social interaction seemed to account for the disorder's recalcitrance. Second, the theory that anxiety and social stress play an etiologic role (the tension-reduction model of alcohol consumption) was not well-supported in much of the experimental literature. Most of the positive findings appeared to be related to laboratory conditions, rather than real-life tension-inducing situations. Third, studies at that time tentatively confirmed the long-held views regarding set and social influence. As children, alcoholics may learn models of heavy drinking behavior from their parents, just as adult alcoholics model their drinking companions' behavior. Since this review, the impact on people's drinking behavior of their expectations about alcohol's effects has also been investigated intensively.

Alcohol and Expectancies

Regarding this line of research, Donovan and Marlatt stated, "An individual's cognitive expectancies concerning the effects of alcohol may exert a greater degree of control over drinking and subsequent behavior than the pharmacological effects of the drug" (Donovan and Marlatt, 1980, 1159). As they summarized the way in which social expectancies operate, specific expectations about alcohol develop through peer and parental modeling, direct and indirect experiences with drinking, and media exposure. A first set of expectations relates to mood alteration. Another expectation is enhanced social interaction and perceptions of control or power. A final group of expectancies about alcohol has arisen from traditional views of alcoholism and applies more to alcoholics than to social drinkers. Alcoholics in particular may expect to feel craving sensations and thus feel compelled to drink.

Development of the "balanced placebo design," which permits an unencumbered view of alcohol's pharmacologic and expectancy-induced effects (Marlatt et al., 1973; Wilson, 1981), has led to a diverse set of studies. The balanced placebo design entails giving alcohol to subjects who believe that they have received a placebo and giving a placebo to subjects who believe that they have received alcohol. The belief that one has consumed alcohol appears to exert a more important influence than consuming alcohol on the following behaviors: subsequent drinking in alcoholics (Marlatt et al., 1973); social anxiety (Wilson and Abrams, 1977); sexual responsiveness (Lansky and Wilson, 1981; Wilson and Lawson, 1976); aggression (Heermans and Nathan, 1983; Pihl et al., 1981); delay of gratification (Abrams and Wilson, 1980); mood states (McCollam et al., 1980); motor abilities (Vuchinich and Sobell, 1978); assertiveness (Parker et al., 1981); and cognitive processes such as attention and recognition memory (Lansky and Wilson, 1981). Generalizations from this research are difficult. Sometimes expectations about the impact of alcohol on behavior are divergent from its actual effects (e.g., sexual responsiveness, mood), while at other times the two converge (e.g., assertiveness; social anxiety). Convergence or divergence of expectations and drug effects probably vary as a function of subject sex, research setting, or experimental design.

BEHAVIORAL TREATMENT OF ALCOHOLISM

Treatment Goals

Until the decade of the 1970s, virtually every alcoholism worker accepted but one treatment goal: total, complete, and absolute abstinence. This goal was based upon the widely held conviction that alcoholism is a physical disease characterized by craving for alcohol during periods of sobriety and loss of control over drinking during periods of intoxication.

There are several good reasons for maintaining abstinence as the sole criterion of successful treatment for alcoholism. The disease model of alcoholism both removes the moral stigma from which alcoholics have long suffered and justifies the abstinence criterion. One cannot obviously endorse providing a sick person with the agent which has caused his or her sickness. Further, abstinence is the easiest of all treatment goals to define and monitor. As well, abstinence is a goal appropriate for all alcoholics. Finally, for those alcoholics whose alcoholism has been accompanied by serious physical sequelae, any treatment goal that does not include abstinence is life threatening.

Given this weight of public and professional opinion, why has another treatment goal—that of controlled social drinking—engendered both public support and public controversy? The concept achieved viability for three reasons. (1) Some alcoholics drink normally, in controlled fashion, either spontaneously or following treatment. (2) Abstinence is not always a component of successful treatment for alcoholism. (3) The disease model of alcoholism does not have firm basis in empirical fact.

A substantial literature, mostly appearing during the last 15 years, now suggests that some abusive drinkers (the precise number and kind remain uncertain) adopt patterns of controlled social drinking either spontaneously or following treatment (Miller and Caddy, 1977). The Rand reports on a national survey of approximately 14,000 clients of 44 fed-erally funded alcoholism treatment centers figure importantly in this literature (Armor et al., 1978; Polich et al., 1981). Among the findings in the 1978 report, some 70 percent of clients completing treatment showed improvement in drinking behavior at 6- and 18-month follow-ups, and at 18 months about one-fourth of the clients had abstained for at least 6 months. At 18 months, most of the improved clients were, however, "either drinking moderate amounts of alcohol—but at levels far below what could be described as alcoholic drinking—or engaging in alternating periods of drinking and abstention" (Armor et al., 1978, v). Among the findings reported in 1981, roughly one in five of the patients who could be interviewed at the four-year mark were judged to be drinking without problems, and they were no more likely than abstainers to manifest concurrent psychiatric symptoms, nor apparently more likely to relapse into problem drinking (Polich et al., 1981).

A variety of explicit behavioral attempts to induce controlled drinking have been reported over the past several years. Most of those identified with these therapeutic approaches claim that their techniques change abusive drinking into controlled social drinking in some subjects for some length of time. The author's own view is that, with one exception (the well-known study by Mark and Linda Sobell discussed below), the outcome data on controlled drinking treatment of chronic alcoholics have not been encouraging. Sufficient data do not exist to justify widespread application of controlled drinking treatment to groups of alcoholic clients. In contrast, more recent research on controlled drinking treatment for problem drinkers (also reviewed below) is more promising.

The traditional view that craving and loss of control invariably accompany abusive drinking has also been questioned. Alcohol given to sober alcoholics in disguised form often fails to induce craving (e.g., Cutter et al., 1970; Marlatt et al., 1973; Merry, 1966), and many alcoholics who have been drinking in uncontrolled fashion can modify their drinking when given appropriate contingent reinforcement (Gottheil et al., 1973; Marlatt, 1978; Nathan and O'Brien, 1971; Strickler et al., 1976).

Another traditional view, that the alcoholic who achieves abstinence will also demonstrate improvement in other areas of functioning, has also been challenged. Pattison (1976) cites an impressive number of studies which show that ". . . the use of total abstinence as the outcome criterion of alcoholism treatment is misleading. It may be associated with improvement, no change, or deterioration in other critical areas of total life health" (180).

The author's view of this controversial matter is that, for a variety of good reasons, abstinence ought to be the goal of treatment for alcoholism. (See Nathan and Niaura [in press] for a detailed consideration of the reasons.) Whether controlled drinking is an appropriate goal for early-stage problem drinkers remains an open question. (See Nathan [1983] for a discussion of this possibility.)

Procedures That Focus on Abusive Drinking

It is ironic that the first procedure to be closely linked with both behavior therapy and alcoholism—*electrical aversion*—is almost certainly ineffective. One reason that electrical aversion has been associated through the years with both behavior therapy and the behavioral treatment of alcoholism was Kantorovich's reported success with electrical aversion more than fifty years ago. Pairing the sight, taste, and smell of beverage alcohol with painful electric shock, Kantorovich reported that 70 percent of his small group of subjects had remained abstinent during follow-up periods ranging from three weeks to twenty months. Control subjects given hypnotic suggestion or medication did not do nearly as well.

The most convincing demonstration of the ineffectiveness of electrical aversion as a treatment for alcoholism was reported by Wilson et al. (1975). After receiving a very large number of electrical aversion conditioning trials extending over several days, their alcoholic subjects were permitted to drink ad libitum in a laboratory setting which neither encouraged nor discouraged consumption. Subjects drank with undiminished enthusiasm, just as they had during a comparable ad libitum period pretreatment, and Wilson and his co-workers concluded that conditioned aversion had not been established.

Covert sensitization aims to induce aversion by imaginal means; the aversive goal is usually nausea (Cautela, 1966; 1970). Covert sensitization has not heretofore been considered effective, because treatment studies used only small numbers of subjects who were followed for brief periods of time and assessed by weak outcome measures. However, a recent report is more adequate methodologically and more convincing clinically (Elkins, 1980). Of 57 chronic alcoholic subjects who entered treatment, 52 remained in treatment for at least six covert sensitization sessions. A variety of physiological correlates of nausea, including respiratory and GSR changes, confirmed nausea induction in 45 subjects. Of this group, 29 developed "conditioned nausea," in which an association was established between alcohol cues (e.g., sight, smell, taste, and swallowing) and the experience of nausea. Mean total abstinence after discharge for this group of subjects was 13.74 months; subjects who did not develop conditioned nausea were abstinent, on average, for fewer than five months.

In the 1940s and 1950s, Voegtlin, Lemere, and their colleagues at the Shadel Hospital in Seattle published a series of reports on the successful use of *chemical aversion* to treat alcoholism. The procedures followed at the Shadel Hospital were described by Voegtlin (1940) and Lemere and Voegtlin (1950). Patients were hospitalized for approximately ten days; the five treatment sessions were spaced on alternate days. Treatment sessions took place in rooms that were specially designed to minimize distractions and maximize visibility of a large array of alcoholic beverages. An emetine-pilocarpine-ephedrine mixture was administered intravenously, producing nausea within two to eight minutes. Immediately prior to initial signs of nausea, the patient was given a drink of his or her preferred beverage to smell, then to taste. Further drinks were given over a thirty-minute to one-hour period, as nausea and vomiting persisted.

Results of the first 13 years of treatment at the Shadel Hospital were based on follow-up data from 4,096 of 4,468 patients treated, a most impressive follow-up of 92 percent. Of these patients, 44 percent had remained totally abstinent over 2 to 13 years, while another 7 percent had relapsed and been successfully retreated. Of patients followed up, 60 percent had been abstinent for one year, 51 percent for 2 years, 38 percent for 5 years, and 23 percent for 10 years.

These outcome data are remarkably similar to those reported more recently by Wiens et al. (1976): 63 percent of 261 alcoholic patients treated by emetine conditioning at the Raleigh Hills Hospital in Portland were abstinent after one year. Another Raleigh Hills Hospital has reported one-year abstinence rates averaging 54 percent. From a low of 36 percent for patients who were younger than 62 years of age, disabled, unemployed, and on Medicare, the rates ranged to a high of 73 percent for patients who were married and employed (Neubuerger et al., 1981; Neubuerger et al., 1982).

Procedures That Focus on Antecedents and Consequences

Contingencies have always been a part of both formal and informal treatment for alcoholism. The alcoholic whose wife refuses to talk, have sex, or cook for him if his drinking continues is being subjected to a punishment contingency. So is the saleswoman who is told that she will lose her job if she continues to drink. Professionals who have limited experience with alcoholics often marvel at the fact that alcoholics continue to drink in the face of such dire consequences. The behavioral explanation of this paradox is twofold. (1) What may seem punishing to an observer may be reinforcing, or at least not punishing, to the alcoholic. (2) A contingency is effective only when it is based on mutual agreement, carefully observed, and consistently carried out. Spouses and employers rarely adhere to contingency contracts as rigorously as they should for maximum effectiveness.

The *community reinforcement counseling* program was developed by Hunt and Azrin (1973) and later modified by Azrin (1976) to provide chronic alcoholic inpatients with behavioral training focusing on long-standing vocational, interpersonal, and familial problems. The alcoholics began to experience family, job, and friends as more reinforcing as they became more successful in dealing with them. These newfound reinforcers were then incorporated into a contingency management program in which the patients, once outside the hospital, had access to them contingent on sobriety. At a six-month follow-up, the eight alcoholics who had received community reinforcement counseling had spent significantly less time drinking, unemployed, away from home, or institutionalized than eight other alcoholics who had received only the hospital's standard therapy program.

Finer-grained analysis of the effects of contingent reinforcement and punishment has been a consistent goal of a research group at the Baltimore City Hospitals. Among the first of the group's efforts to use *natural contingencies* was Bigelow's successful effort to induce abstinence in four hospital employees who were in danger of being fired for drinking on the job (Bigelow et al., 1973). Required by contingency contract to report daily to the hospital's alcoholism treatment unit for disulfiram therapy, the four were told that failure to report would result in no work and no pay. The contingency produced striking improvements in all employees' job performance and attendance. In like fashion, Liebson and his co-workers (1973) drew up contracts with nine heroin addicts who were simultaneously abusing alcohol. The contracts specified that each man would be maintained on methadone, a potent reinforcer, so long as he continued to ingest disulfiram and to maintain abstinence from alcohol. The treatment was a rousing success with a group of patients notoriously difficult to treat: drinking took place on only 1.4 percent of patient days when methadone maintenance was contingent on disulfiram ingestion, but on 19.2 percent of days when it was not.

Broad-Spectrum Procedures

THE IBTA STUDY Psychologists Mark and Linda Sobell in 1970 developed a broad-spectrum behavioral treatment package they called individualized behavior therapy for alcoholics (IBTA). The evaluation study which they subsequently carried out at the Patton State Hospital (California) has become extremely well-known and also very controversial. They found that, regardless of assigned treatment goal (abstinence or controlled drinking), one and two years posttreatment the patients receiving IBTA appeared to be drinking in controlled fashion significantly more frequently than control patients. However, some have raised questions about the adequacy of the study's design and follow-up methodology.

IBTA subjects engaged in a series of "behavior change training sessions" in which they identified the functions of their excessive drinking and alternate, more positive behavior. Nondrinker and controlled drinker experimental groups received the same treatment, except that the latter subjects were trained and practiced in controlled drinking. The sessions thus incorporated four stages: (1) problem identification; (2) identification of alternative responses to drinking; (3) evaluation of alternatives; and (4) preparation to engage in the best behavioral alternative (Sobell, 1978).

First-year outcome data, reported in 1973 (Sobell and Sobell, 1973), revealed that both experimental treatment groups (nondrinkers and controlled drinkers) achieved levels of functioning, including reductions in alcohol-related problems, superior to their respective control groups. These data were based on follow-up information from 69 of the study's original 70 subjects, an impressive follow-up retention rate. At the end of the second follow-up year, the experimental controlled drinkers were continuing to function better than their controls, while the experimental nondrinker subjects were doing better, but not significantly better, than their controls (Sobell and Sobell, 1976). Unexpectedly, subjects in the controlled drinker experimental group reported significantly more abstinent days than nondrinker experimental subjects, for whom abstinence was the sole treatment goal.

A follow-up of the experimental controlled drinkers ten years after they were treated by the Sobells reported that only one of the twenty subjects had successfully controlled his drinking over several years (Pendery et al., 1982). Most had experienced rehospitalization, alcohol-related arrests, and heavy-drinking bouts. It is unfortunate that Pendery et al. failed to report on a parallel follow-up of control subjects. The absence of the latter data makes valid conclusions about the experimental subjects' outcomes impossible. Even though most of the experimental subjects were doing badly ten years later, it is possible that the control subjects had done even worse. An unpublished version of the Pendery et al. paper and media interviews raised additional questions, including the initial random assignment of subjects to experimental and control groups, the frequency of subject follow-up, and the integrity of the Sobells' reports of design, procedures, and outcome.

The seriousness of these charges led the Addiction Research Foundation of Toronto, the Sobells' employer, to appoint a four-person committee of inquiry to look into these allegations. After very thorough consideration of all available documentation from the Sobells' original study, but without the cooperation of Pendery et al., who refused to furnish data from their own follow-up, the committee concluded that the Sobells had carried out the research in the way they reported and that they had not misrepresented the results. By design, the committee did not evaluate a central issue: whether alcoholics can be taught to moderate their drinking.

INTEGRATED BEHAVIOR CHANGE TECHNIQUES In three reports, Volger et al. (1975; 1977a; 1977b) described the use of "integrated behavior change techniques" with groups of alcoholics and problem drinkers. The methods included many of the procedures which had been components of the Sobells' IBTA (Vogler and the Sobells had worked together for a time at the Patton State Hospital).

Four groups of problem drinkers participated in the second trial (Vogler et al., 1977b). From an original pool of 409 subjects, 80 were followed through to the one-year follow-up mark. A group of 23 received the full complement of integrated behavior change techniques, another group (19) received blood alcohol level discrimination training, behavioral counseling, alternatives training, and alcohol education, a third group (21) received only alcohol education, and a fourth group (17) received behavioral counseling, alternatives training, and alcohol education. The treatment goal for subjects in all groups was moderation. Fifty of the 80 subjects completing treatment and follow-up were considered moderate drinkers at the one-year follow-up mark; 3 additional subjects had maintained abstinence over the same period. Overall, subjects had decreased their consumption of absolute ethanol by 50 to 65 percent. Unexpectedly, membership in the four treatment groups was not associated with differential outcomes, raising serious questions about relationships between treatment method and outcome.

MIDDLE-INCOME PROBLEM DRINKERS Pomerleau and his colleagues (1978) at the University of Pennsylvania School of Medicine offered broad-spectrum behavior therapy to a group of problem drinkers who differed from both the problem drinkers and alcoholics treated by Vogler and his colleagues and the chronic alcoholics treated by the Sobells. They were almost certainly more highly motivated for treatment, more intact intellectually, socially, and emotionally, and possessed of greater familial, vocational, and economic resources than the prior groups of broad-spectrum behavior therapy patients studied. Of 32 problem drinkers selected, 18 were randomly assigned to behavioral treatment and 14 to so-called traditional treatment. Treatment, behavioral and traditional, was conducted in groups of 3 to 7 problem drinkers for ninety minutes once a week for three months, then for five additional sessions programmed at increasing intervals for another nine months.

Behavioral treatment consisted of four overlapping phases. A baseline phase involved a detailed drinking history, a treatment fee, a refundable "commitment fee" of up to $300, and instruction on recording consumption, drink by drink, and on identifying situations which led to excessive drinking. The second phase targeted reduction in drinking as an objective. Subjects designated daily quotas for a week's worth of drinking at a time, as well as final treatment goals (abstinence or controlled drinking). Stimulus control and contingency management techniques enabled subjects to identify appropriate and inappropriate drinking circumstances, to delay or interfere with maladaptive drinking patterns, and to increase the likelihood of not drinking in designated situations. In a third phase, behavior therapy focused on altering behavioral problems that had the capacity to affect drinking behavior. Finally, to help patients maintain gains in drinking behavior and social and vocational spheres, a fourth phase encouraged them to develop interests in alcohol-free activities. New friends, rather than old drinking companions, were recommended.

Of 18 patients treated by behavioral techniques, 16 remained in treatment throughout; in contrast, of 14 patients treated by traditional procedures, only 8 remained to the end of the treatment. Drinking rate decreased significantly from screening to the end of the follow-up year in both treatment groups. The fact that significantly fewer behavioral participants dropped out of treatment suggests a modest advantage for behavioral over traditional treatment.

EARLY-STAGE PROBLEM DRINKERS Martha Sanchez-Craig, a psychologist at the Addiction Research Foundation, Toronto, recently reported on a cognitive-behavioral program offered to 70 socially stable, early-stage problem drinkers in good physical health. Following thorough pretreatment assessment, subjects were randomly assigned to a treatment goal of abstinence or of controlled drinking. Each of two therapists taught controlled drinking to half the subjects who were assigned that goal and abstinence to half the subjects in that group. Six weekly individual sessions were required, each lasting less than ninety minutes (Sanchez-Craig, 1980).

During the first three weeks of treatment, subjects in the abstinence group drank on a greater number of days ($p<.05$) and drank more heavily when drinking occurred ($p<.01$). Analysis of the acceptability of the two drinking goals to the subjects indicated that subjects in the controlled-drinking conditions more frequently accepted the assigned goal ($p<.001$). While six-month follow-up data on the 59 subjects who remained in treatment and could be located for follow-up indicated no significant outcome differences between treatment groups, Sanchez-Craig and Annis (1982) concluded that moderate drinking goals are viable with early-stage problem drinkers. The abstinence goal is more often unacceptable to them, and hence moderate drinking may be the only basis on which early prevention efforts may be offered—and followed.

FUTURE TRENDS

The exploration of cognitive mediating processes important in the maintenance of chronic alcoholism, along with procedures for their modification by behavioral means, will increase rapidly over the next few years. The nature of cognitive processes and their influence on adaptive and maladaptive behavior have begun to be studied intensively by behavioral researchers outside (Bandura, 1977; Mahoney, 1974; Meichenbaum, 1977) and within (Marlatt, 1978; Wilson, 1981) the alcoholism arena. No longer will behavioral researchers be content to attribute responsibility for maladaptive drinking solely to external environmental variables. The important additional impact of what alcoholics tell themselves about their drinking and its effect on them will be a continuing research subject. One outcome of basic research findings to date has been their application in the broad-spectrum behavior therapy programs.

More emphasis on primary and secondary prevention of alcohol problems and less emphasis on tertiary prevention will increasingly characterize the field. As elsewhere, behavior therapists working with alcoholics have chosen to concentrate their efforts on the remediation of existing problems. Much less attention has been paid to adolescents at risk for alcoholism or to problem drinkers who might already have begun to acquire the behavioral stigma of alcoholism. Despite the infusion of large sums of money for these programs, we have not developed the ways and means to prevent alcoholism in groups at risk (Nathan, 1983). For this reason, the author is particularly enthusiastic about the efforts of Sanchez-Craig and her colleagues to teach moderate drinking to early-stage problem drinkers (Sanchez-Craig, 1980; Sanchez-Craig and Annis, 1982). Perhaps the targeted effort to work with a risk group in this early phase will yield outcomes superior to those we have achieved up to this time.

Chapter 22

Psychotherapy in the Treatment of Alcoholism
by Sheila B. Blume, M.D.

INTRODUCTION

Thoughtful consideration of the problems and techniques involved in psychotherapy with alcoholic patients raises a series of basic questions. Is a theoretical psychodynamic explanation of alcoholism a necessary condition for successful psychotherapy with alcoholic patients? Must any such psychodynamic construct differentiate alcoholism from other forms of drug addiction? Can the large group of disparate patients loosely termed alcoholics be subclassified in a way that will help us to choose the most appropriate psychodynamic approaches? Where does psychotherapy fit into the overall scheme of alcoholism treatment? How does psychotherapy with alcoholic patients differ from the psychotherapeutic treatment of other disorders?

Addressing these questions is important in an update such as this, since both the medical education and the psychiatric training experiences that most psychiatrists receive are remarkably silent on these issues. Indeed, it is the rule rather than the exception for a practicing psychiatrist to complete residency training without ever having been responsible for the psychotherapeutic treatment of a primary alcoholic patient. Yet we know from population surveys that one out of ten adult Americans who drinks experiences significant alcohol-related problems and that between 20 and 50 percent of medical and surgical hospital admissions are in some way related to drinking.* Thus, alcoholic patients

*Editor's note: In Part III of this volume, Cavanaugh and Wettstein review the available studies on the prevalence of alcohol-related disorders among medical inpatients.

may be found in every medical practice, whether or not they are recognized. Fortunately, appropriate treatment leads to success more often than failure, and few experiences are more satisfying than helping to guide the recovery of an alcoholic patient.

CONCEPTUAL FRAMEWORK FOR PSYCHOTHERAPY WITH ALCOHOLIC PATIENTS

Psychodynamic Constructs

A review of the older literature reveals the general viewpoint that alcoholism, like most other disorders affecting feeling, thought, and behavior, has its roots in early childhood experience (e.g., see Knight, 1938). Among later writers, this view is either tacitly assumed (e.g., Twerski, 1982; Silber, 1982) or articulated (e.g., Zimberg, 1982; Mack, 1981), whether for alcoholism alone or as a general underlying factor in all compulsive drug use (e.g., Kohut, 1977; Khantzian and Treece, 1977). Such views are based primarily on retrospective data gathered in clinical treatment. Unfortunately, however, patient recollections are very often significantly distorted (see the excellent case study by Vaillant, 1981).

An alternative view is supported by Vaillant's large-scale longitudinal studies of alcohol abuse in white males (Vaillant, 1983). The psychopathology of alcohol-dependent patients can be conceptualized as a reaction or an adaptation to the traumatic experience of becoming and being an alcoholic (Bean, 1981; Wallace, 1978). As Bean has described it, "The personality disruption . . . overlies and may partially obscure the original personality, which will reemerge when the alcoholism is treated, with two other developments possibly added. The alcoholic may have permanent or temporary personality destruction on a neurological basis, and he may have massive repair and relearning to do to restore his psychic integrity after the devastating experiences that occur in the lives of alcoholics, much as a stroke victim or concentration-camp inmate will be affected by his experience" (Bean, 1981, 56).

What is the practical importance of these alternative views? The first is that, whatever one's perspective, neither treatment of the underlying nor of the reactive psychopathology alone will cure the alcohol dependence. Once such a dependence is established or the patient is clearly headed in that direction, first attention must be given to interrupting the drinking and establishing a stable state of sobriety (Blane, 1977; Zimberg, 1978; Blume, 1982; Bean, 1981; Khantzian, 1981). The failure to appreciate this important principle has been the single greatest cause of frustration and failure in the psychotherapeutic treatment of alcoholic patients. The second important principle is that resolution of deep psychological conflict is not a necessary condition for achieving stable recovery. The majority of recoveries are achieved without reconstructive psychotherapy, although fundamental changes do occur in attitudes, values, and self-concept, as well as in behavior.

Classification of Patients

Many useful classifications have been proposed. Jellinek (1960), considering alcoholism in its widest sense, classified alcoholics into alpha, beta, gamma, delta, and epsilon groups. Gamma and delta alcoholics were the only subgroups that he considered to be suffering from alcoholism as a disease.

DSM-III offers the diagnoses of Alcohol Dependence (303.9x) and Alcohol Abuse (305.0x) (American Psychiatric Association, 1980). Patients diagnosed under Alcohol Dependence should be approached and treated as outlined in this chapter. Those diagnosed under Alcohol Abuse will be a mixed group of early-stage, predependent alcoholics and patients with a wide variety of other patterns of drinking causing interpersonal and social problems. Clinical judgment must dictate the individual approach. However, where there is a strong family history of alcoholism, and when otherwise in doubt, the safest course will be to assume that the patient is in an early stage of alcohol dependence, to treat him or her as such, and also to make the assumption explicit.*

A third suggested subclassification is between primary alcoholism (without preexisting diagnosable psychiatric disorder) and secondary alcoholism (with either a history of a preexisting psychiatric disorder or such a disorder developing during prolonged abstinence) (Schuckit and Morrissey, 1976). In men, secondary alcoholism is most frequently associated with sociopathic personality disorder, and in women, with affective disorder, usually recurrent depression. An important principle here is that although the primary-secondary distinction will be useful in long-term management, the term secondary does not imply a causal relationship. Treating the psychiatric disorder alone cannot therefore be expected to cure the alcoholism. The alcoholism itself requires specific treatment.

Two other conceptualizations, reactive alcoholism (Knight, 1938) and situational alcoholism, relate the patient's pathological alcohol use to a specific life problem or precipitating event. The same caveat applies. Although attention to such proximal events will be critical in psychotherapy, appropriate direct attention must also be paid to interrupting the drinking itself.

Another important subgroup comprises those patients with other drug dependencies in addition to their alcoholism. The same general approach should be used with these patients, although more general concepts and terms may be applicable, e.g., chemical dependency rather than alcoholism and drug free rather than sober.

These considerations remind us that with alcoholic patients, as with others, our general treatment framework must be adapted to the unique history, reactions, pressures, and motivations of each individual, and that we must never neglect active involvement with all members of the family and attention to immediate life problems. Assessments of the stage of the disease, such as that suggested by Zimberg (1982), and of ego function, such as that of Greenspan (1977), may be of assistance in this respect.

Psychotherapy in the Overall Treatment Context

Table 1 presents a scheme of alcoholism treatment which shows the great variety of settings and combinations in which the psychotherapies may

---

*Preceptor's note: Robins goes into greater detail on the DSM-III diagnoses in her chapter, and Nathan considers some different approaches to the behavioral treatment of alcoholic patients and problem drinkers.

Table 1. Components of Treatment for Alcoholic Patients

Phases	Goals	Modalities	Settings
Identification and Intervention	1. Recognize and define problem 2. Enter treatment	Breaking down rationalization and denial via nonjudgmental confrontation Individual, family, or group psychotherapeutic counseling	Hospital or physician's office Information/referral agency Employee assistance program Drinking driver program School or welfare agency Criminal justice system In- or outpatient medical or psychiatric services
Detoxification	1. Save life 2. Become alcohol and sedative free 3. Enter rehabilitation	Pharmacotherapy Good nursing care Nutrition Individual, family, or group counseling	*Inpatient* Hospital medical unit Freestanding detox unit *Outpatient* Ambulatory detox (clinic or emergency service, private practitioner)
Rehabilitation Motivation Understanding alcoholism Understanding self New ways to handle old problems Emergency plan	1. Change self-concept and attitude 2. Change personality traits 3. Change life-style 4. Restore physical health, nutrition 5. Help for family	Self-help groups Individual and group psychotherapies Marital and family treatment Psychodrama Physical health care Psychiatric management Disulfiram Recreation therapy Spiritual counseling Vocational rehabilitation Legal aid	*Inpatient* Specialized unit (hospital or free-standing) Night hospital Community residence *Outpatient* Clinic Day program Private practice (Plus self-help groups)
Long-Term Follow-Up	1. Prevent relapse 2. Maintain and reinforce new patterns of sober living	As above for Rehabilitation Physician available for help regularly and as needed	*Outpatient* Clinic Private practice (Plus self-help groups)

Source: Adapted from Blume (1982).

be used. The physician's office or the outpatient clinic can be seen as one of the most important settings for the accomplishment of each treatment component.

While the four distinct phases of treatment have differing goals and methods, some form of counseling or psychotherapy is integral to each phase. The time sequence of phases is important. Measures that may be very helpful at a later phase of treatment will be fruitless or counter-productive if applied earlier. For example, such rehabilitative methods as vocational training and formal sex therapy, applied with an alcoholic patient who has not been detoxified and who has not established so-briety, will be unsuccessful. The resulting frustration for patients, fam-ily, and therapist will merely succeed in adding one more failure to each party's list. Similarly, in cases of relapse, rehabilitative changes in living or working arrangements will not stop the drinking. Such changes should be deferred until the relapse is identified appropriately, detoxification has been completed, and the patient is reengaged in the rehabilitation phase of the treatment.

The first phase, identification and intervention, involves helping the patient recognize that his or her drinking is a major cause of the im-mediate and painful presenting life problems, rather than the reverse. The patient also needs to see that impaired control over alcohol use is part of an illness and that treatment is available which will lead to re-covery. Constructive and nonjudgmental confrontation in a work, school, criminal justice, family, or health care setting is frequently required. The alcoholic patient does not often spontaneously seek help stating, "I be-lieve I have a drinking problem." Rather, the patient's drinking may still offer some relief or at least escape from the pain generated by his or her many severe problems, both external and internal. This phase is con-cluded successfully when the patient and, if possible, the family agree to enter treatment specifically for the alcoholism.

The second phase, detoxification, must be complete before rehabili-tation can begin. At the same time, the therapist must make it clear to both the patient and the family that drying out alone is not sufficient treatment for alcoholism. Work on a mutually acceptable long-range treatment plan should begin as soon as the detoxification begins.

Rehabilitation develops progressively in a series of stages later dis-cussed in the context of psychotherapeutic technique and includes sev-eral important components.

1. Continued attention to patient motivation, aimed at developing self-motivation to replace external pressures
2. Education about the nature and course of alcoholism, its effects on the family, and the dangers of other drugs of dependency
3. Increasing self-knowledge, particularly concerning the role of alcohol in the patient's life: as psychoactive drug, as medicine, as weapon, as excuse, and as substitute for other satisfactions
4. Opening new options for handling life problems without alcohol, us-ing social support systems and improved interpersonal relationships
5. Developing a carefully thought out emergency plan—including tele-phone numbers to call and a prearranged way to establish a tempo-rary safe environment—for use in case of unexpected emotional dis-tress which might otherwise lead to relapse

Goals of the rehabilitation phase include helping family members and reestablishing the patient's physical health, as well as improving individual functioning and self-esteem.

Finally, the long-term follow-up phase attempts to consolidate the gains made in rehabilitation and to prevent relapse.

Although the discussion that follows focuses on individual psychotherapy in an outpatient or office practice, much of it applies to other therapies and settings as well. For a discussion of the techniques of group psychotherapy, family therapy, and psychodrama as applied to alcoholism, see Zimberg et al. (1978).

PSYCHOTHERAPEUTIC TECHNIQUE

When it comes to treating patients who are dependent on drugs, including alcohol, most would agree with Wurmser (1977) that one thing is very clear: one cannot do "business as usual." Individual psychotherapy is seldom used alone for alcoholic patients. It is usually combined with education about alcoholism, referral to AA, family intervention with referral to Al-Anon and Alateen, the prescription of disulfiram, and other modalities. Furthermore, the psychotherapy has three important distinguishing phases. The early, middle, and late phases of psychotherapy have different goals, techniques, and problems.

In general, the therapist takes a more active role with an alcoholic patient than with other patients. The therapist is both supportive and educative, on one hand, and confronting, on the other. It is important that the therapist understand the self-loathing, the fragile self-esteem, and the feeling of being trapped by the addiction which underlie the denial or superficial bravado of some alcoholics. In order to plan constructive confrontation, the therapist must have both a conception of the ego disturbances surrounding self-care and regulation of affect in alcohol-dependent patients (Khantzian, 1981; Mack, 1981) and an appreciation of the preferred defense structure of the alcoholic (Wallace, 1978). These understandings of the alcoholic patient are extremely important. Finally, the therapist must adopt an active involvement without accepting ultimate responsibility for the alcoholic's sobriety. Responsibility for sobriety must remain squarely in the patient's lap at all times. Other components of the active role include keeping track of the patient's alcohol and drug intake, aggressive follow-up of missed appointments, and an offer to be one of the available resources in the patient's emergency plan in case of an unexpected and otherwise unmanageable urge to drink (Blume, 1982).

The Early Phase

As with other patients, this phase includes developing a therapeutic alliance, making and discussing a diagnosis, setting goals, and negotiating a therapeutic contract, either implicit or explicit. The alcoholic patient is often initially motivated into treatment by outside forces and may be overtly angry or present with a blank wall of denial. Displaying an understanding of these feelings will help the therapist to establish the relationship of trust that is necessary in assessment, diagnosis, and goal setting (Blane, 1977; Zimberg, 1982). Assessment should include interviews with the family or others or both.

The therapeutic contract should be explicit, setting clear ground rules and expectations for both parties. A goal of abstinence from alcohol and drugs of dependence must be backed up, for example, by the patient's agreement to attend AA, take disulfiram, and so forth. The therapist agrees to help the patient make contact with AA, to oversee the use of disulfiram, to help the patient construct an emergency plan for handling unexpected craving, and to be a resource to call instead of (but not after) taking a drink.

An important maneuver in early-phase psychotherapy is building a cognitive framework in which the patient can make sense out of the disrupting feelings and loss of control he or she is experiencing. The disease concept of alcoholism is the most effective frame of reference here because it relieves guilt over having become an alcoholic without removing the responsibility for cooperating in treatment and remaining abstinent (Blume, 1983). In addition, insights derived from learning theory can be useful in helping the patient achieve initial sobriety (Galanter, 1983).

With an alcoholic patient, the therapist encounters a number of defenses, including denial, projection, all-or-none thinking, conflict minimization, rationalization, obsessional focusing, and a number of others. An example is the early sobriety rationalization, "I can't do that, I might get drunk," which may be used to avoid conflict-laden situations and relationships. Wallace (1978) has presented an excellent discussion of the alcoholic patient's preferred defenses and how they may be used in the service of recovery during the early phase. "The role of the therapist is not to expose, confront, and modify the defenses of the alcoholic client . . . Denial, rationalization, projection, and so forth have for too long been construed in moralistic terms by psychotherapists. In actuality, such mechanisms are perfectly acceptable tactics when used deliberately and selectively for particular purposes. In the case of the alcoholic, these tactics have become part of a preferred defense structure throughout years of alcoholic drinking. For a therapist to try to remove these is equivalent to trying to force water to flow uphill" (Wallace, 1978, 27).

With particular reference to denial in early psychotherapy, Bean has suggested, "It is most effective to empathize with the pain that generated the defense, and to relieve the pain by acknowledging it, offering help, instilling hope, and contradicting despair. When the pain decreases, the defense mechanism can be abandoned. In addition, denial of the dangers of drinking must be confronted, and the patient's need for safety stressed" (Bean, 1981, 91).

Zimberg has summarized the patient's feeling during this early phase of recovery, with the initial motivation from without and the need for external support and control, as "I *can't* drink" (Zimberg, 1978). When the patient develops more stable internal motivation and controls, he or she can say, "I *won't* drink," signaling the arrival at the middle stage of recovery.

The Middle Phase

Once goals have been set, immediate problems have been handled, some degree of internal control has been achieved, and an initial social support system is established, both within the family and through self-help groups, the psychotherapy can proceed to the middle phase. During this phase, problems that have been laid aside earlier are explored and worked through. The patient develops new ways to structure leisure time and to handle feelings and situations that were previously dealt with by drinking. According to the patient's needs, the treatment focuses on trying out new behaviors, from practicing self-assertion to learning patience, from controlling one's temper to expressing anger. Most important, patients learn how to relax, enjoy the pleasures of living, and express affection without a drink. The identification and discussion of feelings and aspects of self-care must receive much attention (Khantzian, 1981). Sexual problems are common in alcoholic patients and will also need attention. Conjoint sessions with a spouse or formal sex therapy may be indicated.

Transference is interpreted during this phase only when necessary to avoid disruption of treatment, and positive transference is encouraged (Blane, 1977). The patient still requires a great deal of positive reinforcement and attention to sobriety. Relapses should be handled not as personal or treatment failures, but as signals to reevaluate the structure that the patient has built for maintaining abstinence and to institute additional measures (for example, disulfiram or a self-help group). This phase of psychotherapy will usually require between six months and a year, although individual needs vary. Blane considers the middle-phase goals accomplished when the patient: "(1) reports spontaneous engagement in new activities, interests, and behavior; (2) handles unique, potentially conflictual situations in an adult and self-satisfying manner; (3) accepts setbacks without becoming anxious or depressed, or without acting-out; (4) knows and experiences feelings as they occur; (5) when conflicted, examines and works through the conflict himself or in a nondefensive way with the therapist" (Blane, 1977, 139).

The Late Phase

Most therapists and patients will elect to conclude treatment at this point, leaving an open door for further help if needed. Some patients, however, will elect to continue in deeper psychoanalytically oriented exploration of conflicts and defenses, leading, in Zimberg's framework to the conflict resolution stage of recovery. Here, the patient can say, "I don't have to drink" (Zimberg, 1978). Patients with specific personality or sexual problems may particularly profit from such treatment. Stable sobriety must, however, be well established before any attempt at deep exploration or interpretation. Otherwise, anxiety generated during the psychotherapy could precipitate relapse. The late phase of therapy may last for an additional year or two. As with termination after the middle phase, late-phase treatment should always conclude with an open invitation to return for consultation if problems arise.

The principles outlined in this chapter are useful for treating patients who suffer from the disease of alcoholism, that is, those who are already alcohol dependent or judged to be developing the dependence syndrome. Very little literature exists concerning psychotherapy with other alcohol abusers. Although the literature has more often discussed behavior therapy for this group, there is no reason to believe that psychotherapy is either inappropriate or ineffective with such patients. Treatment goals and techniques might vary with the overall picture, but close attention to drinking and drug use is always an absolute necessity with substance abusers.

Role Models

Unless the psychotherapist himself or herself is a recovered alcoholic and imparts that information, the patient receiving individual psychotherapy for alcoholism will not automatically have a positive role model for recovery. A role model is an important adjunct to treatment for a variety of reasons. The therapist should attempt to see that the patient meets others who have achieved stable remissions. If self-help groups are unavailable, autobiographies of recovered alcoholics (Allen, 1978; Rebeta-Burditt, 1977) and the book *Alcoholics Anonymous* (1955) may be of value. It is especially helpful early in therapy to introduce the patient to other alcoholics of the same sex, ethnic group, and age group in order to facilitate identification. This is particularly true for alcoholics in under-represented groups, such as Jews (Blume et al., 1980), women, Hispanics, elderly people, blacks, native Americans, and so forth. The psychotherapist should become familiar with the self-help groups in his or her community, for example, AA, Women for Sobriety, Pills Anonymous, Al-Anon family groups, and Alateen. Personal acquaintance with the groups will both facilitate individual referrals and help the therapist to evaluate the patient's reactions to the group experience. Most self-help groups are delighted to cooperate with professionals, will extend a warm welcome to them at open meetings, and will be important allies in treatment.

CONCLUSION

Psychotherapy as an integral part of the treatment of alcoholic patients can be both effective and rewarding, provided the therapist is acquainted with the special principles and techniques involved. Although it is not "business as usual," it is surely the business of our profession.

Chapter 23

Pharmacotherapy in the Detoxification and Treatment of Alcoholism

by Ernest P. Noble, Ph.D., M.D.

INTRODUCTION

Virtually no pharmacopoeia is designed specifically for the treatment of alcohol dependence and the various problems that accompany the misuse of alcohol. In marked contrast, many pharmacologic agents are available and more are developing for the treatment of other mental disorders. Clinical psychiatrists now have at their disposal a broad spectrum of anxiolytic, antipsychotic, and antidepressant drugs. However, with the exception of disulfiram, most of the drugs currently used for the various ramifications of alcoholism have been borrowed from the treatment of other mental disorders.

The problems that the misuse of alcohol engenders are multiple and complex. Ethanol, like other depressant drugs, produces both excitatory and depressant effects on both behavioral and physiological functions.

Its predominant acute effect, however, is depression of brain function. Unfortunately, the resultant impairments in motor coordination, judgment, attention, and other aspects of behavior represent a serious threat to the health and safety of both the drinker and the nondrinker. A systematic search for amethystic (sobering) agents has only recently begun, and while the development of such agents is feasible and testing under laboratory conditions has shown some candidates to be effective, clinical trials on a large scale have so far not been conducted.

Ethanol also has the property of inducing dependence in a significant number of individuals. The development of alcohol withdrawal reactions after cessation of or reduction in drinking have been well characterized (Wolfe and Victor, 1972; Gross et al., 1974). But while a large number of drugs have proven effective in aborting or mitigating withdrawal symptoms, these drugs do have significant side effects, including the liability for cross-dependence with ethanol.

Besides its ability to induce intoxication and dependence, ethanol, when used chronically, affects brain function and behavior in a variety of other ways. A recent review of the world literature (Parsons and Farr, 1981) indicates that a majority of alcoholics suffer cognitive dysfunction as demonstrated by certain visual-spatial and peripheral-motor tasks. While some reversibility in these deficits occurs with abstinence, complete recovery of brain function is rare (DeLuca, 1981; Carlen, 1982). Recent evidence also indicates that alcohol consumption in social drinkers is correlated with cognitive dysfunction (Parker and Noble, 1977; Parker et al., 1980). Currently, no drugs are available for treating ethanol-induced cognitive dysfunction.

Other organic mental disorders associated with prolonged alcohol ingestion include dementia, alcohol amnestic disorder (Korsakoff's syndrome), and alcohol hallucinosis. Again, few or no therapeutic agents are available specifically for treating these disorders.

Finally, a few alcohol-sensitizing drugs are currently used, most notably disulfiram. However, even disregarding the issue of compliance, these drugs have inherent problems.

The brief and selective review in this chapter primarily emphasizes the CNS effects of putative therapeutic agents used in intoxication and detoxification and in the treatment of alcohol problems. More comprehensive reviews of these subjects are available elsewhere (Wallgren and Barry, 1970; Noble et al., 1975; Noble, 1978; Gessner, 1979; Faiman, 1979; Alkana and Noble, 1979).

AMETHYSTIC AGENTS

A quick and safe means to antagonize acute ethanol intoxication could help reduce ethanol-induced harm. For example, amethystic agents[1] might be useful in treating acute ethanol overdose, a condition which has no specific remedy at this time. Such agents might also serve as investigative tools and lead to a better understanding of ethanol's mechanisms of action. In addition, the ability to reverse ethanol's acute effects might ultimately supply valuable insights into the adaptive pro-

[1] *Amethystic* comes from the Greek word amethystos meaning "not drunken." The Greeks believed that the mineral, amethyst, prevented intoxication. *Amethystic* is defined here as "sobering."

cesses that result in alcohol dependence. Finally, since central depression, tolerance, and withdrawal may represent a continuum of ethanol's effects over time, it seems reasonable that aborting or mitigating an initial step in the sequence might interfere with the subsequent changes induced by ethanol.

An obvious criterion for an amethystic agent is that the drug have a high potential as an ethanol antagonist. Although numerous studies report antagonistic interactions between ethanol and other drugs, and several folk remedies purportedly hasten sobriety, no chemicals or techniques are known which, as with the opiate antagonists, unequivocally and completely reverse the central depressant effects of ethanol or other general anesthetics in human beings (Alkana and Noble, 1979). Furthermore, with the exception of dialysis (Marc-Aurele and Schreiner, 1960; Koppanyi et al., 1961; Perey et al., 1965), no method is effective in rapidly eliminating ethanol from the body. As well as possessing antagonistic efficacy, the ideal amethystic agent would (1) restore behavior to predrinking levels without causing marked stimulation or inducing disturbance of natural sleep; (2) have a rapid onset of action and be effective within 15 to 30 minutes after it is taken; (3) have a sufficiently long duration of action so that blood ethanol concentration can fall below 50 mg/dl; (4) have a convenient method of administration with minimal discomfort (oral, sublingual, or via inhalation); (5) have no toxic or cumulative adverse effects either in the presence or absence of ethanol; (6) have a low abuse liability; and (7) be inexpensive and possess a long shelf life.

Once ethanol is administered, two methods are available for reversing its central effects. The first is pharmacokinetic antagonism: the amount of ethanol in the brain may be reduced by decreasing its absorption, altering its distribution, or enhancing its removal. The second method is pharmacodynamic antagonism: the effects of ethanol may be counteracted by antagonizing its actions or effects on the brain.

Pharmacokinetic Antagonism

Several means are available for reducing the rate of ethanol absorption. These generally involve substances or techniques which delay gastric emptying time or reduce gastrointestinal circulation, such as the ingestion of food or the administration of sympathomimetic or anticholinergic drugs (Kalant, 1971). However, once the blood ethanol concentration reaches an intoxicating level (100 mg/dl or greater), the limiting factor in reducing the blood ethanol concentration is the maximum rate at which ethanol can be eliminated from the body. Since this rate is approximately 15 mg/dl per hour (Wallgren and Barry, 1970), it would take several hours to achieve an appreciable reduction in the concentration, even with ethanol absorption blocked. Therefore, absorption blockade alone cannot reverse intoxication rapidly. Reversal must depend upon altered ethanol distribution, increased ethanol elimination, or central-mediated antagonism.

While drugs known to alter ethanol distribution have been studied (McNamee et al., 1975; Eskelson et al., 1976), results concerning reduction of ethanol effects have been inconsistent. Since approximately 95 percent of the ethanol entering an organism is eliminated by oxidation, primarily in the liver, agents that enhance ethanol metabolism could conceivably be of value in reinstating sobriety. The rate of ethanol elimination is determined primarily by the rate of hepatic oxidation of ethanol to acetaldehyde via the enzyme alcohol dehydrogenase (ADH), with the coenzyme nicotinamide-adenine-dinucleotide (NAD) acting as the hydrogen acceptor. The rate of reoxidation of NADH formed during the metabolism of ethanol and acetaldehyde is thought now to be the rate-limiting factor for ethanol oxidation (Lindros et al., 1972). Theoretically, therefore, ethanol metabolism may be enhanced by augmenting the oxidation of NADH to NAD, or perhaps by increasing the NAD-to-NADH ratio by adding exogenous NAD. Unfortunately, exogenous administration of NAD to ethanol-treated rats did not enhance ethanol metabolism (Majchrowicz et al., 1967). Moreover, in another study (Wilson, 1967), while the administration of nicotinamide raised the concentration of NAD in mouse liver, it did not alter the rate of ethanol elimination.

Although numerous other agents have been tested for their amethystic efficacy, including carbohydrates, insulin, proteins, amino acids, glycogen, and glucocorticoids, no known substances can produce the tenfold acceleration in ethanol elimination that is required to reinstate sobriety. Detailed reviews on this subject are available in the literature (Wallgren and Barry, 1970; Noble et al., 1975; Alkana and Noble, 1979). Of all agents tested, fructose appears to be the most effective stimulator of ethanol elimination. Reported accelerations vary from 15 percent to over 100 percent (Lowenstein et al., 1970; Thieden et al., 1972; Damgaard et al., 1973), but the effect is inconsistent. The mechanism underlying the increased rate of elimination is unknown. It may involve a fructose-induced increase in oxidation of NADH to NAD, coupled with inhibited ethanol absorption (Thieden et al., 1972; Clark et al., 1973). In view of the reports indicating that fructose may induce dangerous adverse effects (Cohen, 1972; Levy et al., 1977) and the relatively small degree of acceleration compared with the required tenfold increase, fructose clearly does not represent a practical amethystic agent.

Pharmacodynamic Antagonism

Considerable attention has focused on elucidating a possible link between ethanol's behavioral effects and changes in central catecholamine systems. In general, attenuators of central catecholamine function markedly increase ethanol's depressant effects. For example, pretreatment with α-methyl-para-tyrosine, an inhibitor of catecholamine synthesis, prolonged ethanol sleep time in mice and increased ethanol-induced impairment of psychomotor performance and reaction time in human subjects (Blum et al., 1972; Ahlenius et al., 1973). Similar increases in ethanol-induced depression have been shown with the catecholamine-depleting agent, reserpine (Forney et al., 1962). More recently, a single dose of propranolol ingested by human subjects following alcohol administration significantly increased ethanol's depressant effects on the EEG, divided-attention performance, and inebriation assessments, without increasing ethanol blood concentration (Alkana et al., 1976). On the other hand, L-dopa, used clinically to treat Parkinson's disease and known to increase brain catecholamine levels, has central stimulant properties. The administration of this substance following alcohol administration significantly improved performance in several measures, including platform-balance and divided-attention performance, and it reduced ethanol's depressant effects on the EEG (Alkana et al, 1977). L-dopa and other compounds that increase brain catecholamines, particularly norepinephrine, may thus be useful as amethystic agents.

Recent evidence suggests a role for 3', 5' cyclic adenosine monophosphate (cAMP) in mediating the postsynaptic effects of catecholamine transmitters in several brain regions (Bloom, 1974; Iversen, 1975). Moreover, ethanol induces a dose-dependent decrease in rat cerebral cAMP levels beginning one hour after ethanol ingestion (Volicer and Gold, 1975). Taken together, these results suggest that some of ethanol's depressant effects may be reversed by increasing central cAMP (by blocking its metabolism with inhibitors of phosphodiesterase, the enzyme catalyzing the conversion of cAMP to adenosine monophosphate), and/or by increasing synthesis of cAMP (by stimulation of adenylate cyclase, the enzyme promoting the conversion of adenosine triphosphate to cAMP) (Butcher and Sutherland, 1962).

Caffeine, a methyl xanthine with phosphodiesterase-inhibiting properties (Ritchie, 1970), and caffeine-containing beverages have long been regarded as antagonists to ethanol (Nash, 1966). Research on this drug in human subjects has shown that it antagonizes ethanol's depressant effects as measured by driving-simulator performance (Rutenfranz and Jansen, 1959), balance and motor coordination (Strongin and Winsor, 1935; Newman and Newman, 1956), cognitive capacity (Graf, 1950), and respirator depression (Victor, 1966; Ritchie, 1970). However, the antagonism appears to be concentration dependent and inconsistent (Pilcher, 1911–12; Rutenfranz and Jansen, 1959; Forney and Hughes, 1965). Therefore, despite the several indications of its antagonism, caffeine does not represent a reliable or effective amethystic agent. Amphetamine has also been tested as an amethystic agent, but its antagonistic properties also appear to be concentration dependent and unreliable (Newman and Newman, 1956; Hughes and Forney, 1964), and this agent presents the significant problem of misuse.

Caffeine is not the only drug available that increases central cAMP concentrations. For example, theophylline is a potent phosphodiesterase inhibitor, resembles caffeine structurally, and has pronounced CNS stimulant properties (Ritchie, 1975). Ephedrine also acts as a CNS stimulant and reportedly activates adenylate cyclase through a direct action on catecholamine receptors, as well as by inducing release of central catecholamines (Inness and Nickerson, 1975). Recent studies in man have shown that aminophylline, ephedrine, or a combination of these substances ingested after ethanol significantly reduced ethanol's effects on platform-balance performance and EEG without appreciably altering blood ethanol concentrations (Alkana et al., 1977). However, these drugs neither reduced ethanol's effect on divided-attention and memory performance nor influenced mood or intoxication ratings. Despite the limited antagonism observed, these drugs have encouraging amethystic potential. Higher doses of aminophylline and ephedrine should be tested to see if they can produce a stronger or more complete antagonism.

Considerable interest in naloxone as an amethystic agent has led to a number of recent studies. The administration of naloxone to patients with ethanol-induced coma reportedly reversed the coma in a significant number of individuals (Sorensen and Mattisson, 1978; Mackenzie, 1979; Jeffreys et al., 1980). Controlled studies with normal subjects were generally negative, however, so far as the amethystic properties of naloxone are concerned (Kimball et al., 1980; Catley et al., 1981; Ewing and McCarty, 1981; Mattila et al., 1981; Whalley et al., 1981). Of related interest, some clinical reports have shown that small or moderate doses of naloxone are beneficial in shock due to sepsis (Dirksen et al., 1980; Tiengo, 1980; Wright et al., 1980; Peters et al., 1981), cerebral infarction (Quinn, 1966; Baskin and Hosobuchi, 1981), and hemorrhage (Peters et al., 1981). Naloxone may not be a powerful amethystic agent per se (Dole et al., 1982). Rather, with intoxicated, comatose patients, naloxone's effect may be due to blockade of the vascular actions of the endogenous peptides (endorphin and enkephalin) that are released in patients with cerebral ischemic shock (Gallant, 1981; Dole et al., 1982).

A variety of other substances, including acetylcholine and the related substances, γ-aminobutyric acid (GABA), analeptics, and cations, have been tested both in human subjects and in animals. But thus far these substances alone have not shown great promise as amethystic agents (Noble et al., 1975; Alkana and Noble, 1979).

THE PHARMACOTHERAPY OF THE ALCOHOL WITHDRAWAL REACTION

In the 1950s, major advances were made toward understanding the etiology of reactions that follow alcohol withdrawal. Careful clinical observations (Victor and Adams, 1953; Isbell et al., 1955) established that alcohol withdrawal reactions were caused specifically by cessation of, or reduction in, ethanol ingestion and were not due to toxic or nutritional factors.

Following prolonged alcohol consumption, reduction or cessation of consumption may lead to a minor or major alcohol withdrawal syndrome (Wolfe and Victor, 1972). The minor syndrome, called Alcohol Withdrawal in DSM-III, is characterized by the onset of tremor and diaphoresis, which may appear as early as six to eight hours following the cessation of drinking. These signs may occur alone or with hallucinations or convulsions or both. Patients in the early stages of withdrawal may be mildly disoriented in time and may have difficulty recalling events of the last few days of their drinking sprees. Varying degrees of anorexia, insomnia, autonomic hyperactivity, depressed mood, anxiety, and general weakness are common associated symptoms. Tremor and hallucinations attain their greatest severity, and convulsions attain their peak incidence, between ten and thirty hours after cessation of drinking. These manifestations in patients who show only the minor syndrome subside to a large extent forty to fifty hours after cessation of drinking.

A relatively small proportion of patients experience the major syndrome, called Alcohol Withdrawal Delirium in DSM-III (previously called delirium tremens). The major syndrome has some important distinctions from the minor syndrome. The disorientation is much more profound and is compounded by perceptual disturbances such as gross misinterpretations and misidentifications. Another striking difference is the absence of convulsions during the course of Alcohol Withdrawal Delirium. In most cases, the delirium is preceded by minor withdrawal symptoms, though, and almost one-third of patients have seizure or short bursts of seizures at the outset. When seizures do occur, they always precede the onset of the delirium, and they do not recur once the delirium is established. Other characteristic manifestations of the major syndrome are overactivity of the autonomic nervous system (fever, tachycardia, elevated blood pressure, and severe diaphoresis) and increased psychomotor activity, manifested by restlessness, tremor, and vivid hallucinations. In some patients who go through both the minor syndrome and the major syndrome, the former blends imperceptibly with the latter; in others, the two syndromes are quite distinct.

Once the etiology and characteristics of alcohol withdrawal reactions were established, controlled clinical trials began in the 1960s to test the efficacy of various pharmacotherapies for the minor and the major syndromes. As a consequence of the knowledge developed over the past thirty years, morbidity and mortality from alcohol withdrawal reactions have in the United States declined dramatically compared with rates at the turn of the century (Boston, 1908; Boucharlat et al., 1976).

The consideration of specific chemical agents for alcohol withdrawal reactions must begin with a consideration of some general management issues with individuals undergoing detoxification. First and foremost, a thorough physical examination is necessary, since many alcoholics have in the past received multiple trauma and frequently they have alcohol-induced organ damage. Patients should not be restrained or subjected to sensory deprivation, as these measures could aggravate their withdrawal reactions. While temperatures are usually somewhat elevated during alcohol withdrawal, temperatures of over 101° F are usually of infectious origin and hence require specific treatment. Correction of electrolytes and fluid is often necessary. An assessment of blood electrolytes should be made before instituting corrective measures. Moreover, patients are frequently malnourished and sometimes hypoglycemic, requiring adequate diets and vitamin supplements, particularly B complex. Finally, nausea, headache, and constipation frequently develop following withdrawal from alcohol and require appropriate drug therapy.

The alcohol-barbiturate drugs have thus far been shown to be the most effective agents in the treatment of alcohol withdrawal reactions. These include ethanol, chloral hydrate, paraldehyde, barbiturates, chlormethiazole, and the benzodiazepines. Chloral hydrate (Wilson, 1886) was first used in the 1880s, and within a year of its introduction, paraldehyde (Gugl, 1883) was employed. Paraldehyde remained the primary treatment for alcohol withdrawal reactions for many years (Piker and Cohn, 1937; Block, 1956). The rationale was that substitution of one CNS depressant for another of the same type was necessary in dealing with alcohol withdrawal reactions (Kalinowsky, 1942). Isbell (1967) advanced the substitution rationale more forcefully, taking the position that Alcohol Withdrawal and Alcohol Withdrawal Delirium are reactions to abstinence from alcohol. The principal use that he put forth was, first, to substitute for alcohol one of the hypnotic drugs of the alcohol-barbiturate type, thus reintoxicating the individual, and then, gradually to reduce the dose of the substitute. This substitution method resembles that used in the treatment of barbiturate withdrawal, a procedure which has been elaborated into a careful titration with phenobarbital and pentobarbital (Gessner, 1965).

Benzodiazepines

The benzodiazepines, particularly chlordiazepoxide and diazepam, are currently the drugs of choice for treating Alcohol Withdrawal and Alcohol Withdrawal Delirium (Favazza and Martin, 1974). A number of studies attest to the efficacy of these drugs compared with placebo in controlling the manifestations of alcohol withdrawal (Rosenfeld and Bizzoco, 1961; Koutsky and Sletten, 1963; Sereny and Kalant, 1965; Kaim et al., 1969). Compared with other drugs of the alcohol-barbiturate type, however, the benzodiazepines have generally failed to show greater efficacy (Golbert et al., 1967; Muller, 1969; Thompson et al., 1975; Kramp and Rafaelsen, 1978). The benzodiazepines have nevertheless continued, since their introduction about thirty years ago, as mainstays in the detoxification of the alcoholic person.

Typically, on the first day of detoxification, the dose of chlordiazepoxide or diazepam is titrated until sedation is achieved. On subsequent days, the dose is reduced in steps, according to the patient's degree of intoxication, tremulousness, and insomnia, and the drug is usually discontinued five or six days after it is instituted. Rarely do patients require the benzodiazepines for more than a week. Indeed, prolonged use may lead to toxic manifestations because of the long half-life of chlordiazepoxide and diazepam and their active metabolites (Sellers and Kalant, 1976). Moreover, increasing concern and evidence have developed regarding the alcoholic patient's potential for abusing these drugs (Selig, 1966; Preskorn and Denner, 1977; Kramp and Rafaelsen, 1978).

Paraldehyde

Paraldehyde was for many years the drug most commonly used in treating Alcohol Withdrawal and Alcohol Withdrawal Delirium. Indeed, many studies have shown that paraldehyde, alone or in combination with chloral hydrate, is effective in the treatment of alcohol withdrawal reactions (Thomas and Freedman, 1964; Golbert et al., 1967). Nevertheless, paraldehyde is today used infrequently compared with the benzodiazepines (Favazza and Martin, 1974). The decrease in its use followed some unfavorable publicity due to unexpected, unexplained deaths, apnea (suggesting an overdose effect) (Thompson and Maddrey, 1975; Thompson et al., 1975), episodic violent agitation during induction (Thompson et al., 1975), and "idiosyncratic" toxicity of small doses (Kotz et al., 1938; Burstein, 1943; Baratham and Tinckler, 1964).

Barbiturates

Some physicians in the United States continue to use barbiturates for Alcohol Withdrawal and Alcohol Withdrawal Delirium (Isbell, 1967; Sapira, 1973; Favazza and Martin, 1974), and European physicians have regarded them as the treatment of choice for more than fifty years (Kramp and Rafaelsen, 1978; Hemmingsen et al., 1979). Their use in this country has been limited, however, because of concern that an alcoholic person can readily become cross-dependent upon them. Moreover, the various barbiturates have markedly different onsets and durations of action. These problems are further compounded by the fact that chronic ethanol consumption induces the microsomal-ethanol oxidizing system, which in turn enhances barbiturate metabolism (Misra et al., 1971), leading to low and sometimes unpredictable blood barbiturate levels.

Ethanol

Alcoholics frequently try to mitigate the development of alcohol withdrawal reactions by administering alcohol to themselves. Thus, orally and intravenously administered ethanol has in the past been used for treating Alcohol Withdrawal and Alcohol Withdrawal Delirium (Lereboullet et al., 1960; Golbert et al., 1967). With the advent of the benzodiazepine drugs, however, the use of ethanol as a therapeutic agent has for the most part ceased. Other reasons for its abandonment are ethanol's short duration of action, its narrow range of safety, and increasing recognition of its manifold cytotoxic properties.

Chlormethiazole (clomethiazole)

Chlormethiazole not only resembles the thiazole portion of vitamin B_1, but it is also a metabolite of this vitamin (Bergener, 1966). Its use in the treatment of alcohol withdrawal reactions may be somewhat attributable to the theory that B_1 deficiency plays a part in the pathogenesis of Alcohol Withdrawal Delirium. Furthermore, chlormethiazole is an excellent hypnotic (Lundquist, 1966), and two to three days after cessation of its administration, subjects experience withdrawal reactions (Quinn, 1966; Kryspin-Exner and Mader, 1971; Reilly, 1976).

In Europe, chlormethiazole has achieved some popularity as a therapeutic agent for alcohol withdrawal reactions, and European studies have generally attested to its efficacy (Glatt et al., 1965; Bergener, 1966; Madden et al., 1969; McGrath, 1975). For various nonmedical reasons, however, chlormethiazole is not available in the United States.

Antipsychotic Drugs

With the introduction of the phenothiazines in the 1950s, the new antipsychotic agents were naturally expected to be useful with the various aberrant behavioral states that follow alcohol withdrawal. Initial reports were enthusiastic (Albert et al., 1954; Schultz et al., 1965; Fazekas et al., 1956), but controlled experiments failed to demonstrate the superiority of the phenothiazines over the alcohol-barbiturate drugs (Laties et al., 1958; Johnson, 1961; Thomas and Freedman, 1964; Golbert et al., 1967). Moreover, an even greater concern arose over several adverse consequences of the phenothiazines with patients in alcohol withdrawal. Not only did the phenothiazines have the capacity to reduce the threshold for seizures (Schlichter et al., 1956; Fazekas et al., 1957; Fink and Swinyard, 1960), but excess mortality was observed in subjects undergoing Alcohol Withdrawal Delirium who received these drugs compared with those who were given alcohol-barbiturate drugs (Thomas and Freedman, 1964; Golbert et al., 1967). The experiences were similar with haloperidol, a butyrophenone with proven antipsychotic efficacy (Gross et al., 1974; Gessner, 1979).

Certainly, antipsychotic agents are less effective than the benzodiazepines in prophylaxis against delirium. However, once delirium occurs, the situation is less clear. Some investigators believe that phenothiazines are contraindicated because of the fact that they lower the seizure threshold. Other investigators (Clark, 1983) believe that once frank delirium occurs (in a patient already premedicated with benzodiazepines), haloperidol or chlorpromazine are the drugs of choice, precisely because of their general antipsychotic properties and wide margin of safety. Antipsychotics can also be used safely and effectively in the syndrome known as alcohol hallucinosis (Freedman et al., 1975).

Anticonvulsants

Seizures of the grand mal type are an inherent part of the reaction to alcohol withdrawal (Victor and Adams, 1953; Isbell et al., 1955; Kaim et al., 1969). Moreover, the mortality rate for patients who manifest seizures at the onset of Alcohol Withdrawal Delirium is twice as great as the rate for those who do not (Tavel et al., 1961). While the benzodiazepines or alcohol-barbiturate drugs are usually effective in controlling such seizures, in certain cases the prophylactic use of anticonvulsants in combination with the benzodiazepines may be indicated. In particular, those alcoholics with a previous history of seizures following withdrawal or those with idiopathic epilepsy may benefit during detoxification from receiving diphenylhydantoin in addition to a benodiazepine (Rothstein, 1973; Sampliner and Iber, 1974).

Another anticonvulsant agent, unrelated to the alcohol-barbiturate drugs, is n-dipropylacetate (sodium valproate). This drug, which has been used in Europe, can apparently control a wide spectrum of epileptic disorders. In animal studies, it has raised brain GABA levels (Godin et al., 1969; Simler et al., 1973), and it has been effective in controlling the convulsions that follow the withdrawal of alcohol (Hillbom, 1975; Noble et al., 1976). Clinical studies in Italy have shown favorable results in the treatment of Alcohol Withdrawal and Alcohol Withdrawal Delirium (Bonfiglio et al., 1972; 1977). However, control trials are not yet available in the United States, and the Food and Drug Administration has not approved it for use in treating alcoholics.

Magnesium

Evidence is growing that serum magnesium levels may play an important role in Alcohol Withdrawal and Alcohol Withdrawal Delirium (Flink et al., 1954; Flink, 1971). Low serum magnesium levels are generally associated with increased seizure susceptibility (Anonymous, 1967; Wacker and Parisi, 1968; Seelig et al., 1975).

A very recent Japanese study (Ogata, 1983) showed a progressive decline in serum magnesium levels following withdrawal of alcohol from alcoholics, with the lowest levels achieved 16 to 20 hours after the withdrawal. Interestingly, other serum electrolyte levels showed insignificant changes. The acute change in serum magnesium levels correlated with spikes, short bursts of sharp waves, and paroxysmal discharges in the EEG. Moreover, all the subjects studied showed positive responses to photic stimulation on the EEG at the time of lowest serum magnesium levels. The abnormal EEG changes, including epileptic and photosensitive discharges, returned to normal within 45 hours after the withdrawal of alcohol, corresponding to the time when serum magnesium returned to normal levels.

Parenteral administration of magnesium does not have established efficacy in mitigating the adverse consequences that follow the withdrawal of alcohol. Some have claimed that magnesium administration shortens Alcohol Withdrawal Delirium (Flink, 1956) and lowers the incidence of hallucinations when compared with a control placebo (Beroz et al., 1962). In addition, parenteral administration of magnesium sulfate was reportedly as effective as diazepam in controlling Alcohol Withdrawal (Shulsinger et al., 1977). Others have refuted these reports on statistical or methodological grounds (Wacker and Valee, 1958; Beroz et al., 1962, Gessner, 1979). Clinicians have nonetheless continued to administer magnesium sulfate as a prophylactic agent during the first few days of detoxification (2 cc of 50 percent magnesium sulfate intramuscularly every four hours). The treatment is used especially with patients who show low serum magnesium levels and patients who have in the past experienced severe alcohol withdrawal reactions.*

DRUGS IN THE LONG-TERM TREATMENT OF ALCOHOLISM

Some alcoholic persons may still require pharmacotherapy after detoxification. As a chemical aid to the alcoholic person in overcoming momentary temptations to use alcohol, alcohol-sensitizing drugs have been used for many years and are still widely used. Alcoholic patients experience a variety of dysphoric states, including depression and insomnia, for periods as long as four years after they stop using alcohol (Kissin, 1979). While the judicious use of antidepressants may be necessary in these instances, great care must be exercised in the use of drugs with cross-dependence liability in the alcoholic individual.

Alcohol-Sensitizing Drugs

Alcohol-sensitizing drugs, which produce adverse reactions when alcohol is consumed, include disulfiram and, outside the United States, citrated calcium carbamide. Such agents have been employed as therapeutic tools for a number of years (Kissin, 1977). Most agree that these compounds inactivate aldehyde dehydrogenase in the liver and that disulfiram causes its unpleasant effect when alcohol is consumed because unmetabolized acetaldehyde accumulates (Liebson et al., 1973).

Despite the fact that disulfiram has been used for more than thirty years, its effectiveness remains controversial. Most of the clinical trials have been either uncontrolled or poorly designed (Lundwall and Baekeland, 1971). However, a recent review of various antialcohol programs supported by the National Institute on Alcohol Abuse and Alcoholism concluded that disulfiram has had some degree of therapeutic success (Armor et al., 1976). Moreover, a recent well-designed study showed that the percentage of patients who remained abstinent with disulfiram was twice as large as the percentage remaining abstinent without disulfiram (Fuller, 1976). Furthermore, the patients on disulfiram drank on a smaller number of days, worked more days, and kept appointments more regularly than those who did not receive disulfiram.

Notwithstanding its wide use and some of its benefits, disulfiram use can be problematic. Disulfiram is contraindicated with people who have

*Part V of this volume contains a brief discussion of the use of another group of drugs, the β-adrenergic blockers, with patients undergoing alcohol withdrawal reactions. In his initial discussion of the evidence regarding these agents, Cole reviews several relevant studies of propranolol.

arteriosclerotic heart disease, cirrhosis, kidney disease, diabetes mellitus, and other chronic disorders in which tolerance to acetaldehyde may be low (*Alcohol and Health*, 1971). Reports indicate that disulfiram can cause hepatitis (Keeffe and Smith, 1974; Eisen and Ginsberg, 1975), acute organic brain syndrome (Knee and Razani, 1974; Hotson and Langston, 1976), and convulsions (Price and Silberfarb, 1976). Furthermore, one of its metabolites, carbon disulfide, may play a role in atherosclerosis and other toxic reactions (Rainey and Neal, 1975; Rainey, 1977).

A key factor in the effective use of disulfiram is patient compliance. Methods are now known for determining two products of disulfiram metabolism: carbon disulfide can be detected in breath (Kraml, 1973; Paulson et al., 1977), and diethylamine, in urine (Neiderhiser, 1976; Gordis and Peterson, 1977). Unfortunately, these methods are not yet available for use in rapid screening by practicing clinicians.

Another approach to assuring compliance is implantation. This technique obviates the daily oral ingestion of disulfiram and involves making an incision in the lower abdomen, inserting 100 mg sterile disulfiram trocars, and then suturing the incision. However, disagreement surrounds the question of whether enough disulfiram is released to result in acetaldehyde intoxication (Malcolm et al., 1974; Kingstone and Kline, 1975; Lewis et al., 1975; Wilson, 1975). The disulfiram-ethanol reaction is less acute with this method, but it is more prolonged (Wilson, 1975), and the effect may be more psychological than chemical (Malcolm et al., 1974). Follow-up studies have suggested that the method warrants further investigation (Thorpe and Perret, 1959; Obholzer, 1974; Whyte and O'Brien, 1974).

As is now becoming recognized, poor delivery of disulfiram from implants may be due in part to encapsulation of the implant by fibrotic tissue. To overcome this problem, the disulfiram was embedded in a polylactic glycolic acid matrix before testing its implantation in animals. This resulted in a sustained release of the disulfiram, such that significant levels were released over periods four times as long as with more conventional implants (Phillips, 1983).

As currently used, disulfiram is initially given as a single oral dose of 500 mg daily for one to two weeks and then 250 mg daily as maintenance dose. The use of disulfiram alone, without adjunctive therapy and physician supervision, is strongly discouraged.

Psychoactive Agents

It is now well recognized that depression, attempted suicide, and suicide occur commonly during alcoholics' drinking phases. Various pharmacologic, genetic, psychological, and social explanations have been advanced (Kendell, 1983; Winokur, 1983). What is less well appreciated is that depression, self-destructive behavior, and anxiety are not at all uncommon following alcoholics' cessation of drinking. However, long-term pharmacologic treatment of these symptoms remains controversial (Noble, 1978). Some argue against such treatment because of the risks of abuse, dependence, overdosage, and tolerance development. Others acknowledge these risks but maintain that the treatment can be important and effective.

Few systematic and well-controlled studies have examined the efficacy with alcoholics of the antidepressant tricyclic compounds and monoamine oxidase (MAO) inhibitors. Diverse and sometimes unpredictable effects ensue when alcohol is used in combination with antidepressants. For example, alcohol-amitriptyline combinations have caused enhanced behavioral and psychomotor impairment (Landauer et al., 1969; Seppala et al., 1975), which could be dangerous in driving. On the other hand, a minor antagonistic interaction has appeared between alcohol and nortriptyline (Hughes and Forney, 1963).

Many alcoholics experience fatigue, insomnia, and other symptoms of depression during the initial phase of alcohol withdrawal. Particular care should be exercised during this phase with the tricyclic antidepressants, since they increase the susceptibility for convulsions (Coleman and Evans, 1975–76). Moreover, with a significant percentage of alcoholics who have depressive symptoms at this time, the symptoms are most likely due to an imbalance in the biogenic amine system and will markedly decrease or abate within a few weeks of alcohol withdrawal (Kendell, 1983; Nakamura et al., 1983).

In a small percentage of alcoholics, depression has previously coexisted with alcoholism and has been confounded by the acute effects of alcohol. With this minority of patients, depression becomes fully manifest only during the protracted alcohol withdrawal phase (Kissin, 1979; Kendell, 1983; Nakamura et al., 1983). With such patients, the main medications in the protracted phase are tricyclic antidepressants. However, cardiovascular difficulties are common in alcoholics (Noble, 1978), and certain tricyclic antidepressants produce cardiotoxic effects (Gilman et al., 1980). Caution should therefore be exercised whenever these drugs are administered. Based on available evidence, amitriptyline, protriptyline, and perhaps imipramine may be more dangerous than doxepin or mianserin in patients with cardiac disease (Burrows et al., 1976; Hollister, 1978).

Caution is also advisable with MAO inhibitors, since alcohol has a considerable potential to interact with these drugs (Kissin, 1974; Coleman and Evans, 1975–76). The MAO inhibitors slow the metabolism of alcohol, which causes alcohol intoxication to be greater than expected. Moreover, the MAO inhibitors interact with tyramine, which is found in some alcoholic beverages and the tyramine–MAO inhibitor combination can lead to a hypertensive crisis, with symptoms of nausea and severe headache.*

Lithium carbonate has been proposed as a treatment for depressed alcoholics. In a double-blind study, depressed alcoholics who received lithium had fewer alcoholic episodes than controls (Kline et al., 1974). Although this study could not demonstrate that the alcoholic episodes were related to depression, another study showed that the beneficial effects with lithium occurred only in those alcoholics who were depressed (Merry et al., 1976; Reynolds et al., 1977). Other investigators believe that the purported value of lithium may be related to other effects. Lithium seems to diminish the deterioration of cognitive and psychomotor performance which alcohol causes (Linnoila et al., 1974; Judd et al., 1977),

*Editor's note: In Part V of *Psychiatry Update: Volume II*, Drs. Jonathan O. Cole and Alan F. Schatzberg review the effects and side effects of the various antidepressant drugs, including the newer agents and the tricyclics and MAO inhibitors (pages 472–491). Their chapter concludes with a list of tyramine-containing foods and beverages which should be avoided by patients taking MAO inhibitors.

and it may block euphoria or reduce the desire to drink (Pendery and Huey, 1974; Judd et al., 1977). Despite these observations, the role of lithium in the treatment of alcoholics remains unclear. Moreover, the potentiation of lithium toxicity by ethanol in animals (Ho and Ho, 1978) necessitates additional studies in human subjects before lithium can take a definitive place in the treatment of alcoholism.

Chapter 24

Alcohol Policy: Preventive Options
by Dean Gerstein, Ph.D.

Clinicians must concern themselves with the differential diagnosis and treatment of individual patients. Researchers can best invest their attention in closely focused, precisely defined questions of fact, theory, or method. In contrast, formulators and executors of public policy must work in broad strokes that can be readily understood and broadcast across large and heterogenous groups of citizens.

This chapter outlines a series of analytic, normative, and pragmatic issues that arise in connection with policies designed to help reduce or prevent trouble with alcohol. The chapter sketches the ideas underlying these policies, presents a scheme defining types of policy instruments, and fills out this scheme with some prominent examples of specific preventive policies, covering the principal issues involved in their selection and implementation.

GOVERNING IDEAS ABOUT ALCOHOL

The term *alcohol policy* is broadly defined for the purposes of this chapter and refers to the many roles of governmental and nongovernmental organizations in the prevention and treatment of dependence, abuse, problem drinking, and so forth. Opinions about appropriate alcohol policy are shaped not only by specific ideas about alcohol, but also by general philosophies about the appropriate roles of the state and other social institutions and by practical judgments about how effective various kinds of policies have been in the past. A rationale for alcohol policymaking that seems powerful to one whose attention is fixed on the subject may appear trivial or inconceivable to people who are less involved. A policy will not be viable if it conflicts with a current overall direction of government, requires heavy use of bureaucratic capacities that do not exist or are otherwise invested, or flies in the face of powerful contrary social interests or values. On the other hand, policies often become viable when, aside from any intrinsic argument in their favor, they are consistent with an overall trend in power, make good use of an underused or ambitious institutional instrument, or line up neatly with the aims of a powerful social movement.

Policy must be governed by simple ideas, and exogenous social currents may have much to do with which ideas are best received in a particular time or place, but this does not relieve anyone of the responsibility to think hard and make political choices. At any given time, moreover, we can expect that more than one idea will be afloat. Public as well as private debate will reflect tensions between competing ideas, and every action taken, not only in the realm of politics, but also in the privacy of our clinics, work places, and homes, will reflect to some degree the influence of the policies that governments adopt.

The Wet and Dry Views

Among the small number of powerful alcohol policy ideas discerned by students of such matters in the United States (Levine, 1978; Room, 1974), two of the strongest reach well back into our history. One is the "wet" view that dominated the colonial period (Rorabaugh, 1979).

According to the wet view, drinking is a valued and valuable social custom; overindulgence arises from a flaw in moral character or training; and, if necessary, a good strong dose of public discipline is the appropriate response to excessive or poorly timed drunkenness. Krout (1925) offered evidence of the social value accorded drinking during the colonial period. The early student rosters of Harvard University, which arrayed students' names by social position rather than alphabet, listed innkeepers' sons before clergymen's sons. Also in that era, respected public officials, finished with their terms of office, would often continue their public careers as tavern owners. As two historians have commented, "Men habituated to moral surveillance could thus continue their scrutiny" (Aaron and Musto, 1981, 133).

In contrast stands the "dry" view that began roughly with independence and became dominant in the nineteenth century (Gusfield, 1963; Levine, 1978). According to this view, alcohol (or at least strong liquor) is an addicting poison and threatens to ruin anyone who drinks it; selling or consuming alcohol is basically a public hazard, not only to the health and family life of those who drink, but also to the morality of public and political officeholders, who may be corrupted by saloon ethics and profits; and using the law to restrict or ban the sale of drink is the most appropriate response. The commitment of the Anti-Saloon League to this view and its adoption by electoral majorities in most of the country led, by the eve of World War I, to the Eighteenth Amendment and the subsequent Volstead Act.

The language of the Eighteenth Amendment reveals some careful hedging: it prohibited "the manufacture, sale, or transportation of intoxicating liquors" but did not prohibit purchase or consumption, and it left rulemakers at various levels of government having to decide what kinds of alcoholic beverages were "intoxicating liquors" and under what circumstances they would be so deemed. The concomitant of this fundamental ambiguity, which reflected unresolved conflicts within the dry majority and the wet minority, to say nothing of the implacable opposition between "bone dry" and "prosaloon" extremes, was a patchwork of implementing statutes and enforcement efforts. Instead of making alcohol unavailable, Prohibition controls resulted in a much higher price for alcohol and a lucrative criminal enterprise for its manufacture and sale. Overall per capita consumption dropped by one-third to one-half of its previous rate and liver cirrhosis death rates were halved (Warburton, 1932; Jellinek, 1947; Gerstein, 1981). The price of the Prohibition policy, however, and the economic and political advantages of restoring the industry as a New Deal measure, ultimately overrode its health bonus.

The battle of the wets and the dries still echoes in programs that implement public policy and in private beliefs and practices, even as the old adversaries have receded behind the screen of historical experience. Newer views about alcohol policy reflect an effort to find a workable modern compromise between the old wet and dry views.

Alcoholism as a Disease

First and best-known of the newer views is that alcoholism is a progressive, chronic, addictive disease and that the disease has the following features: (1) vulnerability is confined to a fraction of the population who are, or at least could be, perfectly normal in all other respects, while the rest of the population is virtually immune (Jellinek, 1960); (2) the causes of vulnerability are as yet unclear, limiting our ability to put any preventive measures into effect, except earlier detection; and (3) the disease can be treated successfully with one or more therapeutic methods, the most general aim being complete and lasting abstinence for the alcoholic.

The major policy implications of this conception are that we need to educate the public on recognizing the signs of alcoholism, to reduce ideological and financial barriers to treatment, and to promote research on the causes of vulnerability to alcoholism. The alcoholism movement, a quasi-formal coalition of AA members, various physician caucuses, and affiliates of the National Council on Alcoholism, at first took the stance that no policies other than those related to these limited measures should be supported, lest its priority interest in alcoholism as a disease be lost (Wiener, 1980).

Alcoholic Beverage Control

This second newer view was already strong at the time of Prohibition's repeal and was the principal reason for establishing the current alcoholic beverage control (ABC) system in the United States. In this view, alcohol is considered a popular commodity that cannot and should not be totally suppressed, but that needs to be overseen by a strong regulatory watchdog, since consumer demand for alcohol has been disastrously exploited in the past by greedy merchants and criminals. Eighteen states now have some form of government monopoly over alcoholic beverage sales, and all states have ABC agencies with broad regulatory powers. John D. Rockefeller, Jr., the most influential advocate of control policies in the late Prohibition and early repeal era, put the object of these controls quite simply: take the profit out of alcohol (Fosdick and Scott, 1933; cf. Levine, 1983).

Measured by Rockefeller's yardstick, the goal of alcohol beverage control has not been achieved. The ABC boards today see their primary objectives as the collection of tax revenues or profitable operation of government distribution systems, the holding of licensed retail purveyors to the terms of their licenses, and the maintenance of legal and orderly distribution (Medicine in the Public Interest, Inc., 1976). Enforcement efforts are focused on record keeping and in some states on the strict maintenance of drinking age standards.

Public Health

The final one of these newer views holds that alcohol is benign when used in small quantities, but increasingly damaging and risky to health when drunk to excess. Promotion of public health is the goal, and policy implications include discouragement of excessive consumption through strong public education and consistent limits on marketing instruments (such as advertising), price, and availability, all of which can affect the prevalence of excessive consumption (Bruun et al., 1975).

In recent years, the public health conception has grown increasingly strong despite vocal criticism (Pittman, 1980; United States Brewers Association, 1983). Traditional alcoholism-oriented groups, such as the National Council on Alcoholism (1982), and consumer health activist groups, such as the Center for Science in the Public Interest (Jacobson et al., 1983), have created alliances, and they have been instrumental in legislative and executive public health initiatives at all levels of government. Interest in this view has spread throughout North America and the world (Davies and Walsh, 1983; Institute of Medicine, 1982; Moser, 1979; Single et al., 1981; World Health Organization, 1981).

An important force behind the public health position is the recognition that trouble with alcohol can arise from poorly timed or badly placed drunken episodes which occur in the general population, not specifically among chronic heavy drinkers. Survey results have repeatedly suggested that around half of all intoxication-related incidents of interpersonal violence, legal involvements, accidental trauma, job trouble, and the like occur among the large pool of moderate and light drinkers who average at most four drinks daily (Polich and Orvis, 1979; Clark and Midanik, 1980; Moore and Gerstein, 1981).

The role of groups working against drunk driving, such as Remove Intoxicated Drivers (RID) and Mothers Against Drunk Driving (MADD), is still unclear. The details of the policies which they have supported have for the most part derived from years of research and demonstration programs supported by the National Highway Traffic Safety Administration (1979; Jones and Joscelyn, 1978; Ross, 1983; United States Department of Transportation, 1968). For the most part, these groups have formulated their goals in terms of promoting justice and preventing crime rather than promoting health and preventing disease.

In summary, three more general governing ideas meld the compatible features of the newer public health, beverage control, and alcoholism views and begin to stake out a stable position between the old wet and dry views (Moore and Gerstein, 1981). First, alcohol problems are permanent, because drinking is an important and ineradicable part of our society and culture. Second, alcohol problems tend to be so broadly felt and distributed as to be a general social problem, even though they are excessively prevalent in a relatively small fraction of the population. Third, the possibilities for reducing the problem by preventive measures are modest but real and should increase with experience; they should not be ignored because of ghosts from the past.

TYPES OF PREVENTION POLICIES

Alcoholism is chronic, relapsing, and often accompanied by complicated sequelae, and yet episodes of drunkenness may generate bad effects when nothing one might reasonably call a disease process is present. Therefore, the policy approaches discussed here, while they overlap strongly with a familiar primary prevention concept, are conceived somewhat differently. With a colleague, the author has elsewhere summarized the approaches as follows: *"They are all policies that operate in a non-personalized way to alter the set of contingencies affecting individuals as they drink or engage in activities that (when combined with intoxication) are considered risky . . .* They operate through the remote manipulation [throughout society] of a relevant set of incentives and contingencies: the terms and circumstances under which alcohol is available, the attitudes of people surrounding the drinker, and the benignity of the physical and social environment toward drunkenness" (Moore and Gerstein, 1981, 53).

Three classes of preventive policies are included in this conception. One class of policies aims to regulate *supply* by prescribing the terms and conditions for the availability of alcohol and the places in which to drink it. A second class attempts to influence people's *drinking practices* directly through pedagogical efforts and legal stipulations. The third group of policies seeks to reduce *environmental risk* in order to decrease the damaging consequences of intoxication. The three types of policies are related to each other directly. Supply policies try to regulate the markets for a matched pair of goods and services, alcohol itself and the places where people drink it. Policies on drinking practices presume that alcohol and drinking places are available; they try to influence the ways that people use these opportunities, in terms of how much and how often they drink and what activities are paired with drinking. Finally, policies designed to reduce environmental risk presume that some people will drink to intoxication and put themselves in danger; the object of these policies is to limit the severity of the consequences by making the environment less hostile.

Regulating Supply

Regulation of supply generally aims to isolate criminal elements, to maintain order in drinking places, to limit excessive consumption, and to keep alcohol away from people for whom it is considered especially dangerous, such as children or people engaged in hazardous activities. Typical instruments of supply policy include manufacturing controls, regulation of the ownership, number, location, and retail hours of outlets, taxation, price controls, minimum age or other restrictions on the purchase of alcoholic beverages, and attachment of legal liability to servers of alcoholic beverages (i.e., "dram shop laws", for which see Mosher, 1979; 1983). The most controversial of these instruments in the United States today are price controls and age restrictions.

PRICES AND TAXES   Alcoholic beverage prices can be controlled either directly by fair trade or price support plans or indirectly by ensuring certain minimum price floors with excise taxation. The practical question is whether price controls affect chronic, heavy consumption and episodic intoxication, instead of or in addition to light nonhazardous patterns of drinking.

In general, the weight of evidence affirms that prices do affect heavy drinking practices (Cook and Tauchen, 1984; Davies, 1983; Moore and

Gerstein, 1981). Multiple increases in price through highly restrictive market controls or massive tax impositions have, in various consistent cases, depressed traditional rates of consumption by as much as one half. Smaller changes, such as a 10 percent real price increase, decrease consumption by 5 to 10 percent. Studies of the effects of price increases also show that they generally result in decreased rates of cirrhosis mortality, an indicator of heavy consumption, and auto fatalities, a usable indicator of acute drunkenness (Beaubrun, 1977: Bruun et al., 1975; Cook, 1981; Cook and Tauchen, 1984; Warburton, 1932). These findings confirm that heavy drinkers are not exempt from the laws of supply and demand.

Two arguments concerning taxation are relevant to price-oriented controls: (1) that alcohol taxes are unfair to light and moderate drinkers and (2) that excise taxes on consumer items fall most heavily on the poor, who can least afford them.

Is it fair for all drinkers to be taxed if only some drink dangerously or excessively? The high preventive tax that affects all drinkers is meant to keep people from drinking too much and from putting themselves at greater risk. Since virtually all people who become excessive drinkers were at one time light or moderate drinkers, it is difficult to sustain the notion that light and moderate drinkers are free from the risk of becoming excessive drinkers. Furthermore, the damages wrought by excessive drinking (e.g., injuries due to assaults and accidents) often fall on people who themselves do not usually and did not on that occasion drink excessively but who were unfortunate enough to be around someone who did. Thus the preventive effect of taxes can benefit those who themselves drink safely and who would be even better off if others followed suit. In any case, one-tenth of the drinking population consumes over half the alcohol, so the heaviest drinkers in fact pay most of the tax (Gerstein, 1981).

Do alcohol taxes fall most heavily on the poor and hardly affect the wealthy? In fact, econometric studies suggest that higher taxes on alcoholic beverages result in most people spending little or no more money on drinking, but rather result in most people drinking less for the same expense (Cook, 1981; Harris, 1983). Those who do increase their expenditure appear for the most part to be those who can afford to do so without financial distress. Wealthier people generally spend considerably more on alcohol to begin with, so an increased tax would affect them considerably.

AGE RESTRICTIONS   The debate about age restrictions in the United States has not centered on whether or not age restrictions should exist at all, but on whether the right to purchase alcohol should commence at age 18 or age 21 or somewhere in between. Complicating and dominating this debate are two somewhat different issues, drunken driving accidents and drinking by children under the age of 18 (Wechsler, 1980).

The downward movement of the minimum legal drinking age from 21 to 19 or 18 in roughly half the states during the early 1970s paralleled constitutional reductions in the minimum voting age. The recent tide of reversals in this relatively small age adjustment has been undertaken largely because so many people aged 18, 19, and 20 die in drunken driving accidents, and these newly entitled purchasers are thought to be making alcohol more available to even younger children. The evidence indicates that changes in the legal purchasing age do not greatly change the overall quantity of alcohol consumed by people in the directly affected age group, but that they do considerably affect where these people drink. When purchase is illegal, people in this age group are excluded from bars and other by-the-drink establishments. They therefore spend considerably less time driving to and from such places on the highways and instead do most of their drinking in private places nearer to home. When their status changes, a measurable difference, in the range of 20 to 30 percent, occurs in the rate of auto crash fatalities. For the United States as a whole, this difference adds up to several hundred lives a year. As for the effects on children who are well below the controversial age range, studies tend to show that adjustments in the minimum age do not affect the younger children's drinking behavior (Cook and Tauchen, 1984; Douglass, 1979–80; Hingson et al., 1983; Williams et al., 1983).

This highlights an important dimension of the policy issues surrounding alcohol use. A clear national consensus exists that Prohibition in the 1920s was a mistake. But the great majority of people in the United States still clearly believe in prohibiting alcohol to a large segment of the population (including some voting citizens) because they are too young. This continued endorsement of partial prohibition, along with implementive measures which do not destroy legitimate business, remind us that alcohol is different from other kinds of beverages. Alcohol is too dangerous to be put freely into the hands of those not possessing the skills or the judgment to use it safely and appropriately. But what is safe and appropriate use? What is being done to see that the necessary skills and judgment are there when partial prohibition ends at a person's 18th, or 19th, or 20th birthday? And what measures can or should the government take thereafter to see that these useful faculties are exercised? These are the prominent questions that arise in considering policies that try to shape drinking practices directly.

Shaping Drinking Practices Directly

Adults are on the whole legally licensed to drink. But powerful forces constrain their freedom to use this license. Undoubtedly the most powerful of these constraints are the informal norms that children learn at home and early in life, the norms which they later test, modify, and transmit to each other as adult expectations in families, friendships, and work relations. Whether or not governments undertake to shape drinking practices, these informal social and cultural controls go on operating in everyday life.

If a government does decide to construct a preventive policy focused on drinking practices, a number of difficulties arise. First, at the level of ideals, the government must define the kinds of drinking practices—amounts, frequencies, and occasions for drinking—that are considered safe and appropriate. It must clearly set off those practices that fall outside these boundaries. Yet virtually all national societies are multiethnic, and the sheer variety of drinking customs will mean that no matter where the boundary lines are drawn, there will be uproar somewhere. Inevitably, the boundaries that set off what is not acceptable will exclude ways of drinking that a substantial population considers quite normal, acceptable, and none of the government's business. The same boundaries will also permit some drinking practices that a substantial group will consider outrageous and unusual; they will accuse the government of giving positive assent to behavior that they consider frightening, hazardous, or wrong. The task of drawing boundaries that minimize irreconcilable sources of citizen displeasure is not an enviable one.

Policies can be tuned to create less discord. Not all lines need be drawn with equal force. As an earlier review of this matter suggested, "A line defended by criminal statutes must command wider compliance . . . and be focused on behavior that produces more adverse external effects than a line defended by weaker measures such as economic incentives, civil sanctions, advisory educational programs, or exemplary actions of government . . . Criminal statutes should be sparsely used to discourage only the rarest and most dangerous conduct. Other programs could be used more liberally and establish somewhat more controversial goals" (Moore and Gerstein, 1981, 57–58). Governments have several ways to implement conceptions about safety and appropriateness in drinking practices. The principal means are laws or statutory regulations governing individual conduct, controls over advertising, and education, including information and training programs conducted in the schools, mass media, and elsewhere.

Assuming that the government can find a consensus about which practices are sufficiently hazardous or deviant to merit one or another means of action, it must then face the countervailing considerations of effectiveness and competition for resources. In shaping drinking practices, strong resistance will arise against any effort that tries to move very far beyond discouraging what the informal norms already condemn, or encouraging what these norms already esteem. An effective strategy for overcoming such resistances might, for example, entail strengthening discouragement with effective deterrence or backing encouragement with efficient training. But the government must be prepared to devote time and money to these tasks, possibly at the expense of other tasks. Two familiar policy areas illustrate these issues: laws against drunken driving and classroom education about alcohol.

DRUNK DRIVING AND THE LAW The odds are long against any single episode of drunkenness at the wheel being detected when it occurs: no better than 500 to 1 in very attentive jurisdictions (Borkenstein, 1974; Reed, 1981). The chronic violator who drives intoxicated hundreds of times a year is likely to be caught sooner or later and, if caught once, is likely to be caught again if the violations persist. But most drivers responsible for drunk driving accidents are "first offenders," i.e., have escaped previous police detection (Ross, 1983). Countermeasures must be designed for the large pool of violators as yet unknown to the law. Extra or specially equipped police patrols or roadblocks in the lanes where most serious drunk driving accidents occur can reduce fatal accidents by one-third to one-half, but only if the effort attracts extensive media publicity. Without publicity, much of the preventive effect is lost (Ross, 1983). These efforts are expensive (Levy et al., 1978; cf. Reed, 1981), and there are limits to how many police personnel can be shifted into drunk driving deterrence if the community is also to have police action on assaults, robberies, drug transactions, and so forth. Of the 10 million arrests annually recorded in the FBI annual crime index for the United States, over 1.25 million are for drunk driving (Federal Bureau of Investigation, 1982). (Another 1.25 million are for public drunkenness.)

Considerable sentiment favors increasing current drunk driving penalties or applying the existing statutes with fuller force instead of using plea bargains, diversions to treatment or education, probation, and suspended sentences (Presidential Commission on Drunk Driving, 1983; Governor's Alcohol and Highway Safety Task Force, 1981). But no empty jail cell awaits the drunk driver. Jail space is a scarce, expensive resource that the criminal justice system must marshal carefully. Every decision to imprison one person for any length of time necessarily means delaying or denying imprisonment for some other person convicted of an offense that is legally subject to this sanction. The question is, Shall we free the rapist or thief sooner in order to imprison the drunk driver? To some degree, the answer is clearly yes. But the resource limits on incarcerative responses to crime mean that only a massive mobilization of effort will persuade judges (and jurors, who are usually more lenient than judges) to jail drunk drivers on first or even second offenses, given the rarity of imposing such sanctions for other felony offenses. The evidence indicates that sentencing crackdowns alone have no impact on rates of drunk driving (Ross, 1983). However, in combination with rapid adjudication, more aggressive sentencing can satisfy the aggrieved victims, the survivors, and sympathetic citizens, and it can also reinforce publicity on the morally serious nature of other actions against drunk driving.

EDUCATION, ALCOHOL, AND CHILDREN From their schoolteachers children learn how to work successfully through a series of graded, progressively more difficult lessons, how to remember and make use of such factual knowledge as when Columbus landed in the New World, and how to behave in nonfamily environments. By example, cajolery, and discipline, teachers transmit habits of thought, imagination, civility, and interest in the practical world and its lessons. By system, trial, and error, they can train children in particular numerical and literacy skills. But in the context of prohibition for children and detached professional concern among teachers, what can serve as a lesson plan on safe and appropriate drinking? When other areas of curriculum are considered, a contrast becomes quite clear. Students are not expected to learn how to multiply without practicing multiplication tables, or to learn to read without taking books home for study, and bringing in homework for criticism and praise. If we wish children not to drink at all, this message can certainly be transmitted. But telling children nothing more than "not until you're older" does little to inculcate safe or appropriate behavior once they are older.

The most effective approach begins with the recognition that most children will have to learn for themselves about alcohol and its problems. What they need most in the way of education is the benefit of adult experience and example in gauging the times, places, amounts, and risks involved in drinking and not drinking. Alcohol education for schoolchildren should focus on present situations instead of the distant future. Respect for legal prohibition needs to be stressed for its protective significance (drunkenness is a very poor learning condition), but this should be tempered with respect for children's real experience, which they must interpret and learn to control for themselves. Some experimental programs have relied on peer counseling and example to develop coping skills that are applicable to potential alcohol and drug use situations and have yielded a margin of encouragement for this approach (McAlister et al., 1981; McAlister, 1983).

ADVERTISING A surprising amount of public debate about alcohol centers on the advertising practices of distillers, brewers, and vintners. The manufacturers argue that their main advertising goal is to increase or maintain the market shares of their brands against those of competitors with already established drinkers and that advertising has no impact on the general population's market participation. Critics argue that the major effect of advertising is to increase the overall amount of consumption of all brands and to seduce new, especially young, consumers. Econometric and quasi-experimental studies of variation in advertising expenditures or laws governing advertising generally support the manufacturers' argument on this point (Smart, 1982; Grant et al., 1983).

In a different vein, critics of beverage advertising argue that commercial messages fail to convey important warning information and that they trade on false glamor by associating drinking exclusively with athletics, youth, sex, and success. Virtually no scientific studies have methodically analyzed the content of alcohol advertising as has been done for the content of television programming (Wallack, 1983). The debate over advertising content, health warnings, and labeling is based on the symbolic significance attached to commercial messages and their control and reflects some untested conflicting assertions and presumptions about the long-range impact of these features of advertising.

Reducing Environmental Risk

Even the most strenuous efforts to reduce unsafe or inappropriate drinking practices cannot be expected to eliminate them or to curtail them radically. If we accept this premise, the sensible approach is to design some preventive policies that aim to reduce the damages and the risks brought about by unsafe drunkenness. While some have misinterpreted this approach as "making the world safe for drunks" and have consequently felt uneasy or even outraged, a more accurate expression of the approach is "making the world safer for, and from, people who are affected by alcohol intoxication or other impairments" (Moore and Gerstein, 1981, 100–101).

Strong objections greet proposals that do not directly attack the causes of alcohol-related problems, but instead seem to offer acceptance to excessive or poorly timed drunkenness and seem to make its consequences less stern. Aside from the practical counterpoint that deploring a condition does not make it less real, some sound arguments can be made for the environmental approach. First, protection against the consequences of drunken behavior is not only beneficial to drunks. An intoxicated pilot, mechanic, bus driver, railroad engineer, or switch operator menaces the lives of many others. Second, while drunkenness may have a greater voluntary component than fatigue, absentminded-ness, irritation, or a previous injury, the resulting impairments and associated risks of human error are similar. Measures taken to reduce the harm of drunken mishaps will reduce the harm of the other mishaps.

Finally, ample precedent exists for interventions that reduce illness or discomfort without special regard for the morality or legality of the contributory actions. Preventive as well as therapeutic measures are used to control venereal disease without barriers concerning marital status or particular sexual practices. Neither cigarette smokers nor obese people are denied publicly supported treatment for heart disease. Blood pressure testing and cardiopulmonary resuscitation training are widely encouraged even though many, indeed most, of the people who will benefit from these measures have been indulgent in diet and deficient in physical discipline.

The two principal categories of environmental risk are interpersonal hazards and physical casualties. In regard to the interpersonal hazards, the most common impression about drunkenness and interpersonal conflict is that drunks endanger others. Yet the evidence suggests that intoxication leads more often to victimization *of* the drunk than *by* the drunk. "Rolling drunks" is a substantial criminal pastime. A history of alcoholism can also cost people important life opportunities regardless of their current and prospective state of sobriety.

In regard to physical casualties, since alcohol intoxication tends to make people clumsy and inattentive, it has been implicated to some degree in many kinds of traumas, including drownings, burns, falls, and momentum injuries, notably motor vehicle accidents (Aarens et al., 1977). If everyday materials and machines were made less likely to rip, trip, bludgeon, or burn people who were less than fully efficient (whether due to drunkenness or some other impairment), alcohol-related and other casualties would be fewer. Alcohol-related casualties might be particularly affected, as noted elsewhere, "since alcohol-related casualties tend to be concentrated in the most severe categories—deaths and permanent disabilities" (Moore and Gerstein, 1981, 102).

Among the safety mechanisms that could prevent a large number of alcohol casualties, major examples are the automobile safety devices which increase the crashworthiness of vehicles, such as automatic restraining-belt systems (lap-shoulder loops), air bags (impact-triggered pneumatic barriers), and seat belts. In many crashes, of course, no restraining device could prevent mortal wounding, but it would nonetheless be instructive if news reports of serious traffic accidents would indicate not only the sobriety of the dead and the survivors, but also which of them were wearing seat belts.

Public policy can advance the use of safety devices in a number of ways: by educating consumers to desire them, by sponsoring research and development to improve them, by offering favorable tax incentives or credits, by requiring that manufacturers make them available as paid options, or by requiring all automobiles to have them. A similar range of policy options is available for other safety devices (e.g., household smoke detectors, "dead man" controls on train engines, self-extinguishing cigarettes). People who are broadly concerned with preventing alcohol problems have substantial grounds for taking an interest in these more general safety issues and policies (Mosher and Mottl, 1981).

CONCLUSION

Creating and carrying out alcohol policy will never approach the purity of chess or laboratory science, or provide the direct personal validation and satisfaction that accompany successful clinical intervention. But policies do often have results, which can be better or worse. Well-organized research and informed thinking are often a large part of the difference between better and worse results.

References for Part IV

References for the Introduction

Armor DJ, Polich JM, Stambul HB: Alcoholism and Treatment. New York, John Wiley & Sons, 1978

Institute of Medicine: Alcoholism and Related Problems: Opportunities for Research. Washington DC, National Academy of Sciences, 1980

Orford L, Edwards G: Alcoholism. New York, Oxford University Press, 1977

Perry JC: Disorders associated with borderline personality. Paper presented at the Annual Meeting of the American Psychiatric Association, New York City, 1983

Sobell MB, Sobell LC: Second-year treatment outcome of alcoholics treated by individualized behavior therapy: Results. Behav Res Ther 14:195–215, 1976

Vaillant GE: The Natural History of Alcoholism. Cambridge MA, Harvard University Press, 1983

Vaillant GE, Gale L, Milofsky ES: Natural history of male alcoholism: II. Relationship between different diagnostic dimensions. J Stud Alcohol 43:216–232, 1982

References for Chapter 18

The Diagnosis of Alcoholism After DSM-III

American Psychiatric Association: Diagnostic and Statistical Manual of Mental Disorders, 3d ed. Washington DC, American Psychiatric Association, 1980

Armor DJ, Polich JM, Stambul HB: Alcoholism and Treatment. New York, John Wiley & Sons, 1978

Feighner J, Robins E, Guze S, Woodruff R, Winokur G, Munoz R: Diagnostic criteria for use in psychiatric research. Arch Gen Psychiatry 26:57–63, 1972

Gomberg ES: Prevalence of alcoholism among ward patients in a Veterans Administration hospital. J Stud Alcohol 36:1458–1467, 1975

Helzer JE, Robins LN, Croughan J, Welner A: Renard Diagnostic Interview: Its reliability and procedural validity with lay interviewers. Arch Gen Psychiatry 38:393–398, 1981

Robins LN: The diagnosis of alcoholism after DSM-III, in Research Monographs #5, Evaluation of the Alcoholic: Implications for Research, Theory and Treatment. Edited by Meyer RE, Babor TF. Washington DC, US Government Printing Office, 1981

Robins LN, West PA, Murphy GE: The high rate of suicide in older white men: A study testing ten hypotheses. Soc Psychiatry 12:1–20, 1977

Robins LN, Helzer JE, Croughan J, Williams J, Spitzer R: The National Institute of Mental Health Diagnostic Interview (DIS, Version II). Rockville MD, National Institute of Mental Health, 1979

Robins LN, Helzer JE, Croughan J, Ratcliff KS: National Institute of Mental Health Diagnostic Interview Schedule: Its history, characteristics, and validity. Arch Gen Psychiatry 38:381–389, 1981

Spitzer R, Endicott J, Fleiss J, Cohen J: The Psychiatric Status Schedule: A technique for evaluating psychopathology and impairment in role functioning. Arch Gen Psychiatry 23:41–55, 1970

Spitzer R, Endicott J, Robins E: Clinical criteria for psychiatric diagnosis and DSM-III. Am J Psychiatry 132:1187–1192, 1975

References for Chapter 19

The Course of Alcoholism and Lessons for Treatment

Aamark C: A study in alcoholism. Acta Psychiatr Scand (Suppl 70) 1951

Armor DJ, Polich JM, Stambul HB: Alcoholism and Treatment. New York, John Wiley & Sons, 1978

Blane HT: The Personality of the Alcoholic: Guises of Dependency. New York, Harper & Row, 1968

Cahalan D, Room R: Problem Drinkers Among American Men. New Brunswick NJ, Rutgers Center for Alcohol Studies, 1974

Clark WB: Loss of control, heavy drinking, and drinking problems in a longitudinal setting. J Stud Alcohol 37:1256–1290, 1976

Clark WB, Cahalan D: Changes in problem drinking over a four-year span. Addict Behav 1:251–259, 1976

Costello RM: Alcoholism treatment effectiveness: Slicing the outcome variance pie, in Alcoholism Treatment in Transition. Edited by Edwards SG, Grant M. London, Croom Helm, 1980

Essen Möller E: Individual traits and morbidity in a Swedish rural population. Acta Psychiatr Scand (Suppl 100) 1956

Gerard DL, Saenger G, Wile R: The abstinent alcoholic. Arch Gen Psychiatry 6:83–95, 1962

Glueck S, Glueck E: Unraveling Juvenile Delinquency. New York, Commonwealth Fund, 1950

Goodwin DW: Alcoholism and heredity. Arch Gen Psychiatry 36:57–61, 1979

Goodwin DW, Crane JB, Guze SB: Felons who drink: An 8-year follow-up. Q J Stud Alcohol 32:135–147, 1971

Jellinek EM: Phases of alcohol addiction. Q J Stud Alcohol 13:673–684, 1952

Jellinek EM: The Disease Concept of Alcoholism. New Haven CT, Hillhouse Press, 1960

Kammeier ML, Hoffmann H, Loper RG: Personality characteristics of alcoholics as college freshman and at time of treatment. Q J Stud Alcohol 34:390–399, 1973

Keller M: Problems of epidemiology in alcohol problems. Q J Stud Alcohol 36:1442–1451, 1975

Knupfer G: Ex–problem drinkers, in Life History Research in Psychopathology, vol 2. Edited by Roff M, Robins LN, Pollack H. Minneapolis, University of Minnesota Press, 1972

McCord W, McCord J: Origins of Alcoholism. Stanford CA, Stanford University Press, 1960

Morrison JR: Bipolar affective disorder and alcoholism. Am J Psychiatry 131:1130–1133, 1974

Ojesjo L: Long-term outcome in alcohol abuse and alcoholism among males in the Lundby general population, Sweden. Br J Addict 76:391–400, 1981

Orford J, Edwards G: Alcoholism. New York, Oxford University Press, 1977

Pendery ML, Maltzman IM, West LJ: Controlled drinking by alcoholics? New findings and a reevaluation of a major affirmative study. Science 217:169–175, 1982

Pettinatti HM, Sugerman H, Maurer HS: Four-year MMPI changes in abstinent and drinking alcoholics. Alcoholism: Clin Exp Res 6:487–494, 1982

Polich JM, Armor DJ, Braiker HB: The Course of Alcoholism. New York, John Wiley & Sons, 1981

Powers E, Witmer H: An Experiment in the Prevention of Delinquency. New York, Columbia University Press, 1959

Robins LN: Deviant Children Grown Up: A Sociological and Psychiatric Study of Sociopathic Personality. Baltimore, Williams & Wilkins, 1966

Roizen R, Cahalan D, Shanks P: "Spontaneous remission" among untreated problem drinkers, in Longitudinal Research on Drug Use. Edited by Kandel DB. New York, John Wiley & Sons, 1978

Schilder P: The psychogenesis of alcoholism. Q J Stud Alcohol 2:277–292, 1941

Schlesser MAG, Winokur G, Sherman BM: Hypothalamic-pituitary-adrenal axis activity in depressive illness. Arch Gen Psychiatry 37:737–743, 1980

Simmel E: Alcoholism and addiction. Psychoanal Q 17:6–31, 1948

Sobell MB, Sobell LC: Second-year treatment outcome of alcoholics treated by individualized behavior therapy: Results. Behav Res Ther 14:195–215, 1976

Sundby P: Alcoholism and Mortality. Oslo, Norway, Universitets Forlaget, 1967

Ullman AD: The first drinking experience of addictive and of normal drinkers. Q J Stud Alcohol 14:181–191, 1953

Vaillant GE: Natural history of male psychological health. VIII. Antecedents to alcoholism and "orality." Am J Psychiatry 17:181–186, 1980

Vaillant GE: Natural History of Alcoholism. Cambridge MA, Harvard University Press, 1983

Vaillant GE, Milofsky ES: The etiology of alcoholism: A prospective viewpoint. Am Psychol 37:494–503, 1982a

Vaillant GE, Milofsky ES: Natural history of male alcoholism. IV. Paths to recovery. Arch Gen Psychiatry 39:127–133, 1982b

Vaillant GE, Gale L, Milofsky E: Natural history of male alcoholism. II. Relationship between different diagnostic dimensions. J Stud Alcohol 43:216–232, 1982

Vaillant GE, Clark W, Cyrus C, Milofsky ES, Kopp J, Wulsin V, Mogielnicki NP: The natural history of alcoholism: An eight-year follow-up. Am J Med, in press

Winokur G, Clayton PJ, Reich T: Manic-Depressive Illness. St. Louis, CV Mosby Co, 1969

References for Chapter 20

Genetic and Biochemical Factors in the Etiology of Alcoholism

Begleiter H, Porjesz B: Brain electrophysiology and alcoholism. Advances in Alcoholism II, February 1983

Bloom FE: A summary of workshop discussions, in β-Carbolines and Tetrahydroisoquinolines. Edited by Bloom F, Barchos J, Sandler M, Usden E. New York, Alan R Liss Inc, 1982

Bohman M, Sigvardsson S, Cloninger R: Maternal inheritance of alcohol abuse. Arch Gen Psychiatry 38:965–969, 1981

Bosron WF, Li TK: Genetic determinants of alcohol and aldehyde dehydrogenases and alcohol metabolism. Semin Liver Disease 1:179–188, 1981

Brown JB: Platelet MAO and alcoholism. Am J Psychiatry 134:206–207, 1977

Cahalan D: Problem Drinkers. San Francisco, Jossey-Bass, 1970

Cloninger CR, Reich T: Genetic heterogeneity in alcoholism and sociopathy, in Proceedings of Association for Research in Nervous and Mental Disease, Genetics of Neurological and Psychiatric Disorders. Edited by Kety SS. New York, Raven Press, 1981

Cloninger CR, Christiansen KO, Reich T, Gottesman II: Implications of sex differences in the prevalences of antisocial personality, alcoholism, and criminality for family transmission. Arch Gen Psychiatry 35:941–951, 1978

Cotton NS: The familial incidence of alcoholism. J Stud Alcohol 40:89–116, 1979

Coursey MD, Buchsbaum MS, Murphy DL: Platelet MAO activity and evoked potentials in the identification of subjects biologically at risk for psychiatric disorders. Br J Psychiatry 134:372–381, 1979

Elmasian R, Neville H, Woods D, Schuckit M, Bloom F: Event-related brain potentials are different in individuals at high and low risk for developing alcoholism. Proc Natl Acad Sci 79:7900–7903, 1982

Gerstein DR: Alcohol use and consequences, in Alcohol and Public Policy. Edited by Moore MH, Gerstein DR. Washington DC, National Academic Press, 1981

Goedde HW, Agarwal DP, Harada S: Alcohol metabolizing enzymes: Studies of isozymes in human biopsies and cultured fibroblasts. Clin Genet 16:29–33, 1979a

Goedde HW, Harada S, Agarwal DP: Racial differences in alcohol sensitivity: A new hypothesis. Hum Genet 51:331–334, 1979b

Goodwin DW, Guze SB: Psychiatric Diagnosis. New York, Oxford University Press, 1979

Goodwin DW, Schulsinger F, Moller N, Hermansen L, Winokur G, Guze SB: Drinking problems in adopted and nonadopted sons of alcoholics. Arch Gen Psychiatry 31:164–169, 1974

Greenfield NJ, Pietruszko R: Two aldehyde dehydrogenases from human liver. Isolation via affinity chromatography and characterization of the isozymes. Biochim Biophys Acta 483:35–45, 1977

Harada S, Misawa S, Agarwal DP, Goedde HW: Liver alcohol dehydrogenase in the Japanese: Isozyme variation and its possible role in alcohol intoxication. Am J Hum Genet 32:8–15, 1980

Harada S, Takagi S, Agarwal DP, Goedde HW: Ethanol and aldehyde metabolism in alcoholics from Japan (abstract). 1st International Society for Biological Research in Alcoholism Congress, Munich 1982, Alcoholism: Clin Exp Res 6:298, 1982

Jenkins WJ, Peters TJ: Selectively reduced hepatic acetaldehyde dehydrogenase in alcoholics. Lancet 1:628–630, 1980

Korsten MA, Matsuzaki S, Feinman L, Lieber CS: High blood acetaldehyde levels after ethanol administration. N Engl J Med 292:386–389, 1975

Li TK: Enzymology of human alcohol metabolism, in Alcoholics. Edited by Meister A. New York, John Wiley & Sons, 1977

Li TK, Magnes LJ: Identification of a distinctive molecular form of alcohol dehydrogenase in human livers with high activity. Biochem Biophys Res Commun 63:202–208, 1975

Lieber CS: Metabolism of ethanol, in Metabolic Aspects of Alcoholism. Edited by Lieber CS. Lancaster, MTP Press Ltd, 1977

Lindros KO: Human blood acetaldehyde levels: With improved methods, a clearer picture emerges. Alcoholism: Clin Exp Res 6:70–75, 1982

Lindros KO, Stowell A, Pikkarainen P, Salaspuro M: Elevated blood acetaldehyde in alcoholics with accelerated ethanol elimination. Pharmacol Biochem Behav 13:119–124, 1980

Meisch RA: Animal studies of alcohol intake. Br J Psychiatry 141:113–120, 1982

Morrison C, Schuckit MA: Locus of control in young men with alcoholic relatives and controls. J Clin Psychiatry 44:306–307, 1983

Myers RD, Critcher EC: Naloxone alters alcohol drinking induced in the rat by tetrahydropapaveroline (THP) infused ICV. Pharmcol Biochem Behav 16:827–836, 1982

Myers RD, McCaleb ML, Ruwe WD: Alcohol drinking induced in the monkey by tetrahydropapaveroline (THP) infused into the cerebral ventricle. Pharmcol Biochem Behav 16:995–1000, 1982

Nathan PE, Lisman SA: Behavioral and motivational patterns of chronic alcoholics, in Alcoholism: Interdisciplinary Approaches to an Enduring Problem. Edited by Tarter RE, Sugerman AA. Reading MA, Addison-Wesley, 1976

Pollock VE, Volavka J, Goodwin DW: The EEG after alcohol in men at risk for alcoholism. Science (in press)

Porjesz B, Begleiter H: Evoked brain potential deficits in alcoholism and aging. Alcoholism: Clin Exp Res 6:53–63, 1982

Propping P: Genetic control of ethanol action on the central nervous system. An EEG study in twins. Hum Genet 35:309–334, 1977

Saunders GR, Schuckit MA: MMPI scores in young men with alcoholic relatives and controls. J Nerv Ment Dis 169:456–458, 1981

Schuckit MA: Drug and Alcohol Abuse: A Clinical Guide to Diagnosis and Treatment. New York, Plenum Press, 1979

Schuckit MA: Acetaldehyde and alcoholism: Methodology. Presented at the American College of Neuropsychopharmacology, San Juan, Puerto Rico, 1980a

Schuckit MA: Alcoholism and genetics: Possible biological mediators. Biol Psychiatry 15:437–447, 1980b

Schuckit MA: Self-rating of alcohol intoxication by young men with and without family histories of alcoholism. J Stud Alcohol 41:242–249, 1980c

Schuckit MA: A theory of alcohol and drug abuse: A genetic approach, in Theories on Drug Abuse. Edited by Lettieri DJ, Sayers M, Pearson HW. Washington DC, Food and Drug Administration, Research Monograph 30:297–302, 1980d

Schuckit MA: An overview of "high-risk" studies on alcoholism. Presented at the National Council on Alcoholism Annual Scientific Session, New Orleans, April 14, 1981a

Schuckit MA: Peak blood alcohol levels in men at high risk for the future development of alcoholism. Alcoholism: Clin Exp Res 5:64–66, 1981b

Schuckit MA: Twin studies on substance abuse: An overview, in Twin Research 3: Epidemiological and Clinical Studies, New York, Alan R Liss, 1981c

Schuckit MA: Anxiety and assertiveness in the relatives of alcoholics and controls. J Clin Psychiatry 43:238–239, 1982a

Schuckit MA: The history of psychotic symptoms in alcoholics. J Clin Psychiatry 43:53–57, 1982b

Schuckit MA: A prospective study of genetic markers in alcoholism, in Biological Markers in Psychiatry and Neurology. Edited by Hanin I, Usden E. Oxford, Pergamon Press, 1982c

Schuckit MA: Extroversion and neuroticism in young men at higher and lower risk for alcoholism. Amer J Psychiatry 140:1223–1224, 1983a

Schuckit MA: A study of alcoholics with secondary depression. Amer J Psychiatry 140:711–714, 1983b

Schuckit MA: Alcoholism and other psychiatric disorders. Hosp Community Psychiatry 34:1022–1027, 1983c

Schuckit MA, Duby J: Alcohol-related flushing and the risk for alcoholism in sons of alcoholics. J Clin Psychiatry 43:415–418, 1982

Schuckit MA, Haglund R: Etiological theories on alcoholism, in Alcoholism. Edited by Estes N, Heinemann ME. St. Louis, CV Mosby Co, 1982

Schuckit MA, Rayses V: Ethanol ingestion: Differences in blood acetaldehyde concentrations in relatives of alcoholics and controls. Science 203:54–55, 1979

Schuckit MA, Stockard J: The effects of alcohol on men at elevated risk for future alcoholism. Presented at the National Council on Alcoholism Annual Scientific Session. Houston, Texas, April, 1983

Schuckit MA, von Wartburg JP: Hypothesis: Developing a model of causation for alcoholism (in press)

Schuckit MA, Goodwin DA, Winokur G: A study of alcoholism in half siblings. Amer J Psychiatry 128:1132–1136, 1972

Schuckit MA, O'Connor DT, Duby J, Vega R, Moss M: DBH activity levels in men at high risk for alcoholism and controls. Biol Psychiatry 16:1067–1075, 1981a

Schuckit MA, Engstrom D, Alpert R, Duby J: Differences in muscle-tension response to ethanol in young men with and without family histories of alcoholism. J Stud Alcohol 42:918–924, 1981b

Schuckit MA, Shaskan E, Duby J, Vega R, Moss M: Platelet monoamine oxidase activity in relatives of alcoholics. Arch Gen Psychiatry 39:137–140, 1982

Schuckit MA, Parker DC, Rossman LR: Ethanol-related prolactin responses and risk for alcoholism. Biol Psychiatry (in press)

Sullivan JL, Cavenar JO, Maltibie AA, Lister P, Zung WWK: Familial biochemical and clinical correlates of alcoholics with low platelet monoamine oxidase activity. Biol Psychiatry 14:385–394, 1979

von Wartburg JP: Polymorphism of human alcohol and aldehyde dehydrogenase. Acta Psychiatr Scand (Suppl) 268:179–188, 1980

Watt DC: The search for genetic linkage in schizophrenia. Br J Psychiatry 140:532–537, 1982

Weiner H: A model to estimate the in vivo level of TIQ's in brain during the consumption of ethanol, in β-Carbolines and Tetrahydroisoquinolines. Edited by Bloom F, Barchos J, Sandler M, Usden E. New York, Alan R Liss, 1982

Zeiner R: Acetaldehyde and the risk for alcoholism. Presented at the 20th International Congress on Applied Psychology, Edinburgh, Scotland, July 25–31, 1982

References for Chapter 21

Contributions of Learning Theory to the Diagnosis and Treatment of Alcoholism

Abrams DB, Wilson GT: Self-control of delay of gratification. Rutgers University, 1980 (unpublished manuscript)

Armor DJ, Polich JM, Stambul HB: Alcoholism and Treatment. New York, John Wiley & Sons, 1978

Azrin NH: Improvements in the community reinforcement approach to alcoholism. Behav Res Ther 14:339–348, 1976

Bandura A: Social Learning Theory. Englewood Cliffs, NJ, Prentice-Hall, 1977

Bigelow G, Cohen M, Liebson I, Faillace L: Abstinence or moderation? Choice by alcoholics. Behav Res Ther 10:209–214, 1972

Bigelow G, Liebson I, Lawrence C: Prevention of alcohol abuse by reinforcement of incompatible behavior, Paper presented at Association for Advancement of Behavior Therapy, December 1973

Bigelow G, Liebson I, Griffiths, RR: Alcohol drinking: Suppression by a behavioral time-out procedure. Behav Res Ther 12:107–115, 1974

Bigelow GE, Stitzer ML, Griffiths RR, Liebson IA: Contingency management approaches to drug self-administration and drug abuse: Efficacy and limitations. Addict Behav 6:241–252, 1981

Cahalan D, Cisin IH, Crossley HM: American Drinking Practices. New Brunswick, NJ, Rutgers Center of Alcohol Studies, 1969

Cahalan D, Room R: Problem Drinking Among American Men. New Brunswick, NJ, Rutgers Center of Alcohol Studies, 1974

Caudill BD, Marlatt GA: Modeling influences in social drinking: An experimental analogue. J Consult Clin Psychol 43:405–415, 1975

Cautela JR: Treatment of compulsive behavior by covert sensitization. Psychol Rep 16:33–41, 1966

Cautela JR: Covert reinforcement. Behav Ther 1:33–50, 1970

Conger JJ: Effects of alcohol on conflict behavior in the albino rat. Q J Stud Alcohol 12:1–29, 1951

Conger JJ: Alcoholism: Theory, problem and challenge. II. Reinforcement theory and the dynamics of alcoholism. Q J Stud Alcohol 17:291–324, 1956

Cutter HSG, Schwaab EL, Nathan PE: Effects of alcohol on its utility for alcoholics. Q J Stud Alcohol 30:369–378, 1970

Donovan DM, Marlatt GA: Assessment of expectancies and behaviors associated with alcohol consumption: A cognitive-behavioral approach. J Stud Alcohol 41:1153–1185, 1980

Elkins RL: Covert sensitization treatment of alcoholism: Contributions of successful conditioning to subsequent abstinence maintenance. Addict Behav 5:67–89, 1980

Goodwin DW, Guze SB: Heredity and alcoholism, in Biology of Alcoholism, vol 3. Edited by Kissin B, Begleiter H. New York, Plenum Press, 1974

Gottheil E, Crawford H, Cornelison FS Jr: Alcoholics' ability to resist available alcohol. Dis Nerv Sys 34:80–84, 1973

Griffiths RR, Bigelow G, Liebson I: Assessment of effects of ethanol self-administration on social interactions in alcoholics. Psychopharmacologia 38:105–110, 1974

Griffiths RR, Bigelow G, Liebson I: Effect of ethanol self-administration on choice behavior: Money vs socializing. Pharmacol Biochem Behav 3:443–446, 1975

Heermans HW, Nathan PE: Effect of alcohol, arousal, and aggressive cues on human physical aggression in males. Rutgers University, 1983 (unpublished manuscript)

Higgins RL, Marlatt GA: Effects of anxiety arousal upon the consumption of alcohol by alcoholics and social drinkers. J Consult Clin Psychol 41:426–433, 1973

Higgins RL, Marlatt GA: Fear of interpersonal evaluation as a determinant of alcohol consumption in male social drinkers. J Abnormal Psychol 84:644–651, 1975

Hunt GM, Azrin NH: Community-reinforcement approach to alcoholism. Behav Res Ther 11:91–104, 1973

Lansky D, Wilson GT: Alcohol, expectations and sexual arousal in males: An information processing analysis. J Abnorm Psychol 90:35–45, 1981

Lemere F, Voegtlin WL: An evaluation of the aversion treatment of alcoholism. Q J Stud Alcohol 11:199–204, 1950

Liebson I, Bigelow G, Flame R: Alcoholism among methadone patients: A specific treatment method. Am J Psychiatry 130:483, 1973

McCollam JB, Burish TG, Maisto S, Sobell M: Alcohol's effects on physiological arousal and self-reported affect and sensations. J Abnorm Psychol 89:224–234, 1980

Mahoney MJ: Cognition and Behavior Modification. Cambridge, MA, Ballinger, 1974

Marlatt GA: Drinking Profile: A questionnaire for the behavioral assessment of alcoholism, in Behavior Therapy Assessment: Diagnosis, Design, and Evaluation. Edited by Mash EJ, Terdal LG. New York, Springer, 1976

Marlatt GA: Craving for alcohol, loss of control, and relapse: A cognitive-behavioral analysis, in Alcoholism: New Directions in Behavioral Research and Treatment. Edited by Nathan PE, Marlatt GA. New York, Plenum Press, 1978

Marlatt GA: Drinking history: Problems of validity and reliability, in Evaluation of the Alcoholic: Implications for Research, Theory, and Treatment: National Institutes of Alcohol Abuse and Alcoholism Research Monograph 5. Rockville, MD, National Institutes of Alcohol Abuse and Alcoholism, 1981

Marlatt GA, Donovan DM: Behavioral psychology approaches to alcoholism, in Encyclopedic Handbook of Alcoholism. Edited by Pattison EM, Kaufman E. New York, Gardner, 1982

Marlatt GA, Demming B, Reid JB: Loss of control drinking in alcoholics: An experimental analogue. J Abnorm Psychol 81:233–241, 1973

Marlatt GA, Kosturn CF, Lang AR: Provocation to anger and opportunity for retaliation as determinants of alcohol consumption in social drinkers. J Abnorm Psychol 84:652–659, 1975

Meichenbaum DH: Cognitive-Behavior Modification. New York, Plenum Press, 1977

Mello NK: Behavioral studies of alcoholism, in Biology of Alcoholism, vol 2. Edited by Kissin B, Begleiter H. New York, Plenum Press, 1972

Mello NK, Mendelson JH: Operant analysis of drinking patterns of chronic alcoholics. Nature 206:43–46, 1965

Mendelson JH, Mello NK: Experimental analysis of drinking behavior of chronic alcoholics. Ann NY Acad Sci 133:828–845, 1966

Merry J: "Loss of control" myth. Lancet 1:1267–1268, 1966

Miller WR, Caddy GR: Abstinence and controlled drinking in the treatment of problem drinkers. J Stud Alcohol 38:986–1003, 1977

Nathan PE: Failures in prevention: Why we can't prevent the devastating effect of alcoholism and drug abuse on American productivity. Am Psychol 38:459–468, 1983

Nathan PE, Lisman SA: Behavioral and motivational patterns of chronic alcoholics, in Alcoholism: Interdisciplinary Approaches to an Enduring Problem. Edited by Tarter RE, Sugerman AA. Reading, MA, Addison-Wesley, 1976

Nathan PE, Niaura RS: Behavioral assessment and treatment of alcoholism, in Diagnosis and Treatment of Alcoholism, 2nd ed. Edited by Mendelson JH, Mello NK. New York, McGraw-Hill (in press)

Nathan PE, O'Brien JS: An experimental analysis of the behavior of alcoholics and nonalcoholics during prolonged experimental drinking. Behav Res Ther 2:455–476, 1971

Nathan PE, Titler NA, Lowenstein LM, Solomon P, Rossi AM: Behavioral analysis of chronic alcoholism. Arch Gen Psychiatry 22:419–430, 1970

Neubuerger OW, Hasha N, Matarazzo JD, Schmitz RE, Pratt HH: Behavioral-chemical treatment of alcoholism: An outcome replication. J Stud Alcohol 42:806–810, 1981

Neubuerger OW, Miller SI, Schmitz RE, Matarazzo JD, Pratt H, Hasha N: Replicable abstinence rates in an alcoholism treatment program. JAMA 248:960–963, 1982

Oates JR, McCoy RT: Laboratory Evaluation of Alcohol Safety Interlock Systems. National Highway Traffic Safety Administration, US Department of Transportation Pub. No. HS-800, 927. Springfield, VA, US Nat Tech Inform Serv, 1973

Okulitch PV, Marlatt GA: Effects of varied extinction conditions with alcoholics and social drinkers. J Abnorm Psychol 79:205–211, 1972

Parker JC, Gilbert G, Speltz ML: Expectations regarding the effects of alcohol on assertiveness: A comparison of alcoholics and social drinkers. Addict Behav 6:29–33, 1981

Pattison EM: A conceptual approach to alcoholism treatment goals. Addict Behav 1:177–192, 1976

Penderey ML, Maltzman IM, West LJ: Controlled drinking by alcoholics? New findings and a reevaluation of a major affirmative study. Science 217:169–175, 1982

Pihl RO, Zeichner A, Niaura R, Nagy K, Zacchia C: Attribution and alcohol-mediated aggression. J Abnorm Psychol 90:468–475, 1981

Polich JM, Armor DJ, Braiker HB: Course of Alcoholism: Four Years After Treatment. New York, John Wiley & Sons, 1981

Pomerleau OF, Pertschuk M, Adkins D, Brady JP: A comparison of behavioral and traditional treatment for middle-income problem drinkers. J Behav Med 1:187–200, 1978

Sanchez-Craig M: Random assignment to abstinence or controlled drinking in a cognitive-behavioral program: Short-term effects on drinking behavior. Addict Behav 5:35–39, 1980

Sanchez-Craig M, Annis HM: Initial evaluation of a program for early-stage problem drinkers: Randomization to abstinence and controlled drinking. American Psychological Association Annual Meeting, Washington DC, August 1982

Selzer ML: Michigan Alcoholism Screening Test: Quest for a new diagnostic instrument. Am J Psychiatry 127:1653–1658, 1971

Sobell MB: Empirically derived components of treatment for alcohol problems: Some issues and extensions, in Behavioral Assessment and Treatment of Alcoholism. Edited by Marlatt GA, Nathan PE. New Brunswick, NJ, Rutgers Center of Alcohol Studies, 1978

Sobell MB, Sobell LC: Alcoholics treated by individualized behavior therapy: One-year treatment outcome. Behav Res Ther 11:599–618, 1973

Sobell MB, Sobell LC: Second-year treatment outcome of alcoholics treated by individualized behavior therapy: Results. Behav Res Ther 14:195-215, 1976

Strickler D, Bigelow G, Lawrence C, Liebson I: Moderate drinking as an alternative to alcohol abuse: A nonaversive procedure. Behav Res Ther 14:279–288, 1976

Tharp RG, Wetzel RJ: Behavior Modification in the Natural Environment. New York, Academic Press, 1969

Tracey D, Karlin R, Nathan PE: Experimental analysis of chronic alcoholism in four women. J Consult Clin Psychol 44:832–842, 1976

Vaillant GE, Milofsky ES: The etiology of alcoholism. Am J Psychol 37:494–503, 1982

Voegtlin WL: The treatment of alcoholism by establishing a conditioned reflex. Am J Med Science 199:802–809, 1940

Vogler RE, Compton JV, Weissbach TA: Integrated behavior change techniques for alcoholics. J Consult Clin Psychol 43:233–243, 1975

Vogler RE, Weissbach TA, Compton JV, Martin GT: Integrated behavior change techniques for problem drinkers in the community. J Consult Clin Psychol 45:267–279, 1977a

Vogler RE, Weissbach TA, Compton JV: Learning techniques for alcohol abuse. Behav Res Ther 15:31–38, 1977b

Vuchinich R, Sobell MB: Empirical separation of physiological and expected effects of alcohol on complex motor performance. Psychopharmacology 60:81–85, 1978

Wiens AN, Montague JR, Manaugh TS, English CJ: Pharmacological aversive conditioning to alcohol in a private hospital: One-year follow-up. J Stud Alcohol 37:1320–1324, 1976

Wilson GT: Expectations and substance abuse: Does basic research benefit clinical assessment and therapy? Addict Behav 6:221–231, 1981

Wilson GT, Abrams DB: Effects of alcohol on social anxiety and physiological arousal: Cognitive versus pharmacological processes. Cog Ther Res 1:195–210, 1977

Wilson GT, Lawson DM: Expectancies, alcohol, and sexual arousal in male social drinkers. J Abnorm Psychol 85:489–497, 1976

Wilson GT, Leaf R, Nathan PE: The aversive control of excessive drinking by chronic alcoholics in the laboratory setting. J Appl Behav Anal 8:13–26, 1975

References for Chapter 22

Psychotherapy in the Treatment of Alcoholism

Alcoholics Anonymous. New York, AA World Services Inc, 1955

Allen C: I'm Black and I'm Sober. Minneapolis, CompCare Publications, 1978

American Psychiatric Association: Diagnostic and Statistical Manual of Mental Disorders, 3rd ed. Washington DC, American Psychiatric Association, 1980

Bean MH: Denial and the psychological complications of alcoholism, in Dynamic Approaches to the Understanding and Treatment of Alcoholism. Edited by Bean MH, Zinberg NE. New York, Free Press, 1981

Blane HT: Psychotherapeutic approach, in The Biology of Alcoholism, vol 5. Edited by Kissin B, Begleiter H. New York, Plenum Press, 1977

Blume SB: Alcoholism, in Current Therapy. Edited by Conn HE. Philadelphia, WB Saunders Co, 1982

Blume SB: Disease concept of alcoholism, 1983. J Psychiatr Treatment Eval (in press) 1983

Blume SB, Dropkin D, Sokolow L: The Jewish alcoholic: A descriptive study. Alcohol Health and Research World 4:21–26, 1980

Galanter M: Psychotherapy for alcohol and drug abuse: An approach based on learning theory. J Psychiatr Treatment Eval (in press) 1983

Greenspan SI: Substance abuse: An understanding from psychodynamic, developmental and learning perspectives, in Psychodynamics of Drug Dependence, Research Monograph 12. Edited by Blaine JD, Julius DA. Washington DC, US Department of Health, Education and Welfare, National Institute on Drug Abuse, 1977

Jellinek EM: The Disease Concept of Alcoholism. New Brunswick NJ, Hillhouse Press, 1960

Khantzian EJ: Some treatment implications of the ego and self disturbances in alcoholism, in Dynamic Approaches to the Understanding and Treatment of Alcoholism. Edited by Bean MH, Zinberg NE. New York, Free Press, 1981

Khantzian EJ, Treece JC: Psychodynamics of drug dependence: An overview, in Psychodynamics of Drug Dependence, Research Monograph 12. Edited by Blaine JD, Julius DA. Washington DC, US Department of Health, Education and Welfare, National Institute on Drug Abuse, 1977

Knight RP: The psychoanalytic treatment in a sanitorium of chronic addiction to alcohol. JAMA 3:1443–1448, 1938

Kohut H: Preface, in Psychodynamics of Drug Dependence, Research Monograph 12. Edited by Blaine JD, Julius DA. Washington DC, US Department of Health, Education and Welfare, National Institute on Drug Abuse, 1977

Mack JE: Alcoholism, AA, and the governance of the self, in Dynamic Approaches to the Understanding and Treatment of Alcoholism. Edited by Bean MH, Zinberg NE. New York, Free Press, 1981

Rebeta-Burditt J: The Cracker Factory. New York, Macmillan Publishing Co, 1977

Schuckit MA, Morrissey ER: Alcoholism in women: Some clinical and social perspectives with an emphasis on possible subtypes, in Alcoholism Problems in Women and Children. Edited by Greenblatt M, Schuckit MA. New York, Grune & Stratton, 1976

Silber A: The contribution of psychoanalysis to the treatment of alcoholism, in Alcoholism and Clinical Psychiatry. Edited by Solomon J. New York, Plenum Publishing, 1982

Twerski AJ: It Happens to Doctors Too. Center City MN, Hazelden, 1982

Vaillant GE: Dangers of psychotherapy in the treatment of alcoholism, in Dynamic Approaches to the Understanding and Treatment of Alcoholism. Edited by Bean MH, Zinberg NE. New York, Free Press, 1981

Vaillant GE: The Natural History of Alcoholism. Cambridge MA, Harvard University Press, 1983

Wallace J: Working with the preferred defense structure of the recovering alcoholic, in Practical Approaches to Alcoholism Psychotherapy. Edited by Zimberg S, Wallace J, Blume SB. New York, Plenum Press, 1978

Wurmser L: Mr. Pecksniff's Horse? (Psychodynamics in compulsive drug use), in Psychodynamics of Drug Dependence, Research Monograph 12. Edited by Blaine JD, Julius DA. Washington DC, US Department of Health, Education and Welfare, National Institute on Drug Abuse, 1977

Zimberg S: Principles of alcoholism psychotherapy, in Practical Approaches to Alcoholism Psychotherapy. Edited by Zimberg S, Wallace J, Blume SB. New York, Plenum Press, 1978

Zimberg S: The Clinical Management of Alcoholism. New York, Brunner/Mazel, 1982

Zimberg S, Wallace J, Blume SB: Practical Approaches to Alcoholism Psychotherapy. New York, Plenum Press, 1978

References for Chapter 23

Pharmacotherapy in the Detoxification and Treatment of Alcoholism

Ahlenius S, Carlsson A, Engel J, Svensson T: Antagonism by alpha methyltyrosine of the ethanol-induced stimulation and euphoria in man. Clin Pharmacol Ther 14:586–591, 1973

Albert SN, Rea EL, Duverhy CA, Shea JG, Fazekas JF: Use of chlorpromazine in treatment of acute alcoholism. Med Ann DC 23:245–247, 1954

Alcohol and Health: 1st Special Report to the US Congress on Alcohol and Health. Washington DC, US Government Printing Office, 1971

Alkana RL, Noble EP: Amethystic agents: Reversal of acute ethanol intoxication in humans, in Biochemistry and Pharmacology of Ethanol, vol 2. Edited by Majchrowicz E, Noble, EP. New York, Plenum Press, 1979

Alkana RL, Parker ES, Cohn H, Birch H, Noble EP: Reversal of ethanol intoxication in humans: An assessment of the efficacy of propranolol. Psychopharmacology 51:29–37, 1976

Alkana RL, Parker ES, Cohn H, Birch H, Noble EP: Reversal of ethanol intoxication in humans: An assessment of the efficacy of L-dopa, aminophylline and ephedrine. Psychopharmacology 55:203–212, 1977

Anonymous: Magnesium deficiency. Br Med J 2:195, 1967

Armor DJ, Polich JM, Stambul HB: Alcoholism and Treatment, Report No. R-1739-NIAAA. Santa Monica, Rand Corp, 1976

Baratham G, Tinckler LF: Paraldehyde poisoning: A little-known hazard of post-operative sedation. Med J Aust 2:877–878, 1964

Baskin DS, Hosobuchi Y: Naloxone reversal of ischaemic neurological deficits in man. Lancet 2:272–275, 1981

Bergener M: EEG-changes during treatment of delirium tremens with chlormethiazole. Acta Psychiatr Scand (Suppl) 192:65–85, 1966

Beroz E, Conran P, Blanchard RW: Parenteral magnesium in the prophylaxis and treatment of delirium tremens. Am J Psychiatry 118:1042–1043, 1962

Block MA: The medical treatment of alcoholism. JAMA 162:1610–1619, 1956

Bloom F: To spritz or not to spritz: The doubtful value of aimless iontophoresis. Life Sci 14:1819–1834, 1974

Blum K, Merritt JH, Wallace JE, Owen R, Hahn JW, Geller I: Effects of catecholamine synthesis inhibition on ethanol narcosis in mice. Curr Ther Res 14:324–329, 1972

Bonfiglio G, Fallis S, Pacina A: Terapia della sindrome da soppressione di alcool col sale di sodio dell'acido n-dipropilacetico. Il Lav. Neuropsichiatr 50:115, 1972

Bonfiglio G, Falli S, Pacina A: Proposta di introduzione nella pratica ospedaliera di una nuova sostonza: il dipropilacetico di sodio nella prevenzione e terapia del Delirium Tremens alcoolico. Minerva Med 68:4233–4245, 1977

Boston LN: Delirium tremens (Mania E Potu): Statistical study of 156 cases. Lancet 1:18–19, 1908

Boucharlat PJ, Ledru J, Maitre A, Ratel M, Wolf R: Mais où est passé le delirium tremens. Ann Med Psychol (Paris) 134:557–564, 1976

Burrows GD, Vohra J, Hunt D, Sloman JG, Soggins BA, Davies B: Cardiac effects of different tricyclic antidepressant drugs. Br J Psychiatry 129:335–341, 1976

Burstein CL: The hazard of paraldehyde administration. JAMA 121:187–190, 1943

Butcher RW, Sutherland EW: Adenosine 3′,5′-phosphate in biological materials. J Biol Chem 237:1244–1250, 1962

Carlen PL: Reversible effects of chronic alcoholism on the human central nervous system: Possible biological mechanisms, in Cerebral Deficits in Alcoholism. Edited by Wilkinson DA. Toronto, Addiction Research Foundation, 1982

Catley DM, Lehane JR, Jones JG: Failure of naloxone to reverse alcohol intoxication. Lancet 1:1263, 1981

Clark ER, Hughes IE, Letley E: The effect of oral administration of various sugars on blood ethanol concentrations in man. J Pharm Pharmacol 25:319–323, 1973

Clark WD: Alcohol abuse, in Emergency Medicine. Edited by Kravas T, Warner C. Rockville MD, Aspen Systems Corp, 1983

Cohen R: Effects of fructose on blood-alcohol levels. Lancet 2:1086, 1972

Coleman JH, Evans WE: Drug interactions with alcohol. Alcohol Health and Research World: Experimental Issues, pp. 16–19, Winter 1975-1976

Damgaard S, Lundquist F, Tonnesen K, Hansen F, Sestoft L: Metabolism of ethanol and fructose in the isolated perfused pig liver. Europ J Biochem 33:87–97, 1973

DeLuca J: 4th Special Report to the US Congress on Alcohol and Health. Washington DC, US Government Printing Office, 1981

Dirksen R, Otten MH, Wood CJ, Verbaan CJ, Haalebos MMP, Verdouw PV, Nijhuis GMM: Naloxone in shock. Lancet 2:1360–1361, 1980

Dole VP, Fishman J, Goldfrank L, Khanna J, McGivern RF: Arousal of ethanol-intoxicated comatose patients with naloxone. Alcoholism 6:275–279, 1982

Eisen HJ, Ginsberg AL: Disulfiram hepatoxicity. Ann Intern Med 83:673–675, 1975

Eskelson CS, Myers LE, Calkins CN, Cazee CR: Some aspects of DH-524 (2[3,4-dichlorophenoxy]methyl-2-imidazoline) antagonistic like actions of ethanol intoxication in rats. Life Sci 18:1149–1156, 1976

Ewing JA, McCarty D: Are the endorphins involved in mediating the mood effects of ethanol. Alcoholism 5:148, 1981

Faiman MD: Biochemical pharmacology of disulfiram, in Biochemistry and Pharmacology of Ethanol, vol 2. Edited by Majchrowicz E, Noble EP. New York, Plenum Press, 1979

Favazza AR, Martin P: Chemotherapy of delirium tremens: A survey of physicians' preferences. Am J Psychiatry 131:1031–1033, 1974

Fazekas JF, Schultz JD, Sullivan PD, Shea JG: Management of acutely disturbed patients with promazine (sparine). JAMA 161:46–49, 1956

Fazekas JF, Shea JC, Ehrmantraut WR, Alman RW: Convulsant action of phenothiazine derivatives. JAMA 165:1241–1245, 1957

Fink GB, Swinyard EA: Effects of psychopharmacological agents on experimentally-induced seizures in mice. J Am Pharm Assoc-Sci Ed 49:510–512, 1960

Flink EB: Magnesium deficiency syndrome in man. JAMA 160:1406–1409, 1956

Flink EB: Mineral metabolism in alcoholism, in Biology of Alcoholism, vol 1 Biochemistry. Edited by Kissin B, Begleiter H. New York, Plenum Press, 1971

Flink EB, Stutzman FL, Anderson AR, Konig T, Fraser R: Magnesium deficiency after prolonged parenteral fluid administration and after chronic alcoholism complicated by delirium tremens. J Lab Clin Med 43:169–183, 1954

Forney R, Hughes F: Effect of caffeine and alcohol on performance under stress of audiofeedback. Q J Stud Alcohol 26:206–212, 1965

Forney R, Hulpieu H, Hughes F: The comparative enhancement of depressant action of alcohol by eight representative ataractic and analgesic drugs. Experientia 18:468–470, 1962

Freedman AM, Kaplan HI, Sadock BJ: Comprehensive Textbook of Psychiatry, 2nd ed. Baltimore, Williams & Wilkins Co, 1975

Fuller RK: Evaluation of efficacy of disulfiram (antabuse) for alcoholic veterans. Clin Res 24:568A, 1976

Gallant DM: Isolation of alcohol dehydrogenase. Alcoholism 5:469–471, 1981

Gessner PE: Drug therapy of the alcohol withdrawal syndrome, in Biochemistry and Pharmacology of Ethanol, vol 2. Edited by Majchrowicz E, Noble EP. New York, Plenum Press, 1979

Gessner PK: Alcohol withdrawal. JAMA 193:165–166, 1965

Gilman AG, Goodman LS, Gilman A: Pharmacological Basis of Therapeutics, 6th ed. New York, Macmillan Publishing Co, 1980

Glatt MM, George HR, Frisch EP: Controlled trial of chlormethiazole in the treatment of the alcohol withdrawal phase. Br Med J 2:401–404, 1965

Godin Y, Heiner L, Mark J, Mandel P: Effects of di-n-propylacetate, an anticonvulsive compound, on GABA metabolism. J Neurochem 16:869–873, 1969

Golbert TM, Sanz CJ, Rose HD, Leitschuh TH: Comprehensive evaluation of treatment of alcohol withdrawal syndromes. JAMA 201:113–116, 1967

Gordis E, Peterson K: Disulfiram therapy in alcoholism: Patient compliance studied with a urine-detection procedure. Alcoholism 1:213–216, 1977

Graf O: Increase of efficiency by means of pharmaceuticals (stimulants), in German Aviation Medicine: World War II, vol 2. Washington DC, Department of the Air Force, 1950

Gross MM, Lewis E, Hastey J: Acute alcohol withdrawal syndrome, in Biology of Alcoholism, vol 3 Clinical Pathology. Edited by Kissin B, Begleiter H. New York, Plenum Press, 1974

Gugl: Über Paraldehyd als Schlafmittel. Z Ther 1:153–157, 1883

Hemmingsen R, Kramp P, Rafaelsen OJ: Delirium tremens and related clinical states. Acta Psychiatr Scand 59:337–369, 1979

Hillbom ME: The prevention of ethanol withdrawal seizures in rats by dipropylacetate. Neuropharmacology 14:755–761, 1975

Ho AKS, Ho CC: Potentiation of lithium toxicity by ethanol in rats and mice. Alcoholism 2:386–391, 1978

Hollister LE: Tricyclic antidepressants. N Engl J Med 299:1106–1109; 1168–1172, 1978

Hotson JR, Langston JW: Disulfiram-induced encephalopathy. Arch Neurol 33:141–142, 1976

Hughes FW, Forney RB: Delayed audiofeedback (DFA) for induction of anxiety. JAMA 183:556–558, 1963

Hughes FW, Forney RB: Dextro-amphetamine, ethanol and dextro-amphetamine-ethanol combinations on performance of human subjects stressed with delayed auditory feedback. Psychopharmacologia 6:234–238, 1964

Inness I, Nickerson M: Atropine, scopolamine, and related antimuscarinic drugs, in Pharmacological Basis of Therapeutics, 5th ed. Edited by Goodman LS, Gilman A. New York, Macmillan Publishing Co, 1975

Isbell H: Alcohol problems and alcoholism, in Cecil-Loeb Textbook of Medicine, 12th ed. Edited by Beeson PB, McDermott W. Philadelphia, WB Saunders Co, 1967

Isbell H, Fraser HF, Wikler A, Belleville RE, Eisenman AJ: An experimental study of the etiology of "rum fits" and delirium tremens. Q J Stud Alcohol 16:1–33, 1955

Iselin HU, Weiss E: Naloxone reversal of ischemic neurological deficits. Lancet 2:642–643, 1981

Iversen L: Dopamine receptors in the brain. Science 188:1084–1089, 1975

Jeffreys DB, Flanagan RJ, Volans GN: Reversal of ethanol-induced coma with naloxone. Lancet 1:308–309, 1980

Johnson RM: The alcohol withdrawal syndromes. Q J Stud Alcohol (Suppl) 1:66–76, 1961

Judd LL, Hubbard RB, Huey SY, Attewell PA, Janowsky DS, Takahashi KI: Lithium carbonate and ethanol induced "highs" in normal subjects. Arch Gen Psychiatry 34:463–467, 1977

Kaim SC, Klett TJ, Rothfeld B: Treatment of the acute alcohol withdrawal state: A comparison of four drugs. Am J Psychiatry 125:1640–1646, 1969

Kalant H: Absorption, diffusion, distribution and elimination of ethanol: Effects on biological membranes, in Biology of Alcoholism, vol 1 Biochemistry. Edited by Kissin B, Begleiter H. New York, Plenum Press, 1971

Kalinowsky LB: Convulsions in nonepileptic patients on withdrawal of barbiturates, alcohol and other drugs. Arch Neurol Psychiatry 48:946–956, 1942

Keeffe EB, Smith FW: Disulfiram hypersensitivity hepatitis. JAMA 230:435–436, 1974

Kendell RE: Alcohol and suicide. Substance Alcohol Actions/Misuse 4, 1983 (in press)

Kimball CD, Huang SM, Torget CE, Houck JC: Plasma ethanol, endorphin, and glucose experiment. Lancet 2:418–419, 1980

Kingstone E, Kline SA: Disulfiram implants in the treatment of alcoholism. Some mechanisms of action. Int Pharmacopsychiatry 10:183–191, 1975

Kissin B: Interactions of ethyl alcohol and other drugs, in Biology of Alcoholism, vol 3 Clinical Pathology. Edited by Kissin B, Begleiter H. New York, Plenum Press, 1974

Kissin B: Medical management of the alcoholic patient, in Biology of Alcoholism, vol 5 Treatment and Rehabilitation of the Chronic Alcoholic. Edited by Kissin B, Begleiter H. New York, Plenum Press, 1977

Kissin B: Biological investigations in alcohol research. J Stud Alcohol (Suppl) 8:146–181, 1979

Kline NS, Wren JC, Cooper TB, Varza E, Canal O: Evaluation of lithium therapy in chronic and periodic alcoholism. Am J Med Sci 268:15–22, 1974

Knee ST, Razani J: Acute organic brain syndrome: A complication of disulfiram therapy. Am J Psychiatry 131:1281–1828, 1974

Koppanyi T, Canary J, Maengwyn-Davies G: Problems in acute alcohol poisoning. Q J Stud Alcohol (Suppl) 1:24–36, 1961

Kotz J, Roth GB, Ryon WA: Idiosyncrasy to paraldehyde. JAMA 110:2145–2148, 1938

Koutsky CD, Sletten IW: Chlordiazepoxide in alcohol withdrawal-Intramuscular effects. Minn Med 46:354–357, 1963

Kraml M: A rapid test for antabuse ingestion (ltr.). Can Med Assoc J 109:578, 1973

Kramp P, Rafaelsen OJ: Delirium tremens: A double-blind comparison of diazepam and barbital treatment. Acta Psychiatr Scand 58:174–190, 1978

Kryspin-Exner VK, Mader R: Entzugsdelirium bei chlormethiazolsucht. Wien Med Wochenschr 121:811–815, 1971

Landauer AA, Milner G, Patman J: Alcohol and amitryptyline effects on skills related to driving behavior. Science 163:1467–1468, 1969

Laties VG, Lasagna L, Gross GM, Hitchman IL, Flores J: A controlled trial of chlorpromazine and promazine in the management of delirium tremens. Q J Stud Alcohol 19:238–243, 1958

Lereboullet J, Benda P, Poisson M: Injectable meprobamate. Effective treatment of acute alcoholic psychoses. Press Med 68:473–475, 1960

Levy R, Elo T, Hanenson IB: Intravenous fructose treatment of acute alcohol intoxication. Arch Intern Med 137:1175–1177, 1977

Lewis MJ, Bland RC, Baile W: Disulfiram implantation for alcoholism. Can Psychiatr Assoc J 20:283–286, 1975

Liebson I, Bigelow G, Flamer R: Alcoholism among methadone patients: A specific treatment method. Am J Psychiatry 130:483–485, 1973

Lindros KO, Vihma R, Forsander OA: Utilization and metabolic effects of acetaldehyde and ethanol in the perfused rat liver. Biochem J 126:945–952, 1972

Linnoila M, Saairo I, Maki M: Effect of treatment with diazepam or lithium and alcohol on psychomotor skills related to driving. Europ J Clin Pharmacol 7:337–342, 1974

Lowenstein LM, Simone R, Boulter P, Nathan P: Effect of fructose on alcohol concentrations in the blood of man. JAMA 213:1899–1901, 1970

Lundquist G: The clinical use of chlormethiazole. Acta Psychiatr Scand (Suppl) 192:113–114, 1966

Lundwall L, Baekeland F: Disulfiram treatment of alcoholism. J Nerv Ment Dis 153:381–394, 1971

McGrath SD: A controlled trial of chlormethiazole and chlordiazepoxide in the treatment of the acute withdrawal phase of alcoholism. Br J Addict 70 (Suppl 1):81–90, 1975

Mackenzie AI: Naloxone in alcohol intoxication. Lancet 1:733–734, 1979

McNamee HB, Mendelson JH, Korn J: Fenmetozole in acute alcohol intoxication in man. Clin Pharmacol Ther 17:736–737, 1975

Madden JS, Jones D, Frisch EP: Chlormethiazole and trifluoperazine in alcohol withdrawal. Br J Psychiatry 115:1191–1192, 1969

Majchrowicz E, Bercaw B, Cole W, Gregory D: Nicotinamide adenine dinucleotide and the metabolism of ethanol and acetaldehyde. Q J Stud Alcohol 28:213–224, 1967

Malcolm MT, Madden JS, Williams AF: Disulfiram implantation critically evaluated. Br J Psychiatry 125:485–489, 1974

Marc-Aurele J, Schreiner GE: The dialysance of ethanol and methanol: A proposed method for the treatment of massive intoxication by ethyl or methyl alcohol. J Clin Invest 39:802–807, 1960

Mattila MJ, Nuotto E, Seppala T: Naloxone is not an effective antagonist of ethanol. Lancet 1:775–776, 1981

Merry J, Reynolds CM, Bailey J, Coppen A: Prophylactic treatment of alcoholism by lithium carbonate. A controlled study. Lancet 2:481–482, 1976

Misra PS, Lefèva A, Ishii H, Rubin E, Lieber CS: Increase of ethanol, meprobamate and pentobarbital metabolism after chronic ethanol administration in man and in rats. Am J Med 51:346–351, 1971

Muller DJ: A comparison of three approaches to alcohol withdrawal states. South Med J 62:495–496, 1969

Nakamura MM, Overall JE, Hollister LE, Radcliffe E: Factors affecting outcome of depressive symptoms in alcoholics. Alcoholism 7:188–193, 1983

Nash H: Psychological effects and alcohol-antagonizing properties of caffeine. Q J Stud Alcohol 27:727–734, 1966

Neiderhiser DH, Fuller RK, Hejduk LJ, Roth HP: Method for the detection of diethylamine, a metabolite of disulfiram, in urine. J Chromatogr 117:187–192, 1976

Newman HW, Newman EJ: Failure of dexedrine and caffeine as practical antagonists of the depressant effects of ethyl alcohol in man. Q J Stud Alcohol 17:406–410, 1956

Noble EP: 3rd Special Report to the US Congress on Alcohol and Health. Washington DC, US Government Printing Office, 1978

Noble EP, Alkana RL, Parker ES: Ethanol induced CNS depression and its reversal: A review, in Proceedings of the 4th Annual Alcoholism Conference of the National Institute on Alcohol Abuse and Alcoholism. DHEW Publ No ADM-76-284. Rockville MD, National Institute on Alcohol Abuse and Alcoholism, 1975

Noble EP, Gillies R, Vigran R, Mandel P: The modification of the ethanol withdrawal syndrome in rats by di-*n*-propylacetate. Psychopharmacologia 46:127–131, 1976

Obholzer AM: A follow-up study of nineteen alcoholic patients treated by means of tetraethyl-thiuram disulfide (Antabuse) implants. Br J Addict 69:19–23, 1974

Ogata M: Alcohol withdrawal syndrome: Acute, subacute and chronic phase. Substance Alcohol Actions/Misuse 4, 1983 (in press)

Parker ES, Noble EP: Alcohol consumption and cognitive functioning in social drinkers. J Stud Alcohol 38:1224–1232, 1977

Parker ES, Birnbaum IM, Boyd R, Noble EP: Neuropsychological decrements as a function of alcohol intake in male students. Alcoholism 4:330–334, 1980

Parsons OA, Farr SP: The neuropsychology of alcohol and drug use, in Handbook of Clinical Neuropsychology. Edited by Filskov S, Boll T. New York, John Wiley & Sons, 1981

Paulson SM, Krause S, Iber FL: Development and evaluation of a compliance test for patients taking disulfiram. Johns Hopkins Med J 141:119–125, 1977

Pendery M, Huey L: Lithium and the alcoholic, in Highlights of the 19th Annual Conference. New Orleans LA, Veterans Administration Studies in Mental Health and Behavioral Sciences, March 20, 1974

Perey BFJ, Helle SJ, MacLean LD: Acute alcoholic poisoning. A complication of gastric hypothermia. Can J Surgery 8:194–196, 1965

Peters WP, Friedman PA, Johnson NW, Mitch WE: Pressor effect of naloxone in septic shock. Lancet 1:529–532, 1981

Phillips M: A new implantable system for sustained delivery of disulfiram. Alcoholism 7:119, 1983

Piker P, Cohn JV: The comprehensive management of delirium tremens. JAMA 108:345–349, 1937

Pilcher JD: Alcohol and caffeine: A study of antagonism and synergism. J Pharm Exp Ther 3:267–298, 1911–12

Preskorn SH, Denner LJ: Benzodiazepines and withdrawal psychosis. Report of 3 cases. JAMA 237:36–38, 1977

Price TRP, Silberfarb PM: Convulsions following disulfiram treatment (ltr.). Am J Psychiatry 133:235, 1976

Quinn JT: Oral and intravenous chlormethiazole therapy in the alcoholic withdrawal phase. Acta Psychiatr Scand (Suppl) 192:161–166, 1966

Rainey JM Jr: Disulfiram toxicity and carbon disulfide poisoning. Am J Psychiatry 134:371–378, 1977

Rainey JM Jr, Neal RA: Disulfiram, carbon disulphide, and atherosclerosis. Lancet 1:284–285, 1975

Reilly TM: Physiological dependence on, and symptoms of withdrawal from, chlormethiazole. Br J Psychiatry 128:375–378, 1976

Reynolds CM, Merry J, Coppen A: Prophylactic treatment of alcoholism by lithium carbonate: An initial report. Alcoholism 1:109–111, 1977

Ritchie J: Central nervous system stimulants: II The xanthines, in Pharmacological Basis of Therapeutics, 4th ed. Edited by Goodman LS, Gillman A. New York, Macmillan Publishing Co, 1970

Ritchie J: Central nervous system stimulants: The xanthines, in Pharmacological Basis of Therapeutics, 5th ed. Edited by Goodman LS, Gilman A. New York, Macmillan Publishing Co, 1975

Rosenfeld JE, Bizzoco DH: A control study of alcohol withdrawal. Q J Stud Alcohol (Suppl) 1:77–84, 1961

Rothstein F: Prevention of alcohol withdrawal seizures: The roles of diphenylhydantoin and chlordiazepoxide. Am J Psychiatry 130:1381–1382, 1973

Rutenfranz J, Jansen G: On the compensation of alcohol effects by caffeine and pervitin in a psychomotor task. Int Z Angew Physiol Einchl Arbeitsphysiol 18:62–81, 1959

Sampliner R, Iber FL: Diphenylhydantoin control of alcohol withdrawal seizures. JAMA 230:1430–1432, 1974

Sapira JD: Alcoholism. South Med J 1417–1420, 1973

Schlichter W, Bristow E, Schultz S, Henderson AL: Seizures occurring during intensive chlorpromazine therapy. Can Med Assoc J 74:364–366, 1956

Schultz JD, Rea EL, Fazekas JF, Shea JC: Chlorpromazine in the management of acute alcoholic states. Q J Stud Alcohol 16:245–250, 1965

Seelig MS, Berger AR, Spielholz H: Latent tetany and anxiety, marginal magnesium deficit, and normocalcemia. Dis Nerv Sys 36:461–465, 1975

Selig JW Jr: A possible abstinence syndrome. JAMA 198:951–952, 1966

Sellers EM, Kalant H: Alcohol intoxication and withdrawal. N Engl J Med 294:757–762, 1976

Seppala T, Linnoila M, Elonen E, Mattila MJ, Mäki M: Effect of tricyclic antidepressants and alcohol on psychomotor skills related to driving. Clin Pharmacol Ther 17:515–522, 1975

Sereny G, Kalant H: Comparative clinical evaluation of chlordiazepoxide and promazine in treatment of alcohol-withdrawal syndrome. Br Med J 1:92–97, 1965

Shulsinger OZ, Forni PJ, Clyman BB: Magnesium sulfate in the treatment of alcohol withdrawal: A comparison with diazepoxide, in Currents in Alcoholism, vol 1. Edited by Sexias FA. New York, Grune & Stratton, 1977

Simler S, Ciesielski L, Maitre M, Randrianarisoa H, Mandel P: Effect of sodium *n*-dipropylacetate on audiogenic seizures and brain α-aminobutyric acid levels. Biochem Pharmacol 22:1701–1708, 1973

Sorensen SC, Mattisson K: Naloxone as an antagonist in severe alcohol intoxication. Lancet 2:688–689, 1978

Strongin E, Winsor A: The antagonistic action of coffee and alcohol. J Abnorm Soc Psychol 30:301–313, 1935

Tavel ME, Davidson W, Batterton TD: A critical analysis of mortality associated with delirium tremens: A review of 39 fatalities in a 9-year period. Am J Med Sci 242:18–29, 1961

Thieden H, Grunnet N, Damgaard S, Sestoft L: Effect of fructose and glyceraldehyde on ethanol metabolism in human liver and in rat liver. Europ J Biochem 30:250–261, 1972

Thomas DW, Freedman DX: Treatment of the alcohol withdrawal syndrome. JAMA 188:316–318, 1964

Thompson WL, Maddrey WL: Diazepam or paraldehyde for delirium tremens: In comment. Ann Intern Med 83:279, 1975

Thompson WL, Johnson AD, Maddrey WL, Osler Med. Housestaff: Diazepam and paraldehyde for treatment of severe delirium tremens. A controlled trial. Ann Intern Med 82:175–180, 1975

Thorpe JJ, Perret JT: Problem drinking: A follow-up study. Arch Industr Health 19:24–32, 1959

Tiengo M: Naloxone in irreversible shock. Lancet 2:690, 1980

Victor M: Treatment of alcoholic intoxication and the withdrawal syndrome. A critical analysis of the use of drugs and other forms of therapy. Psychosom Med 28:636–650, 1966

Victor M, Adams RW: Effect of alcohol on nervous system. Res Publ Ass Res Nerv Ment Dis 32:526–573, 1953

Volicer L, Gold B: Interactions of ethanol with cyclic AMP, in Biochemical Pharmacology of Ethanol. Edited by Majchrowicz E. New York, Plenum Press, 1975

Wacker WEC, Parisi AF: Magnesium metabolism. N Engl J Med 278:658–663; 712–717; 772–776, 1968

Wacker WEC, Vallee GL: Magnesium metabolism. N Engl J Med 259:475–482, 1958

Wallgren H, Barry H III: Actions of Alcohol, vol 2. Amsterdam, Elsevier, 1970

Whalley LJ, Freeman CP, Hunter J: Role of endogenous opioids in alcoholic intoxication. Lancet 2:89, 1981

Whyte CR, O'Brien PM: Disulfiram implant: A controlled trial. Br J Psychiatry 124:42–44, 1974

Wilson A: Disulfiram implantation in alcoholism treatment. J Stud Alcohol 36:555–565, 1975

Wilson EC: Ethanol metabolism in mice with different levels of hepatic alcohol dehydrogenase, in Biochemical Factors in Alcoholism. Edited by Maickel RP. Elmsford NY, Pergamon Press, 1967

Wilson, JC: Alcoholism, in A System of Practical Medicine by American Authors, vol 5 Diseases of the Nervous System. Edited by Pepper E. Philadelphia, Lea Brothers, 1886

Winokur G: Alcoholism and depression. Substance Alcohol Actions/Misuse 4, 1983 (in press)

Wolfe SM, Victor M: The physiological basis of the alcohol withdrawal syndrome, in Recent Advances in Studies of Alcoholism. Edited by Mello NK, Mendelson JH. Washington DC, US Government Printing Office, 1972

Wright DJM, Phillips M, Weller MPI: Naloxone in shock. Lancet 2:1361, 1980

References for Chapter 24

Alcohol Policy: Preventive Options

Aarens M, Cameron T, Roizen J, Roizen R, Room R, Schneberk D, Wingard D: Alcohol, Casualties, and Crime. Berkeley CA, Alcohol Research Group, 1977

Aaron P, Musto D: Temperance and prohibition in America: A historical overview, in Alcohol and Public Policy: Beyond the Shadow of Prohibition. Edited by Moore MH, Gerstein DR. Washington DC, National Academy Press, 1981

Beaubrun MH: Epidemiological research in the Caribbean context, in International Collaboration: Problems and Opportunities. Edited by Rutledge B, Fulton E. Toronto, Addiction Research Foundation, 1977

Borkenstein RF, Crowther RF, Shumate RP, Ziel WB, Zylman R: The role of the drinking driver in traffic accidents. Blutalkohol (Suppl 1) 11: 1974

Bruun K, Edwards G, Lumio K, Makela K, Pan L, Popham RE, Room R, Schmidt W, Skog OJ, Sulkunen P, Osterberg E: Alcohol Control Policies in Public Health Perspective. New Brunswick NJ, Rutgers University Center of Alcohol Studies, 1975

Clark WB, Midanik L: Results of the 1979 national survey. Berkeley CA, Alcohol Research Group, 1980

Cook PJ: The effect of liquor taxes on drinking, cirrhosis, and auto accidents, in Alcohol and Public Policy: Beyond the Shadow of Prohibition. Edited by Moore MH, Gerstein DR. Washington DC, National Academy Press, 1981

Cook P, Tauchen G: The effect of liquor taxes on heavy drinking. Bell J Econ 13:379–390, 1982

Cook P, Tauchen G: The effect of minimum drinking age legislation on youthful auto fatalities, 1970–1977. J Legal Studies 13, 1984 (in press)

Davies P: Some empirical grounds for controlling alcohol consumption. Br J Alcohol Alcoholism 17:109–116, 1983

Davies P, Walsh D: Alcohol Problems and Alcohol Control in Europe. New York, Gardner Press, 1983

Douglass RL: The legal drinking age and traffic casualties: A special case of changing alcohol availability in a public health context. Alcohol Health Res World 4:101–117, 1979-1980

Federal Bureau of Investigation: Uniform Crime Reports: Crime in the United States. Washington DC, US Government Printing Office, 1982

Fosdick R, Scott A: Toward Liquor Control. New York, Harper & Row, 1933

Gerstein DR: Alcohol use and consequences, in Alcohol and Public Policy: Beyond the Shadow of Prohibition. Edited by Moore MH, Gerstein DR. Washington DC, National Academy Press, 1981

Governor's Alcohol and Highway Safety Task Force: Report of the Governor's Alcohol and Highway Safety Task Force. Albany NY, Office of the Governor, 1981

Grant M, Plant M, Williams A (eds): Economics and Alcohol: Consumption and Controls. New York, Gardner Press, 1983

Gusfield J: Symbolic Crusade: Status Politics and the American Temperance Movement. Urbana, University of Illinois Press, 1963

Harris JE: Remarks on excise taxation at the conference to review the report Alcohol and Public Policy. Wash ington DC, Committee on Substance Abuse and Habitual Behavior, National Academy of Sciences, May 20–21, 1983

Hingson RM, Scotch N, Mangione T, Meyers A, Glantz L, Heeren T, Lin N, Mucatel M, Pierce G: Impact of legislation raising the legal drinking age in Massachusetts from 18 to 20. Am J Public Health 73:163–170, 1983

Institute of Medicine: Legislative Approaches to Prevention of Alcohol-Related Problems: An Inter-American Workshop. Washington DC, National Academy Press, 1982

Jacobson M, Hacker G, Atkins R: The Booze Merchants. Washington DC, Center for Science in the Public Interest, 1983

Jellinek EM: Recent trends in alcoholism and alcohol consumption. Q J Stud Alcohol 8:1–42, 1947

Jellinek EM: The Disease Concept of Alcoholism. New Haven CT, College and University Press, 1960

Jones RK, Joscelyn KB: Alcohol and Highway Safety 1978: A Review of the State of Knowledge. Springfield VA, National Technical Information Service, 1978

Kissin B, Begleiter H: The Pathogenesis of Alcoholism: Psychosocial Factors (The Biology of Alcoholism, Vol 6). Edited by Kissin B, Begleiter H. New York, Plenum Press, 1983

Krout JA: The Origins of Prohibition. New York, Knopf, 1925

Levine HG: The discovery of addiction: Changing conceptions of habitual drunkenness in America. J Stud Alcohol 39:143–177, 1978

Levine HG: The committee of fifty and the origins of alcohol control. J Drug Issues 13:95–116, 1983

Levy P, Voas R, Johnson P, Klein TM: An evaluation of the Department of Transportation's alcohol safety action projects. J Safety Res 10:162–176, 1978

McAlister A: New approaches to the prevention of alcohol abuse: Children and alcohol. Washington DC, Committee on Substance Abuse and Habitual Behavior, National Academy of Sciences, 1983

McAlister A, Perry C, Killen J, Slinkard LA, Maccoby N: Pilot study of smoking, alcohol, and drug abuse prevention. Am J Public Health 70:719–721, 1981

Medicine in the Public Interest, Inc: The Effects of Alcoholic-Beverage-Control Laws. Washington DC, Medicine in the Public Interest, 1976

Moore MH, Gerstein DR: Alcohol and Public Policy: Beyond the Shadow of Prohibition. Report of the Panel on Alternative Policies Affecting the Prevention of Alcohol Abuse and Alcoholism, National Research Council. Washington DC, National Academy Press, 1981

Moser J: Prevention of Alcohol-Related Problems: An International Review of Preventive Measures, Policies, and Programmes. Geneva, World Health Organization, 1979

Mosher JF: Dram shop liability and the prevention of alcohol-related problems. J Stud Alcohol 40:773–798, 1979

Mosher JF: New direction in alcohol policy: Implementing a comprehensive server intervention policy. Washington DC, Committee on Substance Abuse and Habitual Behavior, National Academy of Sciences, 1983

Mosher JF, Mottl JR: The role of nonalcohol agencies in federal regulation of drinking behavior and consequences, in Alcohol and Public Policy: Beyond the Shadow of Prohibition. Edited by Moore MH, Gerstein DR. Washington DC, National Academy Press, 1981

National Council on Alcoholism: Position statement on prevention and education. New York, National Council on Alcoholism, 1982

National Highway Traffic Safety Administration: Summary of National Alcohol Safety Action Projects. Publication No. DOT HS 804-032, Washington DC, US Department of Transportation, 1979

Pittman DJ: Primary Prevention of Alcohol Abuse and Alcoholism: An Evaluation of the Control of Consumption Policy. St Louis, Washington University Social Science Institute, 1980

Polich JM, Orvis BR: Alcohol Problems: Patterns and Prevalence in the US Air Force. Santa Monica CA, Rand Corporation, 1979

Presidential Commission on Drunk Driving: Final Report. Washington DC, US Government Printing Office, 1983

Reed DS: Reducing the costs of drinking and driving, in Alcohol and Public Policy: Beyond the Shadow of Prohibition. Edited by Moore MH, Gerstein DR. Washington DC, National Academy Press, 1981

Room R: Governing images and prevention of alcohol problems. Prev Med 3:11–23, 1974

Rorabaugh WJ: The Alcoholic Republic: An American Tradition. New York, Oxford University Press, 1979

Ross HL: Deterring the Drinking Driver: Legal Policy and Social Control. Lexington MA, Lexington Books, 1983

Schifrin LG: Societal costs of alcohol abuse in the United States: An update, in Economics and Alcohol: Consumption and Controls. Edited by Grant M, Plant M, Williams A. New York, Gardner Press, 1983

Single E, Morgan P, de Lint J: Alcohol, Society, and the State, Vol 2, The Social History of Control in Seven Countries. Toronto, Addiction Research Foundation, 1981

Smart R: The impact of prevention measures: An examination of research findings, in Legislative Approaches to Prevention of Alcohol-Related Problems: An Inter-American Workshop. Washington DC, Institute of Medicine, National Academy Press, 1982

United States Brewers Association: Federal and state excise taxes and malt beverages: A USBA analysis. Brewers Digest (January):23–36, 1983

United States Department of Transportation: 1968 Alcohol and Highway Safety report. Printed for the Committee on Public Works, 90th Congress, 2d session. Washington DC, US Government Printing Office, 1968

United States Senate, Subcommittee on Alcoholism and Drug Abuse, 96th Congress: Report on Consumer Health Warnings for Alcoholic Beverages and Related Issues. Washington DC, US Government Printing Office, 1979

Wallack L: Television programming, advertising, and the prevention of alcohol-related problems. Washington DC, Committee on Substance Abuse and Habitual Behavior, National Academy of Sciences, 1983

Warburton C: The Economic Results of Prohibition. New York, Columbia University Press, 1932

Wechsler H: Minimum-Drinking-Age Laws. Lexington MA, Lexington Books, 1980

Wiener C: The Politics of Alcoholism: Building an Arena Around a Social Problem. New Brunswick NJ, Transaction Books, 1980

Williams AF, Zador PF, Harris SS, Karpf RS: The effect of raising the legal minimum drinking age on involvement in fatal crashes. J Legal Studies 12:169–179, 1983

World Health Organization: Community Response to Alcohol-Related Problems, Phase I, Final Report. Contract No. ADM 281-78-0028. Rockville Md, National Institute on Alcohol Abuse and Alcoholism, 1981

V

The Anxiety Disorders

Part V

The
Anxiety
Disorders

Authors for Part V

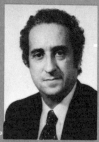

Donald F. Klein, M.D.,
Preceptor

Professor of Psychiatry
College of Physicians and Surgeons
Columbia University
Director of Research
New York State Psychiatric Institute

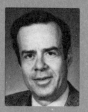

Robert L. Spitzer, M.D.
Professor of Psychiatry
College of Physicians and Surgeons
Columbia University
Chief
Biometrics Research Department
New York State Psychiatric Institute

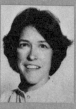

Janet B.W. Williams, D.S.W.
Assistant Professor of Clinical
  Psychiatric Social Work
  (in Psychiatry)
Columbia University
Research Scientist
Biometrics Research Department
New York State Psychiatric Institute

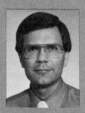

Raymond R. Crowe, M.D.

Professor of Psychiatry
University of Iowa
　Hospitals and Clinics

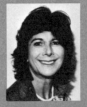

Rachel Gittelman, Ph.D.

Professor of Clinical Psychology
College of Physicians and Surgeons
Columbia University
Director of Psychology
New York State Psychiatric Institute

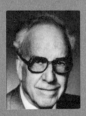

Jerome D. Frank, M.D., Ph.D.

Professor Emeritus of Psychiatry
Johns Hopkins University
　School of Medicine
Johns Hopkins Hospital

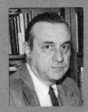

John C. Nemiah, M.D.

Professor of Psychiatry
Harvard Medical School
Psychiatrist-in-Chief
Beth Israel Hospital

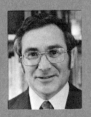

Herbert Benson, M.D.

Associate Professor of Medicine
Harvard Medical School at the
　Beth Israel Hospital

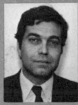

Matig Mavissakalian, M.D.

Associate Professor of Psychiatry
University of Pittsburgh
　School of Medicine
Western Psychiatric
　Institute and Clinic

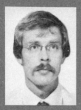

William Coryell, M.D.
Associate Professor of Psychiatry
The University of Iowa

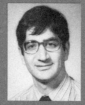

Jack M. Gorman, M.D.
Assistant Professor of
  Clinical Psychiatry
College of Physicians and Surgeons
Columbia University

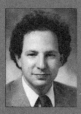

Steven M. Paul, M.D.
Chief
Clinical Neuroscience Branch
National Institute of Mental Health
Alcohol, Drug Abuse and
  Mental Health Administration

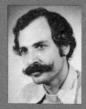

Phil Skolnick, Ph.D.
Laboratory of Bioorganic Chemistry
National Institute of Arthritis,
  Diabetes, Digestive and Kidney Diseases
National Institutes of Health

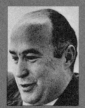

Jonathan O. Cole, M.D.
Chief
Psychopharmacology Program
Co-director
Affective Disease Program
McLean Hospital
Lecturer in Psychiatry
Harvard Medical School

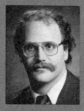

Michael R. Liebowitz, M.D.
Assistant Professor of
  Clinical Psychiatry
College of Physicians and Surgeons
Columbia University
Director
Anxiety Disorders Clinic
New York State Psychiatric Institute

The
Anxiety
Disorders

	Page
Introduction to Part Five *Donald F. Klein, M.D.*	390

The Diagnosis, Epidemiology, and Genetics *of the Anxiety Disorders*	
Chapter 25	392

Diagnostic Issues in
   the DSM-III Classification
   of the Anxiety Disorders
Robert L. Spitzer, M.D.,
Janet B.W. Williams, D.S.W.	

Introduction	392
Overview of the DSM-III Anxiety Disorders	393
Problems and Proposed Solutions for Defining the Disorders	395
Conclusion	402

Chapter 26	402
The Role of Genetics in the Etiology of Panic Disorder *Raymond R. Crowe, M.D.*	
Introduction	402
Epidemiology	403
Basic Genetic Studies	404
Gene Action	407
Conclusion	410

Chapter 27	410
Anxiety Disorders in Children *Rachel Gittelman, Ph.D.*	
Introduction	410
Diagnostic Principles	410
Simple Phobias	411
Separation Anxiety	412
Comment	418

Psychotherapeutic and Behavioral Treatments
for the Anxiety Disorders

Chapter 28   *418*
The Psychotherapy of Anxiety
Jerome D. Frank, M.D., Ph.D.
Introduction   418
Etiologic Considerations   419
Psychotherapeutic Interventions   420
Summary   425

Chapter 29   *426*
Anxiety and Psychodynamic Theory
John C. Nemiah, M.D.
Mise en Scène   426
Janet's Theory of Anxiety   427
Freud's Theories of Anxiety   429
Signal Anxiety and Panic Anxiety   436
Reflections on Theory and Research   438
Some Principles of Treatment   439

Chapter 30   *440*
The Relaxation Response
   and the Treatment of Anxiety
Herbert Benson, M.D.
Historical Precedents   441
Physiological Basis   444
Current Secular Techniques   445
Clinical Trials   447
Summary   448

Chapter 31   *448*
Exposure Treatment of Agoraphobia
Matig Mavissakalian, M.D.
Introduction   448
The Evolution of the Exposure Principle   449
Recent Research   452
Practical Implications   459

The Biology, Biochemistry, and Pathophysiology
of the Anxiety Disorders

Chapter 32   *460*
Mortality After Thirty to Forty Years:
   Panic Disorder Compared with Other
   Psychiatric Illnesses
William Coryell, M.D.
Introduction   460
Methods   460
Results   461
Discussion   464

Chapter 33   *467*
The Biology of Anxiety
  Jack M. Gorman, M.D.
Autonomic Nervous System Physiology   468
Neurotransmitters in Anxiety   471
Provocative Tests   474
Mitral Valve Prolapse   479

Chapter 34   *482*
The Biochemistry of Anxiety:
  From Pharmacotherapy to Pathophysiology
  Steven M. Paul, M.D.,
  Phil Skolnick, Ph.D.
Introduction   482
Benzodiazepines as Selective Anxiolytics   483
The Discovery of Benzodiazepine Receptors   485
Benzodiazepine Receptors and GABA   486
Benzodiazepine Receptor–Mediated "Anxiety"   487
Summary and Conclusions   488

Pharmacotherapies
  for the Anxiety Disorders

Chapter 35   *490*
β-Adrenergic Blockers and Buspirone
  Jonathan O. Cole, M.D.
β-Blockers   491
Buspirone   497
Discussion   501
Summary   502

Chapter 36   *503*
The Efficacy of Antidepressants
  in Anxiety Disorders
  Michael R. Liebowitz, M.D.
Agoraphobia and Panic Disorder   503
Obsessive-Compulsive Disorder   512
Generalized Anxiety Disorder   516
Other Anxiety Disorders   516
Conclusion   519

Unresolved Questions   *519*
  Donald F. Klein, M.D.
Introduction   519
Questions for Future Research   519
Conclusion   525

References for Part Five   *526*

Introduction[†]
by Donald F. Klein, M.D.

HISTORICAL AND CONCEPTUAL BACKGROUND

Psychiatry has gone through a number of developmental phases, molded by the then current understanding of mental functioning, as well as by the techniques available for modifying feeling, thinking, and behavior.

In the nineteenth and early twentieth century, after the great organic successes in understanding general paresis, vitamin deficiencies, endocrinopathies, and senility, it was commonly believed that all mental illnesses would shortly be shown to be due to brain diseases. However, the evidence for organic etiology did not progressively increase in the realms of the schizophrenic, manic, depressive, anxiety, and personality disorders.

By the turn of the century, it became apparent that many mental disorders could be affected positively by psychological methods ranging from hypnosis through abreaction to psychoanalysis. In the absence of convincing evidence for organic causation and any substantially effective organic treatment, and in the presence of apparent psychotherapeutic success and a convincing body of psychotherapeutic theory, it is not surprising that psychiatry swung in the direction of considering cryptogenic mental illnesses as functional disorders. The term *functional disorder* came to mean that the organism has, through experience, developed certain impairments of thinking, feeling, or behavior that are not due to neuropathology per se. Early formative causes are frequently thought of in terms of psychological trauma, or enduring conflicts, or poor learning experiences, or counterproductive identifications, and so forth.

At times, it is argued that since the mind is not some disembodied wraith, but an aspect of brain functioning, all behaviors are biological. Therefore, it is argued, the distinction between organic causation and psychogenesis is simply a semantic error. However, that argument is erroneous, since it blurs the real distinctions between the physiological systems primarily affected by the relevant etiologic variables. The Preceptor and his colleagues have examined this issue elsewhere (Klein, 1978; Wender and Klein, 1981).

Starting in the middle 1950s, there has been a recrudescence of interest in organic aspects as well as possible organic etiologies of mental disorders. The major impetus came from the development of powerful new psychopharmacologic treatments. The effectiveness and apparent specificity of these drugs in schizophrenia and the affective and anxiety disorders in turn generated a new interest in the neglected area of reliable and useful descriptive diagnosis (Klein and Davis, 1969; Klein et al., 1980), most recently shown by DSM-III. Still, one cannot argue deductively that because an emotional derangement is benefited by a medication the etiology is necessarily organic.

†Supported in part by United States Public Health Service Grants, No. MH 30906 and No. MH 33422.

Genetic evidence, and in particular the development of the new adoption studies, speaks most directly to the issue of one type of organic causal factor, heredity. Positive genetic evidence in the areas of schizophrenia, affective disorders, and anxiety disorders has done much to cast doubt upon an exclusively psychogenic view.

In addition, recent progress in the instrumentation necessary for psychophysiological measurements, microbiochemical determinations, and brain imaging has led to striking potentialities for detecting brain disease at a far more dynamic and subtle level than was possible with post mortem histopathology. Nonetheless, our ignorance still far outweighs our knowledge. We usually treat empirically considerably better than our limited knowledge of the basics would allow. Teasing out the complex causal web and comparatively evaluating therapeutic interventions will occupy psychiatric research for many years to come.

As Comte long ago pointed out, scientific development in many different fields seems to go through a number of analogous stages. Initially, there are striking observations. Then patterns are discerned in the observations, and categories or functional relationships are asserted. Up to this point, the scientific method resembles, in going from the particular to the general, the imaginative play of art and literature.

The scientist, however, puts the patterns to the test and moves from hypothesis formation to hypothesis testing. The most powerful form of hypothesis testing occurs with the application of the controlled experimental method. Experience shows that the nonartistic side of the scientific endeavor, by consciously juxtaposing theory and fact, is actually the stage that presents the most revealing observations and stimulates the most striking hypotheses.

This somewhat philosophical introduction has a practical point. Research is the art of the soluble. The scientific health of an area of investigation can be estimated by the number of questions generated that are either answerable in the reasonably near future or call for feasible technical advances in scientific technology and organization. The study of the anxiety disorders has entered a healthy period of rapid growth and development.

To recapitulate, initially the study of anxiety consisted of many striking clinical observations concerning the course and patterning of symptomatology. With the development of psychoanalysis, there was a complex theoretical development that unfortunately did not progress into the phase of empirical hypothesis testing. The reasons for this failure in development are arguable. At least part of the problem is the real difficulty in formulating psychoanalytic hypotheses in such a way as to be testable.

Psychiatry, as an applied science, is particularly responsive to the development of powerful new therapies. The recent burgeoning of research in the anxiety disorders can largely be attributed to the impact of the behavior therapies and psychopharmacologic approaches. Fortunately, both of these methods have proven relatively amenable to experimental approaches so that strong tests of their findings and theories are possible. *Strong tests* simply mean those which enable us to demonstrate that a supposed observation is incorrect or that a belief is false. When this is possible, science is on its way.

THE ANXIETY DISORDERS

The psychopharmacologic revolution had its initial impact on schizophrenia and the manic and depressive disorders, and most recently on the anxiety disorders. One basis for this recent development was the recognition that many anxious patients were remarkably responsive to agents called antidepressants, even when they were not apparently depressed. That antidepressants seem specifically to blockade the apparently spontaneous, unpredictable panic attack, but have little effect on anticipatory anxiety, raised the possibility that anxiety was not a unitary state and that the anxiety disorders should be subdivided with regard to the presence or absence of the spontaneous panic attack. This subdivision has proved useful for diagnosis, physiological provocation and blockade of anxiety states, genetics, and therapeutics, although it is still not entirely accepted. The border between panic and chronic anxiety requires more detailed investigation. That both phenomena are heterogeneous is certainly likely.

The history of medicine is in large measure the history of splitting vaguely defined amorphous illnesses into more rigorously defined syndromes, thus allowing more appropriate care as well as a more effective search for discrete etiologies. We are currently in the midst of this process with regard to the mental disorders in general, and the anxiety disorders in particular.

The chapters in this Part present a comprehensive overview of the tremendous ferment in this area. Due to practical difficulties, the Part does not include material on the clinical utility of the benzodiazepines, but this should not lead the reader to infer any lack of interest in these important agents. This absence is to some degree mitigated by the ready availability of psychopharmacologic texts.

The last chapter discusses a number of unresolved questions that we may all hope will soon be answered. It is included to give the reader a sense of the thrust of the ongoing and forthcoming work in the area of anxiety disorders.

Chapter 25 | Diagnostic Issues in the DSM-III Classification of the Anxiety Disorders
by Robert L. Spitzer, M.D. and Janet B.W. Williams, D.S.W.

INTRODUCTION

Mental disorders with some form of anxiety as the predominant feature have been recognized since antiquity (Celsus, first century A.D.). Only a few years ago, however, were these disorders grouped in a single diagnostic class called Anxiety Disorders (American Psychiatric Association, 1980). This chapter reviews the background to the DSM-III classification of Anxiety Disorders for adults, discusses some problems with the diagnostic criteria, and offers some possible solutions. Such a reexamination is timely. In May 1983, a month before the authors began writing this chapter, the American Psychiatric Association appointed a work group to revise DSM-III. The work group will consider modifications in the criteria for the various disorders and is scheduled to complete the revision, DSM-III-R, by December 1984.

As is well known, the developers of DSM-III decided that when etiology was unknown, classifications would be based on shared descriptive features, rather than on presumed etiologies. Consequently, DSM-III omits the traditional diagnostic class of neuroses. In the neuroses, DSM-II had included categories that were presumed to share the common cause of unconscious conflict arousing anxiety and leading to the maladaptive use of defense mechanisms, which in turn results in symptom formation. What had been the DSM-II neuroses were thus reclassified in DSM-III with other diagnostic categories that shared their essential descriptive features.

Depressive neurosis (renamed Dysthymic Disorder) joined the Affective Disorders; the two types of hysterical neuroses joined Somatoform and Dissociative Disorders; hypochondriacal neurosis joined Somatoform Disorders; and depersonalization neurosis joined Dissociative Disorders. The remaining neuroses (with the exception of neurasthenic neurosis, whose low energy apparently led to its demise), anxiety neurosis, phobic neurosis, and obsessive-compulsive neurosis, are all characterized either by anxiety being the predominant symptom or by anxiety being experienced if the individual attempts to master other predominant symptoms. Two of these three DSM-II categories were further subdivided in DSM-III, and they were joined with a new category, Posttraumatic Stress Disorder, which also involves predominant symptoms of anxiety, to constitute the DSM-III diagnostic class of Anxiety Disorders.

The elimination of neurosis as a diagnostic class from the DSM-III classification was extremely controversial. Since the publication of DSM-III, however, with only a few exceptions (Frances and Cooper, 1981; Lopez-Ibor and Lopez-Ibor, 1983), researchers and clinicians seem to have accepted the concept of Anxiety Disorders as a diagnostic class. Examples of this acceptance include the large number of recent studies in which investigators have used the DSM-III criteria for describing samples of patients with Anxiety Disorders (Klein and Rabkin, 1981; Barlow and Beck, 1984), the proliferation of specialized clinical services organized to treat these disorders, the convening of several major conferences on the subject (Massachusetts General Hospital and Tufts-New England Medical Center conference, Anxiety Disorders, Panic Attacks, and Phobias, in 1982, and the National Institute of Mental Health conference, Anxiety and the Anxiety Disorders, in 1983), and the decision of the Editor of *Psychiatry Update: Volume III* to devote a whole Part to the subject of the Anxiety Disorders.

OVERVIEW OF THE DSM-III ANXIETY DISORDERS

Table 1 lists the eight specific DSM-III Anxiety Disorders, plus the residual undefined category of Atypical Anxiety Disorder. To facilitate understanding of the historical origins of these disorders, they are discussed in four major groups: Phobic Disorders, Anxiety States, Obsessive-Compulsive Disorder, and Posttraumatic Stress Disorder.

Table 1. DSM-III Anxiety Disorders

Phobic Disorders
    Agoraphobia with Panic Attacks
    Agoraphobia without Panic Attacks
    Social Phobia
    Simple Phobia
Anxiety States
    Panic Disorder
    Generalized Anxiety Disorder
    Obsessive Compulsive Disorder
Post-traumatic Stress Disorder
Atypical Anxiety Disorder

Source: American Psychiatric Association (1980).

Phobic Disorders

The essential feature of each phobic disorder is persistent and irrational fear of a specific object, activity, or situation that results in a compelling desire to avoid the dreaded object, activity, or situation (the phobic stimulus). The individual recognizes that the fear is excessive or unreasonable.

In partial accordance with the classification of phobias proposed by Marks (1970), DSM-III subdivided the Phobic Disorders into three types based on differing symptomatology, age at onset, sex ratio, and treatment response. Agoraphobia is distinguished by a marked fear of being alone or of being in public places where escape might be difficult or where help might not be available in case of sudden incapacitation. Social Phobia is characterized by a fear of situations in which the individual may be exposed to scrutiny by others. Simple Phobia covers fears of situations other than those subsumed by Agoraphobia and Social Phobia, such as fears of animals and heights.

Based on Klein's observation that most cases of Agoraphobia begin following the development of what he calls spontaneous panic attacks (Klein, 1981), the typical form of the disorder was called Agoraphobia with Panic Attacks. In order to provide a category for cases of Agoraphobia with no history of panic attacks (although it was not clear if such cases existed), another subtype was added, Agoraphobia without Panic Attacks.

Anxiety States

The syndrome of recurrent panic attacks was recognized as a separate disorder as early as 1871 when DaCosta described the "irritable heart." Then, in 1894, Freud first applied the name anxiety neurosis to the syndrome, separating it from the category of neurasthenia. In DSM-II, however, the category of anxiety neurosis applied to all individuals who experienced generalized anxiety, whether or not the anxiety occurred in discrete attacks of panic; the panic attacks were assumed in DSM-II to be merely symptomatic of a more severe form of the same disorder. Similarly, the ICD-9 category of anxiety states includes "various combinations of physical and mental manifestations of anxiety, not attributable to real danger and occurring either in attacks or as a persisting state" (World Health Organization, 1978, 35).

Klein had demonstrated in the early 1960s that imipramine blocks recurrent panic attacks (Klein, 1964), and he later showed that imipramine has no apparent effect on phobic anxiety that is not associated with panic attacks (Zitrin et al., 1978). Based on Klein's findings, the developers of DSM-III decided that DSM-III should have a separate category for conditions characterized by recurrent panic attacks, and the DSM-II category of anxiety neurosis was divided into two categories. The first category, Panic Disorder, requires recurrent panic attacks (in the absence of Agoraphobia) and corresponds to Freud's original concept of anxiety neurosis. The DSM-III diagnostic criteria for Panic Disorder were based on the Feighner criteria for anxiety neurosis (Feighner et al., 1972).

The second category, Generalized Anxiety Disorder, was newly created for those cases that under DSM-II would have received a diagnosis of anxiety neurosis, but did not have the recurrent panic attacks. This residual category is intended to cover conditions in which there is generalized, persistent anxiety of at least one month's duration, without the specific symptoms of any of the other Anxiety Disorders. When the category was created, no one was quite sure how prevalent such a condition might be and whether it would have a differential treatment response from Panic Disorder.

Obsessive-Compulsive Disorder

This time-honored category was included with the DSM-III Anxiety Disorders because even though the predominant symptoms are obsessions or compulsions, anxiety is experienced if the individual attempts to resist the obsessions or compulsions.

Posttraumatic Stress Disorder

This category was first referred to as traumatic neurosis (Keiser, 1968), and it was included in DSM-I as gross stress reaction. DSM-II, however, had no direct counterpart for this disorder, despite observations of delayed forms resulting from World War II concentration camp experiences. The criteria for the DSM-III category were developed with the help of clinicians who were involved in treating Vietnam War veterans.

PROBLEMS AND PROPOSED SOLUTIONS FOR DEFINING THE DISORDERS

Despite extensive field testing of the DSM-III criteria prior to their official adoption, experience with them since their publication has revealed, as expected, many instances in which they are not entirely satisfactory and need to be revised. The following is a discussion of the problems that investigators, including the authors, have identified in applying the criteria for Anxiety Disorders. Case examples are presented to illustrate the points discussed, and these examples are frequently the very cases that directed attention to a particular problem with the criteria.

Hierarchical Structure of the Classification

Case example: Ms. G. was a 48-year-old mother of three children who was admitted to the hospital for her third episode of severe depression, which met the DSM-III criteria for Major Depression with Melancholia. She reported that following the onset of each of her three depressions, she had terrifying panic attacks, and that she believed these attacks were triggered by the thought that she would never recover. She claimed that she had never had a panic attack when she was not in one of these depressions. Her description of individual panic attacks fulfilled the DSM-III inclusion criteria for Panic Disorder.

The diagnostic classes in DSM-III are hierarchically organized. The assumption underlying the organization is that a disorder high in the hierarchy may have symptoms found in a disorder lower in the hierarchy, but that the reverse would not occur. The hierarchical structure of the classification is operationalized by exclusion criteria which dictate that a diagnosis (in this case, the "excluded diagnosis" of Panic Disorder) not be given if its inclusion symptoms are symptoms of a higher-order disorder (in this case, the "dominant disorder" of Major Depression with Melancholia).

Do the panic attacks of Ms. G. have any diagnostic significance? According to the DSM-III criteria for Panic Disorder, this diagnosis is not given if the panic attacks occur only in the course of, that is, are judged "due to" a major depressive episode. According to DSM-III, and perhaps usual clinical practice, the panic attacks would merely be regarded as associated symptoms of the Affective Disorder and as having no diagnostic significance.

The Epidemiologic Catchment Area Program, sponsored by the National Institute of Mental Health (Regier et al., 1982) is yielding data that call into question the fundamental assumptions that underlie many of the DSM-III hierarchies, particularly those regarding the Anxiety Disorders. Using data from this program, Boyd et al. (1983) found that the presence of a dominant disorder (e.g., Major Depression) greatly increased the likelihood of the presence of a related excluded syndrome (e.g., panic attacks), as would be predicted by the DSM-III hierarchies. However, there was also a general tendency for the presence of any DSM-III syndrome to increase the likelihood of the presence of almost any other DSM-III syndrome. Other research has also challenged the validity of the DSM-III hierarchical principle that gives Affective Disorders precedence over Anxiety Disorders. Leckman et al. (in press), in a large controlled family study of depression, found that the presence of a history of panic attacks in the probands, whether associated with a Major Depressive Episode or occurring at other times, increased the family prevalence of depression, alcoholism, and other anxiety disorders. These data suggest that research, and perhaps clinical practice as well, might be improved by eliminating some of the DSM-III diagnostic hierarchies that prevent the joint diagnosis of different syndromes when they occur together in one episode of illness.

Additional problems arise with some of the hierarchical principles embodied in the exclusion criteria for the Anxiety Disorders. Some exclusion principles are not applied consistently. For example, a psychotic disorder in DSM-III, such as Schizophrenic Disorder, explicitly takes precedence over all of the Anxiety Disorders except Social Phobia and Posttraumatic Stress Disorder. In addition, some of the exclusion criteria confuse differential diagnostic issues with hierarchical issues. The DSM-III exclusion criteria for Agoraphobia, for example, list Obsessive-

Compulsive Disorder and Paranoid Personality Disorder. These two diagnoses were listed because individuals with Obsessive-Compulsive Disorder and Paranoid Personality Disorder are sometimes afraid to go out of their houses alone. However, the need for a differential diagnosis of the symptom of fear of going out of the house should not be confused with a hierarchical principle. The fear of leaving the house, when it stems from a fear of sudden incapacitation, is the hallmark of Agoraphobia, but is not a symptom of Obsessive-Compulsive Disorder or Paranoid Personality Disorder.

Elsewhere (Spitzer and Williams, 1983a), the authors have proposed that the diagnostic hierarchies in the revised DSM-III be limited to a small number of principles that would be consistently applied to all categories. One important consequence of such a change would be that Affective Disorders would no longer preempt a concurrent diagnosis of an Anxiety Disorder. As applied to Ms. G., both Major Depression and Panic Disorder, which in her case could be considered a complication of each major depressive episode, would be diagnosed.

These principles would also mean that Generalized Anxiety Disorder could be given as an additional diagnosis to an individual who concurrently had a depressive disorder. This would respond to the criticism of Shader and Greenblatt (1981) that DSM-III does not recognize the validity of mixed anxiety and depressive states. It would also be in accord with the recent findings by Finlay-Jones and Brown (1981) that individuals who had experienced both severe loss and severe danger developed mixed anxiety and depression states. The application of the traditional diagnostic hierarchy to these cases would have obscured the mixed nature of the disorder. Finally, these principles would also allow the diagnosis of more than one specific Anxiety Disorder for a single episode of illness, which is now prevented by the exclusion criteria.

What would happen under the proposed revision to the combination category of Agoraphobia with Panic Attacks? In the authors' opinion, sufficient clinical evidence indicates that Agoraphobia is usually a complication of recurrent panic attacks to justify a specific revision in the DSM-III classifications of Agoraphobia and Panic Disorder. The category of Agoraphobia without Panic Attacks should remain unchanged, but the diagnoses of Panic Disorder and Agoraphobia with Panic Attacks would be combined into a single category of Panic Disorder with three subtypes: (1) Panic Disorder, Uncomplicated; (2) Panic Disorder with Limited Phobic Avoidance; and (3) Panic Disorder with Agoraphobia (extensive phobic avoidance).

This revision would acknowledge the central role of panic attacks in the typical development of Agoraphobia. It would also provide a subtype of Panic Disorder for cases where an individual avoids one or more activities because of a fear of having panic attacks (e.g., going into restaurants), but where the phobic avoidance is not as extensive as in Agoraphobia. With DSM-III, there is no satisfactory way to diagnose such cases.

Another current problem with the DSM-III classification of Agoraphobia with Panic Attacks is that there is no way to indicate the common clinical condition in which, with psychopharmacologic treatment (or with time), panic attacks have remitted, but the phobic avoidance behavior of the Agoraphobia persists. For example, a 48-year-old housewife with a history of panic attacks and agoraphobia was unable to leave her home unless accompanied by her husband or a friend, even though she had not actually had a panic attack for several years. A new convention could be adopted that would allow for indicating any disorder in remission. With the proposed principles and this convention, such cases would be diagnosed as Panic Disorder with Agoraphobia (panic attacks in remission).

Problems in Defining the Individual Disorders

AGORAPHOBIA

Case example: A 37-year-old former teacher, Mr. M. complained of panic attacks of 11 years' duration which made it impossible for him to work outside of the home. During the last few years, he had accommodated himself to his illness by organizing his life so that he rarely had to leave his house. He had assumed responsibility for taking care of his children while his wife was away at work, he prepared the family meals, and spent several hours each day lifting weights.

According to DSM-III, in order to give a diagnosis of Agoraphobia there must be "increasing constriction of normal activities until the fears [of being alone or in public places] or avoidance behavior dominate the individual's life" (American Psychiatric Association, 1980, 227). Clinically, there seems little doubt that Mr. M. has Agoraphobia. However, since he has made a new life for himself inside his home, it is not clear whether, strictly speaking, the fears or avoidance behavior now "dominate" his life. The ambiguity inherent in the word "dominate" could be overcome by the following proposed rephrasing: ". . . numerous important activities are avoided or endured with dread." With this proposed revision, Mr. M.'s illness would clearly meet the criteria for Agoraphobia.

AGORAPHOBIA WITHOUT PANIC ATTACKS This category requires further study, and the authors know of only two papers that have commented specifically on it. A reliability study of 60 consecutive outpatients at an anxiety disorders clinic found 23 cases of Agoraphobia with Panic Attacks, but not a single case of Agoraphobia without Panic Attacks (Di Nardo et al., in press), raising the issue of the validity of the category. On the other hand, according to Klein (1982), Agoraphobia without Panic Attacks is "regularly associated with episodic dysautonomic experiences, primarily light-headedness and gastrointestinal distress" (85). If Klein's observation is confirmed, the issue then is whether these dysautonomic experiences are fundamentally different from panic attacks or whether they are merely minor forms of panic attacks and thus do not justify a separate diagnostic category.

SOCIAL PHOBIA

Case example: Mr. S., a 43-year-old construction manager and father of two, sought treatment because, "I seem to be afraid of everything, and I have been this way since I was a kid." Two months earlier his symptoms had intensified when he began a new job that required him to have more interaction with other employees. Detailed questioning revealed that his fears all involved situations in which he feared that others might think him incompetent or might be angry with him. For example, he was afraid to change the oil in his car because a new neighbor next door might see him and think that he did not know what he was doing. He was also afraid that while driving his car he might stop at an intersection and another driver would be annoyed with him for stopping. When he was first introduced to someone, he would be so anxious that he could hardly talk. He also complained of numerous physical manifestations of anxiety, such as muscle tension, palpitations, and trouble concentrating.

In DSM-III, a Social Phobia is defined as "a persistent, irrational fear of, and compelling desire to avoid, situations in which the individual may be exposed to possible scrutiny by others [and fears that he or she may act in a way] that will be humiliating or embarrassing" (American Psychiatric Association, 1980, 227). According to this definition, Mr. S. would seem to have many social phobias, yet DSM-III indicates that an individual generally has only one social phobia. This provision was added because the descriptions of prototypical cases usually involved isolated phobias, such as the fear of eating in public or of writing in the presence of others. Apparently, however, the diagnosis has commonly been applied to patients who, like Mr. S., have multiple social situations that they fear and avoid (Amies et al., 1983; Falloon et al., 1981). There seems no valid reason to exclude such cases from the diagnosis, provided that the basic fear is of humiliation or embarrassment rather than, for example, a fear of being harmed, as might be seen in cases of Paranoid Personality Disorder. Therefore, in the proposed revision, the criteria should make it clear that the diagnosis is appropriate even when the phobic situations are numerous and pervasive.

> *Case example:* Mr. T., a fourth-year medical student, came to the student health service complaining of intense anxiety whenever he had to present a patient to his attendings. For days before a presentation, he would ruminate about the possibility that he would be unable to speak coherently and that his anxiety would be obvious to everyone. Recognizing that it would hurt his career if he attempted to avoid case presentations, he always forced himself to go through with them, and usually he found that he was not as anxious as he had expected to be.

Does Mr. T. have a Social Phobia? According to DSM-III, there must be a "compelling desire to avoid" the phobic situation. This leaves unclear the issue of whether the diagnosis can or should be given to individuals who dread entering the phobic situation but force themselves to do so nevertheless. The authors propose that this criterion (which is also in Simple Phobia and Agoraphobia) be changed to the requirement that "the activity is avoided or endured with dread."

SIMPLE PHOBIA

> *Case example:* Ms. B., a 55-year-old woman in good physical health admitted during a community survey that she avoided crossing any streets that were more than two lanes wide because, she said, "I might fall down and be hit by a car." For many years, she had avoided such streets and had changed her shopping and visiting habits so that she could avoid wide streets. She acknowledged that her fear of falling was unreasonable, but denied that this fear and the avoidance activity caused her any distress.

According to DSM-III, an individual with Simple Phobia (and Social Phobia) must have "significant distress because of the disturbance." Yet it is clinically well known that some individuals such as Ms. B. who show phobic avoidance of an important activity may deny any distress because they have altered their lives to adjust to their incapacity. The authors propose changing this criterion to state, "the [feared] activity is important in the context of the individual's life circumstances, or the fear of the activity causes significant distress." With this revision, a diagnosis of Simple Phobia would clearly apply in Ms. B.'s case.

PANIC DISORDER

Case example: Ms. F., a 50-year-old woman, was presented to a case conference. She complained of panic attacks that, according to her, occurred only when she was either in a crowd or in enclosed places such as buses, cars, or elevators, situations that she avoided whenever possible. Typically, she would start to feel uneasy in anticipation of entering one of these situations, and once in the situation, she would experience a panic attack after a few minutes to an hour or sometimes not at all. She denied ever having had an attack while at home.

The staff was divided on Ms. F.'s diagnosis. Some argued that her panic attacks were not "spontaneous," since they occurred only in certain situations, and that the diagnosis should be Simple Phobia. Others argued for a diagnosis of Panic Disorder.

The authors agree with the diagnosis of Panic Disorder. The confusion underlying the diagnosis here is the DSM-III statement that in Panic Disorder the panic attacks are "not precipitated only by exposure to a circumscribed phobic stimulus." The purpose of the DSM-III statement was to exclude from the diagnosis of Panic Disorder panic reactions that inevitably occur in response to a specific phobic stimulus, such as the panic reaction experienced by an individual with a morbid fear of heights. Ms. F. was predisposed to having a panic attack in certain situations, but unlike an individual with a true Simple or Social Phobia, she did not always have an attack in the feared situations. Furthermore, when she did have an attack, it did not occur immediately upon exposure to the phobic stimulus, but after a variable period of time. The criteria for Panic Disorder should be revised to differentiate a panic reaction from a reaction to a circumscribed phobic stimulus, with the statement that the attack must occur at "times other than . . . immediately before or upon exposure to a situation that always causes anxiety or avoidance."

In the authors' experience with interviewing patients whose chief complaint is anxiety, there is rarely any difficulty in distinguishing true panic attacks from periods of intense anxiety. When there is difficulty, an examination of the temporal course of the anxiety experience will usually clarify the situation. In true panic attacks, the peak intensity of the experience always occurs within a few minutes. The revised criteria should therefore include the statement that "the peak intensity of the experience [must be] reached within ten minutes from its onset." This requires that clinicians ask, if the patient has not described the temporal course of the onset of the attack, "How long does it take from when it begins to when it is the worst?"

GENERALIZED ANXIETY DISORDER As already noted, this is a new category in DSM-III, and its description is not based on systematic studies. According to DSM-III, the criteria for the disorder can be met even when the complaints of anxiety are relatively transient (one month's duration). The requirement of only one month's duration makes it difficult to distinguish this category from relatively transient stress reactions, and investigators who have studied this category have generally limited their samples to individuals who have had the symptoms for much longer periods of time (Cloninger et al., 1981; Raskin et al., 1982). The authors therefore propose that the duration requirement be changed to six months during which an individual has been experiencing "nervousness or anxiety," "worry," or "inability to relax."

Another problem with the DSM-III criteria for Generalized Anxiety Disorder is that they only require a single anxiety symptom from each of three out of four areas; thus, an individual who has only "jumpiness," "feeling 'on edge'," and "worry" satisfies the symptom criteria. For a better definition of a syndrome, the new criteria should require the presence of at least 6 of an 18-item index of commonly associated symptoms taken from those currently listed in the DSM-III criteria.

Finally, as discussed previously, the authors propose that Generalized Anxiety Disorder no longer be considered residual to all other specific Anxiety Disorders. Although individuals with circumscribed anxiety syndromes such as Social or Simple Phobia frequently do not have generalized anxiety, some individuals do, and recognizing their associated Generalized Anxiety Disorder might have important treatment implications. Generalized Anxiety Disorder should therefore only be excluded by those other Anxiety Disorders in which persistent anxiety is usually present anyway, i.e., Agoraphobia, Obsessive-Compulsive Disorder, and Posttraumatic Stress Disorder.

OBSESSIVE-COMPULSIVE DISORDER During the development of DSM-III, there was a proposal to subdivide this category according to whether an individual had obsessions alone or had both obsessions and compulsions. As Insel (1982) has noted in a provocative article on this disorder, Sir Aubrey Lewis in 1936 recognized the heterogeneity of the disorder, describing "obsessionals" as being distinct from "compulsives." Nonetheless, at the time that DSM-III was being developed, there seemed to be no compelling reason to subdivide the category. A recent review of psychosocial treatments of Anxiety Disorders (Barlow and Beck, 1984) has indicated that behavioral treatments are often effective when both obsessions and compulsions are present, but not when only obsessions are present. This suggests that it may now be valid to divide the disorder.

POSTTRAUMATIC STRESS DISORDER Much recent research has focused on this category, particularly as it applies to Vietnam veterans (Frye and Stockton, 1982; Atkinson et al., 1982). Based on their experience with Vietnam veterans, Hough and Gongla (1982) have suggested that the DSM-III criteria would be improved by including in the criteria themselves symptoms that are now listed only as associated features, such as rage, explosions of aggressive behavior, fear of aggressive behavior, and impulsive behavior.

Before the publication of DSM-III, Horowitz et al. (1980) completed a study of Posttraumatic Stress Disorder in individuals who had experienced the death of someone close to them and individuals who had sustained personal injuries by violence, accidents, or illnesses. They apparently included individuals even if the stress was not outside the range of normal experience (e.g., bereavement) and found that these individuals also suffered the distinctive syndrome of reexperiencing the trauma. This finding raises the question of whether DSM-III is correct in stating that the essential feature of Posttraumatic Stress Disorder is "the development of characteristic symptoms following a psychologically traumatic event that is generally outside the range of usual human experience . . . [such] as simple bereavement [or] chronic illness" (236).*

CONCLUSION

The DSM-III concept of Anxiety Disorders has been widely accepted, and the diagnostic criteria for the separate disorders have facilitated much research in this area. Beyond the problems discussed regarding the definitions of the disorders and their hierarchical interrelationships are many other diagnostic issues that have not been discussed here. These include evidence for the validity of the Anxiety Disorder categories themselves, the need for a category for Organic Anxiety Syndrome (Mackenzie and Popkin, 1983), and an issue that has plagued nosologists and clinicians for many decades, the relationship between anxiety and depressive states (Gurney et al., 1972; Klerman, 1980; Foa and Foa, 1982). Space has also not permitted discussion of two new standardized diagnostic interview schedules that can be used for diagnosing all of the DSM-III Anxiety Disorders: the Anxiety Disorders Interview Schedule (ADIS) (Di Nardo et al., in press) and the Structured Clinical Interview for DSM-III (SCID) (Spitzer and Williams, 1983b).

Chapter 26 **The Role of Genetics in the Etiology of Panic Disorder**
by Raymond R. Crowe, M.D.

INTRODUCTION

This chapter reviews biological evidence on the etiology of the anxiety disorders from a genetic perspective. The earliest evidence that psychiatric disorders might have a biological basis came from genetically oriented studies which stimulated further research into the biology of these conditions and led to many of the developments in biological psychiatry today. In anxiety disorders we are today where we were ten years ago with affective disorder and schizophrenia. A growing conviction that the anxiety disorders have a biological basis is stimulating a rapid growth in the research into their etiology. This is an appropriate time, therefore, to review what we have learned about the biology of these conditions and where the current research is taking us.

Genetics begins by studying disease in the population and proceeds to ask how genes act at the molecular level to cause the disease. Thus, in approaching the etiology of a disorder, the first questions asked are

*Editor's note: In Part II of this volume, Terr discusses the DSM-III definition of Posttraumatic Stress Disorder, as well as the evolution of the general concept of psychic trauma. While her focus is primarily on children, she also reviews relevant studies of adults.

epidemiologic. How common is the disorder? Are there sex differences? What is the age of onset? Proceeding next to the level of the family, family studies determine whether the illness is familial and therefore likely to be genetic. Studies of twins and adoptees help to separate genetic from environmental influences. Transmission models determine whether various genetic hypotheses can account for the distribution of illness in families and whether other genetic hypotheses can be rejected. Linkage studies use genetic markers to search for linkage between disease and marker, thus implicating a major gene in the transmission of the illness. Finally, biochemical genetics examines the direct effect of genes—the enzymes, neurotransmitters, and receptors which may be responsible for the illness. This chapter follows the foregoing sequence, beginning with population studies and proceeding toward the molecular level in reviewing biological data on the etiology of anxiety disorders.

The review focuses on panic disorder since it has been studied more extensively than the other anxiety disorders and thus serves as a model for the sequence of research questions outlined above and addressed in this chapter. One problem that arises initially in reviewing this particular anxiety disorder is the problem of terminology and classification. Panic disorder has gone by many names over the years—neurasthenia, neurocirculatory asthenia, effort syndrome, and anxiety neurosis, to name a few. Despite the great variety of diagnostic terms, however, clinical descriptions of the illnesses associated with the diverse terms indicate that they all constitute essentially the same condition. Moreover, there is good reason to believe that panic disorder and agoraphobia with panic attacks are the same condition, and together they account for the majority of anxiety disorders in most clinics (Hallam, 1978; Klein, 1981).

EPIDEMIOLOGY

Estimates of the prevalence of panic disorder vary considerably (Marks and Lader, 1973; Carey et al., 1980), even when confined to those studies that specify diagnostic criteria and that can be considered to be defining panic disorder as it is defined today. An early estimate came from personal examinations of 1,214 residents of Framingham, Massachusetts (Kannel et al., 1958). The diagnostic criteria employed were similar to DSM-III in requiring five criterion symptoms, but differed in not requiring the presence of discrete panic attacks. A surprisingly high prevalence of 11.6 percent was reported. A smaller survey using similar criteria and personal interviews estimated a prevalence of 4.7 percent (Cohen et al., 1951). Estimates of lifetime morbidity risk (the percentage of persons who will develop the disease if they live out their lives) can be derived from age-adjusted illness rates found among control relatives in family studies. Using this method, a morbidity risk of 2.1 percent was found based on family histories (Noyes et al., 1978), and a risk of 2.3 percent was found when the majority of the relatives were personally interviewed (Crowe et al., 1983). In contrast, another family study found a rate of only 0.4 percent panic disorder among relatives of normal controls (Gershon et al., 1982). Excluding the highest and lowest rates, the data suggest a rather common disorder with a prevalence in the range of two to five cases per hundred in the population.

Since the sex ratio in clinic populations may reflect referral patterns rather than true epidemiologic differences, it is important that the observations be based on population samples. The available reports are consistent with one another in this regard and indicate a female-to-male ratio of approximately two to one (Kannel et al., 1958; Cohen et al., 1951; Noyes et al., 1978; Crowe et al., 1983).

Panic disorder typically begins in early adulthood. The mean age of onset was 27.5 years in one large series of patients (Wheeler et al., 1950). A recent study of 41 patients meeting DSM-III criteria for Panic Disorder found a similar mean age of onset of 26.3 years, with a standard deviation of 10.4 years (Crowe et al., 1980). Marks and Lader (1973) have observed that anxiety beginning after the age of 40 is commonly part of a depressive disorder, rather than an anxiety disorder.

BASIC GENETIC STUDIES

Family Studies

The familial nature of panic disorder was noted as early as 1869 (Beard, 1869), and a number of subsequent writers have commented on positive family histories. Oppenheimer and Rothschild (1918) were the first to provide data and reported a family history of nervousness in 45 percent of their patients and in 15 percent of their controls. Subsequent family history investigations have examined the percentage of first-degree relatives affected and have consistently reported rates in the range of 15 to 18 percent (McInnes, 1937; Brown, 1942; Cohen et al., 1951; Noyes et al., 1978). The studies have further indicated that half to two-thirds of patients with panic disorder have at least one first-degree relative with a similar condition.

Family history studies are based solely on information obtained from the patient, and in other psychiatric conditions they have been shown consistently to underestimate the true rates of illness in the family members (Andreasen et al., 1977; Thompson et al., 1982). Preliminary findings from family history studies must therefore be confirmed by investigations in which the family members are personally examined. The first such investigation examined 37 offspring of patients with panic disorder and found 49 percent of the offspring had the same condition (Wheeler et al., 1948). More recently, the Saint Louis group has reported preliminary findings on anxiety disorders in their clinic (Cloninger et al., 1981). They found anxiety neurosis in 13 percent of female relatives of patients with anxiety disorder and in 2 percent of male relatives. Moreover, most of the secondary cases found were in the families of probands with the more severe anxiety disorders of panic disorder and agoraphobia.

The author and his colleagues have recently completed a study of the families of 41 probands with panic disorder. In the study, 66 percent of the first-degree relatives were personally examined, and information on the remainder was obtained from those who were interviewed (Crowe et al., 1983). The age-adjusted morbidity risk was 17.3 percent for definite panic disorder and 7.4 percent for probable panic disorder (in which a case had but two or three criterion symptoms and thus did not meet DSM-III criteria). Among these families, the morbidity risk for both probable and definite panic disorder was 24.7 percent, compared with 2.3 percent among the control relatives. Female relatives were affected about twice as frequently as male relatives (33 versus 16.8 percent). Finally, 25 of the 41 families had at least one first-degree relative affected with panic disorder (61 percent).

The findings from family studies thus leave little doubt that panic disorder is a familial condition, as would be expected if it were a genetic trait. But in order to examine the genetic hypothesis further, one must turn from family studies to investigations that can separate genetic from environmental influences.

Twin Studies

Monozygotic (MZ) twins are genetically identical, while dizygotic (DZ) twins are genetically equivalent to ordinary siblings. Therefore, to the extent that environmental influences act on MZ and DZ pairs alike, differences between the two can be assumed to be genetic. Thus a higher concordance rate in MZ than in DZ twins indicates that genetic factors are involved in causing the illness.

Twin studies in anxiety disorders are limited to two investigations. Slater and Shields found 7 of 17 MZ pairs concordant for anxiety disorder (41 percent), compared with only 1 of 28 DZ pairs (4 percent) (Slater and Cowie, 1971). Torgersen (1978) reported similar findings, with 9 of 30 MZ pairs concordant (30 percent) and 5 of 56 DZ pairs (9 percent). In view of the illness rates among first-degree relatives in family studies, one would expect both the MZ and DZ rates to be higher. The difference between the findings of the family and the twin studies may reflect the twin studies' inclusion of a broader group of anxiety disorders. However, the twin studies are consistent with one another, and they imply a genetic explanation for the familial aspect of panic disorder.

The higher concordance rates for MZ than DZ twins imply that heredity is involved in the etiology of anxiety disorders. However, even the MZ concordance rates are far below 100 percent, indicating that environmental causes are operating as well. The twin studies can be accepted as evidence for a genetic factor provided that the environment is assumed to act equally on both types of twins. This critical assumption is difficult to verify because MZ and DZ twins are often treated differently. This weakness of the twin study has led to a method which can more rigorously separate genetic from environmental influences—the adoption study.

Adoption Studies

Adoptees separated from their biological families at birth and reared by adoptive families provide an excellent means for studying genetic and environmental influences independently of one another. Concordance in diagnosis between adoptee and biological relatives supports a genetic etiology, while concordance between adoptee and adoptive relatives supports an environmental one. In psychiatric genetics, a positive adoption study has been the sine qua non for concluding that a disease is genetic. Unfortunately, no adoption studies of anxiety disorder per se are available.

One relevant adoption study entailed a reanalysis of the Danish adoption study of schizophrenia with respect to anxiety disorder in the relatives (Kendler et al., 1981). Interviews with biological and adoptive relatives of both schizophrenic and control adoptees were reviewed for panic disorder and generalized anxiety disorder. Rates of the two disorders were approximately the same, ranging from 8.0 to 10.5 percent in both the biological and the adoptive relatives of schizophrenic and control adoptees, indicating no association between schizophrenia and a family history of anxiety disorder. A study of adoptees with panic disorder would be extremely valuable in determining whether panic disorder is indeed a genetic trait.

Transmission Model Studies

If a disorder is considered to be genetic, then the next question to be answered is how it is inherited. With psychiatric disorders, this question has proved difficult to answer. Certain characteristics of these disorders, such as incomplete penetrance and different illness rates in the two sexes, result in transmission that does not come close to that expected with Mendelian inheritance. To deal with this problem, genetic models have been developed which allow for variations in penetrance. Basically, these models assume that every person has a certain liability to develop the illness and that both genetic and environmental influences contribute to this liability. Persons above a threshold level will manifest the illness while those below it will not. If males and females have different thresholds, then the different rates of the illness in the two sexes can be accounted for.

The author and his colleagues tested the single-major-locus (SML) (Kidd and Cavalli-Sforza, 1973) and the multifactorial polygenic (Reich et al., 1975) threshold models on 41 pedigrees of panic disorder (Crowe et al., 1983). Analysis of data with transmission models is helpful only when one model can be shown not to fit the data and thus excluded. Demonstrating that a model fits does not necessarily mean that it is the mode of inheritance involved.

The SML model gave an acceptable fit to the data $(.05 < p < .10)$. The best-fitting model predicted a gene frequency of .05 resulting in 0.25 percent of the population being homozygotes for the gene, and 9.5 percent being heterozygotes. Forty-six percent of female heterozygotes and 25 percent of male heterozygotes would be affected, the respective rates for homozygotes being 87 percent and 72 percent. The illness prevalence in the population would therefore be 4.5 percent in females and 2.5 percent in males.

The multifactorial polygenic model differs from the SML primarily in assuming that the genetic component is due to multiple genes, each having a small and additive effect. This model also gave a satisfactory fit to the data $(.25 < p < .50)$, but predicted unacceptably high prevalence rates, 17 percent in females and 9 percent in males. However, when the prevalences were fixed at 10 percent for females and 5 percent for males, the model still gave an acceptable fit $(.05 < p < .10)$.

Since neither model could be excluded by the panic disorder data, no conclusions can be drawn about the mode of transmission of panic disorder.

GENE ACTION

Since genes direct the synthesis of protein, a direct product of gene action at the molecular level must ultimately be sought. Although we are still far from realizing this goal, some recent advances which have been made may eventually lead to a better understanding of anxiety at the molecular level. The earliest of these advances derived from observations of lactate metabolism in patients with anxiety neurosis.

Lactate and Anxiety

One of the cardinal symptoms of panic disorder is easy fatigability. This symptom can be verified objectively by measuring oxygen consumption and lactate production during exercise, the former being lower and the latter higher in panic disorder patients than in normal subjects (Cohen and White, 1950).

In 1967, Pitts and McClure reported that infusions of sodium lactate produced typical panic attacks in 13 of 14 patients with anxiety neurosis, but in only 2 of 10 normal control subjects. This effect appeared to be specific to lactate since glucose infusions did not lead to anxiety attacks. Further, adding calcium ion to the lactate infusion prevented panic attacks from developing. These observations led the investigators to propose that intracellularly produced lactate complexes ionized calcium at the nerve cell membrane, producing functional hypocalcemia and leading to the symptoms of a panic attack. Pitts and McClure's theory has been criticized on the grounds that the amount of lactate they infused was insufficient to complex enough ionized calcium to produce hypocalcemia (Grosz and Farmer, 1969). In addition, sodium lactate is rapidly metabolized to bicarbonate when it enters the body, and measurements of blood lactate following lactate infusion failed to show any elevation in lactate levels (Grosz and Farmer, 1972).

Although the Pitts-McClure hypothesis may no longer be tenable, the finding that lactate infusion precipitates panic attacks in patients with panic disorder has been replicated by numerous investigators and cannot be seriously challenged (Kelly et al., 1971; Appleby et al., 1981). Moreover, the observation that the lactate-induced attacks are blocked by imipramine argues that they are true panic attacks (Gorman et al., 1981). Whether the lactate induces panic attacks through a direct chemical action, as Pitts and McClure thought, or by a conditioned phobic response triggered by somatic symptoms of anxiety, as suggested by Ackerman and Sachar (1974), remains unsettled. Nevertheless, lactate-induced panic attacks continue to be a useful biochemical model for studying anxiety.

Mitral Valve Prolapse

Mitral valve prolapse would seem an unlikely candidate for the etiology of an anxiety disorder. It is usually caused by a myxomatous degeneration of the posterior mitral valve leaflet, leading to a midsystolic prolapse of the leaflet and the characteristic midsystolic click heard on auscultation (Devereux, 1979). Mitral prolapse is a familial condition, and in many families it appears to be inherited as an autosomal dominant trait with incomplete penetrance (Devereux et al., 1982). Like panic disorder, it is a common condition, affecting 5 to 10 percent of the population, and women are affected about twice as frequently as men (Devereux, 1979). Wooley (1976) was struck by the similarity of the symptoms of the two conditions and proposed that panic disorder and mitral valve prolapse were in fact the same disease. This hypothesis was easily tested since the echocardiogram provides a noninvasive means of viewing the mitral valve during the cardiac cycle. Several centers have used echocardiography to examine patients with panic attacks and have reported mitral prolapse in 38 to 50 percent, substantially higher than the 5 to 10 percent expected in the general population (Venkatesh et al., 1980; Pariser et al., 1978; Gorman et al., 1981; Grunhaus et al., 1982).

Since mitral prolapse appears to be an autosomal dominant trait in many families, its association with panic disorder might explain the transmission of that condition. This question was examined in a series of 19 families in which all probands had panic disorder and 7 also had mitral prolapse (Crowe et al., 1980). A family study revealed that the two groups of families (those with and those without prolapse) had identical morbidity risks for panic disorder in both sexes and in every class of relative. Moreover, when the two groups of families were analyzed with genetic models, no difference in the patterns of transmission was found (Pauls et al., 1979; Pauls et al., 1980). These findings, coupled with the observation that panic attacks are suppressed by imipramine, regardless of the presence of prolapse, indicate that mitral prolapse patients do not represent a separate subgroup of patients with panic disorder (Gorman et al., 1981).

The real test of the association between panic disorder and mitral valve prolapse is whether the two traits segregate together within families, and this question has been examined in two studies. The first was a family study in which 103 first-degree relatives of patients with mitral prolapse received both echocardiograms and psychiatric interviews (Hartman et al., 1982). Although 33 of the relatives had mitral valve prolapse, only 1 had panic disorder, a rate no higher than that of the relatives without mitral prolapse or that of the general population. The second investigation was a family history study of 50 patients with mitral prolapse (Crowe et al., 1982). The principal finding was that the first-degree relatives of mitral prolapse patients with panic attacks had a 15.7 percent rate of panic attacks, while the relatives of those without panic attacks had a 1.2 percent rate. The panic attacks therefore appeared to be inherited independently of mitral prolapse.

These observations contradict the earlier findings of an association between the two traits, and they indicate that an unselected population of patients with mitral prolapse does not have an increased risk for panic attacks. Whatever is responsible for the association in clinic populations, mitral valve prolapse does not seem to account for the familial transmission of panic disorder.*

Neurophysiology

Gray recently reviewed the neurophysiology of anxiety and proposed a neurophysiological theory of anxiety (Gray, 1981a; 1981b). The effects of

*Editor's note: In a later chapter in this Part, Gorman discusses mitral valve prolapse as an autonomic nervous system illness and explores the connection with panic disorder in light of three current hypotheses. Two of these incorporate genetic factors as independent or interacting variables.

anxiolytic drugs are reasonably homogeneous across species, from fish to mammals, implying that a phylogenetically old neural system must be involved in producing anxiety and that the same system is likely to be involved in anxiety in human beings. Animals react to punishment, signs of nonreward, and novel stimuli with increased vigilance and arousal and behavioral inhibition, a reaction that has been interpreted as anxiety. Anxiolytic drugs suppress this response, as they should if it reflects true anxiety. The system that is most likely involved in this animal model is the septo-hippocampal system with its afferents and efferents, especially the dorsal noradrenergic afferents from the locus coeruleus and serotonergic afferents from the midline raphe nuclei. Lesioning the septo-hippocampal system or its dorsal afferents leads to behaviors which mimic those seen following anxiolytic drug administration.

Gray has suggested that the role of the septo-hippocampal system is to compare actual with expected stimuli (Gray, 1981a; 1981b). As long as the two match, the system operates in the checking mode, but when a mismatch occurs, or when a predicted stimulus is aversive, it switches to the control mode and produces anxiety. In this state, the organism proceeds with heightened vigilance, arousal, and caution until actual and expected stimuli again match and the system returns to the checking mode.

Whether Gray's model proves correct or not, the septo-hippocampal system does appear to be instrumental in anxiety, and genetic variation in the function and activity of the system could account for such anxiety disorders as generalized anxiety disorder and panic disorder.

Biochemistry

The serotonergic system, arising from the midbrain raphe nuclei, and the noradrenergic system, arising from the locus coeruleus, may play a role in regulating anxiety (Hoehn-Saric, 1982). Surgical and pharmacologic manipulations of both systems have direct effects on anxiety in animals. Both systems are affected by the tricyclic antidepressants, which are effective antipanic agents. Finally, both systems are in direct communication with the septo-hippocampal system which, as noted, has been implicated in anxiety. The most exciting advances, however, have occurred in the GABA system.

It has been apparent for some time that the anxiolytic drugs exert their effect through facilitation of GABA (γ-aminobutyric acid), an inhibitory neurotransmitter (Hoehn-Saric, 1982). However, a major advance in our understanding of the biochemistry of anxiety occurred in 1977 with the discovery of benzodiazepine receptors (Squires and Braestrup, 1977; Tallman et al., 1980; Paul et al., 1981). Since this rapidly developing area of research is reviewed elsewhere in this volume,* this discussion is limited to the significance of these advances for the genetics of anxiety disorders.

Briefly, the benzodiazepine receptor appears to act by facilitating the action of GABA. The mechanism for the potentiation of GABA is through an increase in the rate of opening of the chloride channel, allowing more chloride ion to enter the neuron and thus raising its depolarization threshold. Nonbenzodiazepine sedative-hypnotics act directly on the

*Editor's note: See the chapter by Paul and Skolnick.

chloride channel, rather than on the benzodiazepine receptor. The benzodiazepine receptor occurs in at least two forms, abbreviated BZ_1 and BZ_2. The BZ_2 receptor is thought to be more relevant to anxiety than the BZ_1, and in view of Gray's hypothesis, it is interesting that the benzodiazepine receptors in the limbic system are predominantly BZ_2.

Of even greater importance for the etiology of anxiety disorders is the likelihood that an endogenous ligand for the receptor may exist analogous to the endorphins and the opiate receptor. Although this is an area of intense research, to date no ligand has been identified.

CONCLUSION

Our ultimate aim in studying the genetics of a disease is to understand the causal sequence of events and perhaps to intervene therapeutically, as we have in diseases like phenylketonuria. Here, a single gene mutation produces a defective enzyme which is responsible for the illness, and dietary intervention, based on our understanding of the pathophysiology, can prevent the serious consequences of the disease from developing. In psychiatry we are not yet close to such an understanding of any mental illness. But in panic disorder the considerable progress now being made may someday lead to a similar understanding and rational treatment for that condition.

Chapter 27 # Anxiety Disorders in Children
by Rachel Gittelman, Ph.D.

INTRODUCTION

Current psychiatric nomenclature in DSM-III specifies several anxiety disorders with a childhood onset. These include Separation Anxiety Disorder, Avoidant Disorder of Childhood or Adolescence, and Overanxious Disorder. In addition, Simple Phobia, which is listed with the adult Anxiety Disorders, is an important condition to consider in the overall evaluation of childhood anxiety disorders. The adult diagnoses of Panic Disorder, Agoraphobia, and Agoraphobia with Panic Attacks have not been reported in children. Social Phobia, which is also an adult diagnosis in DSM-III, can occur in children.

Overanxious Disorder and Avoidant Disorder of Childhood or Adolescence are new categories in the nomenclature of child psychiatric disorders. Based on the author's clinical experience to date, children with clinical levels of social anxiety meet the diagnostic criteria for Overanxious Disorder. This area and many important specific issues such as age of onset, sex distribution, course, and treatment response await systematic clinical investigation.

Of the five disorders that are of concern in children, only two have received systematic attention: Simple Phobia and Separation Anxiety Disorder. These two disorders are the focus of the following review.

DIAGNOSTIC PRINCIPLES

The problem of defining pathological boundaries pervades psychiatric classification and is especially salient in child psychiatry. Much of the time, children for whom psychiatric services are sought present with behavior that in its mild manifestation would be considered unremarkable and undeserving of costly professional attention. The more severe manifestation of the same behavior, however, understandably calls for knowledgeable intervention. Likewise, though simple phobias and separation anxiety are common in childhood, they may sometimes assume forms that render the child dysfunctional.

The severity of a behavior is not the only criterion for defining abnormality in children; timing is also key. Some characteristics are of no diagnostic relevance early in life, but may be viewed as symptoms later on. An obvious example is enuresis. Similarly, although many forms of anxiety are appropriate developmental responses in early childhood, they may be considered abnormal, even when not severe, when they occur in middle childhood and beyond.

SIMPLE PHOBIAS

Simple phobias involving fears of animals, the dark, injections, and so forth are common in young children. Lapouse and Monk's epidemiologic study indicated a very high rate of specific fears, reported by mothers, for a general population of children between the ages of 6 and 12. Considering only children with several fears, as many as 43 percent were reported to have seven or more fears (Lapouse and Monk, 1958; 1959). Though this rate does indicate that multiple fears are the rule rather than the exception in young children, it does not communicate the impairment associated with the fears. The prevalence of simple phobic disorders is therefore unknown, but likely to be high. From the epidemiologic survey, it seems that children's fears are not significantly associated with other behavioral difficulties, at least not in a general population group. This observation supports the common existence of pure simple phobias in children.

The above-mentioned concerns regarding diagnosis when a trait is very common are therefore relevant to the simple phobias. The degree of functional impairment should guide diagnostic practice. If a boy is so frightened of dogs, for example, that he is terror stricken while outside, even in the absence of imminent threat, then clearly he deserves professional attention for the relief of his misery.

Treatment

It is most unusual for a child to enter treatment because of the presence of simple phobias. Most families accommodate to the child's avoidant behaviors. They do not come to professional attention, but readjust their activities to minimize confrontation between the child and the phobic object.

The phobic children described in the literature are either nonpatients or children whose simple phobias are part of a more generalized maladaptive pattern. The two historical examples are Peter, in whom a rabbit phobia was induced and subsequently treated (Jones, 1924), and Little Hans, whose fear of horses was but one aspect of his extremely fearful behavior, most of which stemmed from separation anxiety (Freud, 1909).

Given the evidence that different childhood fears may emerge at various developmental stages (Bauer, 1980), an age phenomenon would also seem likely to affect the onset of disorders. In turn, the treatment efficacy of psychotherapeutic approaches might vary with age. The expectation would be that younger children should be more responsive to treatment than older children.

An abundant literature describes behavioral treatment strategies. These are the treatments in currency for simple phobic disorders. Whether they are superior to other psychotherapeutic treatments for children with phobic disorders cannot be assumed, since the distinction has not been clear between such psychotherapies for children and for adult phobic patients who have more generalized conditions (Miller et al., 1972; Klein et al., 1983).

SEPARATION ANXIETY

The distress that a child experiences when separated from the person who cares for him or her is a normal developmental phenomenon. After the age of six to eight months, most children will occasionally display some negative affect when separated from the caretaker.

Children's immediate responses to separation have been studied both in the laboratory and in natural environments. Weinraub and Lewis (1977) observed 2-year-old children whose mothers were instructed to walk out of a laboratory room following a 15-minute period of free interaction. Ainsworth (1967) conducted intensive naturalistic observations of West African infants' and toddlers' reactions to minor separation events. The children showed a great deal of variability in the intensity of their distress over normal separation experiences such as the mother stepping out of a room and leaving the child's visual field, or the child being left briefly in the care of someone else.

In animal studies, experimentally induced longer-term separation between offspring and parent typically has resulted in marked alterations in the mother-child relationship. Most investigations of the impacts of longer-term separations on children have dealt with their reactions to such major life-disrupting events as the total removal of the child or a parent from the home.

In such cases, it is difficult to relate the reaction of the youngster to the parent's absence exclusively, without regard for the contribution of other factors. Greatly modified life circumstances or social deprivation might contribute significantly to the behavioral changes observed in the child following such separations. In a comprehensive review of the effects of separation on children's behavior, Rutter (1977) noted that several factors may mitigate the severity of the child's immediate and extended reactions to separation: the type of care given during separation, contact with people familiar and close to the child during the separation period, and the parents' reactions to the child upon being reunited.

Bowlby and Robertson have termed the overt distress the protest phase of the separation reaction. In some cases, when separation continues, protest is followed by withdrawal and sadness, referred to as the despair phase. A final phase is the detachment phase, marked by indifference to the reappearance of the person whose departure originally provoked the reaction, and by an active interest in new caretakers (for a review of this work, see Bowlby, 1969). The first part of this emotional sequence, the protest phase, is the psychological state known as separation anxiety.*

Diagnosis

The fact that separation anxiety can be considered part of children's normal social development may lead to some ambiguity about when it should be considered deviant or pathological.

Pathological separation anxiety manifests itself in three ways. First and most obvious is distress on separation, which in the severe form of the disorder becomes panic. Second, morbid worries about the potential dangers that threaten family integrity are also pathognomonic of the disorder. A final sign of the disorder is homesickness involving missing the home or family members and a yearning to be reunited to a degree which goes beyond usual reactions. These key characteristics of separation anxiety can occur concurrently or independently. They are considered symptoms when they restrict the child's activities or interfere markedly with his or her emotional well-being.

Pathological separation anxiety differs from the many disorders of childhood which tend to follow a chronic course and which have no clear-cut age of onset (i.e., conduct disorders, psychotic or pervasive developmental disorders, attention deficit disorder). Unlike these disorders, pathological separation anxiety often appears suddenly, in a previously well-functioning child who has shown no premorbid signs of unusual separation anxiety, although it can also occur in children with histories of chronic separation anxiety, often of subclinical severity. Also in contrast to the other childhood disorders, separation anxiety may remit spontaneously, leaving the youngster free of difficulties.

The possibility that a child has pathological separation anxiety should not be ruled out just because the child does not always show it when removed from the parent. The instances of separation that evoke distress in the child reflect the pervasiveness of the reaction, not its presence or absence. It is possible for a child to have pervasive but mild anxiety or clearly focal but severe anxiety in response to separation.

Pathological separation anxiety is not restricted to children, but can also occur in adults. Although overt protest on separation among adults is rare, some persons with agoraphobia who do not tolerate staying alone may protest separation in the fear of having a panic attack while unattended. Morbid worries about threats to loved ones and acute homesickness are the typical symptoms of adults suffering from excessive separation anxiety.

Pharmacologic Treatment

THEORETICAL CONSIDERATIONS   If one were to retrace the history of pharmacotherapy for children with behavior disorders, one would generally identify two clear and independent patterns. The first would be the completely serendipitous discovery of the effects of drugs on

*Editor's note: Part II of this volume, "Children at Risk," includes several chapters related to the effects of separation on children. Particularly relevant are the chapters by Wallerstein, presenting data on children's short- and long-term responses to divorce, and by Garmezy, reviewing the work of Rutter and others concerning protective factors.

children's behavior. This is true of the psychostimulant treatment of hyperactive children. The second would be a direct, uncritical transfer of established practice from adult psychopharmacotherapy to children's psychiatric disorders. The use of antidepressants for treating depressed children is an example of this pattern. The investigation of imipramine in childhood pathological separation anxiety is, however, unique in pediatric psychopharmacology. Neither the serendipitous nor the purely empirical adult-child transfer model applies. The historical events that led to a trial of imipramine in children who resisted attending school are summarized briefly because of their wider implications. These events shed light on the relationship of the disorder to adult psychiatric disorders and contribute to a theoretical understanding of the nature of anxiety states in children.

The use of the tricyclic, imipramine, with childhood pathological separation anxiety was prompted by a series of clinical observations that Klein made while studying adult agoraphobic patients (Klein, 1964). Klein postulated that these patients were suffering from a disruption in the biological processes that regulate anxiety triggered by separation. Stimulating this idea was the observation that a large proportion of the adult patients had a childhood history of severe separation anxiety and that their response to initial panic had been clinging, dependent behavior. Assuming then that panic anxiety was a pathological variant of normal separation anxiety, imipramine, which relieved panic anxiety, should be useful in patients whose behavioral difficulties clearly stemmed from their inability to separate from significant others. Following this line of reasoning, Klein predicted that imipramine would be effective with children who have pathological levels of separation anxiety, such as school-phobic children. Thus, although the use of imipramine with school-phobic children followed its use with agoraphobic adults, the practice was derived from a particular model of psychopathology rather than from strict therapeutic empiricism.

DRUG TRIALS WITH TRICYCLICS Two controlled studies of tricyclic treatment with school phobia have appeared, one showing positive drug effects (Gittelman-Klein and Klein, 1971; 1973) and the other showing no significant drug effect (Berney et al., 1981).

Among children who refused to go to school, imipramine was significantly more effective than a placebo (Gittelman-Klein and Klein, 1971; 1973). Children between the ages of 7 and 15 who had been absent from school for at least two weeks or who had been attending intermittently under great duress were considered for the study. If after two weeks of vigorous nonpharmacologic treatment effort the child was still not attending school regularly, he or she was entered in the study.

Forty-five children, 24 girls and 21 boys, were randomly assigned to a placebo or imipramine in double-blind fashion. For a six-week period, 25 received placebo, and 20, imipramine. Dosage ranged from 100 to 200 mg/day, with a mean dosage of 159 mg/day. The patient and the family were seen weekly. (Details of the psychotherapeutic management that accompanied the medication regimen are discussed elsewhere [Gittelman-Klein, 1975].)

After treatment, 24 percent of the 25 children on the placebo reported feeling much better, while 90 percent of the 19 on imipramine reported

Table 1. Children's Self-Ratings of Improvement and
Relationship to School Return

Improvement and School Status	Imipramine (19)[1]	Placebo (25)
Much Improved	17 (90%)[2]	6 (24%)[2]
Back to School	14 (74%)	6 (24%)
Not Back to School	3 (16%)	0 (0)
No Change or Slightly Better	2 (10%)[2]	19 (76%)[2]
Back to School	0 (0)	5 (20%)
Not Back to School	2 (10%)	14 (56%)

[1]Self-rating of one subject missing
[2]$\chi^2 = 18.55$; (p<.000)

a similar degree of symptomatic relief (p<.000) (see Table 1). Although 44 percent of the children on the placebo returned to school, nearly half of these children continued to feel uncomfortable. Only 24 percent of the placebo-treated children were back in school and also feeling well, whereas 74 percent of the imipramine-treated children had this outcome.

Imipramine treatment also had a significant positive effect on somatic complaints, which are viewed as secondary symptoms. Of the 38 children who initially reported having difficulties such as stomachaches, nausea, dizziness, headaches, or vague aches and pains, 82 percent of the 17 on imipramine were relieved of the symptoms, but only 33 percent of the 21 on placebo ($\chi^2 = 9.13$; p<.003).

Imipramine should not be viewed as a treatment that automatically leads to renewed school attendance. Rather, it modifies the child's level of anxiety in response to separation. This modification in affective state may enable the child to return to the classroom. On the other hand, even with imipramine, strong anticipatory anxiety about school attendance may inhibit the child from making the necessary attempts to reenter the school situation.

The onset of separation anxiety disorder in adolescence is often thought to signify the development of schizophrenia or some other severe disorder. This contention is not sustained by these data. Response to medication was unrelated to age; adolescents stood as good a chance as prepuberty children of obtaining relief from their subjective distress. In light of the similar rate of improvement with imipramine in children of different ages, it seems unlikely that the symptoms of younger and older children represent different underlying psychopathologies.

Many children require imipramine doses in the adult range (100 to 200 mg/day). Nevertheless, a daily dose of 5.0 mg/kg of body weight should not be exceeded, since cardiovascular effects are possible at the upper limit of the dose used in adult depression (Hayes et al., 1975; Saraf et al., 1974; 1978; Winsberg et al., 1975). No child in this study responded to less than 75 mg/day.

With ongoing administration of imipramine, the extent to which psychotherapy, counseling, or family treatment is necessary varies with the severity of secondary anticipatory anxiety and avoidance maladaptations and with the parents' response to these behaviors.

Berney et al. (1981) reported a 12-week trial of clomipramine in doses of 40 to 75 mg/day in school-phobic children (the mean daily dose was not indicated). Little change in anxiety was obtained on either the placebo or clomipramine. At the end of the trial, 40 percent of the children were not attending school on their own, and 75 percent still had significant levels of separation anxiety.

The level of clomipramine used by Berney and associates was lower than the 75 mg/day found therapeutically necessary in the imipramine study. Yet clomipramine and imipramine have similar potency. No treatment issue other than dosage, such as diagnostic characteristics or type of psychotherapy, appears to explain the different results in the two tricyclic studies, since placebo effects were almost identical. The clomipramine study should not be considered conclusive, therefore, since it used an inadequate dosage.*

OTHER COMPOUNDS Frommer (1967; 1968) has reported that the monoamine oxidase (MAO) inhibitor, phenelzine, is superior to imipramine with phobic children. Frommer's findings on the clinical efficacy of tricyclic drugs and MAO inhibitors may be an artifact of the different doses recommended for each class of drugs. For children 8 to 10 years old, the recommended dose of a MAO inhibitor is proportionately higher than that for tricyclics (30 mg/day vs. 75 mg/day respectively) (Frommer, 1968).

Clinical reports on the therapeutic effects of other agents have also appeared. Chlordiazepoxide has been claimed to have marked beneficial effects in school-phobic children (D'Amato, 1962; Kraft, 1962; Skynner, 1961). Diphenhydramine has been reported of value in young children with "pure anxiety" (Fish, 1960). Finally, claims have been advanced for the efficacy of amphetamines (Fish, 1960; 1968) and sulpiride (Abe, 1975) in school-phobic children.

UNRESOLVED ISSUES Although imipramine was shown to be effective with children who had separation anxiety, the drug cannot be claimed to have a specific effect on this disorder. Conceivably, imipramine could ameliorate all types of anxiety in children, whether they had simple phobias, performance anxiety, or some other type of anxiety. On the other hand, Zitrin et al. (1983) have had relevant findings which indicate that imipramine is ineffective in adults with simple phobias.

A study of rhesus monkeys treated with imipramine or placebo indicated that imipramine may be effective in altering the pattern of behavior associated with separation in these animals. After about three weeks of imipramine treatment, four drug-treated monkeys had less self-

*Editor's note: In *Psychiatry 1982 (Psychiatry Update: Volume I)*, Dr. Joaquim Puig-Antich reviews the efficacy of imipramine and dosage issues with depressed children (pages 291–292). In Volume II, Dr. James M. Perel discusses the age-related pharmacokinetics of tricyclics (pages 497–498).

directed behavior in response to separation and more environmentally oriented behavior than four placebo-treated monkeys (Suomi et al., 1978). Response to separation in animals is believed to provide a useful model of clinical depression in humans, but it seems to have more face validity as a model of response to separation.

Behavioral Treatments and Psychotherapy

Treatments based on conditioning or learning principles are widely used in children with school phobia due to separation anxiety disorder. (The interpretation that school refusal is a symptom of anxiety might be rejected by behaviorists, who would argue instead that the refusal is the disorder.) In vivo desensitization, or forcing the child into school, has been described, as have more gradual desensitization procedures. Numerous case studies have described the clinical management of anxious children, but only one systematic study has appeared.

Miller and colleagues (1972) studied 67 children between the ages of 6 and 13 who were suffering from phobias, primarily school phobias. The children received systematic desensitization or psychotherapy consisting of psychodynamically oriented play therapy for 24 sessions over an eight-week period, or they were placed on a waiting list. The children in the treatment groups received additional clinical interventions as needed, such as assertion training, and their parents were offered therapy when indicated. The parents of children who were not treated were informed that their child's condition was serious enough to require professional attention and that the child had been placed on a waiting list. Children were evaluated at the end of treatment and were also followed up six weeks later. Staff ratings did not distinguish between treated and untreated children. In contrast, parents' ratings of severity and a parent scale of fear symptoms showed significant advantage for the treated children at the end of treatment and at follow-up. No difference appeared between the outcomes of the children who received behavioral therapy and children treated with psychotherapy.

Treatment seemed to have been effective only in the children below the age of 10. Among the younger group, 96 percent improved with treatment, and 57 percent did so without treatment. Among the children 11 and above, 45 percent improved with therapy, and 44 percent improved without therapy. The clinical view that anxiety symptoms in older children signal more serious pathology probably stems from a relative lack of malleability in the clinical status of older children.

As the authors noted, the fact that parents, but not staff, reported treatment effects may be the result of parents' expectations. They may have had biased perceptions of their children, or, reflecting cognitive dissonance, they may have adjusted their views of their children's progress to fit the effort made in undergoing treatment. Unfortunately, we have no way of knowing whether the parents or the clinicians were accurate in their evaluations.

Many other reports of therapy have appeared, but they consist almost exclusively of single case reports (for review, see Ollendich and Mayer, 1982). Similarly, case reports of interpretative therapy in anxious children have appeared (i.e., Sperling, 1967), the most notable of these being Freud's (1909) report on Little Hans.

COMMENT

Empirical study of childhood anxiety disorders and their treatment is very limited. Clinical experience has clearly shown that even where imipramine is helpful, as in severe separation anxiety, psychotherapeutic involvement with the child and family is necessary. Furthermore, the efficacy of imipramine has been studied only in conjunction with psychotherapeutic efforts. It would therefore be misleading, and probably inaccurate, to attribute the same level of efficacy to the drug without other concomitant treatment.

The concept of separation anxiety that led to the use of imipramine follows an ethological model (Bowlby, 1973) which conceives of separation anxiety as an evolutionarily adaptive mechanism that does not require learning. This model implies an intrinsic process in children with severe separation anxiety. Such a view contrasts sharply with the communication model which holds that the child's anxiety is a response to the mother's neurotic needs (Eisenberg, 1958). If the communication model were correct, the therapeutic effect of imipramine would have to be interpreted as protecting the child from the mother's needs. Since this would be a most unusual drug effect, the drug effect argues for the intrinsic presence of a disorder in the child. Nonetheless, environmental influences may still play an important role in the various aspects of separation anxiety, such as its severity, specific form, and maintenance. Pathological separation anxiety may thus result from an interaction between a biological predisposition in the child and a family setting that facilitates the expression of that predisposition. The same interactional model may be active in the child who develops pathological levels of social anxiety or simple phobias.

Chapter 28 # The Psychotherapy of Anxiety
by Jerome D. Frank, M.D., Ph.D.

INTRODUCTION

The term anxiety easily creates confusion in the psychiatric literature. *Anxiety* can refer either to a conscious and specific mental state or to a theoretical construct postulated as the unconscious source of a wide range of psychopathological symptoms that may or may not be accompanied by conscious anxiety (Freud, 1920; Horney, 1937; Sullivan, 1953). In this chapter, the author does not attempt to navigate these deep and treacherous theoretical waters, but uses the term anxiety only to refer to that conscious mental state which signals the actual presence or anticipation of danger to one's bodily or personal integrity. The state is characterized by uneasiness and apprehension, typically accompanied by signs of autonomic discharge such as tachycardia, dry mouth, increased sweating, trembling, and feelings of weakness.

Since danger is an omnipresent feature of the human condition, almost everyone has experienced periods of anxiety. If the person perceives the danger to be mild—for example, the possibility of failing an examination—anxiety may be accompanied by a feeling of exhilaration and may stimulate increased efforts to deal with the danger. At the other extreme, a perceived immediate and overwhelming danger—for example, an automobile bearing down and out of control—may evoke panic and paralysis.

Descriptively, according to DSM-III (American Psychiatric Association, 1980), the conscious manifestations of anxiety fall into three basic categories: the Phobic Disorders, including Agoraphobia, Social Phobia, and simple irrational fears; the Anxiety States, including panics (which are often associated with agoraphobia), Generalized Anxiety Disorder, and Obsessive-Compulsive Disorders;[1] and Posttraumatic Stress Disorder. Finally, anxiety may be a manifestation of Adjustment Disorder with Anxious Mood. This last category is used for anxiety reactions that are briefer and milder than those in the first three categories and that are linked to an identifiable stressor.

To come to psychiatric attention, the anxiety must be severe enough to interfere with a person's ability to function and usually must also be inappropriate in strength or intensity to the apparent danger. Examples include panics without apparent source, phobias of innocuous objects or situations, or persistent generalized anxiety.

Anxiety symptoms alone, however, do not generally constitute a sufficient incentive to bring people into psychotherapy. In addition, a person must be demoralized, must feel so incompetent as to despair of being able to cope unaided with his or her difficulties (DeFigueiredo and Frank, 1982). An example suggesting that even severe anxiety symptoms alone do not bring people to seek psychiatric help is the finding that patients with panic attacks do not come to treatment until an average of 12 years after the onset of the first symptom. In other words, they do not appear until the anxiety has become so pervasive and severe that it has demoralized them (Shader et al., 1982). A few patients, to be sure, will seek psychiatric help for their anxiety symptoms without also being demoralized; they will have heard that certain psychotherapeutic procedures are specific for these symptoms, just as a person may seek a medical remedy for the relief of a particular complaint.

ETIOLOGIC CONSIDERATIONS

Since human beings are open biopsychosocial systems in which perturbations of any part can affect the rest, the etiology of anxiety symptoms involves an interplay of constitutional and biographical determinants. Constitutional factors seem to determine which organs are the most reactive to the sense of danger, whether it be the stomach or the heart, and perhaps also the general threshold for experiencing anxiety. Some persons are obviously able to withstand stronger threats than others without becoming anxious. The biological determinants of special organ vulnerabilities and general susceptibility to anxiety remain obscure.

A person's life experiences determine the personal meanings of events, and these meanings are usually the most important determinants of anxiety. A person's sense that a current event is dangerous depends on his or her interpretation of it, which in turn depends largely on the remembered experience of previous seemingly similar events. Enough ex-

[1]Since obsessive-compulsive disorders are generally not accompanied by conscious anxiety except when interrupted by some intervention, they lie outside the self-imposed boundaries of this chapter.

periences of failure can create a general sense of demoralization, coupled with a fear of being unable to cope with future situations as well as situations that one is currently facing (Frank, 1982).

Different theories of psychopathology emphasize different etiologic roles for a person's life experiences. For example, Bowlby stresses the importance of a secure attachment to protective figures in very early life, when separation would literally mean death. It is initially through the basis of confidence in attachment figures that the individual finds the courage to tackle and cope with challenges. If these figures are rejecting or inconsistent, an individual develops persistent or excessive anxiety about their availability. This "anxious attachment" would obviously provide a fertile soil for the development of psychopathology (Bowlby, 1975).

Since human beings are social creatures, every person's important life experiences involve other persons whose responses may influence the susceptibility to anxiety and the forms of its manifestations. Furthermore, the responses of others to the symptoms themselves may exacerbate the symptoms. Anxiety is contagious and mutually reinforcing, so that anxious family members can intensify the anxiety of the patient. The anxiety of others may lead them to be overprotective, which undermines the patient's sense of self-efficacy by depriving him or her of opportunities to encounter and master challenges. Alternatively, other people may react to the anxious patient with rejection or inconsistency, which perpetuates attachment anxiety.

PSYCHOTHERAPEUTIC INTERVENTIONS

In considering the role of psychotherapy in anxiety states, it is important to keep clearly in mind the distinction between the causes of psychiatric symptoms and their meanings or functions. The causes of anxiety symptoms may range anywhere from biological vulnerabilities to misinterpretations of external events or internal stimuli. Their meanings, however, are always the same. All anxiety symptoms are responses to experiences which the patient perceives as potentially or actually dangerous, often including the anxiety symptoms themselves.

Psychotherapy functions entirely at the level of meanings. Its tools are usually words, and sometimes bodily exercises, which have symbolic connotations. Procedures of all therapeutic schools seek to change the meanings of the anxiety-producing experiences from dangerous to innocuous. Besides providing direct relief in this way, since human beings are open systems in which biological, psychological, and social realms continually interact, changing the meanings of certain stimuli from dangerous to innocuous may also alter the biological responses to them. Thus, even when the major cause of traumatic anxiety states is sheer physiological exhaustion, the underlying neurophysiological processes can often be resolved by strictly psychological means. It was commonplace during World War II to relieve flashbacks and nightmares following severe combat experiences by inducing an altered state of consciousness in which the patient could relive the experience in the context of a highly supportive environment. Initially, amobarbital was used to achieve this state (Grinker and Spiegel, 1945), but usually it could be accomplished equally well by light hypnosis. An almost ludicrous example is that of the soldier who after a harrowing jungle experience had nightmares of being pursued by Japanese soldiers. Under light hypnosis he reexperienced the episode and was told simply to shout at the Japanese and they would run away. He did, they ran off, and the nightmares did not recur.

Chronic posttraumatic anxiety states often produce severe demoralization with accompanying dependence on compensation and resentment at this dependency. In addition, after breaking down under severe stress, the patient may lose the sense of basic trust in the safety of the environment, leading to paranoid fearfulness and suspiciousness (Kardiner, 1959). These symbolic aspects are sometimes amenable to psychotherapy.

Finally, the symbolic component of panic attacks is amenable to psychotherapy even if psychotherapy cannot prevent the occurrence of the attacks themselves. Some patients, if they can change the perception of the panic state from a life- or sanity-threatening occurrence to one that is harmless and always transient, can resume essentially normal functioning despite persistence of the attacks (Weeks, 1977).

Different hypotheses regarding the major causes of anxiety underlie the psychotherapeutic interventions of the different psychotherapeutic schools. To oversimplify greatly, behavioral therapies view anxiety as the end result of a conditioning process and seek to desensitize the person to the anxiety-producing stimuli (Stampfl and Levis, 1967; Wolpe, 1958). According to cognitive therapies, the thinking of the anxious patient is dominated by themes of danger, and the therapeutic procedures seek to combat these cognitions (Beck, 1976). Existential psychotherapies regard anxiety as the inevitable response to the recognition of the essential meaninglessness and transitoriness of human existence, to be counteracted by a totally open and nondefensive therapeutic encounter that in some sense involves a merging of patient and therapist (Havens, 1974). Analytic schools attribute anxiety to unresolved unconscious conflicts which can be resolved, with relief of the concomitant anxiety, by being brought to conscious awareness (Freud, 1920).

The extent to which the effectiveness of psychotherapies depends on their underlying theoretical orientation remains unknown. Indeed, effectiveness may be largely unrelated to theory. Different approaches may seem differentially effective with certain symptoms, but this differential may be due more to the relative plausibility of different procedures to the patient and the therapist than to the relative correctness of their theories of causation. A patient with circumscribed symptoms would probably regard focused therapies, whether cognitive or behavioral, as more plausible than open-ended explorations, while a patient suffering from a diffuse sense of existential anxiety might experience more hope from an intimate encounter with an existentially oriented therapist. Analogously, patients who believe that their symptoms are manifestations of unconscious conflicts would find an exploratory analytic approach to be the most plausible.*

Since any differences among the various therapies in their ability to combat anxiety are small at best (Smith et al., 1980; Shapiro and Shapiro, 1982), the following discussion considers the general principles ap-

*Editor's note: In Part I of this volume, Lazarus echoes these thoughts in his discussion of the "bridging and tracking" principles in multimodal therapy. Readers with a particular interest in cognitive therapy may want to refer to Rush's chapter, also in Part I.

plicable to all psychotherapeutic schools rather than the possible special indications and effects of particular strategies and tactics.

Shared Components of Psychotherapies

Regardless of specific conceptualizations or techniques, all forms of psychotherapy include some components to combat the sense of present or impending danger that characterizes all forms of anxiety. One way to identify some of these components would be to ask yourself what qualities you would seek in a guide if you were a tenderfoot about to embark on an exploration into unknown territory with various unknown dangers. Two qualities you would certainly want in a guide would be trustworthiness and competence. You would expect to be able to rely fully on the guide's concern about your welfare. Since you would not be personally acquainted, your confidence that the guide would maintain this concern would depend on your knowledge of his or her professional training and standards.

With respect to competence, you would want the guide to be thoroughly familiar with the terrain and how to cope with the hardships and dangers you might meet. In addition, you would hope that this competence would extend to a knowledge of your own strengths and vulnerabilities, for example, how far you could carry a canoe and whether or not you could swim.

PROFESSIONALISM OF THE THERAPIST Considering the psychotherapist in terms of this analogy, the therapist's ability to combat anxiety in the patient rests in the first instance on an ability to convey that he or she has the patient's interest at heart. The therapist must take the patient seriously and be concerned about his or her welfare. This attitude springs from the therapist's professional training and standards, not from any momentary feelings about the patient. Showing concern for the patient's welfare does not necessarily imply liking or condoning the patient's actions, but simply continuing to be interested no matter how self-damaging or shocking the patient's revelations might be.

Second, the good therapist conveys both knowledgeability and competence. The therapist is well informed about the relevant theoretical issues and has mastered the therapeutic procedures. Perhaps most important, the good therapist is an expert at understanding the patient's communications and at conveying this understanding to the patient.

Several features of professional training may enable the therapist to combat the patient's anxiety more effectively than family members or friends. Being both knowledgeable and competent, the therapist can provide more precise and useful support than the undiscriminating reassurance that families are apt to offer. The therapist is also more able to help the patient to reconceptualize symptoms in ways that diminish anxiety. Because the therapist has a professional role, the patient can rely on being treated with steadfast interest and discretion and can trust in not being a subject of gossip. The therapist, furthermore, avoids becoming entangled in the vicious circles that trap families. Keeping free from anxiety, the therapist neither increases the patient's anxiety through contagion nor overprotects the patient. At the same time, the therapist will not reject the patient because of being hurt, offended, or shocked by what the patient has revealed. This relieves the patient of the burden of having to protect the therapist, and also of the fear of driving the therapist away. In short, the therapist is consistent and predictable. These qualities, of course, are very similar to those Bowlby describes as facilitating the creation of a secure attachment.

THE PROFESSIONAL SETTING Perhaps the single most important anxiety-allaying property of the therapist as a professional is the ability to create an atmosphere in which the patient feels increasingly free to open up. Such an atmosphere is facilitated by the therapeutic setting. The essential aspect of the setting is that it conveys a sense of security. The therapist's presence is a guarantee that no matter how upset the patient becomes, he or she will not be allowed to go out of control or do any harm. In addition, in dyadic therapy the therapist is a guarantor that nothing the patient says, no matter how sensational or shocking, will go beyond the confines of the room. In conjunction, these two aspects of the setting greatly facilitate the patient's ability progressively to reveal hidden fears and other feelings.

ABILITY TO LISTEN It is hard to overestimate the anxiety-allaying power of the therapist's ability simply to listen in an understanding way. A good example of this was the middle-aged woman who had a crippling social anxiety based on the delusion that her nose was growing and that this was obvious to everyone. This type of symptom is often considered to have an ominous prognosis. Her symptom had started in adolescence, preventing her from attending school dances, and it had reached the point that, for the four years before she came to the clinic, she had been unable to work, and for two-and-a-half years, she had been essentially confined to her home. Her adolescent children did the shopping for her, hung up the laundry, and so forth. Eventually, she sought help from a plastic surgeon, who, of course, referred her to the psychiatric clinic. Her understanding was that she had been referred so that the clinic could advise the surgeon to perform the operation.

A medical student interviewed her for over an hour and tried, apparently in vain, to convince her that her problem was a psychological one. She left vowing to go back to her surgeon. Six days later, she called the clinic to speak to the medical student, saying that she just had to tell him how much better she felt. She was now able to leave the house and talk to people face-to-face; she no longer required her daughter to hang up the laundry; she was about to look for a job; and she no longer felt so concerned about her nose. She added that she was convinced of the desire to help her by the amount of time and concern that was given her.

Being suspicious of such a quick cure of a serious problem, the author called this patient eight months later, and she added some details. She had indeed been very distressed by the interview and on leaving had felt that she was going crazy. Then her head suddenly cleared, and, as she put it, she decided that she wanted to live. Her nose, she said, was now a little thing, whereas it had once been the most important thing in her life. Curiously, she did not mention the efforts to persuade her that her problem was psychological, but instead dwelt on her conviction that the clinicians wanted to help her and on their encouraging her to talk. When asked what had helped her, she first mentioned the plastic surgeon: "He stood by me so much. He seemed like a friend to me, someone I could talk to." She added, "I loved the medical student. He had a feeling I wanted to talk, and he let me talk."

SHARED FEATURES OF THERAPEUTIC PROCEDURES The therapist's trustworthiness and competence do more than allay anxiety. They provide the leverage to motivate the patient to participate in whatever procedures the therapist believes to be specifically therapeutic.

Two shared features of all therapeutic procedures may be particularly relevant. First, they are emotionally arousing, and emotion seems necessary to provide the motive power for changes in attitude and behavior. In the insight-oriented therapies, permitting repressed thoughts and feelings to enter consciousness has this effect. In existential therapies, the encounter itself by definition is highly emotionally charged, as is the experience of fear-arousing situations or fantasies in the behavior therapies.

Second, all therapeutic procedures combat anxiety by reinforcing the patient's sense of self-efficacy or mastery. Merely discovering that one can withstand the situations or emotions that one had fearfully sought to avoid has this effect. In addition, all therapies provide a conceptual framework by which the patient can label and order his or her experiences, strengthening a chief means that all human beings have for gaining control over themselves and their environments. Behavior therapies add an additional anxiety-combating component through their experiences of success. Commonly, these experiences occur with the patient progressively mastering graded tasks presented by the therapist. In the abreactive or flooding types of therapies, the very discovery that one can withstand at full intensity those emotions one once thought intolerable engenders strong feelings of success. Whatever the source of experiences of success, they give the patient courage to tackle and master progressively more anxiety-arousing tasks, whether at the subjective or the behavioral level.

Group Acceptance and Group Therapies

Since human beings are social creatures who in the first few years of life are totally dependent for their survival on the benevolence of others, the fear of separation or isolation is a very severe psychological source of anxiety. Whether symbolic or actual, finding oneself in a minority of one often produces anxiety because it implies danger of rejection by the group. If the isolated person can find just one ally, however, the anxiety sharply diminishes (Asch, 1951). The therapist, regardless of school, combats anxiety by being such an ally. Patient and therapist form a group of two, based initially on their shared perception of the sources of the patient's difficulties and what is to be done about them. The therapist also serves as a bridge between the patient and the larger group to which they both adhere, whether it be a particular school of therapy or society at large. As a representative of this group, the accepting therapist facilitates the patient's reintegration into it.

In this connection, the healing rituals of preindustrial societies can relieve anxiety more powerfully than the dyadic treatments of Western societies, because so much of their therapy is specifically directed toward reintegrating the patient into the family and the tribe and toward preparing them to receive the patient again. Properly managed, therapeutic groups in Western societies can perform the same function, albeit to a lesser degree. Interestingly, many of the new therapeutic schools, such as primal scream, provide follow-up groups which the patients are encouraged to attend regularly, thereby maintaining the sense of group cohesiveness and reinforcing the concepts and rituals which both the patient and the group believe are the means of allaying the patient's symptoms (Janov, 1970).

In theory at least, groups should be especially effective in counteracting social anxiety by convincing the patient that the revelation of hidden thoughts and feelings does not lead to rejection. Therapeutic groups, however, as compared with dyadic therapy, do have one potential disadvantage in this respect. Group pressures may cause the patient to reveal secrets before he or she feels sufficient group support to risk such revelations; consequently, stress may outrun support in early meetings, causing the patient to drop out of the group.

Interaction of Psychotherapy with Anxiolytic Drugs

For many patients, the combination of anxiolytic medications with psychotherapy may be more effective than either alone. Since other chapters in this Part deal with medications, it is sufficient here to note that, like psychotherapeutic maneuvers, medications carry meanings for the patient that can facilitate or impede progress.

If the patient interprets medication as a means of controlling anxiety which in turn enables better coping with feared situations or fantasies and the mastery of previously avoided situations, then medication can facilitate therapeutic progress by raising hopes and enhancing the sense of self-efficacy. As the patient achieves these gains, medication can eventually be discontinued.

On the other hand, the patient can come to rely on medication as the essential source of relief. This perception weakens the patient's incentives to develop more effective ways of coping with anxiety-arousing fantasies or situations. The result is a vicious cycle. The patient's perception of dependency on the medication undermines the sense of self-efficacy. The more incompetent the patient feels, the greater the anxiety, leading to increasing dependence on the drugs. In prescribing medication, the psychotherapist must keep in mind such potential negative effects and be ready to combat them.

SUMMARY

The experience of anxiety is elicited by the perception of actual or threatened danger to the integrity of the person. It thus involves biological, psychological, and social components. Group or individual psychotherapy can beneficially alter the psychological and social components directly. The psychotherapist allays the patient's anxiety basically by being a caring, competent, and trustworthy ally and guide, thereby offering a secure attachment figure. In addition, the therapeutic procedures of all schools can raise the patient's hopes and enhance feelings of self-efficacy thereby enabling him or her to learn and use more effective ways of dealing with anxiety-arousing situations. For many patients, group approaches may be more effective than dyadic ones in combating anxieties related to feelings of isolation. Although psychotherapy cannot directly ameliorate physiological symptoms that have nonpsychological causes, as in the case of panic attacks, changing the meaning of these symptoms through psychological means may enable the patient to feel and function considerably better in spite of their persistence. Anxiolytic medications can facilitate or impede psychotherapy depending on how the patient interprets their purpose.

Chapter 29

Anxiety and Psychodynamic Theory
by John C. Nemiah, M.D.

Despite the venerable history of anxiety as a scourge of humankind, the modern scientific study of the disorder dates back only a little more than a century. It is the task of this chapter to review the development and nature of the psychodynamic view of anxiety as a clinical phenomenon. In the course of this review, anxiety is considered both as the central symptom of a psychiatric syndrome in its own right and also as a pivotal factor in the processes of psychological conflict that lead to a variety of other psychiatric symptoms. And these psychological concepts are considered in relation to the more recently discovered biological aspects of anxiety disorders.

MISE EN SCENE

Let us begin with the examination of a patient suffering from severe, disabling anxiety. In *Obsessions and Psychasthenia*, Pierre Janet (1903) described the clinical problem of Cs.

> [A woman of 38, Cs.] was a remarkable example of anxiety neurosis in the diffuse form of the disorder. . . . During her youth, she already gave evidence of being easily excitable—that is to say, simple emotions often got in the way of her carrying out simple actions. She was, for example, very timid. When she attempted to do things in public (which, as we know, are the most difficult of all), she would experience a sensation of suffocation, her heart would pound, and she could neither say nor do what she wanted to. These disturbances were not, however, considered to be particularly serious, and she remained simply an impressionable person until she was 30. At the age of 31, she had her third child. She was recovering from a difficult delivery, which had occurred two days before, when the attendant made an unlikely and stupid blunder. As she stood looking at the patient's baby, she suddenly began to scream and cried out, "Madame! he doesn't seem to be breathing! Is he dead?" Needless to say, the baby was merely sleeping quietly and began to howl when his mother grabbed him up violently. She herself was thrown into complete confusion and felt an alteration in her entire being that she could not describe. . . .
>
> For several months the patient remained in a dreadful state; she was ceaselessly anxious, sighing and incapable of applying herself to anything. She gradually improved, however, especially when she recovered her physical health several months after the delivery. A year later she consulted her doctor for some pains she was experiencing. He quite innocently requested a urine sample for analysis. "Why?" she asked, al-

ready frightened. "I want to know whether there is albumin present," the doctor replied. This word, which vaguely recalled to her the illness of a neighbor, had the same baneful effect as the phrase uttered previously by the attendant: headaches, generalized uneasiness, attacks of anxiety. She could scarcely get back home, and from that point her illness recurred in full force.

Let us examine the state in which she now finds herself. The illness appears to progress in small stages. The symptoms are not continuously present. The patient is often calm enough, sleeps reasonably well during the night, although she claims the contrary; she eats adequately, and though she has neurasthenic digestive complaints, she digests her food tolerably well. From time to time you will find her playing checkers or dominoes with her attendant in the most innocent manner in the world. But at intervals the scene changes: a dozen times a day . . . you will observe the patient to be extremely agitated. She cannot stay put in one place; she gesticulates and pounds on the furniture. Simultaneously her face is flushed, she appears to breathe with difficulty, is short of breath, and her heart beats violently. But above all internal sufferings are added to these physical symptoms. She constantly complains, "Oh! I've got such a headache in the back of my head and my temples! I have such a pain in my neck, my throat, my stomach, my heart, my belly! I'm lost, I shall never get well, I'm going to die! Help me!" and so on. Nothing whatsoever can quiet these jeremiads and these cries. They are shrill enough to upset a whole household, and they last two or three hours at a stretch. Then the patient gradually calms down and is unconcerned about what has happened or the exhaustion of the attendants. She then remains reasonably quiet, though she remembers everything, and then in a half hour she begins all over again. This is the kind of life the patient has led and has inflicted on her relatives over the course of many years (Janet, 1903, vol. 2, 86–88 [translated by the author]).

Janet's patient, as her history unfolds in his graphic description of her travails, shows us many of the affective and somatic features of those acute accesses of anxiety that constitute "panic disorder." She reveals the chronic, debilitating course that patients with anxiety disorders are often fated to follow. She raises, moreover, certain central questions about the nature of anxiety. Where does anxiety belong in the panoply of emotional disorders? What is its role and function in the human psychic structure? What is its source and etiology? An answer to these questions can be approached through a consideration of the modern historical development of the concept of anxiety.

JANET'S THEORY OF ANXIETY

Hysteria and Dissociation

Janet's clinical studies began at a time when psychiatric clinicians were struggling to make diagnostic sense out of the disorderly jumble of symptoms to which their patients were prey. When he began to work in Charcot's clinic at the Salpêtrière toward the end of the nineteenth century, Janet found (like Freud) that Charcot had brought a degree of order to the definition and understanding of major hysteria. Janet's clinical psychological studies (begun even before his move to Paris) were initially focused on patients with predominantly hysterical disorders manifested in disturbances of sensorimotor functions and in pathological alterations of consciousness. From his observations he had developed his

initial theoretical formulations of dissociation, devised to explain the remarkable clinical manifestations of patients with amnesias and multiple
personalities, as well as the related hypnotic phenomena to which such
patients were readily susceptible (Janet, 1889; 1907). He was well aware
that large segments of mental contents, both cognitive and affective, could
escape from voluntary recall—that is, they could become *dissociated* from
consciousness. At the same time, he recognized that these dissociated
mental contents remained active in the patient's "subconscious mind"
(we would now say "unconscious"), but could return in a fragmentary
form as consciously experienced ego-alien symptoms. Janet was also
aware that the dissociated mental elements were often painful memories of past emotionally traumatic events.

Psychasthenia and Nervous Energy

In the course of Janet's investigations at the Salpêtrière, the range of his
attention expanded beyond patients with hysterical disorders to include
individuals with a wide variety of neurotic symptoms including anxiety,
fatigue, obsessions, phobias, and multiple somatic complaints. To this
diverse congeries of symptoms Janet attached the label "psychasthenia," and in his ultimate classification neurotic disorders were limited to two major diagnostic categories, hysteria and psychasthenia.

Janet's increasing clinical experience eventually led him to an
explanatory hypothesis to account for the diversity of symptoms he had
observed (Janet, 1903). Central to his thesis was the concept of nervous
(or mental) energy. The primary function of this postulated energy was
to bind together all the elements of mental functioning (cognitive, affective, sensory) into a unified whole under the coordinating control of the
ego (experienced as a sense of self and of reality). The ego, in turn, as
master of the entire mental apparatus, directed its energies to the performance of volitional acts that enabled the individual to adapt to the
environment and to enter into mature human relationships. Emotional
disorders resulted from changes in the quantity and action of the nervous energy. These changes were the immediate and primary source of
a whole train of pathological psychic processes manifested clinically as
psychiatric symptoms. Let us turn our attention briefly, therefore, to the
nature of the changes and their sequelae.

Pathogenesis of Symptoms

The total quantum of nervous energy in each individual varies, Janet
proposed, according to the demands made upon it. Serious physical illness (Janet makes not infrequent references to typhoid fever) or emotionally stressful events result in a lowering of the quantity of mental
energy; if it becomes seriously depleted, the binding power it affords
the ego will be compromised so that the ego loses control over certain
psychological processes of which it is normally master. One striking result of this disintegration is the dissociation of ideas that underlies hysterical symptom formation. The weakened ego cannot keep memories
and their related affects bound together in an organized system completely available to consciousness, and it loses the power of direction
over specific sets of mental associations which in turn fall away from
conscious recall and conscious awareness. These then take up an auton-

omous existence of their own outside the realm of consciousness, and thus, as dissociated mental complexes, they produce changes in physical and mental functioning in the form of ego-alien hysterical symptoms.

The pathogenesis of the myriad symptoms of psychasthenia is similarly related to a lowering of nervous energy, without, however, involving the mechanism of subconscious dissociated ideas. It reflects instead the direct effect of diminished "psychic tension." The most immediate manifestation of a lowering of energy is the patient's experience of easy fatigability and generalized lassitude. In addition, as the binding power of the ego is increasingly compromised, a disorganization of the psyche leads to the autonomous discharge of mental elements lower in the hierarchy of the mental structure. Imagination escapes the control of the ego's synthesizing, rational adaptive thinking and takes the form of debilitating obsessions and phobias. Similarly, lower automatic centers, free from the governance of hierarchically higher functions, discharge independently to produce all of the somatic and psychic symptoms of anxiety. The pathological process is further compounded by the fact that the energy formerly employed in the service of the ego's highest adaptive functions, once these are disrupted, finds an outlet over the lower pathways of discharge and intensifies their peripheral effects.

Hereditary Factors

Finally, it should be noted, Janet attributed the ultimate etiology of neurotic symptoms to a hereditary disposition. Most people have sufficient nervous energy to withstand the buffets of illness and emotional trauma. Even though these accidents of life cause the expenditure of a specific sum of nervous energy, a sufficient amount remains to enable the ego to maintain its organizing, binding adaptive functions. Certain individuals, however, are born with a genetically determined inadequacy of nervous energy, which predisposes them to neurotic disorders. These may appear spontaneously because of the inherent genetic insufficiency of nervous energy, or they may follow illness and emotional trauma that have brought the already inadequate quantity of energy down below the critical level which the ego requires to maintain its central organizing function. This then results in the secondary pathological disaggregation and autonomous discharge of lower psychic elements that have been described above.

FREUD'S THEORIES OF ANXIETY

Defense Hysteria and Psychological Conflict

This brief account of Janet's observations and concepts provides us with the background for understanding the climate of clinical ideas within which Freud worked and for appreciating the contributions to the theory of symptom formation that Freud made in the early years of his study of the psychoneuroses. During his visit to Charcot's clinic in the 1880s, Freud found that recognition had already been given to the role of unconscious mental elements in the production of ego-alien symptoms which symbolically represented the underlying dissociated ideas. Like Janet, Freud was concerned with explaining the etiology of the dissociation that initiated the chain of processes that led to the appearance of hysterical symptoms. In his earliest psychoanalytic writings, Freud introduced the term "defense hysteria," which carried the germ of an important new theoretical idea (Freud, 1894; Breuer and Freud, 1895). Mental elements (especially memories and their associated affects), Freud postulated, are lost to voluntary recall because they are *actively pushed from conscious awareness* so that the ego may avoid experiencing the unpleasant emotions (shame, disgust, fright) associated with the memories. Here was born the original and innovative concept of *psychological conflict*, which formed the departure point for the subsequent elaboration of all psychoanalytic theory. We must therefore examine its nature and implications in somewhat greater detail.

Freud's theoretical formulation is different from Janet's. According to Janet, dissociation results from the passive falling away of mental events from an ego that is too weak to keep them under control. In Freud's view, on the contrary, dissociation occurs when the ego has the active strength to exclude undesirable mental elements from its conscious awareness. Janet's explanatory model of symptom formation is that the mental apparatus falls apart under the deadweight of its component parts when the energy that binds it together is diminished. Freud's model conceives of a mental apparatus whose elements are held together within a dynamic equilibrium of conflicting forces. Janet's model is that of a disintegrating structure whose component parts, once loosened from central control, function autonomously and without design in an anarchy of psychological disorganization. Freud's theoretical scheme conceives of a tightly organized, complex psychic structure which enables the orderly processing and discharge of internal emotional arousal through external behaviors that in turn represent compromise formations arising from the conflicting forces of the internal psychic apparatus. Freud's model can be generalized to apply to all behavior, normal and abnormal. Janet's is relevant only to pathological symptoms. Freud's model moves; Janet's is static.

Anxiety Neurosis

We should note yet another difference between Freud and Janet. Both initially based their explanatory theories on their observations of hysterical patients and their symptoms. When they went further afield to investigate neurotic symptoms beyond the hysterical, each was forced to expand his diagnostic and theoretical ideas about neurotic illness. Janet, as we have seen, divided the neuroses into two major categories, hysteria and psychasthenia, the latter being a diagnostic portmanteau for all those psychological symptoms not specifically hysterical in nature. Freud, on the other hand, early in the course of his study of the neuroses argued that anxiety had specific clinical features that merited its being considered a separate nosological entity. In a long and detailed clinical paper, he presented a careful phenomenological description of acute and chronic anxiety that has hardly been improved on in modern writings (Freud, 1895b). At the same time, he proposed an explanation of its pathogenesis that modified the earlier formulation of symptom formation based on his observation of hysterical disorders.

Freud had explained the formation of hysterical symptoms within the framework of psychological structure and conflict described briefly above.

Memories of traumatic events (especially those that were sexual in nature), he suggested, are excluded from consciousness along with their affective component. Though unconscious and unavailable to voluntary recall, the memories, driven by the force of the affect attached to them, return to consciousness in the form of an ego-alien hysterical symptom that is shaped by and symbolically represents the underlying unconscious material.

Freud's explanation of the pathogenesis of anxiety was notably different. As with hysterical symptoms, he proposed, anxiety is related to the sexual drive, but unlike the hysterical symptom it does not derive from the memory of a sexually traumatic experience. Instead, it is the direct result of accumulating sexual tension that is undischarged in normal sexual intercourse and directly transformed into pathological anxiety. Furthermore, the elaborate psychic structure that mediates the formation of hysterical symptoms plays no part in the production and clinical emergence of anxiety. In Freud's words, *"The anxiety neurosis . . . has a sexual origin . . . ,* but it does not attach itself to ideas taken from sexual life; properly speaking, it has no psychical mechanism. Its specific cause is the accumulation of sexual tension, produced by abstinence or by unconsummated sexual excitation" (Freud, 1895a, 81). "[T]he anxiety which underlies the clinical symptoms of the [anxiety] neurosis can be traced to *no psychical origin. . . . The mechanism of anxiety neurosis is to be looked for in a deflection of somatic sexual excitation from the psychical sphere, and in a consequent abnormal employment of that excitation. . . . * Anxiety neurosis . . . is the product of all those factors which prevent the somatic excitation from being worked over psychically. The manifestations of anxiety neurosis appear when the somatic excitation which has been deflected from the psyche is expended subcortically in totally inadequate reactions" (Freud, 1895b, 107–109).

Because of this signal difference in the mechanisms of hysterical and anxiety symptom formation, Freud called anxiety neurosis an "actual neurosis," that is, a neurosis whose symptoms were the result of immediately present causal factors rather than of painful memories of *past* traumatic events. Although in his view the production of anxiety did not involve the operation of psychic processes, Freud did postulate that, once undischarged libido had been directly transformed into anxiety, the anxiety could become secondarily attached to memories of places and objects with which the outbreak of anxiety had been associated, leading to the psychological symptom of a phobia. "In the case of agoraphobia," he wrote, " . . . we often find *the recollection of an anxiety attack,* and what the patient actually fears is the occurrence of such an attack under the special conditions in which he believes he cannot escape it" (Freud, 1895a, 81). We shall return to these early formulations of the nature and genesis of anxiety in a later discussion of the relationship between biological and psychological concepts of anxiety. But first, we must review the emergence of Freud's concept of signal anxiety.

The Topographical Model of Psychological Functioning

During the first decade of Freud's analytic investigations, he consolidated his ideas of psychological conflict and its relationship to symptom formation. Early in his clinical studies, he came to recognize that painful memories of actual past traumatic events were not the primary source of conflict. By the turn of the century, he had replaced this formulation with the so-called topographic model of psychological functioning. In this model, the ego and its self-preservative instincts are in opposition to the libidinal drive, which, along with its associated fantasies and affects, is rendered unconscious by the force of repression. Barred from full and open expression, the libido maintains a steady pressure against the repressive forces of the ego, but it can achieve only a partial discharge of its biologically maintained driving force in the form of compromise symptoms and behavior that disguise its nature and goals. Of particular importance, Freud maintained in this model his theoretical notion that consciously experienced anxiety is produced by the transformation of the repressed, undischarged sexual drive into the somatic and psychic manifestations of the anxious state.

ANXIETY AND PSYCHOLOGICAL DEFENSES At the same time Freud modified his original idea that this transformation involved *no* psychological processes. In *The Interpretation of Dreams*, which was published in 1900, he wrote:

> There is no longer anything contradictory to us in the notion that a psychical process which develops anxiety can nevertheless be the fulfillment of a wish. We know that it can be explained by the fact that the wish belongs to one system, the *Ucs.* [the Unconscious], while it has been repudiated and suppressed by the other system, the *Pcs.* [the Preconscious]. Even where psychical health is perfect, the subjugation of the *Ucs.* by the *Pcs.* is not complete; the measure of suppression indicates the degree of our psychical normality. Neurotic symptoms show that the two systems are in conflict with each other; they are the products of a compromise which brings the conflict to an end for the time being. On the other hand, they allow the *Ucs.* an outlet for the discharge of its excitation, and provide it with a kind of sally-port, while, on the other hand, they make it possible for the *Pcs.* to control the *Ucs.* to some extent. It is instructive to consider, for instance, the significance of a hysterical phobia or an agoraphobia. Let us suppose that a neurotic patient is unable to cross the street alone—a condition we rightly regard as a "symptom." If we remove this symptom by compelling him to carry out the act of which he believes himself to be incapable, the consequence will be an attack of anxiety; and indeed the occurrence of an anxiety-attack in the street is often the precipitating cause of the onset of an agoraphobia. We see, therefore, that the symptom has been constructed in order to avoid an outbreak of anxiety; the phobia is erected like a frontier fortification against the anxiety (Freud, 1900, 580–581).

What is of special note here is the suggestion that anxiety, whatever its source, is a painful affect and motivates defensive actions on the part of the individual to be preserved from the distress of experiencing it, in the example cited here the defensive mechanism of phobic avoidance. In the famous case history of Little Hans, Freud (1909) elaborated in considerable detail on the vicissitudes of anxiety as it motivates a variety of defensive operations. From then on, the idea of psychological defenses was an important element of the analytic theoretical structure. It was not, however, until the publication of *Inhibitions, Symptoms and Anxiety* in 1926 that Freud made a radical change in his conception of the nature and source of anxiety, a change that was part of an even greater revision of his theoretical formulation as he moved from the *topographical* to the *structural* model of psychic organization.

The Structural Model of Psychological Functioning

We need not go through all the steps in Freud's thinking that led to this major revision. Suffice it to say that the earlier topographical conception of ego instincts pitted against libidinal instincts gave way to the now familiar view of a psychic structure composed of ego, superego, and id. In the new model, the id is seen as the source of the instincts (libidinal and aggressive) and the ego as a set of regulating and executive functions that control and canalize the expression of the instincts in conformity with the sanctions of the superego and the dictates of external reality. Anxiety is no longer merely transformed libido, but is an independent mental element in its own right. As an ego affect, anxiety represents the ego's response to the internal danger that arises when an id impulse threatens to escape from the ego's control; the ego's response is to strengthen its defensive operations (repression and auxiliary defenses) in order to contain and offset the increased pressure for discharge of the underlying drive. In this new scheme, anxiety is no longer a secondary result of the repression of the drives (especially the libido); it is instead the primary motivating force for the erection of repression and other ego defenses. Anxiety, in other words, plays a central role in maintaining the psychic equilibrium by functioning as a *signal* to the ego of impending internal danger. This notion of *signal anxiety* is a pivotal concept in the modern psychoanalytic view of the formation of neurotic symptoms, and we may now observe a patient who demonstrates its nature and function.

An Illustrative Case

Mabel G. was a 27-year-old mother of three children, two boys aged 4 and 2½ respectively, and an infant daughter, who was only three weeks old. Shortly after the birth of her daughter, the patient had been admitted to the hospital for dysthymic reaction characterized by depression, loss of interest in her usual activities, feelings of being "all washed up" and "a failure in life," and wishes that she were dead. The symptoms had begun during her last pregnancy, were intensified after moving to a new apartment that deprived her of the close contact with her mother on whom she relied for support, and had become sufficiently disabling after the delivery of her new infant to require hospitalization. Despite her complaints of depression, the patient showed no retardation, spoke readily and feelingly, and related well to her physician. During a diagnostic interview, after describing her depressive symptoms, the patient said, "I'm as nervous as anything, you know." Asked to describe her "nervousness," the patient replied:

Patient: Well, I'm nervous like I want to walk around all the time, you know. And I feel like I might lose control of myself. And I get pains in my arms and hands. I just got a fear to me.

Doctor: How do you think you'll lose control?

Patient: I don't know, doctor. God! I don't think I'd ever harm anybody or anything!

Doctor: In what way?

Patient: In any way, you know. Do you think there's any hope for me, doctor? Because I've got those three little kids at home. That's the only thought that comes to my head is my babies. I think of them all the time, doctor . . . I don't like to see anybody harm them. I'm the type of girl, if anybody yells at them, I don't say anything to them. I take it all to heart. I don't yell back at the person that's yelling at them. I just take my children away.

Doctor:	How do you mean, you "take it to heart?"
Patient:	I take everything to heart. If anybody says anything to my kids, it bothers me. I take everything to heart. I just don't let it brush off my shoulders. I think about it.
Doctor:	You don't talk back to them?
Patient:	Oh, no! I'd never fight back, doctor. I never did. My husband says that's why I'm here, because I let everybody bother me.
Doctor:	Do you ever feel like talking back?
Patient:	Once in a while I used to feel like I'd like to talk back to them, but I wouldn't. I would suddenly be quiet and I'd walk away . . . (Pause) I just get scared I might lose control.
Doctor:	What do you think would happen if you lost control?
Patient:	It's just when I get the pains in my hands and arms, I say to myself, "God forbid if I should ever lose control of myself!" What would happen?—because I get so nervous.
Doctor:	What are you afraid of?
Patient:	I don't know, doctor. It's just a feeling that comes over me . . . I was even telling my husband last night, "God! What if anything should happen? If I should lose control of myself." And he said, "It's just foolish thinking." He tries to comfort me. I think of my children all the time, doctor. That's why I've got as much bother as I have with my nerves. I just think of them all the time, saying to myself, "If something should happen to me, what will happen to the kids?" Thoughts like that. That's the only thing I've got in my head, that I'll lose control of myself. I don't know why.

By the patient's own account, her "nervousness," which appears as distressing to her as her feelings of depression, is a chronic state of anxious apprehension without evidence of acute attacks of panic. When asked directly what she is afraid of, the patient is unable to specify the reason for her anxiety, but her associations are interesting and suggestive. She *doesn't* think she would harm anybody. She *doesn't* like to see anyone harm her children. She *never* fights back. In this negative way she introduces the idea of aggression, with repeated references to her children. From these observations one infers that the patient's anxiety stems from an underlying aggressive impulse toward her children, of which she is consciously unaware. This is, however, only inference, for there is no direct evidence from the patient that such an impulse exists within her. Indeed, when one questions her further about her children, her feelings toward them are strikingly the reverse in character. She has, for example, never punished them for anything. "I can't punish them, doctor," she says. "It hurts me to punish them. I just can't do it. I can't face up to hitting them. Even my husband, he'll tell you. Even my sisters say the same thing about me. I'm too good to them. I let them run my life, and yet I can't help it. I don't hit them. They can do anything, and I won't hit them. I know I should, but I can't. . . . I make too many sacrifices for them—that's what my husband says. I never went out or anything. I never left them with anybody. I always stayed in the house."

What the patient appears to be describing here is the defense of reaction formation, that conscious stance of leaning over backward to behave in a manner that is the polar opposite of the underlying drive in the other direction. The patient's family, even the patient herself, recognize that her altruistic behavior toward her children is unduly exaggerated, though she has no conscious awareness of the aggression that appears to be behind it. On the basis of his inference that the patient was in fact defending herself from underlying aggression toward her children, the doctor finally asked her, "Do you ever get mad at your kids?"

Patient: No, no! I never get mad at them.

Doctor: You never get angry at them?

Patient: Now that I'm thinking of it, I might have got angry at my older one—you know, yelled at him . . . Since I had the new baby, he'd go over near the bassinet to look at it. I'd start yelling at him because I didn't want him near it.

Doctor: Why?

Patient: I didn't want him to touch the new baby. I was afraid he might pinch it or go for its eyes. . . . And the two of them had the blanket over the baby's head the day before I came into the hospital. They put the blanket right over the baby's face, and I thought I'd collapse, I was so nervous and upset over it. I started crying. I couldn't control myself. She could have smothered to death.

Here we find the patient admitting that she *has* been angry—at her older boy. And then, although she expresses no resentment of her own at the new baby, she recounts her fears of what her children might do to harm, even kill, the baby. In the light of this new information, the doctor asked the patient, "Have *you* had any thoughts about hurting her?"

Patient: Oh, no! God, no!

Doctor: Or about the boys?

Patient: Well, I wasn't happy while I was carrying the baby. I managed to call my husband home from work and tell him I was going to kill myself. He was scared, you know, because I was so down in the dumps.

Doctor: Did you ever have thoughts about hurting your boys?

Patient: I'd say I did, but I never did hurt them, doctor. I used to say to my husband, "I'll kill them"—just like that. Like I'd say I'd kill myself. But I never hurt them.

Doctor: What would put that thought in your mind?

Patient: I don't know. It just came out of me. I didn't have no plan that I was going to put them in the bathtub, or something. It was just that the thought came out, that's all.

Doctor: To put them in the bathtub?

Patient: No! Like you were saying—if you want to plan something, say, like in the bathtub, or something like that. No—I had no plans on what I was going to do. But I was more disgusted with myself.

Doctor: What were you thinking about with the bathtub? What would you do?

Patient: Who, me?

Doctor: Yes.

Patient: That was just a saying. I had no thoughts in my mind, doctor, when I said "bathtub." I would think more of doing harm to myself than I do to them. I would rather hurt myself than them.

Let us observe the process and sequence of events as they evolved in this interview. Initially, although in direct association to her symptom of anxiety the patient introduces the notion of her harming others, neither she nor the doctor can see that she actually *wishes* to do harm. The existence of such a wish is, at the start, only an inference, a hypothesis, derived from the content of what she says. Toward the end of the interview, during which the doctor has followed the patient's leads and has focused on her indirect references to aggressive thoughts and behavior, the patient at length admits directly to a hostile impulse of her own toward her boys ("I used to say to my husband, 'I'll kill them' "), followed by a somewhat more veiled reference to doing something to them in the bathtub. In this momentary glimpse of her fantasies, we find confirmatory evidence of the correctness of our initial hypothesis that the patient harbors aggressive impulses and thoughts.

Aggression is clearly a source of great concern and anxiety for the patient. This is particularly noticeable at the end of the interview when the patient becomes quite exercised after mentioning her harmful wishes toward her boys. The aggressive impulse finally surfaces here momentarily, arouses anxiety, and immediately leads to several defensive operations in rapid succession: (1) the patient retracts the statement about the bathtub—she undoes it; (2) she attributes the imagery to the doctor—projection; and (3) she turns the aggression inward on herself ("I would rather hurt myself than them"), a defense mechanism that frequently plays a role in the appearance of clinical depression. Although this is perhaps the most striking example of the intimate interplay of impulse, anxiety, and defense, it is evident throughout the interview— in the patient's marked yet exaggerated anxiety for her baby's life when her boys covered her with the blanket, in her attribution to her older son of the impulse to "go for its eyes," in her characteristic pattern of reaction formation against aggression.

Anxiety emerges throughout as a *signal* of internal danger as the aggressive impulse rises (often in response to an external stimulus) and threatens to erupt into consciousness. At the same time, as a painful conscious affect, the anxiety motivates the ego to reinforce its defenses against the anxiety-provoking impulse in order to protect itself from experiencing discomfort. Anxiety, in its role as signal, thus acts as a sensitive governor to keep the balance of psychic forces in an intact, functioning equilibrium.

SIGNAL ANXIETY AND PANIC ANXIETY

In the clinical history and course of Mabel G.'s illness, although her anxiety varied quantitatively in response to the internal and external stresses to which she was subjected, it at no time reached the intensity of panic. This is perhaps not surprising, since almost by definition *signal anxiety* is a modulated affect kept within tolerable limits by the defensive functions it arouses. In the analytic model, *panic anxiety* results when the ego's response to signal anxiety fails and the psychic equilibrium breaks down. When the underlying impulse is of sufficient strength to overwhelm defenses that are inadequate for the task of modifying and containing it, the ego experiences a sense of total helplessness and is flooded with disorganizing panic that demolishes its capacity to function. Signal anxiety, in other words, is constructive, whereas panic anxiety is destructive.

Psychodynamic and Biological Views of Anxiety

In the psychodynamic view, signal and panic anxiety, despite the differences in their effects on the ego, are qualitatively the same and differ only quantitatively. Recent studies, however, suggest that panic may be both phenomenologically and biologically distinct from the milder forms of anxiety (Group for the Advancement of Psychiatry, 1975; Klein and Fink, 1962). Not only are the two types of anxiety differentially responsive to tricyclic antidepressants and benzodiazepines, but clinical histories frequently reveal no environmental or inner psychological precipitants of panic attacks, which appear to arise quite spontaneously. This has led Sheehan (1982) to suggest that panic is an entirely endogenous disorder "associated with a biochemical abnormality in the nervous system" (156). Klein, moreover, has pointed to the fact that patients who suffer from spontaneous panic attacks gradually develop a milder anticipatory anxiety about experiencing further panic, which leads secondarily to avoidance behavior, notably agoraphobia (Klein and Rabkin, 1981).

These modern formulations are curiously reminiscent of Freud's earliest views of acute anxiety attacks. Freud, it will be recalled, proposed that such attacks had "no psychical origin" and that "no psychical mechanism" was involved in their production. Although he attributed their source to the abnormal accumulation of libido rather than to a specific chemical abnormality, his theoretical explanation of the appearance of panic was biological in nature. This explanation differed markedly from his model of hysterical symptom formation, which involved a complex psychological structure of conscious and unconscious psychic mechanisms. Freud, furthermore, anticipated modern ideas about agoraphobia when he related its genesis to "the recollection of an anxiety attack" and the fear of its recurrence "under the special conditions in which [the patient] believes he cannot escape it" (Freud, 1895a, 81).

Alexithymia and the Psychosomatic Process

In Freud's ideas we also find the forerunner of modern hypotheses concerning psychosomatic symptom formation. Recent clinical investigations of classical psychosomatic illnesses (e.g., peptic ulcer, ulcerative colitis, rheumatoid arthritis) have defined a behavioral syndrome (termed "alexithymia" by Sifneos [1972]) that is commonly found in patients with these disorders. Alexithymia is characterized by two psychological features. (1) Alexithymic individuals are unable to describe their feelings in words and cannot differentiate one feeling from another. (2) Their thought content is notable for its preoccupation with concrete *external* persons, objects, and events, and for the absence of fantasies determined by inner feelings and impulses (the *pensée opératoire* of Marty and de M'Uzan [1963]). The thought content is, in other words, stimulus-bound rather than drive determined.

Extensive clinical examples of alexithymia have been given elsewhere (Nemiah, 1978; 1984; Nemiah and Sifneos, 1970). Suffice it to say that the mental processes of alexithymic individuals differ markedly from those of patients with neurotic disorders and conflicts. The latter (as can be seen from the clinical material given above) have a rich inner life consisting of clearly differentiated feelings, of fantasies, of memories, and of mental associations organized in a psychic structure whose elements are partly conscious and partly unconscious. Their symptoms, conscious thought processes, and behavior are, in part at least, the result of compromise formations arising from the conflicting forces of the various parts of the psychological structure. Alexithymic individuals, on the contrary, appear to be quite lacking in this rich psychological life. Their responses during an interview are remarkable for their aridity, shallowness, and drab banality, and their lack of "psychological mindedness" often elicits in the interviewer a sense of frustration mixed with boredom. In contrast to the neurotic patient, their behavior is *not* the product of the conflicting forces of a psychic structure, but is the manifestation of a *lack* of psychological structure resulting both from the absence of a capacity to elaborate fantasy and from an inability to experience, recognize, define, and differentiate feelings.

PANIC AS A PSYCHOSOMATIC SYMPTOM   As a result of their defective psychological apparatus, alexithymic individuals process the internal arousal produced by environmental stress in a different manner from neurotic patients. In the latter, as we have seen, external stressful stimuli activate a complex set of psychological mechanisms, partly conscious and partly unconscious, that result in elaborate psychic compromise formations. In alexithymic persons, the arousal secondary to external stress, lacking that structure, is directly short-circuited into somatic dysfunctions mediated ultimately via the hypothalamus over the endocrine and autonomic nervous system.

This *deficit model* of psychosomatic symptom formation has a remarkable resemblance to Freud's theoretical formulation of the mechanism underlying the production of anxiety attacks, both in postulating a lack of involvement of higher psychic processes and in invoking a direct shunting of inner arousal into somatic channels. As postulated elsewhere (Nemiah, 1984), it suggests that, in some patients at least, the panic attack may be the generic prototype of psychosomatic disorders, involving a generalized autonomic discharge in contrast to the selective activation of specific autonomic and other pathways that appear to underlie discrete psychosomatic disorders. The deficit model also has some similarity to Janet's theoretical model; in particular it has an affinity to his concept that, secondary to the dissolution of higher psychic functions, functions lower in the psychological hierarchy escape from control and, discharging autonomously, result in a variety of psychiatric symptoms, including pathological anxiety.

REFLECTIONS ON THEORY AND RESEARCH

The alexithymic deficit model of psychosomatic symptom formation provides a useful framework for explaining the production of panic attacks as these are conceived of in current biological formulations. The model is congruent with the clinical observation that many patients with panic attacks are unable to associate them with any psychological precipitant and that the attacks appear to be entirely autonomous and unrelated to the psychological processes associated with signal anxiety. Three cautions, however, should be raised about an uncritical acceptance of this hypothetical model.

First, patients with panic attacks have not been examined with the specific goal of determining whether they exhibit the more general characteristics of alexithymic behavior. Such examinations should be included systematically in the current clinical investigations of panic anxiety in order to explore further the validity of the hypothesis.

A second caution pertains to the pathogenesis of panic attacks. Some patients who initially are unable to provide any clues as to the precipitants of their panic attacks will upon more extensive psychological investigation become aware of anxiety-provoking inner drives and fantasies that were initially hidden from consciousness by powerful psychological defenses. One cannot with certainty rule out the presence of underlying psychic mechanisms on the basis of an initial history alone that, by relying merely on direct questioning about symptoms, symptom checklists, and a superficial survey of possible internal and external stresses, fails to reveal psychological precipitants of the attacks. It is possible that the panic attack is the final common product of diverse underlying mechanisms. In some, it may be the result of complex psychological processes; in others, it may represent the direct discharge of arousal over autonomic channels without any higher psychic elaborations. Such a possibility is consonant with the clinical observation that a specific psychosomatic symptom (e.g., ulcerative colitis) is associated with and constitutes the final common path of different internal psychological mechanisms (Karush and Daniels, 1969). Here again, further clinical investigation, guided by a knowledge of psychodynamic principles, is required to elucidate the problem of pathogenesis.

Finally, it should be pointed out, the alexithymic hypothesis suggests that panic attacks are a response to external environmental stress and are not merely an autonomous, endogenous, biologically determined central nervous system storm.

SOME PRINCIPLES OF TREATMENT

With the advent of behavior therapy, pharmacotherapy, and treatment measures using a variety of relaxation techniques, the management of patients with anxiety, especially in the form of panic attacks with or without the secondary elaboration of agoraphobia, has been immeasurably improved. Psychodynamic psychotherapy, including psychoanalysis, has been notoriously unsuccessful with many patients suffering from panic and a variety of phobic disorders. There are at least two reasons for this failure.

Clinical experience suggests that once a phobia has been erected as a learned response which helps the patient to avoid being flooded with anxiety, the phobia itself persists with a life of its own, even though psychotherapy may have resolved the underlying conflicts that created the initiating anxiety. With the advent of behavior therapy, powerful tools have become available for dismantling the phobic structure by relearning. In combination with relaxation techniques and such specific measures as flooding, behavior therapy has been able to help patients to modify the anxiety itself, with resulting significant symptomatic relief.

Similarly, the more recent introduction of the use of antidepressant medication, especially for panic attacks, has brought about dramatic improvement in the symptoms and functioning of patients who had been severely incapacitated for years. One may reasonably postulate that medication for such patients restores the chemical balance in the systems underlying anxiety production that, for whatever reason, are pathologically sensitive to anxiety-producing stimuli and overreact with a symptomatic intensity that is totally disorganizing to the individual.

Where, then, do psychodynamic psychotherapy and psychodynamic concepts fit into the overall management of patients with anxiety disorders? It should be clearly recognized at the start that psychodynamic insight psychotherapy is of limited applicability for patients with psychiatric disorders. To be able to use such treatment effectively, patients must have a degree of psychological mindedness, a capacity for introspection, the ability to experience and tolerate painful affects, and a motivation for psychological change. To determine whether a patient fulfills these criteria for psychodynamic psychotherapy, he or she must be evaluated with techniques that are themselves based on psychodynamic knowledge and understanding. A psychodynamic assessment of every patient with anxiety appears to be in order as a means of exploring the illness and helping to decide the appropriate measures to be included in the treatment plan.

If the patient does not meet the criteria for dynamic psychotherapy, if, for example, a patient with panic attacks is clearly alexithymic, it would be pointless to embark on a course of insight psychotherapy. Here the treatment of choice would involve medication, behavior therapy, and relaxation techniques, and any psychotherapy would be limited to supportive measures.

On the other hand, if evaluation proves the patient to be a good candidate for the techniques of insight psychotherapy, these techniques should be seriously considered. For the patient with lower and tolerable degrees of chronic anxiety, such psychotherapy may be sufficient in itself. For patients with disabling panic attacks or stubborn phobic symptoms, a combination of treatment approaches is indicated. Medication designed to combat the major symptoms should be prescribed, in conjunction with insight psychotherapy aimed at resolving the psychic conflicts that contribute to the production of the anxiety.

Finally, it cannot be too strongly emphasized that both biological and psychodynamic factors must be taken into account in the clinical evaluation and treatment of every patient with anxiety. To polarize our clinical and scientific thinking and to restrict ourselves to either a biological or a psychodynamic view of anxiety or of the anxious patient is to limit our vision and to compromise the patient's opportunity for recovery.

Chapter 30 **The Relaxation Response and the Treatment of Anxiety**
by Herbert Benson, M.D.

The relaxation response is hypothesized to be a coordinated physiological reaction brought about by the stimulation of hypothalamic regions. It results in generalized decreased sympathetic nervous system activity (Benson et al., 1974; Benson, 1975). This chapter describes the historical precedents, the physiological basis, and the clinical usefulness of the relaxation response.

HISTORICAL PRECEDENTS

The elicitation of the relaxation response is associated with subjective experiences that constitute an altered state of consciousness (Dean, 1970). The subjective states have been described as feeling at ease with the world, a sense of well-being, and peace of mind. Others have described ecstasy, clairvoyance, beauty, and a totally relaxing experience. The techniques and practices used to attain this state have had varied aims: peace with oneself, transcendence from the physical, an inner awareness of oneself, union with God. No one technique can claim uniqueness. As William James (1958) stated, "To find religion is only one out of many ways of teaching unity; and the process of remedying inner discord is a general psychological process."

Even though the subjective experiences are described in different ways, marked similarities between the techniques used to achieve the altered state of consciousness strongly support the existence of a common physiological basis, which is hypothesized to be the relaxation response. Moreover, people have experienced this altered state throughout all ages and in both Western and Eastern cultures. To evoke the relaxation response, four elements appear to be necessary: a quiet environment, decreased muscle tone, a passive attitude, and a mental device, i.e., a word, sound, prayer, or phrase repeated audibly or silently (Benson et al., 1974; Benson, 1975). The repeated mental device and passive attitude are crucial (Hoffman et al., 1982).

Western Mystical Practices

Many of the techniques that elicit the relaxation response are presented in a religious context. In the West, a fourteenth century treatise entitled *The Cloud of Unknowing* described how to attain the altered state of consciousness that is required to achieve alleged union with God (Progoff, 1969). According to an anonymous author, this goal could not be reached in the ordinary levels of human consciousness, but rather by use of "lower" levels which could be attained by eliminating physical activity and all worldly distraction. To do away with extraneous thoughts, a single-syllable word, such as God or love should be repeated. "Choose whichever one you prefer, or, if you like, choose another that suits your taste, provided that it is of one syllable. And clasp this word tightly in your heart so that it never leaves it no matter what may happen. This word shall be your shield and your spear. . . . With this word you shall strike down thoughts of every kind and drive them beneath the cloud of forgetting. After that, if any thoughts should press upon you . . . answer him with this word only . . . and with no other words" (Anonymous, quoted in Progoff, 1969, 76–77). There will be moments when "every created thing may suddenly and completely be forgotten. But immediately after each stirring, because of the corruption of the flesh, it [the soul] drops down again to some thought or deed" (Anonymous, quoted in Progoff, 1969, 68).

The Third Spiritual Alphabet was written in the tenth century by Fray Francisco de Osuna and also deals with the altered state of consciousness (Osuna, 1931). "Contemplation requires us to blind ourselves to all that is not God" (viii), and you must ignore all else and "quit all obstacles, keeping your eyes bent on the ground" (293–294). A short, self-composed prayer repeated over and over again or simply saying no to thoughts when they occur are two suggested methods. Fray Francisco wrote that such an exercise would make the practitioner more efficient in all tasks and the tasks more enjoyable. He noted that all men, especially the busy, should be taught this meditation as a retreat and refuge when faced with stressful situations.

Saints John and Terese, the famous fifteenth century Christian mystics, describe the major steps to achieve the mystical state, which include ignoring distractions, usually by repetitive prayer (Anonymous, 1954; Saint Terese, 1901).

In the Byzantine church, Christian meditation and mysticism became well developed and were known as the Hesychasm (Norwich and Sitwell, 1966). In the fourteenth century, this method of repetitive prayer was described at Mount Athos in Greece by Gregory of Sinai. The technique has survived in modern Catholicism and is called the Prayer of the Heart or the Prayer of Jesus. The prayer allegedly dates back to the beginning of the Christian era and was called a secret meditation. It was transmitted from older to younger monks through an initiation rite with these instructions: "Sit alone and in silence. Lower your head, shut your eyes, breathe out gently, and imagine yourself looking into your own heart. Carry your mind, i.e., your thoughts, from your head to your heart. As you breathe out, say 'Lord Jesus Christ, have mercy on me.' Say it moving your lips gently, or simply say it in your mind. Try to put all other thoughts aside. Be calm, be patient and repeat the process frequently" (French, 1968, 10).

Similar practices are found in Judaism. The works of Rabbi Abulafia were published in the thirteenth century, and his thoughts became a major part of Jewish cabalistic mysticism (Scholem, 1967). Abulafia believed that since our sensory perceptions and emotions are concerned with the finite, the soul's life is finite. We therefore need a higher form of perception which, rather than blocking the soul's deeper regions, opens them. Believing that an "absolute" object was necessary to meditate upon, Rabbi Abulafia found this in the Hebrew alphabet and developed a mystical system that contemplated the letters of God's name. As one historian described Abulafia, "immersed in prayer and meditation, uttering the divine name with special modulations of the voice and with special gestures, he induced himself in a state of ecstasy in which he believed the soul had shed its material bonds, and, unimpeded, returned to its divine source" (Bokser, 1954, 9).

Scholem compared Rabbi Abulafia's teachings to Indian traditions.

[Abulafia's] teachings represent but a Judaized version of that ancient spiritual technique which has found its classical expression in the practices of the Indian mystics who followed the system known as *Yoga*. To cite only one instance out of many, an important part in Abulafia's system is played by the technique of breathing; now this technique has found its highest development in the Indian *Yoga*, where it is commonly regarded as the most important instrument of mental discipline. Again, Abulafia lays down certain rules of body posture, certain corresponding combinations of consonants and vowels, and certain forms of recitation. . . . The similarity even extends to some aspects of the doctrine of ecstatic vision, as preceded and brought about by these practices (Scholem, 1967, 139).

The same basic elements that elicit the relaxation response in these practices of Christianity and Judaism are also found in Islamic mysticism or Sufism (Trimingham, 1971). Dhikr is the method employed. The person excludes distraction by constantly repeating God's name, either aloud or silently, or by rhythmic breathing. Music, musical poems, and dance are also employed, since they can enhance the states of ecstasy. An initiate receives the *wird*, a secret or holy sound that is repeated in conjunction with rhythmic exercises, coordinated movement, and control of breathing.

Eastern Religious Practices

In the main, the relaxation response elicited by religious techniques was not a part of the routine practice in Western religions, but rather a part of the mystical traditions. In the East, however, the meditational practices which elicited the relaxation response were developed much earlier and became a major element in religion as well as in everyday life. In the sixth century B.C., the Indian scriptures, the Upanishads, stated that individuals might attain "a unified state with the Brahmin [the deity] by means of restraint of the breath, withdrawal of the senses, meditation, concentration, contemplation and absorption" (Organ, 1970, 303).

A multitude of Eastern religions and ways of life, including Zen and Yoga and their many variants, elicit the relaxation response. The techniques employ both mental and physical methods and include the repetition of a word or sound, a quiet environment, the exclusion of meaningful thoughts, and the adoption of a passive attitude. Zen Buddhism uses a Yoga-like technique of coupling respiration with a count to ten, i.e., one on inhaling, two on exhaling, and so on to ten. With practice, one stops counting and "follows the breath" (Johnston, 1971, 78).

Taoism and Shintoism are major religions of China and Japan. One method of prayer in Shintoism consists of sitting quietly, inspiring through the nose, holding inspiration for a short time, and expiring through the mouth, with the eyes directed toward a mirror at their level. A priest repeats ten numbers or sacred words throughout the exercise, pronouncing them according to religious teachings (Herbert, 1967). "It is interesting that this grand ritual characteristic of Shintoism is doubtlessly the same process as *Yoga*" (Fujisawa, 1959, 23). Taoism, as well as using methods similar to those of Shinto, employs concentration on nothingness to achieve absolute tranquility (Chang, 1963).

Secular Methods

Secular techniques also exist for eliciting the relaxation response. Gazing upon an object and keeping attention focused upon that object to the exclusion of all else is a method which many have used (Lowell, 1892; Underhill, 1957). The nineteenth century "nature mystics" elicited the relaxation response by immersion in the quiet of nature. Wordsworth stated that when his "mind was freed from preoccupation with disturbing objects, petty cares, little enmities and low desires," he could then reach a state of equilibrium, which he described as "a wise passiveness" or "a happy stillness of the mind" (Spurgeon, 1970, 61). Anyone, Wordsworth believed, could deliberately induce this condition by a type of relaxation of the will. Thoreau attained such feelings by sitting alone with nature for hours. Indeed, Thoreau had compared himself to a Yogi (Sanborn, 1894). Many other such experiences may be found in Johnson's *Watcher on the Hills* (1959).

PHYSIOLOGICAL BASIS

The hypothesis that a physiological response, the relaxation response, underlies this altered state of consciousness is supported by objective data (Benson et al., 1974; Benson, 1975). The physiological changes are consistent with generalized decreased sympathetic nervous system activity. Oxygen consumption and carbon dioxide elimination are uniformly and significantly decreased. Respiratory quotient is unchanged. There is, in addition, a simultaneous decrease of heart and respiratory rates and a marked lowering in arterial blood-lactate concentration. Slow α-wave activity is intensified with occasional theta waves on the electroencephalogram. Muscle blood flow stabilizes (Levander et al., 1972). These physiological changes are distinctly different from those observed during quiet sitting or sleep and characterize a wakeful hypometabolic state (Beary and Benson, 1974).

Even though the physiological changes of the relaxation response are consistent with decreased sympathetic nervous system activity, the plasma norepinephrine does not decrease during its elicitation (Michaels et al., 1976). Indeed, others have even found increased levels of plasma norepinephrine in subjects who regularly elicit the relaxation response (Lang et al., 1979). Some recent physiological experiments by the author and his colleagues have resolved this apparent paradox in which either unchanged or increased plasma norepinephrine levels are coupled with physiological changes consistent with lower sympathetic nervous system function (Hoffman et al., 1982). Experimental and control subjects were exposed to graded orthostatic and isometric stress during monthly hospital visits. Between visits, the experimental subjects practiced a technique that elicited the relaxation response, while the control subjects simply sat quietly for an equivalent period of time. Heart rate and blood pressure responses to the graded stresses did not differ in either group between visits. Plasma norepinephrine levels in the experimental group, however, were significantly higher in response to the graded stresses after they had regularly elicited the relaxation response for one month. In the control group, plasma norepinephrine levels did not change from their baseline values. These results were then replicated in a crossover experiment carried out with the control group in the subsequent month. In other words, after the control group crossed over and elicited the relaxation response regularly, heart rate and blood pressure responses were again unchanged, but plasma norepinephrine levels were significantly higher. The repeated elicitation of the relaxation response thus resulted in increased plasma norepinephrine levels that were not reflected in increased heart rate or blood pressure responses. These observations are consistent with reduced norepinephrine end-organ responsivity. An important feature of these changes in sympathetic responsivity is the fact that they had a carry-over effect, lasting longer than the actual period during which the mental relaxation-response exercise was performed.

Hess described physiological changes similar to those constituting the relaxation response and termed them the trophotropic response (Hess and Brugger, 1943; Hess, 1957). In his Nobel Prize–winning work, Hess electrically stimulated the anterior hypothalamic areas of the cat brain and induced physiological changes like those later noted during the elicitation of the relaxation response in man. Even though Hess's work is more than 25 years old, most consider it still valid (Morgane, 1979). His pioneering investigation established that electrical stimulation of subcortical areas of the brain was associated with a wide variety of behavioral and physiological patterns that were much more complex than simple reflexes. The remarkable refinements in technique since Hess's initial studies have allowed much more localized areas of stimulation without the spread of electrical stimulus and also more precise identification of the anatomical site being stimulated. Others, not Hess, believe that his work represented evidence for the presence of discrete "centers" in the diencephalon and limbic areas of the brain (Morgane, 1979). Hess interpreted his results as representing patterned neuronal circuits, not isolated centers. The author and his colleagues hypothesize that the activation of neuronal circuits that Hess described as the trophotropic response in the cat is consistent with the elicitation of the relaxation response in human subjects.

These physiological changes are opposite to those of the reaction originally described by Cannon in 1941, which he termed the emergency response and which is popularly called the fight-or-flight response. Hess stated, "Let us repeat at this point that we are actually dealing with a protective mechanism against overstress . . . and promoting restorative processes. We emphasize that these adynamic effects are opposed to those reactions which are oriented toward increased oxidative metabolism and utilization of energy" (Hess, 1957, 40).

The physiological changes of the relaxation response occur during the practice of Zen and Yoga as well as transcendental meditation (Anand et al., 1961; Bagchi and Wenger, 1957; Hoenig, 1968; Karambelkar et al., 1968; Onda, 1965; Sugi and Akutsu, 1968; Wallace, 1970; Wallace et al., 1971). Oxygen consumption, respiratory rate, and heart rate decrease. Skin resistance increases as does the production of α waves.

CURRENT SECULAR TECHNIQUES

Among the secular techniques that elicit the relaxation response are autogenic training, progressive muscular relaxation, and hypnosis.

Autogenic training is a technique of medical therapy which was designed to elicit the trophotropic response of Hess (Luthe, 1969; 1972). The technique includes six "Standard Exercises." Exercise 1 focuses on feelings of heaviness in the limbs, 2 on the cultivation of a sense of warmth in the limbs, 3 on cardiac regulation, 4 on passive concentration on breathing, 5 on warmth of the upper abdomen, and 6 on coolness in the forehead. An absolute essential is the subject's attitude toward the exercises; this attitude must not be intense and compulsive, but rather of a quiet, "let it happen" nature. The physiological changes of the relaxation response occur during the practice of autogenic training. Respiratory rate, heart rate, and muscle tension decrease, and skin resistance and production of α waves increases (Luthe, 1969).

Progressive muscular relaxation is a technique in which discriminative control over skeletal muscle is increased so that a subject can induce very low levels of tonus in the major muscle groups (Jacobson, 1938). The practitioner assumes a supine position in a quiet room. A passive attitude is deemed essential because mental images induce slight, measurable tensions in muscles, especially those of the face and eyes. Changes similar to those of the relaxation response take place. Oxygen consumption, heart rate, and electromyographic voltages all decrease (Warrenburg et al., 1980). These physiological changes are indistinguishable from the changes achieved by the practice of a simple meditative technique that elicits the relaxation response (Warrenburg et al., 1980).

Hypnosis is an artificially induced state characterized by increased suggestibility (Gorton, 1949; Barber, 1961). The subject is believed to be in the hypnotic state when he or she manifests a high level of response to test suggestions such as amnesia, hallucination, anesthesia, muscle rigidity, and posthypnotic suggestion. The procedures for self- and hetero-hypnotic induction and those for eliciting the relaxation response appear to be quite similar (Walrath and Hamilton, 1975; Morse et al., 1977; Benson et al., 1981). In addition, before hypnotic phenomena are experienced, during either traditional or active induction, the physiological state is comparable to the relaxation response. Heart rate, respiratory rate, and blood pressure decrease (Benson et al., 1981). There is also increased α in the electroencephalogram (Melzack and Perry, 1975). After these physiological changes occur, the individual proceeds to experience hypnotic phenomena such as perceptual distortions, age regression, posthypnotic suggestion, and amnesia, phenomena not characteristically associated with the elicitation of the relaxation response.

A Simple Secular Technique

A simple nonreligious technique was developed in the laboratory of the author and his colleague. The method incorporates the four elements common to a multitude of historical techniques. The use of the technique results in the same physiological changes that the author and his colleagues first noted using transcendental meditation as a model (Beary and Benson, 1974). Instructions for this technique follow.

1. Sit quietly in a comfortable position and close your eyes.
2. Deeply relax all your muscles, beginning at your feet and progressing up to your face. Keep them deeply relaxed.
3. Breathe through your nose. Become aware of your breathing. As you breathe out, say the word one silently to yourself. For example, breathe in, then out saying "one"; breathe in, then out saying "one"; etc. Continue for ten to twenty minutes. You may open your eyes to check the time, but do not use an alarm. When you finish, sit quietly for several minutes, at first with closed eyes, and later with opened eyes.
4. Do not worry about whether you are successful in achieving a deep level of relaxation. Maintain a passive attitude and permit relaxation to occur at its own pace. Expect other thoughts. When distracting thoughts occur, ignore them by thinking "Oh well" and continue repeating "one." With practice, the response should come with little effort. Practice the technique once or twice daily, but not within two hours after any meal, since the digestive processes seem to interfere with the subjective changes.

The relaxation response should not be confused with simple relaxation. During simple relaxation, that is, sitting quietly, the physiological alterations of decreased oxygen consumption, carbon dioxide production, and respiratory rate do not occur (Benson et al., 1974). On the other hand, when the instructions that elicit the relaxation response are followed, these parameters significantly decrease.

Two essential elements are the adoption of a passive attitude and the repetition of a word or phrase. In teaching the method, the author and his colleagues currently choose the repeated word, sound, prayer, or phrase to conform to the belief system of the patient. Catholic patients frequently choose the Prayer of the Heart; Protestant patients, a short phrase from either the Lord's Prayer or the Twenty-third Psalm; Jewish patients, Shalom or Shamah Israel. Others use the number one or the word love or peace. The instructions are the same; only the repetition changes. Although the physiological changes are similar, with any technique that elicits the relaxation response compliance is markedly enhanced when the belief system of the patient is considered.

CLINICAL TRIALS

The elicitation of the relaxation response is hypothesized to alter the sequence of events by which stressful stimuli lead to increased sympathetic nervous system activity. The relaxation response may prevent the elicitation of the emergency response. At a cognitive level, the regular practice of a behavior such as prayer may change the belief or perception of what is a potentially stressful event, and the sequence of sympathetic nervous system activation may be mitigated or may even not be initiated. Furthermore, the regular elicitation of the relaxation response reduces peripheral responsiveness to secreted norepinephrine: more norepinephrine is required to bring about increases in heart rate and blood pressure.

Clinical trials of the therapeutic usefulness of the relaxation response were initiated, since increased sympathetic nervous system activity is believed to initiate or exacerbate several cardiovascular and immunological disease states. The relaxation response has been demonstrated to lower blood pressure in hypertensive patients (Benson, 1977; Lehmann and Benson, 1982), to alleviate cardiac arrhythmias (Benson et al., 1975; Lown et al., 1977), and to reduce pain (Kabat-Zinn, 1982). The efficacy of the relaxation response as a therapy in several immunological disorders is currently under investigation (Borysenko, 1982).

The relaxation response is useful in the treatment of anxiety. In a study of 32 patients, change in anxiety was determined by three types of evaluation, psychiatric assessment, physiological testing, and self-assessment (Benson et al., 1978). After elicitation of the relaxation response, 31 percent of the patients showed improvement by psychiatric assessment, and 63 percent were improved on self-assessment. No consistent changes occurred in the physiological measurements of blood pressure, oxygen consumption, and heart rate. The conclusion from this study was that techniques for eliciting the relaxation response are simple to use and effective in the treatment of anxiety.

A prospective controlled investigation established the usefulness of the relaxation response in the treatment of anxiety-related symptoms including headache, nausea, diarrhea, excessive worry, nervous habits such as biting fingernails, difficulty getting to sleep, and so forth (Peters et al., 1977a; 1977b). This experiment was conducted at the corporate offices of a manufacturing firm and investigated the effects of daily relaxation-response breaks on five self-reported measures of health, performance, and well-being. For 12 weeks, 126 volunteers filled out daily records and reported biweekly for additional measurements. After 4 weeks of baseline monitoring, they were divided randomly into three groups. Group A was taught a technique for producing the relaxation response, Group B was instructed to sit quietly, and Group C received no instructions. Groups A and B were asked to take two 15-minute relaxation breaks daily. After an 8-week experimental period, the greatest mean improvements on every index occurred in Group A, the least improvements occurred in Group C, and Group B was intermediate. Differences between the mean changes in Groups A and C reached statistical significance (p<.05) on four of five indices: anxiety-related symptoms, illness days, performance, and sociability-satisfaction. Improvements on the happiness-unhappiness index were not significantly different among the three groups. The relationship between the amount of change and the rate of practicing the relaxation response was different for different indices. Somatic symptoms and performance responded with less practice of the relaxation response than did behavioral symptoms and measures of well-being. Overall, while less than three practice sessions per week produced little change on any index, two practice sessions per day appeared to be more than necessary for many individuals to achieve positive changes.

SUMMARY

The relaxation response is a physiological state associated with decreased sympathetic nervous system activity. It is the physiological counterpart of the emergency or fight-or-flight response. Under different guises, the relaxation response has been elicited by mankind throughout the ages. It may be elicited by following simple instructions, and its daily practice is useful in counteracting physiological and pathophysiological states in which increased sympathetic nervous system activity is undesirable.

Chapter 31

Exposure Treatment of Agoraphobia

by Matig Mavissakalian, M.D.

One can hardly ever master a phobia if one waits till the patient lets the analysis influence him to give it up . . . One succeeds only when one can induce them . . . to go about alone and to struggle with their anxiety while they make the attempt.

—Sigmund Freud

INTRODUCTION

Now, more than sixty years later, Freud's suggestion has been confirmed: exposure of patients to the stimuli which induce their phobic anxiety is crucial in the successful treatment of phobias. Indeed, the seemingly fruitful conclusions of nearly 25 years of behavioral research are that the different treatment modalities all share exposure to the phobic situation as their common active ingredient and that the various trappings of each treatment are simply different ways of structuring patients' therapeutic "struggle with their anxiety."

Behavioral approaches have their roots in experimental psychology and learning theory. Simply put, classical conditioning theory states that phobic anxiety is a conditioned response elicited by the phobic situation (the conditioned stimulus). Escape from the phobic situation develops and is maintained because it is reinforced through anxiety reduction (negative reinforcement). Moreover, successful avoidance of the phobic situation conserves the anxiety (Solomon and Wynne, 1954) and thus perpetuates the phobia. Because this theory emphasizes both phobic anxiety and avoidance, it is commonly referred to as the two-factor theory (Mowrer, 1939). The purely operant paradigm, on the other hand, conceives of symptomatic behavior in terms of freely emitted behaviors that produce, and are in turn affected by, environmental consequences. Accordingly, the major behavioral aim in the treatment of phobias (e.g., to decrease avoidance and/or increase approach behavior) can be accomplished by directly reinforcing approach behavior or by removing all reinforcers for avoidance behavior, or both.

Although the shortcomings of learning theory, particularly in regard to the origin of phobic disorders, have been recognized (Rachman, 1976; 1977), these paradigms have nevertheless inspired fertile clinical research and have led to breakthroughs in treatment. This chapter does not attempt an extensive review of the behavioral treatments of agoraphobia, since much of the relevant material has been covered exhaustively in several recent publications (Emmelkamp, 1982; Jansson and Ost, 1982; Mathews et al., 1981; Mavissakalian and Barlow, 1981b). Rather, the chapter briefly outlines the development of behavioral treatments, highlighting the evolution of the exposure principle, and attempts to define an integrated clinical approach to the treatment of agoraphobia.

THE EVOLUTION OF THE EXPOSURE PRINCIPLE

Systematic Desensitization

A landmark in the development of effective treatments of phobias occurred in 1958 with the publication of Joseph Wolpe's book, *Psychotherapy by Reciprocal Inhibition*. Wolpe reported on the successful treatment of 90 percent of a large sample of mixed neurotic patients, mostly phobic, with a new technique termed systematic desensitization. Central to the development of this technique was the principle of countercIconditioning: "If a response inhibitory to anxiety can be made to occur in the presence of anxiety-evoking stimuli, it will weaken the connection between these stimuli and the anxiety responses" (Wolpe, 1958). Another important principle in desensitization was the systematic arrangement of fear-provoking stimuli along a carefully constructed hierarchy, proceeding from the least severe to the most severe, so as to provoke only minimal anxiety. Thus, deep muscle relaxation, the anxiety antagonist, could occur and successfully suppress the anxiety provoked by the phobic stimulus at each step. Finally, the desensitization procedure assumed that gains made in imagination would generalize or transfer quasi-automatically to the real situation (Wolpe, 1963).

Early reviews of the effectiveness of desensitization in treating clinical phobias suggested that about half of the patients improved markedly, compared with only a quarter of controls treated with traditional therapies (McConaghy, 1970); agoraphobics seemed to respond less well than simple phobics (Gelder and Marks, 1966; Gelder et al., 1967; Marks et al., 1968; Marks and Gelder, 1965; Yorkston et al., 1968). A thorough review of the literature emphasizing psychophysiological findings with desensitization, however, failed to find direct evidence "for one of the central postulates of reciprocal inhibition theory, that relaxation reduces or prevents the autonomic anxiety responses associated with the phobic imagery" (Mathews, 1971, 87). Rather, the characteristic decrement in arousal that took place with repeated presentations of phobic stimuli was more parsimoniously conceptualized as habituation. Thus, in this physiological model of desensitization, relaxation would assume the role of ensuring that anxiety or arousal would stay beneath the critical level "above which a repetitive stimulus would not be accompanied by any habituation; instead, level of arousal would become higher with each successive stimulus producing a positive feedback mechanism" (Lader and Mathews, 1968, 412–413).

Flooding in Imagination

Stampfl, working from a slightly different perspective, reported on a technique termed implosion (Stampfl, 1967; Stampfl and Levis, 1967), which in one move did away with the principles of hierarchical presentation and relaxation that underpinned the systematic desensitization procedure. Also called flooding in imagination (Marks, 1972), the implosion procedure required patients to imagine entering their most phobic situations and to experience the most feared consequences until these imagined experiences ceased to provoke anxiety. The deliberate induction of high levels of anxiety by the inclusion of horrifying consequences in the imaginal presentation was initially thought to be important. Later studies demonstrated that although an anxiety response may be essential (Chambless et al., 1979), the induction of extreme anxiety is not necessary (Foa et al., 1977; Hafner and Marks, 1976; Mathews and Shaw, 1973; Watson and Marks, 1971). Habituation with this procedure was demonstrated, and it was frequently found necessary to prolong the period of continuous exposure lest premature termination (e.g., while the patient is still highly aroused) lead to further sensitization (McCutcheon and Adams, 1975). The duration of exposure attracted much research, and Marshall, Gauthier, and Gordon (1979) conducted a comprehensive review of the importance of prolonged exposure. They concluded that "exposure duration . . . appears to be most accurately defined by the subject's return to baseline responding, and this is most satisfactorily determined by a trained observer or perhaps the absence of the stress reported by the subject" (Marshall et al., 1979, 245–246).

A series of early studies with imaginal flooding showed that the procedure can be effective in the treatment of phobic disorders and that with agoraphobia it may even be preferable to systematic desensitization (Chambless et al., 1979; Marks, 1972). However, studies comparing imaginal flooding with systematic desensitization yielded confusing and contradictory overall results (Mavissakalian and Barlow, 1981a). Differing lengths of total treatment and variations of exposure duration among studies certainly contributed to this confusion. But perhaps the most confounding issue was practice in the real situation, which was later shown to be perhaps the most potent therapeutic variable. In retrospect, the major development emanating from these studies was their contribution to a growing interest in a pure extinction model for fear reduction, wherein phobic anxiety would gradually diminish with unreinforced exposure. Predictably, the next wave of research investigated whether the imaginal phase of treatment could be altogether eliminated by initiating the treatment with exposure to the real situation.

Exposure In Vivo

A number of studies with desensitization in clinical and nonclinical populations had shown that the successful elimination of fears in imagination does not transfer readily to the real situation and that in vivo exposure is a more effective fear-reducing modality than imaginal exposure (Agras, 1967; Barlow et al., 1969; Dyckman and Cowan, 1978; Sherman, 1972). An early and thought-provoking study compared systematic desensitization and flooding in imagination (eight sessions), followed by practice in vivo (four sessions), and showed parity between the treatments (Gelder et al., 1973). These investigators also observed that while anxiety in response to the imaginal situation decreased during the imaginal phase of treatment, anxiety anticipatory to being in the real situation did not decline until the in vivo treatment began (Mathews et al., 1974). In addition to commenting on the superiority of in vivo treatments, these authors suggested that imaginal treatments may have a potentiating effect on subsequent in vivo exposure.

Two studies have sought to determine the relative and combined effectiveness with agoraphobia of flooding in vivo and flooding in imagination. Emmelkamp and Wessels (1975) found that following 4 ninety-minute sessions, administered over what appears to be a ten-day period, improvement in phobias with the in vivo procedure was clearly superior to the effects with the imaginal flooding procedure, while the effects of the combined procedures were intermediate. The second study (Mathews et al., 1976; Johnston et al., 1976) used a longer duration of treatment and assigned 36 female agoraphobic patients (1) to 16 weekly sessions of in vivo flooding, (2) to 16 weekly sessions of combined imaginal and in vivo flooding, or (3) to 8 sessions of flooding in imagination followed by 8 sessions of flooding in vivo. The results did not show potentiation of in vivo flooding by imaginal flooding. Indeed, no difference was found among any of the three treatments either on the weekly measures of phobic anxiety or on the outcome measures obtained at the midtreatment, posttreatment, and 6-month follow-up assessments.

The important conclusion drawn from these two studies was that in vivo treatment had a more potent immediate effect, but had no more potent long-term effect, compared with flooding in imagination. A major difference between these two studies was that in the latter, all patients received systematic instructions encouraging them to enter phobic situations between the sessions (e.g., self-directed in vivo exposure). Could it be that differences between in vivo and imaginal treatments disappear when sufficient time and opportunity are provided for patients to confront phobic situations and to practice in vivo exposure on their own? Could it be that practice between sessions is the main determinant of outcome in agoraphobia and that imaginal or in vivo procedures are equivalent ways of bringing this about? These were essentially the questions which Mathews and colleagues raised and which influenced the most recent wave of research in self-directed exposure treatments (Mathews, 1977).

RECENT RESEARCH

Self-Directed Exposure

McDonald et al. (1979) randomly assigned 19 agoraphobic patients either to four exposure planning sessions or to four control sessions (discussions of marital, family, and social difficulties). The experimental condition consisted of exposure homework tasks that required patients to enter into and remain in phobic situations hitherto avoided (e.g., prolonged in vivo exposure), and it effected significant improvements in phobias compared with the control condition. This difference was maintained at one-month follow-up. In a second study, the effects of exposure instructions were compared with the effects of avoidance instructions in a balanced crossover design with 13 phobic and 4 obsessive-compulsive patients (Greist et al., 1980). The exposure instructions were similar to those in the previous study, and the avoidance instructions required that the patients consistently avoid all contact with stimuli which evoked fear or rituals. Despite the short experimental phases (one week), the investigators found that phobias improved with the exposure instructions and became somewhat worse with the avoidance instructions. These results underscored the therapeutic effectiveness of self-directed exposure instructions and raised the possibility that a number of agoraphobic patients may be able to treat themselves successfully if given appropriate instructions.

Mathews and colleagues (1977) enhanced the impact of instructions by using carefully prepared manuals for both patient and spouse. The manuals provided information on the nature of agoraphobia, emphasizing the role of habitual avoidance in maintaining the fears, and presented the therapeutic rationale for self-directed in vivo exposure practice. Twelve agoraphobic patients were instructed and required to practice exposure on their own or with the help of their spouses. The therapist visited the patient's home at a decreasing rate in the first month of treatment essentially to supervise early attempts at exposure and to advise the spouse on appropriate ways of supporting the patient's efforts. With an average of only seven hours in actual treatment for each patient, the method resulted in marked improvements on clinical and behavioral measures of agoraphobia, and the degrees of improvement were by and large comparable in size to those achieved with previous therapist-assisted treatments from the same center.

A second controlled study compared the same home-based procedure, now termed programmed practice, with a control "problem-solving" condition matched to the exposure treatments in all procedural aspects except for rationale and instructions regarding in vivo practice (Jannoun et al., 1980). The results showed that programmed practice was superior to the problem-solving treatment and thus replicated the previous findings on the effectiveness of self-directed exposure.

Finally, in a most recent study, Mathews and colleagues showed that programmed practice manuals alone, without any direct contact between patient and therapist, effect substantial changes and also that it may not always be necessary to include a partner in the self-directed practices of agoraphobic patients (Mathews et al., 1981). Adequate rationale and instructions for self-directed exposure therefore seem to be important active ingredients, and for many agoraphobic patients may be the only therapeutic intervention required.

Although most studies reviewed have given instructions for prolonged exposure, several studies suggest that more graduated exposure methods can also be effective in treating agoraphobia. Variously called successive approximations, shaping, or reinforced practice, these methods emphasize gradually increasing the patient's approach behavior in the phobic situation. Patients are instructed to enter phobic situations until they become uncomfortably tense, at which time they are allowed to retreat with the expectation that they will immediately return to the phobic scene and try to do a little better each time. Once they conquer a situation, they move on to the next using the same gradual approach. A series of studies employing single-case experimental methodology demonstrated the therapeutic effectiveness of reinforced practice (Agras et al., 1968; Agras et al., 1969; Crowe et al., 1972; Leitenberg et al., 1970). Furthermore, Everaerd et al. (1973) provided strong evidence that the shaping method and the prolonged exposure method can be equally effective in the treatment of agoraphobia.

These findings suggested that important factors other than habituation may mediate the therapeutic effectiveness of exposure (Mathews, 1977). Bandura (1977) and Rosenthal and Bandura (1978) suggested that exposure is best considered a quantitative variable rather than an explanatory construct. These investigators proposed that the common mechanism of action in all successful exposure therapies of phobias is an increase in the level of self-efficacy, which basically means an individual's perceived effectiveness in dealing with feared situations. According to them, four main sources of information contribute to self-efficacy. The most powerful of these is actual behavioral experience in the feared situation (exposure), since information derived from this experience is most relevant and salient. A second source of information includes the vicarious experience of observing others cope with the feared situation (modeling effects). A third source is the frequency of the therapist's verbal persuasion and encouragement about the patient's ability to deal with the feared situation. A final source is the actual level of physiological arousal, which patients often use to judge their degree of anxiety and hence their ability to deal with the feared situation. In this model, exposure to feared situations is not seen as therapeutic in itself except to the extent that it facilitates the processing of information in the other three categories, which in turn enhances a patient's perceived self-efficacy in dealing with the situation. Others have argued that exposure may not even be a necessary condition in all instances of fear reduction (De Silva and Rachman, 1981).

Whatever the mechanisms involved, little doubt exists today that treatments based on prolonged exposure and habituation are effective (Marks, 1981). The weight of the evidence in the studies reviewed here and elsewhere is that 60 to 70 percent of agoraphobic patients improve

Table 1. 2 × 2 Analyses of Covariance Between Flooding, Imipramine, Combined Flooding and Imipramine, and Control Conditions

Major Posttreatment Measures	F Ratios			
	Main Effects	Medication Effects	Flooding Effects	Interaction Effects
Global Assessment of Severity	4.83**	8.06**	2.77*	<1
Total fear score (Fear Questionnaire)	3.36*	2.70	4.76*	1.52
Agoraphobia subscore (Fear Questionnaire)	4.05*	3.03*	5.58*	1.52
Clinical scale of phobic anxiety and avoidance	3.26*	2.40	4.79*	2.91
Beck Depression Inventory	3.31*	6.62**	<1	2.04
Subjective Units of Discomfort	3.23*	1.65	5.09*	2.43

Source: Reprinted from Mavissakalian M, Michelson L: Agoraphobia: Behavioral and pharmacological treatment (N = 49). Psychopharmacology Bulletin 19: 116–118, 1983.
Notes: *p<.05
      **p<.01

to a marked degree with in vivo exposure treatments, whether or not the treatments are administered in combination with imaginal methods, whether sessions are conducted individually or in groups, and whether treatment is conducted at the clinic or with minimal therapist contact (Emmelkamp, 1982; Jansson and Ost, 1982; Marks, 1981; Mathews et al., 1981; Mavissakalian and Barlow, 1981b). Whether exposure is sufficient, however, is an interesting question which recent findings at the University of Pittsburgh begin to address.

Combined Treatments

IMIPRAMINE, FLOODING, AND EXPOSURE   The author and a colleague assessed the relative and combined effectiveness of imipramine and in vivo flooding in chronic nondepressed agoraphobic patients, employing a 2 × 2 factorial design (Mavissakalian and Michelson, 1982; 1983a; 1983b). The control condition consisted essentially of programmed practice alone (e.g., rationale and instructions for self-directed in vivo prolonged exposure), and the three experimental groups in addition received therapist-assisted in vivo flooding, imipramine, or a combination of these two. The treatment phase consisted of 12 weekly sessions. Table 1 shows the posttreatment results for 49 patients randomly assigned to the imipramine (14), flooding (12), combined (12), and control (11) conditions. As can be seen, 2 × 2 analysis of covariance revealed significant main effects on: (1) a 5-point clinician rating of global assessment of severity; (2) the total fear score and the agoraphobia subscore of the Fear Questionnaire (Marks and Mathews, 1979); (3) a 9-point clinical scale of phobic anxiety and avoidance; (4) the Beck Depression Inventory (BDI) (Beck et al., 1961); and (5) measures of subjective units of discomfort assessed on a 9-point analogue scale in the course of a standardized behavioral assessment. Significant imipramine effects (average dose 125 mg/day; standard deviation 66.6) were obtained on the global assessment of severity, the agoraphobia subscore, and the BDI, while flooding had a more generalized significant effect on phobic measures but not on BDI.

Post hoc Newman-Keuls analysis at posttreatment revealed that flooding, imipramine, and the combination of the two were equivalent and were each significantly more effective than the control condition. Findings were similar for percentages of patients meeting the criteria for high end-state functioning, an a priori operational definition of near asymptomatic functioning which entailed simultaneous clinician and patient ratings of severity of condition, which required minimal or no phobic anxiety, and which measured avoidance on clinical and direct behavioral measures. Using these criteria, 73 percent (8/11) of the flooding group, 77 percent (10/13) of the imipramine group, 73 percent (8/11) of the combined group, and 33 percent (3/9) of the control treatment group had high end-state functioning. (Five patients, 1 in each experimental group and 2 in the control group, could not be classified due to missing data.) Log-linear $2 \times 2 \times 2$ chi-squares (BMD P3F) did not yield significant main or interaction effects, suggesting that the effectiveness of self-directed in vivo exposure is equally enhanced by the addition of imipramine, flooding, or the combination of the two. Because of the relatively small sample size and the realization that the unclassifiable patients could change statistical significance, these results should be considered tentative. However, the raw data suggest that the clinical effectiveness of self-directed in vivo prolonged exposure instructions is considerably enhanced by the addition of imipramine, therapist-assisted flooding, or the combination. Thus, considered together, these three treatments were significantly superior to the control ($\chi^2 = 5.344$; $p = .02$), and the same strong trend was evident even after the control group with high end-state functioning was increased by arbitrarily assigning the two unclassified control patients ($\chi^2 = 3.166$; $p = .07$).

All patients in this study received a weekly diary with careful and systematic instructions to record their daily out-of-the-home activities throughout the 12-week treatment phase. The diaries included the following information: date, time-out, time-in, whether alone or accompanied, maximum anxiety experienced at each outing, distance from home, time spent at destination, and whether the outing was a practice session or just part of the patient's normal routine. (Practice was defined as an outing undertaken solely for the purpose of practicing self-directed in vivo exposure.) Since all patients in all groups were given therapeutic instructions, the diaries provided an excellent opportunity to investigate the role of self-directed in vivo prolonged exposure in agoraphobia. More specifically, data from the diaries enabled the investigators to explore the hypothesis that the enhanced therapeutic effectiveness of pharmacotherapy or therapist-assisted flooding may be mediated through increased frequency and duration of self-directed exposure. However, a series of analyses showed that none of the be-

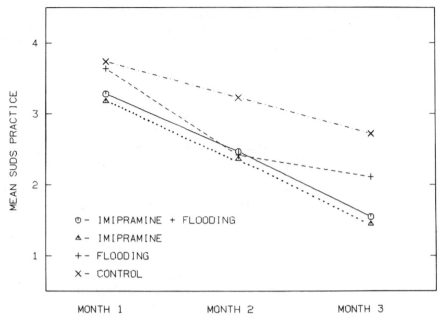

Figure 1. Subjective anxiety (subjective units of discomfort, or SUDS, range 0–8) during in vivo practice at months 1, 2, and 3 (N=49)

havioral diary variables, such as number of outings, number of alone outings, number of practice sessions, and time spent in these activities, differentiated treatment groups or discriminated high end-state functioning patients. The data did establish that patients in all groups complied with instructions to practice exposure (e.g., five sessions of approximately ninety minutes per week). Level of anxiety (Subjective Units of Discomfort, or SUDS), during outings in general and during practice in particular, was the only diary measure that consistently and significantly differentiated the effective treatments and the high-functioning patients (see Figure 1).

DISCUSSION What are the implications of these findings? First, it appears that agoraphobic patients comply with instructions for self-directed prolonged exposure. Second, self-directed exposure, although effective, may not be sufficient in a large proportion of agoraphobic patients. Third, the addition of imipramine or flooding appears to enhance the therapeutic effectiveness of self-directed exposure, and the combination treatment does not seem to add to the effects of the individual treatments. Fourth, the mechanism of this enhancement does not appear to be due to increased numbers of practice sessions or time spent in practice. And finally, enhanced habituation may possibly be a factor in the potentiation of therapeutic effectiveness with imipramine or therapist-assisted flooding.

That many mediating factors, including psychophysiological and cognitive processes, may impede the process of habituation and interfere with emotional processing has been recently recognized (Rachman, 1980). Thus, if one interprets the "positive feedback mechanism" postulated by Lader and Mathews (1968) in their physiological model of phobic anxiety and habituation to mean the experience of panic, it would raise the possibility that imipramine's antipanic effect might have successfully blocked this occurrence and thereby have enhanced habituation (Mavissakalian, 1982). Although this question has not been directly addressed, evidence from biochemical studies of anxiety induced by lactate infusion suggest that both MAO inhibitors and imipramine can effectively block both provoked and spontaneous panic attacks (Appelby et al., 1981; Kelly et al., 1971). The antidepressant may have been useful in yet another way, since recently Foa (1979) has suggested that depression may impede the process of habituation (in obsessive-compulsive patients). Considerable controversy surrounds the mode of action of antidepressants in agoraphobia, but a recent analysis of the existing literature led Marks (1983) to contend that their therapeutic effect may be mediated through their antidepressant properties. (Recall, though, that patients meeting criteria for major depression were not included in the investigation by the author and his colleague.) Whether through independent or related mechanisms, imipramine seems to have a global ameliorative effect on mood (e.g., depression, panic, and anxiety) (Mavissakalian, 1983). Whether this in turn facilitates habituation in agoraphobic patients is an interesting hypothesis in need of confirmatory testing.

In a likewise speculative vein, demonstrating the process of habituation under the controlled and reassuring circumstances created by the therapist's presence may have increased perceived self-efficacy and emotional processing and have offset the likelihood that catastrophic thoughts may heighten arousal to levels prohibiting habituation (Lader and Mathews, 1968). In addition, the overall avoidant attitude, the concern with security cues, and the tendency to employ distracting thoughts can virtually block effective exposure even when the patient is in the actual phobic situation. Unfortunately, very little research has been conducted on the cognitive and attitudinal factors that may mediate or accompany the changes resulting from exposure treatment of agoraphobia.

COGNITIVE THERAPY AND EXPOSURE To date, three controlled studies have investigated the relative and combined effectiveness of cognitive therapy and exposure in vivo (Emmelkamp et al., 1978; Emmelkamp, 1979; Williams and Rappoport, 1983). Cognitive therapy failed to yield significantly greater improvement compared with practice alone and did not have a potentiating effect on exposure in vivo. All three studies, however, suffered from limited treatment duration, which probably prohibited opportunities for patients in the cognitive conditions to integrate and practice their newly learned cognitive coping strategies in the natural environment. Indeed, none of these studies encouraged patients receiving cognitive therapy to practice exposure in real situations, and in one case this was specifically prohibited (Williams and Rappoport, 1983). All of these studies also used Meichenbaum's Self-Statement Training (SST) (Meichenbaum, 1975; 1977). SST is a rational process of cognitive restructuring that endeavors to replace self-defeating cognitions by positive self-statements in preparing for, confronting, and coping with phobic situations, as well as in reinforcing their achievements. Although proven effective as an anxiety-management strategy (Barios and Shigetomi, 1980), SST may not be the cognitive strategy of choice in the treatment of agoraphobia.

The author and his colleagues (Mavissakalian et al., 1983) recently conducted a study comparing SST with Paradoxical Intention (PI) (Frankl, 1960; 1975), which had received encouraging reports of its effectiveness as a cognitive treatment for agoraphobia (Gertz, 1962; 1967; Ascher, 1981). The primary reason for choosing these two cognitive strategies was their diametrically opposed specific instructional sets. In contrast to SST, PI has an intuitive and experiential quality, instructing patients from the beginning to try and increase their anxiety and become as panicky as possible. A major aim of this study, therefore, was to explore the differential effects, if any, of these two cognitive instructional sets in agoraphobia and to assess whether the so-called specific instructions do in fact have "cognitive specificity."

Twenty-four patients with chronic agoraphobia were randomly assigned to PI or SST consisting of 12 weekly, ninety-minute group sessions, with four patients per group. All patients in all groups were given the therapeutic rationale and instructions for self-directed in vivo exposure and were told that the specific cognitive strategy they were about to learn was intended to help them carry out their self-directed practices. A comprehensive assessment battery was administered at pretreatment, midtreatment (6th week), posttreatment (12th week), and at six-month follow-up. In addition to clinical outcome measures, the battery included continuous recordings of spontaneous self-statements made by patients during a behavioral avoidance test. These statements were subsequently categorized as neutral (task irrelevant), self-defeating, or coping cognitions and were subsequently analyzed. Outcome results revealed that the PI group was significantly superior to SST at posttreatment. However, at the sixth-month follow-up, the two treatments were equivalent, primarily due to the SST group "catching up" with the PI group.

Although this study could not address the relative contribution of cognitive restructuring and exposure, the differential rates of improvement between the SST and PI groups suggested a certain cognitive specificity, which was also apparent on the cognitive measures. Self-defeating cognitions were reduced in both treatments, but they were not always replaced by new types of coping statements. The coping statements typical of the SST group (seemingly familiar to agoraphobics as judged by their presence at pretreatment) remained unchanged from their pretreatment levels with SST, while similar statements were gradually eliminated in the PI group. This suggested that while patients in the SST group did apply the prescribed treatment, the patients in the PI group made active changes in habitual ways of thinking. However, the PI group's statements may have simply been less amenable to verbalization due to their intuitive quality.

Clearly, further elucidation is needed regarding the role of cognitive factors in the treatment of agoraphobia. These preliminary findings suggest that cognitions can make a difference, if not in outcome, at least in the speed at which agoraphobic patients improve. Perhaps the early superiority of PI in this study was due to its ability to focus the patients' attention on their fears, whereas the deliberative and rational approach of SST may have unwittingly distracted the patients or may even have seemed prematurely self-reassuring to them.

PRACTICAL IMPLICATIONS

The principal aim of treatments for agoraphobia is to decrease and eliminate avoidance behavior, and self-directed in vivo exposure to phobic situations may well be the final common pathway in all successful treatments. The simplest and most cost-effective strategy would therefore instruct and encourage patients to do just that, and the evidence suggests that at least one-third of chronic agoraphobic patients would successfully treat themselves without requiring additional treatments.

The clinician often sees patients who are either unwilling or unable to practice self-directed exposure. With these patients, the intermediate goal would focus on persuading them to engage in in vivo exposure. In addition to traditional methods of persuasion, imaginal exposure, therapist-supervised in vivo exposure sessions, or both may successfully achieve this aim. As suggested earlier, specific cognitive strategies, particularly Paradoxical Intention, may also be helpful in this regard.

An alternative approach would be to reduce panic attacks with antidepressants (Mavissakalian, 1982). Since agoraphobic patients do not readily distinguish between the experience of spontaneous panic attacks or panic experienced in the phobic situation, it can be easily seen how out-of-the-blue panic can sensitize, reinforce, and maintain phobic avoidance and how its successful suppression can encourage and motivate the patient to attempt exposure in vivo. As tentatively suggested earlier, the antidepressants may enhance habituation and hence the therapeutic effectiveness of self-directed exposure. It would be tempting, therefore, to suggest that all agoraphobic patients who do not have clear contraindications for antidepressants should be prescribed such medication (Liebowitz and Klein, 1982). On the other hand, in addition to the well-known inherent risks with antidepressant therapy and the observation that agoraphobic patients are generally poor pill takers, antidepressants may be altogether unnecessary in at least one-third of these patients. Furthermore, while the effectiveness of exposure without antidepressants has been demonstrated, no convincing evidence has to date shown that antidepressants without exposure will reduce avoidance behavior in agoraphobic patients (Mavissakalian, 1983). Indeed, the only published study which controlled for the effect of exposure found that phenelzine and placebo were equally ineffective in reducing phobias in a mixed group of agoraphobics and social phobics (Solyom et al., 1981). Finally, high relapse rates have been associated with antidepressant therapy, whether it was the primary treatment or was used in combination with supervised in vivo flooding sessions (Mavissakalian, 1982; Zitrin et al., 1980).

Considering these issues and the observation that early improvement in treatment (Mathews et al., 1981) is by far the most reliable predictor of outcome in agoraphobia, a more conservative approach seems reasonable. Treatment would begin with programmed practice, perhaps coupled with paradoxical intention, and imipramine would be added only for those patients who fail to show early signs of improvement. In addition to the obvious advantage of avoiding unnecessary interventions, this approach would also minimize exaggerated attributions of success to the adjunctive drugs or to the therapist.

Further research must be done to clarify the relative benefits of exposure and antidepressant treatments and the preferred methods of combining them. Moreover, even with the combined method, a number of patients will fail to improve. With these patients, personal and interpersonal factors may play an all-important role and require focal therapeutic attention (Chambless and Goldstein, 1982). Further clinical observations and research are also very much needed in this area, to study individual differences and their implications for the exposure treatments of agoraphobia.

Chapter 32 **Mortality After Thirty to Forty Years: Panic Disorder Compared with Other Psychiatric Illnesses**
by William Coryell, M.D.

INTRODUCTION

The excess mortality which attends severe psychiatric illness (Babigian and Odoroff, 1969; Innes and Millar, 1970; Rorsman, 1974) varies in nature according to diagnosis. Some patients with untreated mania, for instance, die from exhaustion (Derby, 1933), while this rarely accounts for premature death among alcoholics. They die instead from accidental causes or from organ failure due to poor nutrition or the direct effects of alcohol. The premature deaths due to infection previously noted in schizophrenic patients have been attributed to institutionalization (Tsuang et al., 1980). Individuals with antisocial personality more often die from homicide, those with drug dependence from overdose, and those with primary depression by suicide.

Patients within the broad category of severe neurosis also experience excess mortality (Sims and Prior, 1978). However, as with the other psychiatric conditions mentioned above, excess mortality may vary according to specific diagnoses within the category. The relatively recent appearance of fully operational subdivisions of "neurosis" has permitted us to explore this possibility.

METHODS

The data presented in this chapter describe mortality associated with three of the more common conditions formerly listed under the neuroses (American Psychiatric Association, 1968): Briquet's syndrome, obsessive-compulsive disorder, and panic disorder. To obtain the necessary samples, the author and his colleagues applied research criteria to the charts of consecutively admitted patients whose discharge diagnoses suggested one of these three diagnoses; for obsessive-compulsive disorder and Briquet's syndrome, the Feighner et al. (1972) criteria were used, and for panic disorder, DSM-III (American Psychiatric Association, 1980). Screening began with patients who had been admitted when the University of Iowa Psychiatric Hospital opened in 1924. In the case of Briquet's syndrome patients, screening proceeded through those admitted in 1950. Intake for obsessive-compulsive and panic disorder groups was extended through 1954 and 1955 respectively. Each patient so selected was matched by age, sex, and date of admission to a patient with primary unipolar depression (Feighner et al., 1972). Patients were excluded from either group if hospital records noted a medical illness judged likely to influence mortality.

Most of these charts contained not only the patients' addresses, but also the full names and addresses of many first-degree relatives. Attempts to locate patients therefore began with this information, and they were, in the end, successful in 90 percent of cases. Death certificates were then obtained from the appropriate clerks of court and were presented in random sequence to the author who then classified the cause of death into one of the five categories described by Tsuang et al. (1980): unnatural cause (including suicide), circulatory system disease, neoplasm, infectious disease, and other causes. The three samples, collected sequentially, were followed up from 1979 through 1982 (Coryell, 1981a; Coryell, 1981b; Coryell et al., 1982). Although the depressed control groups overlapped somewhat with those described in earlier mortality studies (Tsuang and Woolson, 1977), they did not overlap with each other.

Raters blind to the mortality data also reviewed the charts of panic disorder patients and their depressed controls and recorded educational level, socioeconomic status, marital status, age, drinking history, history of tobacco use, and condition at discharge. Chart material describing these patients after discharge was also reviewed to determine whether the patient recovered or improved during a follow-up period averaging 5.5 ± 8.6 years. Relationships among these variables have been described elsewhere (Coryell et al., in press).

Using a method devised by Woolson et al. (1978), the author's group then calculated the expected age- and sex-specific death rates for each decade of follow-up. When expected values were five or more, the difference between observed and expected values was tested using the χ^2 statistic; otherwise, a Poisson distribution was used.

An additional cohort of inpatients with panic disorder has been selected by screening all admissions from 1970 through 1980. Although 101 of the discharge diagnoses specified an anxiety disorder, only 33 met DSM-III criteria for panic disorder. Over 90 percent of these patients were located in 1983. (Results for this cohort are presented separately.)

RESULTS

Panic disorder, obsessive-compulsive disorder, and Briquet's syndrome cohorts had similar ages at admission (see Table 1); but sex distributions differed markedly. Because men accounted for less than 10 percent of the Briquet's syndrome patients, they were excluded from mortality analysis. In contrast, the majority of inpatients with panic disorder were men. Compared with the other groups, the panic disorder cohort and the matched control group had a somewhat later median date of admission and therefore a shorter median length of follow-up. Efforts to locate patients were quite successful in all groups.

Table 1.   Age, Sex, and Follow-Up Success by Diagnosis

	Number admitted	Median age at admission	Percent female	Percent located	Median years of follow-up
Briquet's Syndrome	76	32	100	92.1	42
Primary Unipolar Depression	76	32	100	93.4	43
Obsessive-Compulsive Disorder	44	26	65.9	88.6	40
Primary Unipolar Depression	44	29	65.9	88.6	40
Panic Disorder	125	29	38.4	90.4	35
Primary Unipolar Depression	125	30	38.4	89.6	34

Table 2.   Expected and Observed Deaths in Males by Diagnosis and Decade

Diagnosis	Decade 1925–1934	1935–1944	1945–1954	1955–1964	1965–1974
Panic Disorder (N=71)					
Expected deaths	0.05	0.62	1.99	4.79	4.40
Observed deaths	0	2	2	8	13
Standardized mortality ratio	0.00	3.23	1.01	1.67	2.95**
Primary Unipolar Depression (N=67)					
Expected deaths	0.02	0.48	1.64	3.91	4.50
Observed deaths	0	4	5	1	10
Standardized mortality ratio	0.00	8.33**	3.05*	0.25	2.22*
Obsessive-Compulsive Disorder (N=44)					
Expected deaths	0.16	0.40	0.96	2.32	2.96
Observed deaths	0	1	0	0	4
Standardized mortality ratio	0.00	2.50	0.00	0.00	1.35
Primary Unipolar Depression (N=44)					
Expected deaths	0.05	0.14	0.35	0.65	0.63
Observed deaths	2	0	2	1	3
Standardized mortality ratio	40.0*	0.00	5.71	1.53	4.41

Notes: *p<.01
             **p<.001

Male patients with panic disorder exhibited excess mortality during the last decade of follow-up (see Table 2). Their controls with primary depression, in contrast, manifested excess mortality early in follow-up.

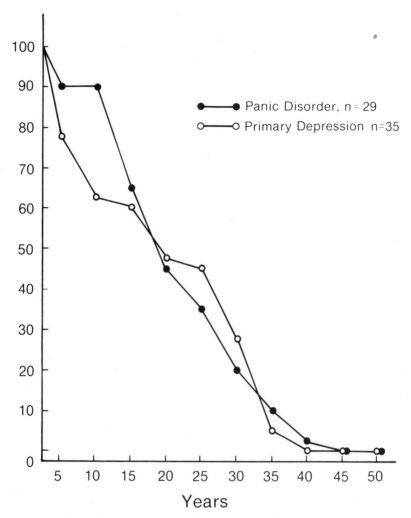

Figure 1. Males who died during follow-up: survival by diagnosis and year of follow-up

Thus, men with panic disorder who died during follow-up did so later than did men with primary depression. While 38 percent of the affective disorder deaths occurred in the first ten years after discharge, only 10 percent of the panic disorder deaths occurred during that time (see Figure 1).

In further contrast to the men with panic disorder, men with obsessive-compulsive disorder exhibited no excess mortality (see Table 2). The numbers involved, though small, were sufficient to show statistically significant excess mortality in the depressed controls.

The group of men with panic disorder and their depressed control group both had an excess number of unnatural deaths (see Table 3). Only the men with panic disorder exhibited excess cardiovascular mortality, however.

Women with panic disorder showed no significant excess in overall

Table 3. Expected and Observed Mortality in Males by Cause and Diagnosis

Cause of Death	Panic Disorder		Primary Unipolar Depression (matched)	
	Expected	Observed	Expected	Observed
Unnatural	1.32	5*	1.22	8*
Circulatory system disease	6.0	12*	5.16	8
Neoplasm	1.8	1	2.01	4
Infectious disease	1.0	1	0.12	1
Other	1.5	3	1.48	4

Note: *p<.01

mortality, though their depressed controls did. In this respect, the women with panic disorder resembled the women with obsessive-compulsive disorder and those with Briquet's syndrome (Coryell, 1981a); neither of these two groups showed excess mortality. Two of the female patients with panic disorder died from unnatural causes, compared with the expected number of 0.31, but this was significant at only the .03 level.

Panic disorder patients who died unnatural deaths did not differ from the remaining panic disorder patients on any of the variables tested (educational level, etc.) Matched patients with primary unipolar depressions who died unnatural deaths were similarly compared with those who did not, and again, no significant differences were found. Furthermore, in none of these comparisons were there strong trends suggesting that large sample sizes would have produced significant results.

Among the 30 of 33 panic disorder patients located in the cohort admitted in the 1970s, one patient had died. This death occurred in a 48-year-old male patient and resulted from a myocardial infarction.

DISCUSSION

Male patients with panic disorder experienced excess mortality, while those with obsessive-compulsive disorder did not. Thus, the importance of psychiatric diagnosis in mortality studies, previously illustrated in the contrast between Briquet's syndrome and primary depression, extends to subdivisions within the neuroses.

These findings are contrary to those of Wheeler et al. (1950), and the reasons for this contrast have been offered elsewhere (Coryell et al., 1982). Briefly, Wheeler et al. (1950) based their mortality analysis entirely on population statistics; they included no psychiatrically ill reference group. Although they calculated expected numbers of deaths in several ways, the resulting numbers were considerably higher than would be predicted by the method of calculation used in the present analysis. Nonetheless, the expected deaths reported here do not seem excessively low, since two of the diagnostic groups (Briquet's syndrome and obsessive-compulsive disorder) were shown to have no excess mortality.

The pattern of mortality differed in certain ways among the panic disorder patients, however. While the men with panic disorder and their depressed control group both had an excess of unnatural deaths, only the panic disorder group had a significant excess of cardiovascular deaths. Furthermore, excess mortality manifested relatively soon after discharge in panic disorder patients. These differences raise questions of both practical and theoretical significance.

First, what are the possible explanations for the cardiovascular mortality among male panic disorder patients, twice that predicted by population statistics? The alleged association between mitral valve prolapse and panic disorder is probably the least likely explanation. Recent work has attributed this apparent association to the selection bias operating in clinic populations (Hartman et al., 1982; Crowe et al., 1982). Furthermore, none of these deaths were attributable to functional arrhythmia.

Alcoholism very often coexists with anxiety neurosis in men (Woodruff et al., 1972). While this study's screening criteria excluded patients with alcoholism at the time of discharge, there was ample follow-up time for them to develop this problem later. In turn, alcoholism may have produced cardiomyopathy or the propensity to cerebrovascular accidents which may follow drinking bouts in younger men (Lee, 1979; Taylor, 1982). Yet none of the death certificates for male panic disorder patients listed cardiovascular accidents or cardiomyopathy as a cause of death (see Table 4).

In a similar vein, tobacco use could have mediated excess cardiovascular mortality. Salmons and Sims (1981) have shown that neurotic patients are as a group more likely to smoke than are surgical controls or members of the general population. When they do smoke, they also inhale more deeply and smoke more of the cigarette. In this study, the panic disorder and affective disorder groups did not differ on the proportions noted in the charts as using tobacco, but the chart method of ascertainment is probably insensitive. Furthermore, a higher proportion of panic disorder patients may have become heavy smokers during follow-up. Thus, tobacco remains a possible factor in the cardiovascular mortality seen in these patients.

At least one study has reported a link between anxiety neurosis and subsequently manifest hypertension (Noyes et al., 1978). At a six-year follow-up, 31 percent of anxiety neurotics compared with 14 percent of age- and sex-matched surgical controls had recorded blood pressure readings in excess of 140/90 and had been given antihypertensive medications. In 19 of 21 anxiety neurotics with hypertension, the hypertension was diagnosed two or more years after the onset of anxiety symptoms. Patients with clinically significant hypertension at the outset were not excluded, however, and in some of these patients, the anxiety neurosis symptoms may themselves have been an early manifestation of hypertension. In turn, patients treated for hypertension are more likely to enter the referral system and are more likely to receive psychiatric treatment for coexisting symptoms of anxiety. In other words, subjects in the community with coincidental panic disorder and hypertension are more likely to receive treatment for either illness than subjects with either condition singly. Thus, the apparent association between hypertension and panic disorder may be an artifact of referral patterns.

Two aspects of the present study do not support the hypertension explanation. First, patients with a history of treatment for hypertension were excluded from follow-up. Second, the artifactual selection bias should operate for other psychiatric illnesses, but several other diagnostic groups were followed in like manner, and no excess in cardiovas-

Table 4. Cardiovascular Deaths Among Males with Panic Disorder

Cause of death	Age at death	Years after admission
"Massive coronary occlusion" "Old coronary occlusion—6 yrs." "Minor CVA—14 months"	38	15
"Cardiac arrest" "Ischemia of the heart" "Coronary arteriosclerosis and hypertensive heart disease"	45	14
"Coronary occlusion"	46	13
"Acute coronary thrombosis"	56	12
"Coronary occlusion"	58	18
"Renal failure" "Arteriosclerotic heart disease" "Hypertensive vascular disease"	58	21
"Heart failure" "Arteriosclerotic heart disease"	61	26
"Coronary occlusion" "Arteriosclerotic heart disease"	61	17

"Acute myocardial failure with
  infarction"
"Convulsive seizure due to brain
  disorder"
	63	32

"Polycythemia vera"	66	36
"Myocardial infarction" "Arteriosclerotic heart disease"	67	35

"Marked pulmonary edema sec-
  ondary to advanced coronary
  artery disease"
	74	42

cular mortality emerged for these groups. In addition, the follow-up by Sims and Prior (1982) noted no differences in baseline physical findings between neurotics who subsequently died from cardiovascular causes and those who survived.

Table 5.   Ratio of Suicides to All Deaths by Sex and Diagnosis (%)

	Panic Disorder	Obsessive-Compulsive Disorder	Briquet's Syndrome	Primary Unipolar Depressed[1]
Males	4/22 (18.2)	0/5 (0)	—	8/34 (23.5)
Females	2/8 (25.0)	0/4 (0)	1/30 (3.3)	7/54 (13.0)

[1] All matched groups combined

The possibility that chronic anxiety neurosis leads to hypertension and thus to excess cardiovascular mortality is an intriguing one. Further exploration of this possibility will require a careful selection of subjects. On the one hand, an artifactually high association between physical illness and psychiatric symptoms may result from referral patterns; this must be avoided by excluding patients with treated physical illness likely to affect mortality and by using control patients in whom such selection factors are equally likely. On the other hand, the exclusion of patients with any sign of physical illness (i.e., borderline high blood pressure) will produce an artificially healthy group which cannot be validly compared with the general population.

Suicide, the other cause of excess mortality among patients with panic disorder, accounted for 6 (19.4 percent) of the 31 deaths among both sexes (see Table 5). As was probably the case with cardiovascular mortality, other factors may have intervened. In this case, secondary depression, alcoholism, environmental stressors, or any combination of these three factors may have immediately preceded many of these suicides. A similar caveat, however, is appropriate for any variable found to be predictive of suicide in the long run.

The lengthier follow-up studies of primary affective disorder, those in which at least 25 percent of the sample have died, have shown remarkable agreement; approximately 15 percent of the deaths involved suicide (Guze and Robins, 1970). In the present study, 27 percent of the primary affective disorder patients had died by follow-up; of these, 31 or 17.0 percent had died by suicide. Thus, the suicide rate for the primary affective disorder patients in this study is quite consistent with other long-term follow-ups. There are no follow-ups of panic disorder of similar length. The suicide pattern described here for panic disorder patients may or may not turn out to be typical. For the time being, clinicians should be aware that panic disorder may imply as much risk for suicide as primary affective disorder.

Chapter 33 # The Biology of Anxiety[†]
by Jack M. Gorman, M.D.

After years of neglect, studies of the biochemical and physiological basis of the anxiety disorders now proliferate. The most interesting areas in-

†This work was supported in part by National Institute of Mental Health Grants, No. MH 33422 and No. MH 30906, and a Research Scientist Development Award No. MH 00416-51.

clude (1) studies of autonomic nervous system physiology in anxiety, (2) studies of the role of neurotransmitters in anxiety, (3) the use of provocative agents to produce anxiety reactions, and (4) the association of mitral valve prolapse and panic disorder. This chapter presents a review of these four topics, highlighting the areas of current investigation and the directions for future research.

AUTONOMIC NERVOUS SYSTEM PHYSIOLOGY

A traditional belief holds that anxious patients have abnormal autonomic responses to various stimuli, perhaps indicating underlying dysfunction of the autonomic nervous system. These abnormalities have generally been believed to cause an increase in sympathetic activity (Mirsky, 1973), and the parameters studied include heart rate, other cardiac functions, peripheral blood flow, and electrodermal response. Investigators have chosen these functions because so much is known about their control by the autonomic nervous system.

Studies focus on baseline differences between patients and normal subjects, with the aim of discerning a basic autonomic disorder in anxiety. Attempts are also made to determine whether anxious people have abnormal responses to a variety of stimuli. As Meyer and Reich (1978) noted, "There is some evidence which allows us to conclude that anxious subjects' physiological responses continue to rise during the presentation of the stressful stimuli and even *after* the *termination* of the stimulus presentation. This would explain the slower peaking and slower return to baseline when anxious subjects are compared to normals" (178).

A major problem in interpreting the physiological studies is their almost complete lack of diagnostic specificity. Anxiety is generally treated as homogeneous; subjects who would meet modern criteria for panic disorder, generalized anxiety disorder, social phobia, or adjustment disorder with anxious mood are indiscriminately grouped together.

Cardiac Function

Studies of heart rate show faster basal rates in anxiety-disordered patients than in normal subjects, less cardiac deceleration after a stressful stimulus, greater cardiac awareness, and more beat-to-beat variability.

White and Gilden showed in 1937 that patients with "anxiety state" had faster heart rate than normal subjects, while Kelly and Walter (1968) found the resting heart rates of 41 patients with chronic anxiety state to be 97.34 compared with only 73.72 for a group of 60 normal subjects. Several other groups have also found tachycardia associated with anxiety (Lader and Wing, 1966; Glickstein, 1957). One study used 24-hour ambulatory monitoring of EKG and reported positive correlations through the day between stress and increased heart rate (Roth et al., 1976). Similarly, patients with neurocirculatory asthenia, a condition that overlaps various categories of anxiety disorder, had significantly more tachycardia and arrhythmias during routine activities and sleep than did normal subjects (Tzivoni et al., 1980).

A second, fairly consistent finding about cardiac function is that anxious patients show less heart rate deceleration immediately after a stressful stimulus (Hart, 1974). Because parasympathetic innervation to the sinus node is responsible for slowing heart rate, this finding may indicate lessened vagal tone.

Anxious patients appear more aware of their heartbeats than normal controls (Tyrer et al., 1980). Schandry (1981) concluded, "in the light of the present data, it seems that higher self-reported anxiety is due to higher perception of physiological processes rather than to actual level of autonomic arousal" (487).

The use of sophisticated computer analyses increases the possibility of detecting subtle cardiac abnormalities. For example, Montgomery (1977) had groups of highly anxious and minimally anxious male college students perform a problem-solving test under stressful and nonstressful conditions. Although average heart rate did not discriminate the two groups or the two conditions, an analysis of second-by-second changes in cardiac rate revealed that greater heart rate variability was a sensitive index of anxiety level. Grayson and colleagues (1980) studied second-by-second heart rate changes in patients meeting research criteria for obsessive-compulsive disorder and found that different forms of stress provoked specific patterns of heart rate variability. Quantitative analysis of cardiac beat-to-beat fluctuations may be the most sensitive physiological tool for determining the reactions of the sympathetic, parasympathetic, and renin-angiotensin systems (Akselrod et al., 1981). Although anxiety disorder is often considered a state of increased sympathetic tone, the findings of impaired cardiac deceleration following stressful stimuli and of greater beat-to-beat fluctuation implicate the parasympathetic system.

Peripheral Blood Flow

During stress, peripheral blood flow is preferentially shunted toward the muscle beds at the expense of skin, kidney, and splanchnic circulation. Finger pulse volume, essentially measuring skin flow, declines, while forearm or leg blood flow, measuring muscle perfusion, increases. The tone of the peripheral vessels is controlled by both α- and β-adrenergic receptors. Hence, clues about the autonomic nervous system during anxiety can be gleaned from patterns of peripheral blood flow.

Bloom and colleagues (1976) reported decreased finger volume to be very sensitive to levels of experimentally induced anxiety. By the same technique, Knight and Borden (1979) found highly anxious patients more vasoconstricted than normal subjects immediately prior to public speaking. Studying forearm blood flow, on the other hand, Kelly consistently found more vasodilation in anxious patients than in normal controls at rest, during mental arithmetic tests, and during sodium lactate–induced panics (Kelly, 1966; Kelly et al., 1971).

One could speculate that during anxiety—or in anxious patients even at rest—there is increased α-adrenergic tone to peripheral vessels in the skin and splanchnic beds, causing vasoconstriction there and a reciprocal vasodilation in the muscle beds. Orthostatic stress testing of these patients, a method of provoking α-adrenergic response, could help to clarify this.

Electrodermal Response

Electrodermal response has been studied for decades as a measure of autonomic arousal in anxious patients. In general, this parameter has three main versions: tonic level, spontaneous fluctuation, and stimulus-provoked response.

Skin conductance level (SCL) is a tonic parameter of electrodermal response. With increased sweating, SCL increases, thus providing a general and relatively nonspecific marker of arousal. SCL has generally been found higher in anxious patients than in normal controls. Bond and colleagues (1974) found a mean conductance level of 13.5 for patients during a passive test, compared with 8.0 for normal subjects. Connolly (1979) demonstrated that SCL becomes systematically higher when subjects are exposed to an individualized phobic stimulus.

Examination of an SCL record, with the patient in a resting state, reveals a varying number of spontaneous fluctuations above baseline. A greater number of spontaneous fluctuations implies more autonomic instability. In 1932, Odegaard noted that highly anxious patients gave very active and unstable SCL records; Solomon and Fentress (1934) made a similar finding. During the passive task experiment by Bond and colleagues (1974), chronic anxious patients had an average of 4.8 skin conductance fluctuations per minute compared with 3.5/min for normal subjects, a significant difference. Chattopadhyay and associates (1980) did a similar study in which 12 anxious patients showed an average of 5.3 fluctuations/min compared with only 1.0/min for a group of normal subjects. Toone et al. (1981) also found a greater number of spontaneous fluctuations in both "anxiety state" patients and schizophrenic patients than in normal subjects during a sensory stimulation test.

When presented with a novel or stressful stimulus, all subjects show an increase in SCL called skin conductance response. With repeated presentation of the same stimulus, the skin conductance response diminishes, a phenomenon called habituation. Patients with anxiety disorder appear to habituate more slowly than normal subjects. In perhaps the most elegant examination of this process, Lader (1967) divided 90 patients with anxiety disorder into five groups: (1) anxiety with depression, (2) anxiety state, (3) agoraphobia, (4) social phobia, and (5) simple phobia. The five groups were not discriminated on the basis of panic attacks, and about two-thirds of the patients in each group had weekly "panic attacks." The 90 anxious patients were compared with 75 normal volunteers. Subjects were administered twenty consecutive auditory stimuli, and SCL was recorded. Lader used a complex scoring system for habituation, dividing subjects into "habituators" and "nonhabituators." Habituators were equally common among patients in the first four groups of anxious patients, and a sharp difference appeared between these four groups and both the fifth anxious group (simple phobia) and the normal group (these latter two groups had significantly more habituators). Furthermore, the results showed a significant correlation (r = .49) between habituation rate before behavioral desensitization treatment and positive clinical outcome after treatment (p < .01) (Lader et al., 1967). An important feature of this study was its use of diagnostic subgroups of anxiety disorder, clearly indicating that not all anxiety-disordered patients react alike.

The physiological basis behind electrodermal response has only recently been addressed. The autonomic innervation to sweat glands involves sympathetic nerves with acetylcholine as the neurotransmitter, a unique situation. By giving intradermal injections of carbachol to anxious patients and normal controls, Iskandar et al. found that a greater number of sweat glands were capable of being stimulated in anxious

Table 1. Physiological Abnormalities in Anxious Patients

Parameters	Findings
Cardiac function	Increased basal rate
	Decreased deceleration after stress
	Increased beat-to-beat fluctuation
	Increased cardiac awareness
Peripheral blood flow	Increased muscle flow
	Decreased skin, renal, splanchnic flow
Electrodermal response	Increased skin conductance level
	Increased spontaneous fluctuation
	Decreased habituation rate

patients than in the normal group (Iskandar et al., 1980). This suggests that anxious patients have a primary hypersensitivity to parasympathetic agonists.

A major criticism of the physiological experiments reviewed so far is the paucity of hypothesis-testing research. Table 1 summarizes the findings in these areas. While the results show fair agreement that heart rate is higher in anxious patients, finger pulse volume diminished, skin conductance higher, and so forth, only recently have investigators speculated on the specific reasons for these findings. Although sympathetic overstimulation has long been assumed, many of the findings suggest diffuse parasympathetic abnormalities. More detailed study is clearly needed.

NEUROTRANSMITTERS IN ANXIETY

Central Noradrenergic Effects

A well-studied neurotransmitter system hypothesis of anxiety disorder links increased central noradrenergic turnover and increased locus coeruleus discharge to the generation of human anxiety. The locus coeruleus, located in the pons, contains approximately 50 percent of the brain's noradrenergic neurons and sends fibers to a wide area of the brain, including the cerebral cortex, hippocampus, amygdala, septum, and hypothalamus (Grant and Redmond, 1981).

Redmond conducted a series of experiments in which electrical stimulation of primate locus coeruleus produced fear reactions indistinguishable from human anxiety (Redmond, 1977). Furthermore, surgical ablation of the locus coeruleus made the animals appear indifferent to stressful stimuli.

Drugs known to decrease locus coeruleus firing and to diminish central noradrenergic turnover in animals—clonidine, morphine, diazepam, and propranolol—decrease anxious behavior in animals (Redmond, 1979). In human beings, clonidine reliably blocks the signs and symptoms of the opiate withdrawal syndrome (Gold et al., 1979), a condition that somewhat resembles acute anxiety. However, clonidine has only partial and transient efficacy in blocking the spontaneous panic attacks of patients with panic disorder (Liebowitz et al., 1981). Tricyclic antidepressants, such as imipramine, which are highly effective in blocking spontaneous panic attacks, appear to curtail locus coeruleus firing (Nyback et al., 1975), although this is not yet certain.

The benzodiazepines decrease central noradrenergic turnover and locus coeruleus firing in rats (Grant et al., 1980). However, the relationship between the locus coeruleus and the recently discovered benzodiazepine receptor has yet to be elucidated.

Drugs known to provoke anxiety reactions in human subjects, such as piperoxane and yohimbine, clearly cause increased noradrenergic turnover in rats (Redmond, 1979).

Another strategy for measuring central noradrenergic turnover and locus coeruleus activity involves measurement of 3-methoxy-4-hydroxyphenylglycol (MHPG) in plasma and urine. Levels of MHPG, a major noradrenergic metabolite, may reflect central as opposed to peripheral noradrenergic activity, although this remains controversial (Elsworth et al., 1982). Only a few studies of MHPG level in anxiety have been performed to date. Working with 24 depressed female patients, Sweeney et al. (1978) found a high correlation ($r = .71$) between urinary MHPG level and state anxiety ($p < .001$).* Beckman and Goodwin (1980) observed a similar relationship. Most recently, Ko and colleagues (1983) suggested that an increase in plasma MHPG can be provoked in agoraphobic patients exposed to phobic stimuli.

Other Neurotransmitters

Other neurotransmitter systems studied in patients with anxiety include the dopamine, peptide, histamine, choline, and adenosine systems. Hoehn-Saric (1982) reviewed the field and suggested a role for the serotonergic system in anxiety generation. In monkeys the locus coeruleus contains serotonergic as well as noradrenergic nuclei (Mason and Fibiger, 1979). (The role of the GABA'ergic system, linked to the benzodiazepine receptor, is discussed elsewhere in this volume.)**

Catecholamine Levels

While central increases in noradrenaline turnover may play a key role in anxiety generation, most investigations find that peripheral increases in adrenaline, rather than noradrenaline, accompany anxiety states. In reviewing this work, Frankenhaeuser (1971) commented, "Situations characterized by novelty, uncertainty and change usually produce a rise in adrenaline secretion, the magnitude of which is closely related to the intensity of the subjective stress reactions evoked by the stimulating condition" (257). Dimsdale and Moss (1980) collected plasma catechol-

*Editor's note: In Part V of *Psychiatry Update: Volume II*, Dr. Joseph J. Schildkraut and his colleagues review their findings regarding urinary MHPG levels and depression (pages 457–471), and they also report on a study of patients with moderate to severe anxiety states (page 463)
**Editor's note: See the following chapter by Paul and Skolnick.

amines through an indwelling ambulatory catheter to permit sampling during natural stress. This method contends with problems raised by the rapid secretion and short plasma half-life of the catecholamines. The study found that public speaking more than doubled adrenaline levels (from 117 pg/ml to 336 pg/ml), while plasma noradrenaline levels increased by only 50 percent (from 583 pg/ml to 919 pg/ml). The exact reverse occurred during physical exercise.

Matthew and his group (1980) studied peripheral catecholamine levels in anxious patients. They found that patients with generalized anxiety disorder had higher pretreatment plasma levels of adrenaline (56.42 pg/ml) and noradrenaline (514.50 pg/ml) than normal controls (26.86 pg/ml and 232.26 pg/ml respectively). Biofeedback treatment of the patients with generalized anxiety disorder led to significant reductions in plasma adrenaline (from 56.42 pg/ml to 39.0 pg/ml) and noradrenaline (from 514.50 pg/ml to 402.71 pg/ml); but no such reductions were found in normal controls given the same treatment. However, these investigators made no correlations between catecholamine level and degree of anxiety either pre- or posttreatment.

The peripheral catecholamine data is obviously conflicting, some studies showing an increase in both noradrenaline and adrenaline and most in adrenaline alone. Although this inconsistency in findings could be due to differences in collection methods and assay, it is almost certainly due to differences in the diagnostic categories under study.

Monoamine Oxidase Levels

Another strategy for assessing neurotransmitter status by peripheral measurement is to assay platelet monoamine oxidase (MAO) levels. Matthew and his group (1981) studied twenty patients with generalized anxiety disorder and an equal number of normal subjects before and after biofeedback treatments. Mean platelet MAO level for the patients was 9.42 (mMoles/4 $\times 10^8$ plts/hr) compared with 6.94 for controls before treatment; the level in the patient group fell significantly after treatment to 7.66, while the normal group showed no significant posttreatment decrease. Similarly, Davidson and colleagues (1980) found consistently higher platelet MAO levels in patients with depression secondary to anxiety than in patients with primary depression. In another study, MAO levels were higher in agoraphobic patients than in normal subjects (Yu et al., 1982). Table 2 summarizes some of the work in the area of neurotransmitters.

Table 2.   Neurotransmitter Abnormalities in Anxious Patients

Levels Measured	Findings
Central noradrenaline	Increased turnover
Central serotonin	Increased activity
Plasma and urinary MHPG	Increased
Plasma adrenaline	Increased
Plasma noradrenaline	Possibly increased
Platelet MAO	Increased

PROVOCATIVE TESTS

A variety of pharmacologic agents routinely provoke anxiety in human subjects. Many of these are autonomic nervous system agonists, affecting the β-adrenergic system (e.g., epinephrine and isoproterenol), the α-adrenergic system (e.g., yohimbine), or the parasympathetic system (e.g., mecholyl and physostigmine). In preliminary trials in the laboratory of the author's group, carbon dioxide appears to be a specific provocative agent for panic attacks in patients with a history of panic disorder. Sodium lactate is the most clearly specific of the provocative agents, inducing panic attacks in most subjects with panic disorder but rarely in normal controls. The author and his colleagues have found that this effect is blocked by chronic imipramine treatment (Rifkin et al., 1981). Table 3 summarizes the actions of these different agents.

Table 3. Responses to Provocative Agents

Agents	Responses
β-Adrenergic Agents	
Epinephrine	Anxiety reaction, possibly specific to patients with anxiety disorder
Isoproterenol	May provoke anxiety attacks in patients, but not in normal subjects
α-Adrenergic Agents	
Yohimbine	Anxiety, specificity questionable
Cholinergic Agents	
Mecholyl	Anxiety in phobic patients
Physostigmine	Anxiety, specificity unknown
Hyperventilation	
Room air hyperventilation	Occasional panic
Carbon dioxide	Panic attacks, possibly specific to panic disorder patients
Sodium lactate	Panic attacks, probably specific to panic disorder patients

β-Adrenergic Agents

Because patients undergoing anxiety attacks exhibit many features partially mediated by β-adrenergic function—tachycardia, tremulousness, sweating—investigators administer β-adrenergic agonists to provoke anxiety. One investigator went so far as to conclude, "β-Adrenergic agonists (epinephrine, isoproterenol) or metabolic products of their action (lactate) will reliably produce (with dose qualification) anxiety symptoms and anxiety attacks in susceptible subjects (anxiety neurotics) but not in matched normal controls" (Pitts and Allen, 1982, 145). In a series of studies done in the 1930s by Lindemann and Finesinger (1938;

1940), epinephrine was administered to a group of patients who would likely be classified today as panic disorder patients. The investigators found that such patients had a specific anxiety response to epinephrine. Basowitz and associates (1956) injected epinephrine in normal volunteers and concluded, "There is a correspondence of psychological and somatic changes perceived by each subject under epinephrine with those singularly typical of this reaction in previous situations of anxiety"(104). Frankenhaeuser and Jarpe (1962), disputing the specificity of epinephrine, have stated, "The emotional reactions appeared to be of the 'as-if' type, i.e., the subjects feeling *as if* they were afraid, anxious, etc., rather than experiencing the genuine emotions" (28).

The issue remains clouded whether epinephrine specifically produces anxiety in patients with anxiety disorder, thereby presumably interacting with abnormally sensitive β-receptors, or if it is a nonspecific agent capable of making anyone anxious.

While epinephrine has weak α-adrenergic stimulating effects in addition to its predominant β-agonist action, isoproterenol is a pure β-adrenergic stimulant. There is some evidence that patients with anxiety disorder may be more sensitive to the effects of isoproterenol than normals. The use of isoproterenol as a provocative agent was begun by Frohlich and colleagues (1969), who studied a group of patients with a condition called hyperdynamic β-adrenergic circulatory state. The patients were primarily young patients and had increased left ventricular ejection rates (but not necessarily increased heart rate), occasional systolic hypertension, often a systolic ejection-type murmur, and bounding arterial pulse. The syndrome has reportedly been successfully treated with propranolol. During intravenous infusion of isoproterenol, patients with this syndrome experienced increased cardiac awareness, exaggerated pulse response, and "emotional outbursts" that may resemble panic attacks. Normal controls had none of these reactions at the doses of isoproterenol used. A small group of patients presenting to an emergency room in the midst of acute anxiety attacks proved to experience these attacks during isoproterenol infusion (Easton and Sherman, 1976) and to experience long-term relief from propranolol. A strain of "congenitally nervous pointer dogs" also showed hypersensitivity to intravenous isoproterenol (Newton et al., 1978). Most recently, Schmidt and Elizabeth (1982) induced anxiety and tachycardia in patients with panic disorder, but not in normal controls, with isoproterenol.

None of the isoproterenol infusions were conducted under double-blind conditions. Also, despite the fact that intravenously infused isoproterenol produces CNS effects (Goldstein and Munoz, 1961), the extent to which the drug crosses the human blood-brain barrier has never been clarified. Therefore, isoproterenol, like epinephrine, may act as a nonspecific stressor or may produce CNS effects by altering blood flow to the cerebral cortex, not by interacting with central receptors.

α-Adrenergic Agents

The only drug influencing the α-adrenergic system studied systematically in the provocation of anxiety is yohimbine. This α2-antagonist binds to the α-adrenergic autoreceptor, increasing the amount of neurotransmitter secreted by the presynaptic neuron. Yohimbine clearly increases central noradrenergic turnover and acts as a stimulant to locus coeruleus discharge.

In two well-designed studies, intravenous administration of yohimbine produced a clear-cut anxiety syndrome (Holmberg and Gershon, 1961; Garfield et al., 1967). In the first of these, 15 schizophrenics, 20 "mental hospital patients with mixed diagnoses," and 9 normal volunteers were given 0.5 mg/kg yohimbine over five minutes. The drug produced anxiety and autonomic arousal in the subjects that correlated with baseline levels of anxiety, regardless of diagnosis. Hence, the most anxious patients responded with the most anxiety to yohimbine. In the second study, 12 psychiatric patients received separate intravenous infusions of yohimbine, epinephrine, and saline. The authors reported that the yohimbine-induced state resembled clinical anxiety more than the epinephrine-induced state.

One might conclude from these studies that yohimbine, interacting with locus coeruleus function and increasing central noradrenergic turnover, represents a good pharmacologic model for human anxiety. However, in the studies described, imipramine potentiated the anxiogenic effects of yohimbine. Because imipramine is the most consistent antipanic drug yet discovered (for both spontaneous and lactate-induced panics), the fact that yohimbine-induced anxiety is worsened by imipramine casts doubt on the possibility that the yohimbine-induced state actually resembles spontaneously occurring panics.

Nevertheless, some trials of yohimbine infusion in patients with specific anxiety disorders might prove interesting. A study administering an α_1-antagonist, such as prazosin, ought to be considered.

Cholinergic Agents

As discussed earlier, the assumption that anxious patients are uniformly in a state of sympathetic hyperactivity is debatable. Unfortunately, pharmacologic investigation of the parasympathetic nervous system has been neglected.

Lindemann and Finesinger (1938) found that the parasympathetic agonist mecholyl produced anxiety in patients with histories of "definite phobias and concrete fears" (363). Doryl, another parasympathetic agonist, did not produce anxiety in normal volunteers in another study (Dynes and Tod, 1940).

Janowsky and colleagues (1982) administered physostigmine, the acetylcholinesterase inhibitor, to forty psychiatric inpatients pretreated with methscopolamine. Methscopolamine blocks the peripheral cholinergic receptors so that enhancement of acetylcholine levels by physostigmine occurs centrally only. According to Janowsky et al., the patients routinely experienced anxiety. The congenitally nervous pointer dogs mentioned earlier are said to be "parasympathetically dominated" (Reese, 1979). Some symptoms of clinical anxiety, such as nausea, vomiting, and diarrhea, are under parasympathetic control. Gellhorn and Loofbourrow (1963) concluded, "It follows . . . that emotional excitement of this type which in man we designate as fear, anger, and rage, elicits both sympathetic and parasympathetic discharges" (70–71).

Hyperventilation

Many patients complain of dyspnea and rapid breathing during anxiety attacks. Sighing respirations have been routinely noted in anxious patients. Some researchers assume that hyperventilation, by inducing respiratory alkalosis, causes panic attacks (Lum, 1975), while others assume that hyperventilation is merely a consequence of the CNS events that begin an anxiety attack (Missri and Alexander, 1978). Very few studies have been conducted in which anxious patients are shown to have panic attacks after being instructed to hyperventilate (Van Dis, 1978). The fact that the common practice of having an anxious patient breathe into a paper bag often aborts the attack by reversing hypocapnia does not prove that respiratory alkalosis caused the anxiety in the first place. All this procedure may be demonstrating is that correction of one outcome of a panic attack is sufficient to arrest the ongoing process.

To explore this issue further, the author's group designed an experiment in which patients with anxiety and normal volunteers were placed in a clear plastic head canopy and shut off from outside air, so that the composition of inspired gases could be exquisitely controlled. After a baseline period of breathing room air, the subjects were given a mixture of 5 percent carbon dioxide in room air to breathe for 20 minutes or until an anxiety attack occurred. Although this amount of carbon dioxide approximately tripled minute ventilation, alkalosis did not develop because of the continuous addition of carbon dioxide. In fact, most subjects became very slightly acidotic due to the buildup of carbon dioxide. After another baseline period of breathing room air, the subjects then hyperventilated room air at about 30 breaths per minute for 15 minutes, or until they became too fatigued to continue, or until a panic attack occurred. Under this condition respiratory alkalosis rapidly occurred in all subjects.

If hyperventilation produces anxiety attacks by the induction of respiratory alkalosis, most patients with panic disorder would be expected to have panic attacks during the room-air hyperventilation phase of the experiment. The carbon dioxide challenge phase would then serve as a control situation to rule out the possibility that simply the suggestive effect of the setting, in addition to breathing fast, could provoke a panic attack.

To the surprise of the author's group, 7 of 13 panic disorder patients had anxiety attacks during the carbon dioxide challenge phase, but only 3 of 13 during the room-air hyperventilation phase. Four normal controls did not have panic attacks under either condition (Gorman et al., 1983b).

These results were difficult to interpret until the author's group learned from Svensson that carbon dioxide inhalation, starting at just 3 percent in room air, provokes dose-dependent increases in rat locus coeruleus discharge (Elam et al., 1981). This suggests that carbon dioxide inhalation may be a specific provocative test for panic disorder. Whether imipramine will block the carbon dioxide–induced panic as it does the lactate-induced panic is still unknown.

Sodium Lactate Infusion

Cohen and associates (1947) noted that patients with neurocirculatory asthenia, who experienced anxiety attacks during or immediately after vigorous physical exercise, developed higher levels of blood lactate than normal controls while walking or running. Although this could simply have been due to differences in physical conditioning, this finding stimulated Pitts and McClure (1967) to administer intravenous sodium

Table 4.	Responses to Sodium Lactate Infusion	
	Panic	*No Panic*
Panic disorder patients	31	12
Normal controls	0	20

$\chi^2 = 31.00$; $p \le .001$

lactate to patients with anxiety neurosis, postulating that high levels of blood lactate may provoke panic in susceptible patients. Indeed, sodium lactate produced panic attacks typical of the patients' naturally occurring panic attacks, while normal controls did not experience panic. This finding has been well replicated under double-blind conditions (Fink et al., 1970; Kelly et al., 1971).

It is now a widely accepted fact that intravenous racemic sodium lactate administered in doses of 10 ml/kg of 0.5 molar lactate over twenty minutes provokes panic in a majority of patients who have panic disorder or agoraphobia with panic attacks, but rarely in normal controls. Table 4 shows the results of sodium lactate infusions in the laboratory of the author's group (Michael R. Liebowitz, personal communication, 1983).

Of great interest are theories that attempt to explain why lactate provokes panic in susceptible patients. One set of hypotheses asserts that some aspects of the metabolic conversion of lactate provokes the attack. Lactate is metabolized to pyruvate, some of which enters the tricarboxylic acid cycle and is ultimately transformed into bicarbonate. Although Pitts (1971) believed that the production of alkalosis by the increase in bicarbonate might be responsible for panic, the finding of the author's group that those patients who become extremely alkalotic during hyperventilation trials do not panic argues against this idea. An extensive search for the possible metabolic product of lactate responsible for panic is now underway in the laboratories of the author's group and others.

Another hypothesis involves the fact that lactate infusion results in a reduction of serum ionized calcium, which may produce neuromuscular irritability. Support for this theory came from the finding that the addition of calcium carbonate to lactate reduced the severity of panic in patients previously shown to be sensitive to lactate alone (Pitts and Allen, 1979). On the other hand, Pitts and Allen (1979) reported giving panic disorder patients infusions of the powerful calcium chelator EDTA almost to the point of producing frank tetany, but no panic attacks occurred. Also, the author's group has infused D-lactate, which is metabolically inert but capable of lowering ionized calcium levels as vigorously as L-lactate. D-lactate in preliminary trials is not panicogenic. This also casts doubt on the hypocalcemia theory.

A final hypothesis, also promoted by Pitts, holds that lactate interacts with hyperactive β-adrenergic receptors (Pitts and Allen, 1982). However, pretreatment with intravenous propranolol immediately prior to lactate infusion failed to abort panic in six patients previously shown to have the capacity to panic during lactate infusion (Gorman et al., 1983a).

Increased levels of carbon dioxide and increased levels of lactate are both indicators of a relative oxygen deficit. The author and his colleagues have speculated that the various forms of panic-attack provocation may trigger an anoxia detector that is hypersensitive in panic disorder patients, creating a perceived need to flee. A panic attack is then an adaptive mechanism gone awry.

The question, Why does sodium lactate produce panic? will involve several laboratories in coming years.

MITRAL VALVE PROLAPSE

The finding that patients with panic disorder and agoraphobia have a high incidence of mitral valve prolapse (MVP), originally thought just an odd quirk of nature, may provide clues to the biology of anxiety. Because MVP is transmitted genetically and appears to be part of a syndrome involving autonomic nervous system dysfunction, understanding why it occurs in so many patients with anxiety disorder may be of great importance.

The Association Between MVP and Panic

DaCosta first hinted at an association between a specific cardiac lesion and anxiety disorder in 1871 when he described a syndrome characterized by attacks of chest pain, palpitations, headache, and "giddiness," along with the physical finding of an unusual systolic murmur which was difficult to characterize. In 1919, Lewis reported virtually the same condition as "the soldier's heart and effort syndrome," and said it occurred mostly in "nervous people." In fact, Wood in 1941 considered DaCosta's syndrome, or soldier's heart, to be a cardiac disease specifically associated with psychiatric disturbance. In 1972, Cohen and White renamed the same condition "neurocirculatory asthenia."

Wooley argued convincingly that all of these disorders, from DaCosta's syndrome to neurocirculatory asthenia, actually describe MVP (Wooley, 1976). In the late 1970s, Pariser and colleagues (1978) described several cases of patients who had spontaneous panic attacks and also had MVP. Since then, systematic studies have shown an incidence of MVP in patients with panic disorder or agoraphobia ranging from 39 percent to 50 percent (Grunhaus et al., 1982; Gorman et al., 1981c). Estimates of the incidence of MVP in the healthy, asymptomatic population range from 6 to 21 percent (Markiewicz et al., 1976; Brown et al., 1975; Darsee et al., 1979).

While MVP clearly seems to be more prevalent among patients with panic disorder, the reverse is not the case. Kane et al. (1981) failed to find a higher incidence of panic attacks in patients with documented MVP than in patients referred for echocardiogram who had negative cardiac findings. Similarly, Hartman and colleagues (1982) studied a group of first-degree relatives of patients with MVP referred to cardiologists. The incidence of panic attacks in the first-degree relatives with MVP only approximated that of the general population.

At first, it was assumed that patients with panic disorder and MVP have panic attacks caused by the abnormal valve itself. However, although some patients with MVP do experience symptoms of palpitations, chest pain, and syncope (Devereux et al., 1976), most are asymptomatic. Furthermore, as Table 5 shows, there is actually poor overlap between symptoms commonly referable to MVP and the symptoms of a panic attack.

Table 5. Comparison of Symptoms: Mitral Valve
Prolapse and Panic Disorder

Symptoms	Mitral Valve Prolapse	Panic Disorder
Fatigue	+	–
Dyspnea	+	+ +
Palpitations	+ +	+ +
Chest pain	+ +	+
Syncope	+	–
Choking	–	+ +
Dizziness	–	+ +
Derealization	–	+ +
Paresthesias	–	+ +
Hot/cold flashes	–	+ +
Sweating	–	+ +
Fainting	–	+ +
Trembling	–	+ +
Fear of dying, going crazy, losing control	–	+ +

Key: + + = symptom often present
+ = symptom occasionally present
– = symptom rarely present

. Further refuting the idea that MVP is sufficient to cause panic are four additional findings. (1) Patients with panic disorder and MVP respond to sodium lactate infusion with panic attacks at the same rate and in the same fashion as do panic patients who do not have MVP (Gorman et al., 1981b). (2) Patients with both MVP and panic disorder respond to imipramine with alleviation of panic attacks in exactly the way that patients with panic disorder alone respond (Gorman et al., 1981c). (3) In a group of patients with panic disorder and MVP, imipramine treatment led to complete clinical remission of panic attacks, but repeat echocardiograms after successful treatment proved that each patient still had MVP (Gorman et al., 1981a). (4) A family study of 50 probands with MVP showed that panic attacks and MVP segregate independently (Crowe et al., 1982), a finding opposite to what would be expected if prolapsed mitral valves caused panic attacks.*

MVP as an Autonomic Illness

An interesting aspect of the association between MVP and panic disorder is the possibility that both MVP and panic disorder are part of a general syndrome involving primary autonomic nervous system dysfunction. Evidence that MVP patients have autonomic nervous system abnormalities comes from numerous studies. Boudoulas and colleagues (1979) collected 24-hour urinary epinephrine and norepinephrine levels and plasma total catecholamine levels from 18 symptomatic MVP patients and found them to have higher adrenergic tone than a group of

*Editor's note: In his chapter, Crowe reviews these findings further and explores several other possible genetic effects in panic disorder.

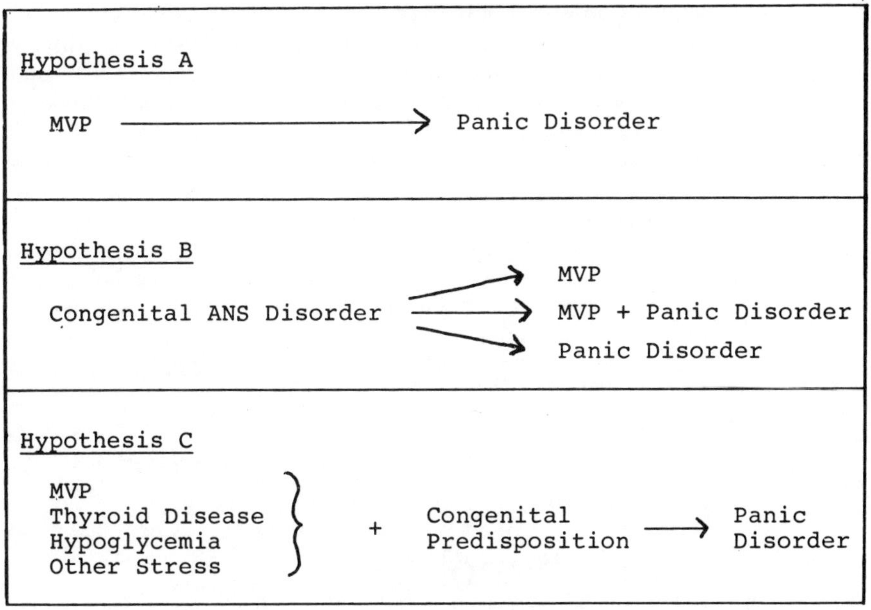

Figure 1. Three current hypotheses for understanding the relationship between mitral valve prolapse and panic disorder

normal subjects. Similarly, Gaffney and associates (1979) studied 19 women with MVP and 16 healthy female controls with the diving reflex, phenylephrine infusion, and the lower body negative pressure test. Measurements of cardiac output, heart rate, blood pressure, and forearm blood flow were made during each procedure. The results indicated decreased parasympathetic, increased α-adrenergic, and normal β-adrenergic tone and responsiveness in the patients. Gaffney has also shown that some patients with MVP have abnormal responses to orthostatic stress (F. Andrew Gaffney, personal communication, 1983), while orthostatic hypotension has been implicated as the "cause" of some symptoms of mitral valve prolapse (Santos et al., 1981).

Coghlan and colleagues (1979) administered standard Valsalva maneuver tests and a postural test to 44 patients with MVP and 15 normal controls, measuring blood pressure, heart rate, and respiratory rate. Clear dysfunctional responses were found in the patients, postulated by the group to represent abnormal central modulation of baroreflexes. Neuroendocrine and cardiovascular tests of 20 symptomatic patients with MVP showed higher 24-hour urinary total catecholamine levels and shorter electromechanical systole in the patients, the latter also a measure of increased adrenergic tone (Boudoulas et al., 1980). Finally, Pasternac and associates in two studies found increases in both urinary and plasma catecholamines in patients with MVP (Pasternac et al., 1979; 1982).

Figure 1 schematically outlines three possible explanations for the high incidence of MVP in panic disorder patients. Hypothesis A, that MVP causes panic, seems unlikely in view of the treatment, sodium lactate, and genetic data already described. Hypothesis B contends that both MVP and panic disorder are part of a general and probably congenital syndrome of ANS dysfunction. Patients would theoretically inherit MVP or panic disorder or both. Hypothesis C postulates that MVP may be one of a number of autonomic stressors capable of interacting with a genetic predisposition to panic disorder. Other such stressors may include thyroid disease, hypoglycemia, or life-threatening events. While this hypothesis would appear the most likely, no definitive data exist. A fourth possibility, which the author's group considers remote, is that panic attacks, by inducing repetitive bouts of tachycardia, actually cause MVP.

This survey has touched upon some of the psychobiological aspects of anxiety that are currently under investigation. Significant advances in diagnosis and in biochemical and physiological technology have recently enhanced our ability to uncover the basic mechanisms of the pathological anxieties. From the knowledge we are now beginning to acquire, more specific and rational treatments should emerge.

Chapter 34

The Biochemistry of Anxiety: From Pharmacotherapy to Pathophysiology

Steven M. Paul, M.D. and Phil Skolnick, Ph.D.

INTRODUCTION

Anxiety is a broad behavioral concept related to fear, but it is usually distinguished from fear by the unconscious nature of the precipitating stimulus. The precise definition of anxiety often depends upon both the theoretical and practical context in which it is being considered. Anxiety, like fear, is a normal component of human emotion with adaptive and perhaps even evolutionary significance. On the other hand, anxiety can become incapacitating and thus maladaptive to the overall functioning of the organism.

To the psychiatrist, anxiety is a common presenting symptom that is associated with many neurotic states, as well as with depression and schizophrenia. In certain patients, however, anxiety is the primary symptom, and many of these individuals are subsequently diagnosed under current nosology (American Psychiatric Association, 1980) as suffering from an anxiety disorder. This classification scheme undoubtedly includes a variety of heterogeneous clinical states, such as simple phobias, agoraphobia with or without panic attacks, obsessive-compulsive disorders, and generalized anxiety disorders. The underlying pathophysiology of these clinical states may or may not be related. Therefore, when studying the possible neurobiological mechanism(s) of anxiety, it is important to distinguish between "normal" and "pathological" anxiety. In some cases, the pathological state may simply result from a quantitative extension of the normal state (e.g., the continuum from normal anxiety to a generalized anxiety disorder), while other conditions (e.g., agoraphobia and panic) may represent qualitatively unique behavioral states that are typically not seen in healthy individuals.

Evidence that the various anxiety disorders may in fact represent separate and distinct clinical entities (with their own etiologic and pathophysiological factors) derives from several sources, including recent genetic and epidemiologic studies (Carey and Gottesman, 1981). The most impressive evidence, however, is the differential sensitivity of these disorders to pharmacologic intervention. While the benzodiazepines are found more effective in the treatment of generalized anxiety disorders (Greenblatt and Shader, 1974), tricyclic antidepressants and monoamine oxidase inhibitors are shown to be more effective in the treatment of agoraphobia with or without panic attacks (Klein, 1964; Sheehan, 1982). These observations support the contention that the underlying disturbances in the particular disorders lie in different neurochemical systems. Thus, an understanding of the specific neurochemical and neurophysiological mechanism(s) of action of the various antianxiety drugs could provide some insight into the biochemical bases of anxiety. Such studies, while still in their infancy, have proven useful, and several testable biochemical hypotheses have emerged over the past few years.

Perhaps the single most important factor contributing to the rapid advances in this area is the recent progress in unraveling the molecular mechanism(s) of action of the major class of anxiolytic drugs, the benzodiazepines (for review, see Skolnick and Paul, 1982). Benzodiazepines are now known to produce their anxiolytic actions by first interacting with a specific neuronal protein (the benzodiazepine receptor) that is functionally associated with a recognition site (receptor) for the major inhibitory neurotransmitter in brain, γ-aminobutyric acid (GABA). Although the precise structural relationship between benzodiazepine and GABA receptors has not been established, it is almost certain that the benzodiazepine-GABA-receptor complex exists in association with other regulatory proteins, including the chloride channel or ionophore (Skolnick and Paul, 1982). In addition, strong evidence indicates that many chemically unrelated anxiolytics, including the barbiturates, propanediol carbamates, and ethanol,[1] may produce their anxiolytic actions (like the benzodiazepines) via an interaction with the benzodiazepine-GABA-receptor complex, and ultimately therefore through the enhancement of GABA-mediated chloride permeability. Furthermore, work over the past two years has revealed a number of novel high-affinity benzodiazepine-receptor ligands (Braestrup et al., 1980) that produce in animals and human beings behavioral effects which are essentially opposite to those of the benzodiazepines (Schweri et al., 1982; Braestrup et al., 1982). Several lines of evidence support the idea that these compounds produce an "anxiogenic" action (Ninan et al., 1982), thus suggesting that the benzodiazepine-GABA-receptor complex may be involved in the pathogenesis of anxiety.

BENZODIAZEPINES AS SELECTIVE ANXIOLYTICS

The most common drugs used in the treatment of anxiety are the benzodiazepines, and these compounds are still among the most com-

---

[1]Sedatives such as ethanol and barbiturates produce a variety of pharmacologic effects, and both ethanol and the barbiturates share at least some pharmacologic properties with the benzodiazepines (e.g., "anticonflict" actions in animals). There is now evidence that the anxiolytic actions of barbiturates and ethanol may be mediated via an indirect effect on the benzodiazepine-GABA-receptor complex (Skolnick and Paul, 1982; Paul et al., 1981). Nevertheless, the general sedative and anesthetic properties of the barbiturates and ethanol are probably not mediated through a specific benzodiazepine-GABA-receptor mechanism(s), since these agents produce a variety of membrane effects when administered at pharmacologically relevant concentrations.

monly prescribed of all medications (Tallman et al., 1980). Benzodiazepines have been shown to have "anxiolytic" actions in both animals and
human beings. In animals, benzodiazepines produce potent effects on
a variety of conditioned and unconditioned behaviors. In general, the
benzodiazepines are selective in "releasing" behaviors that are ordinarily suppressed by punishment (Geller and Seifter, 1960; Lippa et al., 1979).
In one such test, animals were deprived of food, water, or both, and
then given access to a sucrose solution delivered through an electrified
drinking spout. When hungry or thirsty rats were placed in this so-called
conflict situation, they generally responded to the punishment by not
eating or drinking. Thus, the number of shocks taken by the untreated
animals was relatively low. Animals given benzodiazepines, on the other
hand, increased their eating or drinking even during periods of punishment. A quantitative measure of the anticonflict activity of benzodiazepines is the increase in the number of shocks taken by the animal. The
conflict paradigm may represent a useful animal model of human anxiety since the clinical actions of benzodiazepines also appear to involve
a decrease in the behavioral and physiological (i.e., autonomic and endocrine) response to frustration, fear, and punishment. Furthermore, the
relative potencies of a large series of benzodiazepines in producing anticonflict actions in animals was highly correlated with their potencies
as anxiolytics in human subjects (Lippa et al., 1979).

The extent to which benzodiazepines are specific and selective as anticonflict agents in animals (and as anxiolytics in human beings) is important if an understanding of their neurochemical mechanisms of action is to yield important information about the underlying neurobiology
of anxiety. Several lines of evidence support the specificity of these drugs
as anticonflict and anxiolytic agents. First, benzodiazepines produce their
anticonflict effects in animals (as well as their anxiolytic effects in human beings) at doses well below those that produce sedation. In fact,
sedation will nonspecifically decrease both punished and nonpunished
responses in the conflict test and will therefore antagonize the observed
anticonflict actions of anxiolytic drugs. Furthermore, the tolerance which
has been shown to develop in regard to the sedative actions of benzodiazepines during chronic administration does not develop in regard to
either their anticonflict actions in animals (Stein et al., 1973) or their
anxiolytic actions in human beings (Greenblatt and Shader, 1974). Second, at anxiolytic doses benzodiazepines are devoid of any significant
antipsychotic or antidepressant activity, although they will frequently
reduce the symptoms of anxiety in schizophrenic or depressed patients
(Rickels, 1978). Third, a variety of psychotropic drugs including stimulants, antidepressants, antipsychotics, and opiates, have been tested as
anticonflict agents and have been found to be without significant activity at pharmacologically relevant doses. In addition, drugs which specifically block or enhance noradrenergic, dopaminergic, cholinergic, or
glycinergic neurotransmission fail to produce or alter anticonflict activity
in animals. Other drugs, however, which show cross-dependence with
the benzodiazepines, including the barbiturates, propanediol carbamates, and ethanol, produce anticonflict and anxiolytic actions in a variety of species, albeit at relatively high doses. The fact that benzodiazepines are effective anxiolytics at very low doses, many being active in

low microgram per kilogram doses in human subjects,[2] is especially significant since this separates them from the other minor tranquilizers and indirectly implies a very specific locus of action.

THE DISCOVERY OF BENZODIAZEPINE RECEPTORS

Early experimental evidence from both behavioral and electrophysiological studies supported a role for central GABA'ergic and serotonergic pathways in the pharmacologic actions of benzodiazepines (Koe, 1979). Nevertheless, until 1977 very little definitive data existed on the mechanism(s) of action of these drugs. In that year, two groups of investigators discovered high-affinity, saturable, and stereospecific binding sites for benzodiazepines in membranes derived from the CNS of a variety of species including human subjects (Squires and Braestrup, 1977; Mohler and Okada, 1977). These observations sparked a flurry of activity since for the first time they indicated a highly specific locus of action for these drugs in the brain. Furthermore, strong suggestion that these binding sites were indeed pharmacologic receptors came from the excellent correlations between the potencies of a large series of benzodiazepines in displacing ^{3}H-diazepam binding from these sites in vitro and their potencies as anticonflict agents in animals and as anxiolytics in human beings. We now know that the reversible binding of benzodiazepines to the benzodiazepine receptor initiates a cascade of neuronal events that results in the major pharmacologic (anxiolytic) actions of these drugs. Several of the critical biochemical steps following the binding of benzodiazepines to their receptor, such as regulation of chloride ion channel permeability, have also been delineated (Study and Barker, 1982).

Subsequent studies by many laboratories have confirmed and extended the initial findings on the importance of benzodiazepine receptors in mediating the pharmacologic actions of benzodiazepines. Several groups (e.g., Williamson et al., 1978) have also demonstrated the presence of benzodiazepine receptors using in vivo labeling techniques and have shown that the potencies of various benzodiazepines for displacing the specific binding of ^{3}H-diazepam or ^{3}H-flunitrazepam in vivo is also highly correlated with their behavioral and clinical potencies (Chang and Snyder, 1978). Using a variety of lesioning techniques, benzodiazepine receptors have been shown to be localized almost exclusively to neurons, and predominantly to areas of synaptic contact (Bosmann et al., 1978). Interestingly, although an excellent correlation exists between the occupation of benzodiazepine receptors by various benzodiazepines in vivo and their behavioral effects in animals, only about 25 percent of benzodiazepine receptors need be occupied to yield a complete pharmacologic effect (Paul et al., 1979). The physiological significance, if any, of "spare" receptors for the benzodiazepines is not yet clear. Nevertheless, small changes in receptor number or affinity may be physiologically relevant, such as the changes seen in the Maudsley reactive rat (Robertson et al., 1978) or following the development of "kindled" epileptogenic foci (McNamara et al., 1980).

Benzodiazepine receptors are widely distributed in brain, with the

[2]In human subjects, benzodiazepines such as the triazolobenzodiazepines, triazolam and alprazolam, are active at doses as low as 5 to 10 μg/kg!

highest densities being present in phylogenetically younger areas such as the cerebral cortex (Young and Kuhar, 1979). Subcortical areas such as the hippocampus and amygdala also contain relatively high densities of benzodiazepine receptors, while the phylogenetically older areas such as the pons and medulla have fewer receptors. However, in contrast to many other drug and neurotransmitter receptors, the relative difference in benzodiazepine-receptor density among various brain regions is relatively small and does not vary by more than an order of magnitude. This rather diffuse distribution of benzodiazepine receptors suggests that they may in fact regulate a number of neuronal events.

Several investigators have attempted to localize the anticonflict (anxiolytic) actions of benzodiazepines to a specific brain region. Preliminary results suggest that the local injection of benzodiazepines into the amygdala (Scheel-Kruger and Petersen, 1982), hippocampus, or midbrain raphe (Tallman et al., 1980) in rats can mimic the anticonflict effects of parenterally administered benzodiazepines. This approach will undoubtedly prove useful in delineating the neuroanatomical pathways which mediate the anticonflict actions of benzodiazepines in animals and hopefully define an analogous system in human beings. Since these studies further suggest that only a small population of benzodiazepine receptors are involved in the anxiolytic actions of the benzodiazepines, it seems reasonable to assume that a similar discrete population of receptors would be involved in the pathogenesis of anxiety.

BENZODIAZEPINE RECEPTORS AND GABA

Shortly after the discovery of benzodiazepine receptors, it was recognized that the affinity of the receptor for various benzodiazepines could be increased both in vitro and in vivo by the presence of GABA, the major inhibitory neurotransmitter in brain. This observation has now been confirmed by many laboratories and represents the first demonstration of a functional interaction between GABA and benzodiazepine receptors (Tallman et al., 1980). The finding also supports early electrophysiological and pharmacologic evidence that benzodiazepines selectively enhance the inhibitory effects of GABA on neuronal excitability (Haefely et al., 1975; Costa et al., 1975). It is now generally accepted that benzodiazepine receptors are functionally and structurally coupled to the GABA receptor, and that along with an associated chloride channel, they together form a "supramolecular receptor complex," whose ultimate function is to regulate the transport or permeability of chloride across neuronal membranes (Skolnick and Paul, 1981).

In the unstimulated state, neuronal membranes are relatively impermeable to chloride ions. However, when GABA activates its receptor, the chloride channel allows chloride ions to move more readily from the extracellular space to the inside of the neuron. The net effect of enhanced chloride permeability is to increase the negative potential across the neuronal membrane, making it less excitable (hyperpolarization). Thus, GABA inhibits neuronal excitability. When applied alone to neurons, benzodiazepines produce very little effect on chloride permeability (Study and Barker, 1982). In the presence of GABA, however, benzodiazepines markedly potentiate the GABA-stimulated increases in chloride permeability. This effect appears to be due to an increase in the frequency of GABA-mediated openings of chloride channels, not to an enhanced conductance of chloride by each channel.

Other sedative-hypnotic drugs may also produce their anxiolytic effects through the "benzodiazepine-GABA-receptor complex," although not by interacting directly with the recognition site for benzodiazepines (Skolnick et al., 1981; Olsen, 1981). Barbiturates, for example, appear to interact directly with a chloride channel coupled to benzodiazepine receptors, resulting in an increase in the time, rather than the frequency, of channel opening. In this way, barbiturates (like benzodiazepines) enhance GABA-mediated chloride permeability; but their direct, rather than allosteric, effects on chloride channels probably explain their far greater toxicity when compared with the benzodiazepines. The common action of benzodiazepines and barbiturates in enhancing GABA-mediated chloride permeability is also believed to explain the ability of these drugs to substitute for one another, both as anxiolytics and in the development of cross-dependence.

Over the past several years, a number of novel and chemically unrelated anxiolytics have been developed, and several have been shown to be relatively free of sedation at therapeutic doses. In virtually every instance, these drugs have been shown to interact with one or more sites on the benzodiazepine-GABA-receptor complex (Paul and Skolnick, 1982), which has accordingly been proposed as a common site of minor tranquilizer action (Paul et al., 1981). The benzodiazepine-GABA-receptor complex is a prime candidate for studies on the neurobiological bases of anxiety.

BENZODIAZEPINE RECEPTOR–MEDIATED "ANXIETY"

Although the evidence is overwhelming that the benzodiazepine-GABA-receptor complex mediates the anxiolytic actions of benzodiazepines and perhaps of most, if not all, minor tranquilizers, the possibility that this receptor is somehow involved in the pathogenesis of anxiety has until recently been only speculative (Paul and Skolnick, 1981). In 1980, during their attempts to isolate an endogenous ligand for the benzodiazepine receptor, Braestrup and colleagues (1980) isolated from human urine a novel high-affinity benzodiazepine-receptor ligand that was subsequently identified as β-carboline-3-carboxylic acid ethyl ester (β-CCE). Although initially believed to be naturally occurring, β-CCE has since been artifactually produced by a Pictet-Spengler condensation of tryptophan during the extraction process. Although β-CCE cannot therefore be considered an endogenous ligand, its extremely high affinity for the benzodiazepine receptor, coupled with its unique pharmacologic properties, have made it and chemically related β-carboline derivatives extremely valuable tools for studying the benzodiazepine receptor. Unlike benzodiazepines, β-CCE has no anticonvulsant or anticonflict activity in animals, but instead blocks the anticonvulsant, anticonflict, and sedative-hypnotic actions of benzodiazepines (Tenen and Hirsch, 1980; Cowen et al., 1981). These observations were the first indication that compounds such as β-CCE could be developed that would antagonize the pharmacologic properties of benzodiazepines. Since the initial discovery of β-CCE, recent discoveries have identified several other β-carboline derivatives, as well as novel benzodiazepines (e.g., Ro15-1788) and chemically unrelated compounds (e.g., CGS 8216), that antagonize all of the pharmacologic (including anxiolytic) actions of the benzodiazepines (Hunkeler et al., 1981; Czernik et al., 1982).

More recently, a rather surprising series of experiments demonstrated that several benzodiazepine-receptor antagonists, including β-CCE, have potent intrinsic pharmacologic properties of their own. Because of the rapid metabolism of β-CCE in rodents (Schweri et al., 1984), the behavioral effects of the β-carboline esters are less robust than in primates (Ninan et al., 1982) including human beings (Dorow et al., 1983). β-CCE, for example, when administered to rhesus monkeys produces dramatic behavioral effects which include piloerection and generalized "arousal." Higher doses of β-CCE result in behavioral "agitation" (struggling in the restraint chair), which is accompanied by marked autonomic and endocrine changes, including an immediate rise in heart rate and blood pressure. Activation of the hypothalamic-pituitary-adrenal axis also occurs following β-CCE administration. Plasma concentrations of adrenocorticotrophic hormone (ACTH), cortisol, and the catecholamines, epinephrine and norepinephrine, are all significantly increased following administration of β-CCE at doses as low as 100 μg/kg. That the effects of β-CCE are mediated via the benzodiazepine-receptor complex is supported by their complete blockade following pretreatment with benzodiazepines such as diazepam as well as the specific benzodiazepine-receptor antagonist Ro15-1788 (Ninan et al., 1982; Insel et al., 1984).

The behavioral, physiological, and endocrine effects of β-CCE in subhuman primates are reminiscent of those seen in extremely anxious patients and in animals or human subjects exposed to anxiety-provoking situations (Rose and Sachar, 1981). The reversal of β-CCE's effects by benzodiazepines supports the hypothesis that this syndrome may represent a reliable pharmacologic model of human anxiety. It is, however, impossible to demonstrate the presence or absence of anxiety in any animal other than the human being. Therefore, a key question is whether the β-CCE-induced syndrome is a valid model of anxiety—and, if so, what kind of anxiety?

Several lines of evidence support the validity of the "benzodiazepine-GABA-receptor model" of anxiety. For one, the symptoms of generalized anxiety disorders which were obtained from epidemiologic studies of anxious patients (American Psychiatric Association, 1980) are selectively ameliorated by benzodiazepines (see Table 1). Not coincidentally perhaps, the major pharmacologic properties of benzodiazepines (muscle relaxant, anxiolytic, and hypnotic) are essentially mirror images of the major symptoms reported by patients with generalized anxiety disorders. Furthermore, when Dorow and associates (1983) administered a β-carboline derivative chemically similar to β-CCE (FG 7142) to human volunteers, the subjects showed symptoms of motor tension, autonomic hyperactivity, and extreme apprehension. Subjectively, these effects were interpreted as being identical to severe anxiety, with "inner tension, excitation, and sensations of physical disturbance," and as in the monkey studies, the symptoms were accompanied by increases in blood pressure, heart rate, and plasma cortisol. In one subject, these symptoms were so severe that intravenous lormetazepam was administered; all symptoms were reported to subside within a few minutes.

SUMMARY AND CONCLUSIONS

The results of these behavioral and biochemical studies suggest that the benzodiazepine receptor recognizes at least three separate classes of drugs (see Figure 1). The first class includes compounds such as the benzodiazepines which facilitate GABA-mediated chloride conductance re-

Table 1. Effects of Benzodiazepine-Receptor Agonists and Antagonists on the Symptoms of Anxiety

DSM-III Criteria for Generalized Anxiety Disorder	Benzodiazepine Agonist Effects	Benzodiazepine Active Antagonist Effects
Motor Tension		
Shakiness, jitteriness, trembling	↓	↑
Muscle aches, tension	↓	↑
Fatigability	—	—
Fidgeting, restlessness	↓	↑
Autonomic Hyperactivity		
Heart pounding, racing	↓	↑
Dizziness	—	—
Light-headedness	↓	—
High respiratory rate	?	—
Paresthesias	?	—
Upset stomach	?	↑
Frequent urination	?	↑
Sweaty, cold, clammy hands	—	—
Flushing	—	—
Apprehensive Expectation		
Anxiety	↓	↑
Fear, worry	↓	↑
Anticipation of misfortune	↓	↑
Vigilance and scanning		
Insomnia	↓	↑

Notes: Adapted from Greenblatt and Shader (1974) (agonist effects) and from Dorow et al. (1983) and Mendelson et al. (1982) (antagonist effects).

Key: ↓ = decrease in symptoms
↑ = production of symptoms
— = not known
? = possible effect

sulting in an anxiolytic action. The second class represents selective benzodiazepine antagonists which act as competitive receptor antagonists and which, when administered alone, have no pharmacologic actions at moderate doses. Selective benzodiazepine-receptor antagonists such as Ro15-1788 (Hunkeler et al., 1981) and CGS 8216 (Czernik et al., 1982) antagonize the effects of benzodiazepines (agonists) as well as "active" benzodiazepine-receptor antagonists like β-CCE which have intrinsic activity of their own (Ninan et al., 1982). The latter compounds represent the third class of benzodiazepine-receptor ligands. β-CCE and related β-carbolines have been shown to bind to benzodiazepine receptors and to inhibit GABA-mediated chloride conductance (Polc et al., 1981), an effect that is essentially opposite to that of the benzodiazepines.

Although the ultimate clinical expression of "anxiety" may involve a variety of neurotransmitter systems, the results detailed in this chapter underscore a critical role for the benzodiazepine receptors and the GABA receptors both in the amelioration of anxiety by anxiolytic drugs and in its development by anxiogenic compounds such as β-CCE. Since GABA

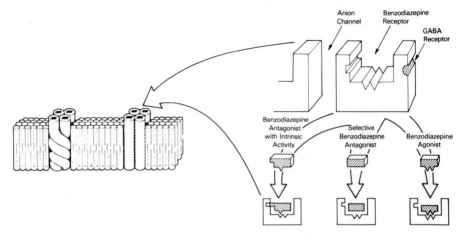

Figure 1. Proposed model of benzodiazepine GABA receptor complex, showing separate domains for agonist, antagonist, and active antagonist (inverse agonist) binding on the benzodiazepine-recognition site. An associated GABA receptor and chloride channel are functionally and perhaps structurally associated with the benzodiazepine receptor. A variety of anxiolytic drugs, including the benzodiazepines, barbiturates, triazolopyridines, and propanediol carbamates, appear to interact with one or more components of this complex.

has been estimated to be an inhibitory neurotransmitter at as many as 30 percent of the synapses in brain, a variety of neurotransmitter systems would probably be altered by enhanced inhibition or disinhibition of this system. Consequently, we may be able to develop anxiolytic drugs that attenuate one or more symptoms of anxiety by affecting a specific neurotransmitter system that is "downstream" in the neuronal circuitry mediating anxiety (Insel et al., 1984). A central question remains, however. Does a primary defect in benzodiazepine-receptor-modulated GABA'ergic neurotransmission have a critical role in the development of human anxiety, in the diagnosable clinical anxiety disorders, or in both? It is apparent that we now have the tools to conduct the studies which will enable us to answer these questions.

Chapter 35 *β*-Adrenergic Blockers and Buspirone

by Jonathan O. Cole, M.D.

For many years, the drug therapy of anxiety disorders has essentially meant choosing from among a growing series of benzodiazepines. These drugs are generally quite safe, as active medications go, and more effective than placebo (Altesman and Cole, 1983). They do have a variety of problems, however, which have caused both public and professional concern (Cole et al., 1981), including overuse, abuse, physical and psychic dependence, and behavioral toxicity. This has led to a search for alternative drug therapies which might be safer, less abusable, and generally more effective or specifically more effective with particular patients or with particular kinds of anxiety disorders. The effects of antidepressant drugs on panic agoraphobia and related disorders are covered elsewhere in this volume.* This chapter reviews the pharmacology and potential effectiveness of several available "different" antianxiety drugs: the group of β-adrenergic blocking drugs, of which propranolol is the best studied, and buspirone, a novel nonbenzodiazepine drug with no obvious similarities to the benzodiazepines either in its structure or in its presumptive mechanisms of action.

β-BLOCKERS

Controlled studies of these drugs in anxiety have been reported periodically since 1965; between twenty and thirty relevant studies are available for review, depending on the criteria used for considering a study relevant (Cole et al., 1979). The most recent reviewers (Pitts and Allen, 1982; Hayes and Schulz, 1983) present intriguing differences in their conclusions. Pitts and Allen (1982), by far the most enthusiastic, asserted that "no negative report has ever been made—every study of β-adrenergic blockade in the treatment of anxiety has found considerable improvement in symptoms consequent to medication." They believe that these drugs are "the treatment of choice for somatic anxiety," somatic anxiety being controlled "immediately," while psychological anxiety is relieved after three to six weeks' continued therapy.

Hayes and Schulz (1983), on the other hand, covered essentially the same literature and stated, "The data reviewed does not support the routine use of propranolol in treating anxiety states" (109). They admitted, however, that propranolol might be useful in patients with physical, especially cardiovascular, symptoms who have failed to respond to benzodiazepines. These reviewers concluded that the "lack of valid scientific data" make β-blockers "among the least useful drugs in treating anxiety disorders" (109).

Probable Mechanism of Action

All commercially available β-blockers have, not surprisingly, the ability to block β-adrenergic receptors in the body. Some are cardioselective, blocking β_1-receptors at lower doses than they block β_2-receptors (e.g., nadolol, atenolol), while others (e.g., propranolol, oxprenolol, pindolol) work about equally on both types of receptors. They all can slow heart rate, suppress ectopic heartbeats and lower blood pressure, usually without causing orthostatic hypotension. The nonselective β-blockers can also cause bronchial constriction and interfere with the body's response to hypoglycemia. β-Blockers, or at least propranolol, also have an antitremor action which is effective with anxiety-related tremors, tremor produced by isoproterenol, a pure β_1-agonist, and familial and lithium tremors. The cardiac effects of β-blockade are primarily peripheral, while the antitremor effects may be either peripheral or central or both (Cole et al., 1979).

*Editor's note: See the next chapter by Liebowitz.

The simplest way of conceptualizing the effects of β-blockers in anxiety disorders is that they should reduce heart rate and suppress arrhythmias, relieving the somatic anxiety symptoms of cardiovascular origin, and should also reduce tremor associated with anxiety. One would therefore predict that β-blockers should be most effective in anxiety states with the above manifestations and that they might be totally ineffective in pure psychic anxiety or in somatic anxiety manifested by muscle spasm, diarrhea, or urinary frequency.

However, there are β-receptors in the brain, though their role is unclear, and some β-blockers, again particularly propranolol but also oxprenolol, have a membrane-stabilizing effect which could be related to their putative central actions. Other β-blockers have mixed agonist-antagonist properties believed to make them more cardioselective (e.g., practolol, pindolol, alprenolol, acebutol).

If adequate controlled studies were available on a range of β-blockers in a range of anxiety states, we might be able to discriminate the specific contributions of their varied pharmacologic properties to their potentially varied antianxiety effects. Unfortunately, the available literature fails to provide the necessary data, and it is, as shown below, an odd literature at best. One obvious reason for this is the fact that the β-blockers were developed by the drug companies as cardiac drugs, and no company to date has made a major effort to prove their efficacy in anxiety or any other psychiatric condition. Most studies of their efficacy in anxiety states have been conducted on small patient samples, often with short treatment durations of one or two weeks, often at a fixed dose of the drug, and usually with equivocal results.

If any of the drugs had been studied in a large multicenter study with both placebo and benzodiazepine control treatments for four- to six-week treatment periods and with dosage adjustment to optimal therapeutic response, we might be in better shape to answer the most obvious and important questions, which are: (1) Are β-blockers more effective than placebo in anxiety disorders in general or in any specific anxiety disorder? (2) Do β-blockers have only a limited antianxiety effect based on their known cardiac and antitremor actions?

The Evidence

Some of the early studies, mainly by cardiologists, focused on the effects of β-blockers in patients with cardiac symptoms but without major cardiac disease, conditions often called "effort syndrome," "cardiac neurosis," "DaCosta's syndrome," or "hyperdynamic β-adrenergic circulatory state." Besterman and Friedlander (1965), Nordenfelt (1965), and Turner et al. (1965) all reported that propranolol reduced tachycardia and palpitations, and with a few such patients propranolol acutely reduced anxiety and discomfort.

Nordenfelt et al. (1968) in fact did a double-blind crossover study of alprenolol (320 mg/day) and placebo, two weeks on each treatment, in a study involving 14 patients with "nervous heart complaints." Pitts and Allen in their 1982 review reported on a chi-square analysis of the data from this study. Patients improved more with drug than placebo on a variety of symptoms, including palpitations, chest pain, oppression, breathlessness, sweating, tremor, nervousness, dizziness, fatigue, headache, mild depression, and gastrointestinal symptoms. Twelve of the 14 patients preferred the active drug, while the 2 who preferred placebo had nausea on the active drug, but noted similar decreases in autonomic symptoms.

Both Frohlich et al. (1969) and Easton and Sherman (1976) described severe cardiac symptoms and panic (probably panic attacks) produced by isoproterenol in patients who had similar spontaneous symptoms and who improved on propranolol but not on placebo. Although it is hard to be certain, the patients in both studies probably had Panic Disorder by DSM-III criteria, and this raises the possibility that β-blockers may be useful in suppressing recurrent panic attacks, as well as in controlling the more chronic symptoms of cardiac anxiety.

Propranolol has also been studied with the cardiovascular symptoms, tremor, and anxiety occurring during alcohol withdrawal (Carlsson, 1969; Zilm et al., 1976). The predicted physiological effects were demonstrated. Carlsson and Johnson (1971) studied 44 patients during alcohol withdrawal, half on 160 mg of propranolol, half on placebo, and found that the drug significantly decreased subjective anxiety and tension; however, all of these patients also received chlormethiazole, a weak sedative, and some received diazepam.

In a more recent and similar study of patients during acute alcohol withdrawal (Sellers et al., 1977), the results were complex, but propranolol alone or in combination with chlordiazepoxide was not clearly better than placebo during a six-day study. Propranolol doses examined were 40 mg/day alone or with chlordiazepoxide 100 mg, propranolol 160 mg alone, chlordiazepoxide 100 mg alone, and placebo. Unfortunately, the study assigned only six patients to each of the five treatments, making for muddy, slightly positive findings. Low-dose propranolol alone and chlordiazepoxide alone looked most effective, while the combination, surprisingly, was never better than placebo.

Recent unpublished reports suggest that isoproterenol, as well as lactate infusions, *can* elicit panic attacks in patients with panic disorder (LaPierre,). Sheehan has commented that in his clinical work with patients who have endogenous anxiety with panic attacks, propranolol is sometimes useful, but less regularly so than antidepressant drugs (David Sheehan, personal communication, 1983).

OPEN STUDIES One way to approach the study of the possible efficacy of a drug in psychiatry is through the large-scale open study, which can help to develop ideas on how the drug should be used, at what dose and with what kinds of patients. Only two such studies are available on β-blockers. Suzman (1976) reported on the use of propranolol with 513 anxious patients whose symptoms were mainly somatic. Half were referred by other physicians primarily for somatic complaints, while the other half had generally failed on previous benzodiazepine therapy. Suzman used a hyperventilation stress test as a measure of β-blockade. A wide range of symptoms were reported to improve, including panic attack symptoms, hyperventilation, and related symptoms, but also fatigue, weakness, headache, gastrointestinal and genitourinary complaints, as well as the more predictable symptoms such as palpitation and tremor. Doses were usually between 80 and 320 mg/day, but were sometimes as high as 1200 mg/day. Patients with predominantly psychic complaints required higher dosages than those with somatic complaints.

Hawkings (1975) used either propranolol or oxprenolol in an open study involving 104 patients. He found the best results with patients who had somatic anxiety symptoms and those who had not previously been on benzodiazepines, about 85 percent improvement in both groups, excluding those who dropped out due to side effects. Patients with mental anxiety, anxiety with depression, and phobic anxiety (not further defined) did less well but were helped. The median propranolol dose was 120 mg/day, the maximum 320 mg/day.

These two studies permit the inference that propranolol's clinical use, over extended periods and at clinically adjusted doses, is of substantial benefit in anxiety disorders, with somatic symptoms perhaps responding better at lower doses.

CONTROLLED STUDIES Controlled studies, in contrast, have almost always used fixed doses for short one- to two-week periods, and have often used crossover designs. Granville-Grossman and Turner (1966) studied the effects of 80 mg of propranolol vs. placebo with 16 patients who had undefined anxiety. Clinician judgments of overall improvement and decreased somatic anxiety reached statistical significance. Tyrer and Lader (1974a) did a most elaborate three-treatment crossover study involving 12 patients, 6 with predominantly psychic anxiety and 6 with mainly somatic anxiety. Each patient received titrated doses of propranolol (120 to 360 mg/day), diazepam (6 to 18 mg/day), or placebo for two weeks, each in counterbalanced order. Propranolol was superior to placebo only with the somatically anxious patients, while diazepam was preferred overall in both patient groups.

Kellner et al. (1974) reported a similar double-blind crossover trial with 22 chronically anxious outpatients, comparing propranolol, 40 to 80 mg/day, with placebo. They reported a weak effect favoring propranolol, observed as trends on most of their 35 measures, and statistical significance being reached only on clusters of items that assessed somatic or psychic anxiety. Tanna et al. (1977) reported on an overly complex crossover study that compared propranolol at two doses, 40 mg/day and 120 mg/day, and placebo. The 28 anxious patients received each treatment for one week after an initial "wash-out" placebo week. Again, propranolol at the higher dose looked a bit better on most measures, reaching statistical significance only on fatigue, shakiness, and initial insomnia. All patients met RDC criteria for anxiety neurosis which require both panic attacks and chronic anxiety symptoms.

Hallstrom et al. (1981) did another complex crossover study involving 24 patients who had "excessive anxiety for at least six months" (not otherwise defined). All patients received two weeks each of propranolol (average 180 mg/day), diazepam (average 7.5 mg/day), placebo, and propranolol and diazepam combined at identical mean dosages. Diazepam and the combination were superior to propranolol and placebo on the somatic anxiety factor of the Hamilton Anxiety Scale. Only the combination was superior to all other treatments on a target symptom score unique to each patient. The only other evidence in favor of propranolol was that, for both propranolol alone and the combination, the psychic anxiety factor of the Hamilton and the target symptom score improved significantly more in those patients with the greater decrease in heart rate (over 7.5 beats per minute). This study produced no evidence that propranolol reduced somatic anxiety scores, as measured rather nonspecifically on the Hamilton Anxiety Scale.

Kathol et al. (1980) reported on another double-blind crossover study comparing two weeks on propranolol (160 mg/day) with placebo. The 26 patients had various DSM-III anxiety disorders, chiefly Panic Disorders and Agoraphobia with Panic Attacks, generally of several years' duration. Propranolol was superior to placebo on the anxiety and interpersonal sensitivity scales of the Symptom Check List (SCL), 90-item version, and on self-ratings of global severity and improvement. Neither the somatic scale of the SCL-90 nor the Hamilton Anxiety Scale showed any drug-placebo differences. Patients with agoraphobia and panic attacks improved the most, while patients with panic alone did less well. There was a trend for decrease in heart rate to correlate with improvement on propranolol.

Wheatley (1969) studied 105 anxious patients in a multiphysician general practice and found 90 mg of propranolol a day and a lowish dose of 30 mg of chlordiazepoxide a day to be essentially equivalent in clinical efficacy. Chlordiazepoxide was superior for symptoms of sleep disturbances and depression, and about one-third of the patients were "symptom free" on both drugs. The absence of a placebo group makes this study hard to evaluate.

One small inconclusive study of ten anxious patients compared 160 mg a day of D-propranolol, the weaker β-blocker of the two chemicals in racemic propranolol, against placebo (Bonn and Turner, 1971). The finding of no differences suggests, but does not prove, that the antianxiety effect of propranolol may be due to β-blockade.

Oxprenolol, the only other β-blocker to be studied at all well in anxiety disorders, is similar to propranolol in its pharmacology, being a nonselective β-blocker with membrane-stabilizing properties. It was equivalent to propranolol in one controlled study (Becker, 1976), but this study unfortunately lacked a placebo group.

Two studies have compared oxprenolol with diazepam and placebo, both using fixed doses of 240 mg of oxprenolol and 15 mg of diazepam. Burrows et al. (1976) conducted a three-week trial (without a crossover for once) with about twenty patients per treatment group. All groups improved, but both active drugs were superior to placebo only in the third and last week of the study. At that point, investigator ratings, but not patient ratings, showed a trend favoring the benzodiazepine over the β-blocker. Johnson et al. (1976) did an identical study, except that only half as many patients were assigned to placebo as to the active drugs. Thirteen patients completed the study on diazepam, 11 on oxprenolol, and 5 on placebo. Diazepam was superior to both other treatments at the end of the first week. On psychic anxiety symptoms, after three weeks diazepam was superior to placebo, and oxprenolol was intermediate and not significantly different from either diazepam or placebo. On somatic anxiety symptoms, all three treatments were equivalent at the third and last week. McMillin (1975) compared 240 mg of oxprenolol with 15 mg of diazepam, each for a week in a crossover study with patients made anxious by events in Northern Ireland. The two drugs were equivalent in efficacy.

Acute Stress

The lay press has reported that β-blockers improve musical performance or reduce examination "nerves," and one does find musicians who routinely use propranolol for this purpose. Again, the simplest assumption would be that the β-blocker would decrease tachycardia and tremor and thereby improve a performance which would otherwise be impaired by the symptoms arising from anxiety over the stressful situation.

Early open studies include that of Imhof et al. (1969), who observed that 40 mg of oxprenolol given before competitive ski jumping decreased "emotional" tachycardia and tensions. Studying psychology students about to take an exam, Brewer (1972) compared placebo and a single administration of propranolol, at a dose previously determined to slow heart rate down to 55 to 65 beats per minute. He found no decrement in performance and "some" benefit with the more anxious students.

Krishnan (1975) randomly assigned students to single preexam doses of oxprenolol (80 mg) or diazepam (4 mg). He found no differences in subjective anxiety experienced during the exam, but students on diazepam tended to get less good grades than predicted by the professor, while students on oxprenolol did slightly better than predicted. Eisdorfer et al. (1970) found that 10 mg of propranolol, as compared with placebo, improved elderly male volunteers' learning of word lists; the drug blocked the heart-rate and plasma free fatty acid increases seen in placebo subjects due to the stress.

Tyrer and Lader (1974b) compared effects of single doses of diazepam (5 mg), racemic propranolol (120 mg), and D-propranolol (120 mg) on normal subjects stressed by electric shocks, shocks plus isoproterenol inhalation, and exposure to individually selected phobic stimuli. Only diazepam decreased subjective anxiety; unfortunately, the D-propranolol decreased pulse rate, vitiating its utility as a non-β-blocking control substance. Gottschalk et al. (1974) found 60 mg of propranolol, as compared with placebo, decreased "anxiety" as measured in a five-minute verbal sample, before, but not after, a stressful interview. Cleghorn et al. (1970) did a similar study, giving propranolol intravenously, and found no effect on anxiety in a verbal sample, in this case following hypnotically induced stress. Nakano et al. (1978) found propranolol (40 mg) to reduce heart rate, but not subjective anxiety, attributable to difficult psychological testing. Krope et al. (1982) compared a single dose of a β-blocker (5 or 10 mg) in two studies, each with about fifty students. Pulse was decreased by the drug, but it did not affect self-rated anxiety or performance.

Two rather detailed studies have been carried out with music students performing before audiences (stage fright). Brantigan et al. (1982) compared propranolol (probably 40 mg) vs. placebo double-blind in two groups, one of 13 subjects in Nebraska and one of 16 subjects in New York. They gave the medication 90 minutes before the performances, and used a crossover design, adding a tape recording to the audience in the second performance to avoid the decrease in stress response often seen with repeated exposure. Professional judges evaluated the performances in both groups, but only in New York were the propranolol sessions judged to be significantly superior. Heart rate decreased, and salivary flow increased significantly on the drug, and nervousness, anxiety, tremor, sweating, and a variety of technical aspects of performance were improved. James et al. (1978) compared oxprenolol (40 mg) and placebo, studying 24 string musicians in a crossover study. During the second session of the crossover, they observed no drug-placebo differences except in heart rate, but during the first session they found significant improvements in anxiety measured on two global ratings, in observer ratings of tremor, and in two of several technical measures of musical performance. Facial pallor was increased by the drug, and subjects felt less tremor and stiffness.

Two studies (Gaind et al., 1975; Hafner and Milton, 1977) have administered a β-blocker or placebo double-blind while patients underwent in vivo exposure to phobic stressors as part of behavior therapy. In both studies, the β-blocker hindered clinical response to the treatment program, though anxiety was reduced during the sessions themselves.

BUSPIRONE

Buspirone was synthesized in the early 1970s as one in a series of azaspirodecanedione compounds with psychotropic activity in animals (Temple et al., 1982). It has no obvious structural relationship with any known psychoactive drug (see Figure 1). A review of buspirone is timely, since it may be marketed in the near future, and it has been shown to be equivalent in potency to diazepam with anxious outpatients.

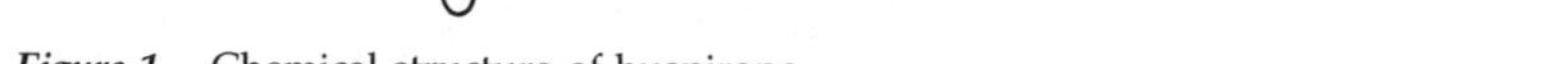

Figure 1. Chemical structure of buspirone

Pharmacology

Buspirone has a unique and complex pharmacology. It has no effect on benzodiazepine receptors, on γ-aminobutyric acid (GABA) receptors, or on a wide variety of other receptors, including adrenergic, histaminic, and muscarinic sites. It does not block reuptake of biogenic amines or GABA. Buspirone shares with dopamine blockers a weak activity at serotonin-binding sites. It has a high activity at dopamine receptors, displacing both dopamine agonist and antagonist ligands equally well (Riblet et al., 1982).

In laboratory animals, buspirone causes sedation only at very high dosages. At lower dosages, it blocks the conditioned avoidance response briefly, but has a prolonged effect on behavioral conflict paradigms; it has a brief neuroleptic-like effect and prolonged anxiolytic-type effects. It tames rhesus monkeys effectively without inducing ataxia. It is as potent in antianxiety tests as diazepam without the malcoordination or muscle weakness seen with diazepam. It acts like a neuroleptic on some systems, blocking apomorphine-induced stereotypy and emesis. It increases the activity of dopaminergic neurons in the basal ganglia even more dramatically than do neuroleptics at any dose. On the other hand, it does not induce catalepsy in rodents at any dose and reverses neuroleptic-induced catalepsy effectively (Riblet et al., 1982). In animals with unilateral lesions in the substantia nigra, it acts like a weak dopamine agonist inducing contralateral turning. In peripheral arteries, it acts as a dopamine agonist. On the quantitative electroencephalogram in the cat, buspirone resembles apomorphine and piribedil, not neuroleptics or benzodiazepines.

In human beings, buspirone can increase blood prolactin, a dopamine-blocking effect, but it increases growth hormone, a dopamine-agonist effect (Meltzer and Fleming, 1982). In an early open trial with schizophrenic patients at very high doses of up to 1000 mg a day, buspirone neither caused parkinsonism or dystonia nor improved the patients' psychopathology, suggesting that it does not act as a typical neuroleptic in human beings.

The pharmacokinetics of buspirone are complex. Buspirone itself is rapidly destroyed in the body, yielding a large number of metabolites. A 5-hydroxylated metabolite is present in some quantity and has a longer half-life; it does not bind to postsynaptic dopamine receptors (Temple et al., 1982).

All this suggests that buspirone acts on dopamine systems in a variety of contradictory ways, an agonist in many, an antagonist in others. So far, the agonist properties seem more important, and the usual neurological side effects of neuroleptics which presumably precede tardive dyskinesia are not seen either in animals or in human beings.

Clinical Studies

Goldberg and Finnerty (1979) conducted the earliest study of buspirone in anxiety, involving 56 adult outpatients with "a primary diagnosis of anxiety neurosis." Patients were randomly assigned, double-blind, to buspirone, diazepam, or placebo, with individual capsules containing 5 mg of either drug. Dosage was titrated clinically, with average doses being just under 20 mg a day for either active drug. Patients had to have a score over 20 on the Hamilton Anxiety Scale and 9 or higher on the Covi Anxiety Scale at baseline. Both physicians' and patients' global improvement ratings showed significant drug-placebo differences at four weeks, the planned duration of the study. By end-point analysis, the Hamilton Anxiety Scale ratings differentiated between drug and placebo at the p<.001 level on almost all items and on all factors. Self-ratings on the SCL-56 were equally sensitive to drug effects. No significant differences between buspirone and diazepam were reported, but weak trends on most self-report and Hamilton Anxiety Scale measures favored buspirone.

Rickels et al. (1982) did an essentially identical study, involving 240 anxious outpatients and identical mean dosages of active drugs during the last two weeks of the four-week study. Moderate to marked improvement was observed in 60 percent of patients on diazepam, 57 percent of patients on buspirone, and 15 percent of patients on placebo. The two drugs were equally effective on most measures, and both were significantly more effective than placebo. Diazepam was more effective than buspirone on the somatic anxiety factor of the Hopkins Symptom Check List and on the vigor factor of the Profile of Mood States (POMS). Buspirone was more effective on the anger-hostility, confusion, and fatigue factors of the POMS. Diazepam also caused significantly more fatigue, reported as a side effect, than buspirone and somewhat more sedation. Buspirone tended to cause more dizziness and headache.

In another study by Goldberg and Finnerty (1982), involving 56 patients with the same design described above, both diazepam and buspirone were more effective than placebo (p<.001) on Hamilton Anxiety Scale measures. POMS and SCL measures were equally sensitive to drug-placebo differences.

Wheatley (1982) conducted a trial run in a variety of general practitioners' offices, involving over forty patients each on buspirone, diazepam, and placebo. The results included no significant buspirone-placebo differences, though all three treatment groups showed improvement over the three-week study. Patients on placebo showed no further significant improvement after the first week, but patients on both active drugs continued to improve over the three weeks. On the Hamilton Anxiety Scale, the patients on buspirone were less symptomatic than those on placebo only at the end of the third week.

Two studies have reported comparisons of buspirone with a benzodiazepine without a placebo group. Buspirone and chlorazepate were essentially equivalent in a double-blind four-week study involving 130 patients, with 3 out of 4 patients on buspirone (Goldberg and Finnerty, 1982). Buspirone was superior to chlorazepate on the anger-hostility, confusion, depression, and fatigue factors of the POMS and on the interpersonal sensitivity and tension factors of the SCL-56. There was a trend (p=.07) for buspirone to be superior to the benzodiazepine on the somatic anxiety factor of the Hamilton Anxiety Scale. In the other comparative study, Feighner et al. (1982) compared buspirone and diazepam at average dosages of about 15 mg a day with patients meeting DSM-III criteria for Generalized Anxiety Disorder. Buspirone was superior to diazepam only on the impaired cognition factor of the SCL-56 and the confusion and fatigue factors of the POMS. Only about 40 percent of the patients in each drug group were judged improved on doctors' or patients' ratings. Diazepam caused significantly more side effects, mainly sedation.

In a review of side effect data pooled from several studies, Newton et al. (1982) reported that buspirone overall causes fewer side effects than diazepam, most strikingly in the area of fatigue, and a 10 percent incidence of depression was noted on diazepam (vs. 3 percent for buspirone) in the 180 patients on each therapy. Nervousness was the only side effect occurring significantly more often with buspirone than with diazepam (9 percent for buspirone vs. 2 percent for diazepam). Nervousness, headache, and dizziness were more frequent on buspirone than on placebo. Against chlorazepate, buspirone caused more nausea, while chlorazepate caused more depression and drowsiness.

Psychological Effects

Lader (1982) compared single doses of 10 mg and 20 mg of buspirone with 10 mg of diazepam and with placebo in a study involving 12 normal volunteers in a double-blind Latin-square design, with all subjects receiving all treatments. On analogue mood scales, all active drugs produced more sedation than placebo one hour after drug ingestion; sedation on 20 mg of buspirone lasted three hours, and subjects on that dose felt less "contented." Both diazepam and the higher dose of buspirone caused dizziness. These treatments, but not the 10 mg of buspirone, slowed reaction time at one hour; only diazepam impaired performance on the digit symbol substitution test (DSST).

In a second and related study, seven days of treatment three times a day with 5 mg of diazepam, 5 or 10 mg of buspirone, and placebo were compared (Lader, 1982). Diazepam impaired DSST performance, tapping speed, and symbol copying more than placebo, while buspirone had much less effect on these measures at either dose. Tolerance developed to the dysphoric effects of the higher buspirone dose, while drowsiness was the main symptom on diazepam.

Mattila et al. (1982) compared the effects of single doses of buspirone (10 mg and 20 mg), lorazepam (2.5 mg), and placebo, with and without alcohol (1 g/kg body weight), in 12 healthy students. Without alcohol, all three drugs were sedative, the higher dose of buspirone being dysphoric. Only lorazepam impaired coordination relative to placebo. Alcohol was euphoriant alone (with placebo) and with lorazepam, while in combination with the higher dose of buspirone the net effect was still dysphoric. Lorazepam, but not either dose of buspirone, increased the adverse effects of alcohol on performance.

Moskowitz and Smiley (1982) gave either diazepam (15 mg/day), buspirone (20 mg/day), or placebo for nine days to groups of 16 subjects on each treatment. Alcohol was added on the ninth day (0.85 g/kg for men, 0.72 g/kg for women). Subjects were tested on a complex computer-run driving simulator and on a divided-attention task. After the initial dose (10 mg of diazepam, 10 mg of buspirone, or placebo), buspirone was related to even better performance than placebo on some measures, while the diazepam impaired performance. On the eighth day, before the A.M. dose, subjects on diazepam were slightly impaired; after the A.M. dose, diazepam impaired performance even more than after the first dose on the first day, while subjects on buspirone showed better performance than placebo subjects. When the drugs were taken with alcohol on the ninth day, the differences between diazepam and buspirone were exaggerated in favor of buspirone.

In summary, buspirone can be sedative and dysphoric, especially after single doses of 20 mg, but it is less likely to impair performance than benzodiazepines, and it does not potentiate the effects of alcohol as do benzodiazepines.

Abuse Liability

Buspirone does not produce evidence of physical dependence in rats even at 200 mg/kg per day for 22 days. It does not substitute for phenobarbital in physically dependent mice. It is not identified as similar to oxazepam or pentobarbital in rats trained to discriminate these drugs from placebo in choice tests. Animals had difficulty learning to discriminate the buspirone state from saline (Riblet et al., 1982). Monkeys trained to self-administer cocaine intravenously would not work to self-inject buspirone (or oxazepam) (Balster and Woolverton, 1982). Thus, in animal models buspirone neither produces nor sustains physical dependence of the barbiturate type; benzodiazepines do have these effects. Abuse and dependence liability appear low in animal test systems.

The author and his colleagues (1982) compared two doses of buspirone (10 mg and 40 mg) with two doses of diazepam (10 mg and 20 mg), one dose of methaqualone (300 mg), and placebo in a study involving 36 volunteers with a history of casual recreational sedative use. Treated in groups of six, subjects received all six treatments in a Latin-square design. The major measures of drug effect were a reduced version of the Addiction Research Center Inventory and global measures of "street" value and of the subject's interest in taking the drug again. Overall, methaqualone was the most euphoriant agent tested, with 20 mg of diazepam next in effect, and both treatments were sedative. Buspirone at 10 mg was indistinguishable from placebo, while 40 mg of buspirone was sedative but quite unpleasant. These findings are compatible with Lader's (1982) evidence that single doses of 20 mg of buspirone caused unpleasant effects in normal volunteers. To the extent that this human model predicts illicit abuse, it seems unlikely that drug abusers will find buspirone a pleasurable euphoriant drug.

DISCUSSION

Given the limitations of the available published literature, buspirone appears more likely to be a useful nonbenzodiazepine drug for the treatment of anxiety disorders than either propranolol or oxprenolol. Since none of the three drugs have been seriously or extensively studied with groups of carefully diagnosed anxious patients, no clear conclusions can be reached about their relative efficacy in generalized anxiety disorder versus panic disorder or panic agoraphobia.

Buspirone seems likely to be about as effective as diazepam or chlorazepate with somewhat different and fewer side effects in anxious outpatients. It seems unlikely to be a euphoriant drug popular with illicit drug abusers, since doses above those used in the treatment of anxiety are predominantly dysphoric. Buspirone does not cause the impairment in cognitive and psychomotor functioning usually seen early in treatment with benzodiazepines and does not potentiate the psychological effects of alcohol. Whether buspirone will have any utility in panic disorders remains to be seen. Whether it will be a useful substitute for benzodiazepines with patients who have become accustomed to taking such drugs for prolonged periods is also not yet known. Buspirone's mixed and complicated effects on dopamine systems in the brain raise the specter of tardive dyskinesia, but the major brain effects appear so far to be dopaminergic and thus opposite to those seen with the antipsychotic drugs.

The β-blockers studied most extensively to date, propranolol and oxprenolol, show continuing modest evidence of antianxiety effects, both in unselected anxious outpatients and in at least a few patients with panic attacks. In the usual studies where doses of propranolol range from 40 to 180 mg a day for periods of two weeks or less, the drug is often more effective than placebo on some clinical measures, but these studies have not shown it to be as effective as diazepam. The question remains whether longer treatment titrated to higher doses and clear physiological evidence of β-blockade (decreased heart rate) would yield more positive findings. Available studies suggest that propranolol is sometimes, but not always, more effective in somatic anxiety, usually undefined, but even here propranolol is not more effective than diazepam. The combination of propranolol and a benzodiazepine has been examined in only two studies and with equivocal results.

The effects of oxprenolol and propranolol on anxiety seem broader than the predictable decreases which should occur in tachycardia and tremor. Even as used in acute stress, β-blockers appear to have inconsistent but often positive effects on stage fright in musicians, and these effects go beyond simple physiological effects on heart functions or tremor. Since the effects are chiefly seen only on the first of two exposures to stress, one wonders why musicians continue to use propranolol before performances over longer periods and whether more than placebo effects are occurring.

The efficacy of the more cardioselective β-blockers in anxiety is essentially unstudied.

Overall, the β-blockers appear safe in doses recommended for use in cardiac conditions, and they may be worth trying with selected patients who have anxiety syndromes when other drugs have failed or are contraindicated. One would guess that they would be more useful with patients who have cardiac symptoms like tachycardia or tremor, but again this may be a wrong hunch. Propranolol and, presumably, oxprenolol are contraindicated for patients with asthma or bronchial disease, Raynaud's disease, and probably insulin-dependent diabetes. The cardiospecific or mixed antagonist-agonist β-blockers may be less dangerous for such patients but should be tried with caution. β-Blockers *can* cause depression (Cole et al., 1979), but this is quite rare in the author's clinical experience.

Much better designed, larger, longer, and more diagnostically precise clinical research needs to be done both with the β-blockers and with buspirone before their real places in the treatment of the anxiety disorders can be defined. If, as expected, buspirone becomes available for prescription use in the next year or so, clinicians will have a still larger choice of drugs to try with anxious patients who require pharmacotherapy. Perhaps one or more of the β-blockers will emerge as generally useful as well, although at the moment propranolol is the best studied and seems the sensible choice if a β-blocker is to be used.

SUMMARY

β-Blockers have been extensively studied in anxiety disorders, but most studies are small and brief and involve crossover designs. Propranolol and probably oxprenolol have some antianxiety effects on both somatic and psychic anxiety, but at the doses and durations studied neither drug appears to be as effective as diazepam. Buspirone, the new nonbenzo-diazepine antianxiety drug, appears to be as effective as diazepam and less liable to be abused. It seems to act via dopamine systems in the brain. Neither the β-blockers nor buspirone have been shown to be clearly preferable to or more effective than benzodiazepines, but they may offer useful alternative drug therapies for anxious patients. Neither propranolol nor buspirone have been shown specifically effective for panic disorder and panic agoraphobia versus generalized anxiety disorder.

Chapter 36

The Efficacy of Antidepressants in Anxiety Disorders
by Michael R. Liebowitz, M.D.

While the recent introduction of the DSM-III classification of Anxiety Disorders represents a distinct advance for empirically based diagnostic practice, much remains to be learned about effective treatment for the various primary anxiety disorders. Both the tricyclic compounds and the monoamine oxidase (MAO) inhibitors have been found effective with patients who have spontaneous panic attacks (Klein, 1964; Zitrin et al., 1983; Sheehan et al., 1980), and these findings have rekindled interest in the possible efficacy of these and other so-called antidepressants in all of the DSM-III Anxiety Disorders. This chapter reviews current knowledge of antidepressant drug therapy of agoraphobia, panic disorder, obsessive-compulsive disorder, generalized anxiety disorder, posttraumatic stress disorder, social phobia, and simple phobia.

AGORAPHOBIA AND PANIC DISORDER

Agoraphobia and panic disorder are discussed jointly because of the centrality to almost all cases of the former and to all of the latter of spontaneous, or unprovoked, panic attacks, which are the hypothesized principal target of drug treatment. The travel restrictions characterizing agoraphobia usually come about as a consequence of panic attacks (in DSM-III, these cases are called Agoraphobia with Panic Attacks); however, these restrictions may continue even after the spontaneous panic attacks have subsided, so that the agoraphobic patient has only situationally bound panic or even no ongoing panic attacks at all. Furthermore, occasional cases of agoraphobia may arise without panic attacks (in DSM-III, Agoraphobia without Panic Attacks). Thus, it is crucial to assess the current status of panic attacks in agoraphobic patients before equating them with panic disorder patients, who by definition still suffer spontaneous panic attacks.

Tricyclics

PLACEBO-CONTROLLED TRIALS The most common subtype of agoraphobia, called Agoraphobia with Panic Attacks in DSM-III and formerly called phobic anxiety, is an example of a diagnosis elucidated by a treatment. Administering imipramine, chlorpromazine, and placebo in a double-blind study with a large psychiatric inpatient population in the early 1960s, Klein and Fink (Klein, 1964; 1967) found imipramine highly effective in blocking panic attacks, in contrast to both placebo and chlorpromazine (the latter was given to a very small number of patients who had a uniformly negative reaction) (see Table 1). In contrast to its marked antipanic effect, imipramine seemed to reduce only slightly the patients' fears of having more panic attacks, which Klein referred to as "anticipatory anxiety." Patients still required "firm direction and support" to overcome their phobic avoidance.

This unexpected antipanic effect of imipramine was substantiated by Klein and colleagues in two later studies. One of these was a 26-week study that compared the effects of imipramine plus behavior therapy (primarily systematic desensitization), imipramine and supportive therapy, and placebo plus behavior therapy (Zitrin et al., 1983). The subject population consisted of patients who had agoraphobia with panic attacks, specific phobias without panics, and mixed phobias with both circumscribed phobias and panic attacks. As hypothesized, a drug-placebo difference was found for the patients with agoraphobia and with mixed phobia but not the patients with specific phobias; thus, imipramine was of benefit only for those patients with spontaneous panic attacks. Another study comparing imipramine and placebo involved 76 agoraphobic patients, all of whom also received a course of group exposure in vivo. Significant imipramine effects were found for panic attacks, primary phobia, and global outcome (Zitrin et al., 1980).

These studies did not include patients with panic attacks but no travel restrictions who would fit the DSM-III criteria for Panic Disorder. While data from open clinical trials with imipramine (Muskin and Fyer, 1981) and with clomipramine (Gloger et al., 1981) suggest that these patients also benefit from tricyclics, no controlled drug trials have been reported yet involving patients with panic attacks but no phobias. One reason for this may be that most patients with panic attacks develop at least some limited patterns of avoidance. The DSM-III Panic Disorder category obscures this distinction by lumping together those patients who have panic attacks and limited avoidance and those who have panic and no phobic avoidance. Subdivision of this category is recommended for DSM-IV.*

COMPARATIVE TRIALS Many patients with panic attacks fail to benefit from benzodiazepines prior to responding to tricyclics. In addition, in the one controlled study comparing a tricyclic with a standard dose of a benzodiazepine in an agoraphobic population, McNair and Kahn (1981) found imipramine superior to chlordiazepoxide for panic and depressive and phobic symptoms. However, since the mean dosages in this eight-week study were relatively low (55 mg of chlordiazepoxide and 132 mg of imipramine), it is unclear if higher doses of benzodiazepines would be more effective. Since a recent open trial suggests that the newly marketed benzodiazepine, alprazolam, blocks panic attacks in higher equivalent doses than have been studied with the older benzodiazepines (Sheehan, 1982), the efficacy of the other benzodiaze-

Table 1. Controlled Trials of Tricyclics in Agoraphobia or Panic Disorder

Study (Year)	Sample	Design	Daily Dosage*	Duration	Final Outcome	Limitation
		PLACEBO-CONTROLLED TRIALS				
Klein (1967)	Mixed inpatient sample N = 311	Imipramine vs. chlorpromazine vs. placebo	IMI up to 300 mg CPZ up to 1200 mg	6 weeks	Imipramine superior to CPZ or placebo for phobic anxiety	Diagnoses made retrospectively in first half of sample
Zitrin et al. (1983)	Mixed phobic sample N = 218	Imipramine + behavior therapy vs. imipramine + supportive therapy vs. placebo + behavior therapy	IMI up to 300 mg Mean dose IMI 204 mg	26 weeks	Imipramine superior to placebo in agoraphobics and mixed phobia with panic attacks	All patients also received some form of psychotherapy
Zitrin et al. (1980)	Agoraphobics with panic attacks N = 76	Imipramine + in vivo exposure vs. placebo + in vivo exposure	IMI up to 300 mg	26 weeks	Imipramine superior to placebo in panic attacks, primary phobia, and global outcome	No patient treated without concomitant behavior therapy

Table 1. Continued

Study (Year)	Sample	Design	Daily Dosage*	Duration	Final Outcome	Limitation
Sheehan et al. (1980)	Panic attacks plus phobias N=57	Imipramine vs. phenelzine vs. placebo	IMI up to 150 mg PHEN up to 45 mg	12 weeks	Both drugs superior to placebo. Phenelzine superior to imipramine on 2/13 scales	Modest dosages. Concomitant psychotherapy for all patients. Modest sample size
			COMPARATIVE TRIALS			
McNair and Kahn (1981)	Agoraphobics and mixed phobics with panic attacks N=36	Imipramine vs. chlordiazepox-ide	IMI up to 200 mg CHLORD up to 80 mg Mean Doses: IMI 132 mg CHLORD 55 mg	8 weeks	Imipramine superior on panic and depression	Modest dosages. Proportion of patients responding to treatment not given
Marks et al. (1983)	Agoraphobics N=45	2 × 2 design: Imipramine vs. Placebo and exposure vs. relaxation	IMI up to 200 mg Mean dose IMI 124 mg (week 6); 158 mg (week 14)	28 weeks	No significant imipramine effect	Modest dosages. Concomitant therapy. Includes previous drug failures

*Note: Final study week; scheduled dosages indicated by "up to"; actually administered doses (if available) denoted by "mean" or "median" pines in treating panic attacks requires further study to see if alprazolam's antipanic effects are unique.

Also demonstrated to be helpful for agoraphobia is behavior therapy, the most efficacious form of which appears to be in vivo exposure (Mathews et al., 1981). Comparing behavior therapy and the tricyclic studies of agoraphobia is difficult, however, because the behavior therapy literature does not give attention to panic attacks, either as a baseline diagnostic feature or as an outcome variable.

Marks and colleagues have recently reported on a study which used a 2 × 2 design to compare imipramine (up to 200 mg/day for 28 weeks), placebo, therapist-aided exposure, and therapist-aided relaxation for 45 agoraphobic patients (Marks et al., 1983). In their design, relaxation was regarded as the placebo behavior therapy. However, patients in all groups also received systematic self-exposure homework, including an instruction manual, which blurs the treatment contrasts. Overall, no significant effects were found for imipramine, while significant but limited effects were found for therapist-aided exposure.

Marks et al. concluded that self-exposure homework is a powerful therapeutic device, that imipramine adds nothing for agoraphobic patients who are not depressed, and that therapist-aided exposure is helpful for some patients. One limit on the generalizability of these conclusions is that the medication dosages were low; mean doses of imipramine were 124 mg at week 6, 158 mg at week 14, and not reported at week 26. (Mean drug plasma levels were in the antidepressant range, but were inflated by several outliers.) In addition, a number of patients previously refractory to antidepressants were taken into the study. Also, among the patients counted as dropouts were two who showed rapid improvement with imipramine. One other interesting point is that ten patients were put on imipramine during the ad lib treatment follow-up period, including eight patients who had been on imipramine before. The investigators did not mention whether these eight individuals had deteriorated when taken off medication the first time.

MAO Inhibitors

Following clinical reports of the benefits of MAO inhibitors for phobic anxious patients (West and Dally, 1959; Sargant and Dally, 1962; King, 1962; Kelly et al., 1970), a number of controlled studies were initiated (see Table 2). Tyrer et al. (1973) compared the effects of phenelzine and placebo on 32 agoraphobic and social phobic patients in an eight-week study. Of the many variables measured, only patient-rated secondary phobias and psychiatrist-rated overall outcome showed phenelzine superior to placebo. It should be noted, however, that while the maximum allowed dosage of phenelzine in this study was 90 mg, mean dosage for the whole study was only 38.5 mg. Unfortunately, mean final dosages were not reported. Another difficulty in this study is the fact that results for agoraphobic and social phobic patients were not reported separately, and it is unclear how many patients of either diagnostic subtype also suffered panic attacks.

Lipsedge et al. (1973) compared iproniazid and placebo in a 2 × 3 design in which some of their sixty agoraphobic patients also received methohexitone-assisted or standard desensitization. Maximum dosage was 150 mg/day, and the study lasted eight weeks. Patients on iproni-

Table 2. Controlled Trials of MAO Inhibitors in Agoraphobia or Panic Disorder

Study (Year)	Sample Completers	Design	Daily Dosage*	Duration	Final Outcome	Limitation
Tyrer et al. (1973)	Agoraphobia and social phobia N=32	Phenelzine vs. placebo	Up to 90 mg/day Mean dose for whole study 38.5 mg	8 weeks	Few drug-placebo differences. Phenelzine superior to placebo on secondary phobias (patient-rated) and overall outcome (psychiatrist-rated)	Outcome of agoraphobics and social phobics not reported separately. Unclear if patients had panic attacks
Lipsedge et al. (1973)	Agoraphobia N=60	2 × 3 design: Iproniazid vs. placebo; Methohexitone-assisted systematic desensitization vs. standard desensitization vs. no desensitization.	Up to 150 mg	8 weeks	Iproniazid superior to placebo on anxiety but not avoidance reduction	One-third of patients had prior Rx with other MAO inhibitors. Unclear if agoraphobics had panic attacks
Solyom et al. (1973)	Agoraphobia, social phobia, or specific phobia N=30	Flooding vs. phenelzine plus brief psychotherapy vs. placebo plus brief psychotherapy	Up to 45 mg/day	3 months	Flooding produced greater decrease on Wolpe-Lang Fear Survey than phenelzine. Phenelzine had greater antianxiety effects than other treatments. Significant phenelzine-placebo difference in reduction of phobia, neurotic symptoms, and social maladjustment. Six of six patients stopping phenelzine relapsed by 2-yr follow up	Only phenelzine vs. placebo assessed blindly. Results not presented separately for different types of phobias. Presence of panic attacks at baseline not specified or rated

Study	Diagnosis	Design	Dosage	Results	Comments
Mountjoy et al. (1977)	Anxiety neurosis N=36 Agoraphobia or social phobia N=22 Depressive neurosis (not discussed here)	Phenelzine plus diazepam vs. placebo plus diazepam	Phenelzine up to 75 mg/day Diazepam 5 mg TID	4 weeks	Few drug-placebo differences. Phenelzine plus diazepam superior on social phobia scale for all phobic patients. Placebo plus diazepam superior on Hamilton Anxiety scale in anxiety neurotics	Heterogeneous sample. Duration short. Small Ns for different treatment groups within each diagnosis. Panic attacks not rated at baseline or completion
Sheehan et al. (1980)	Panic attacks plus phobias N=57	Imipramine vs. phenelzine vs. placebo	IMI up to 150 mg PHEN up to 45 mg	12 weeks	Both drugs superior to placebo. Phenelzine superior to imipramine on 2/13 scales	Modest dosages. Concomitant psychotherapy for all patients. Modest sample size
Solyom et al. (1981)	Agoraphobia or social phobia N=40	2 × 2 design: Phenelzine vs. placebo; Exposure vs. no exposure	Up to 45 mg/day	6 weeks	Phenelzine superior to placebo on anxiety reduction during exposure. Exposure superior to nonexposure on several measures. No significant differences between exposure and phenelzine	Data not reported separately for two types of phobias. Low phenelzine dose. Lack of control for exposure. Panic attacks not specified or rated.

Note: Final study week; dosage scheduled indicated by "up to"; actually administered dose (if available) denoted by "mean" azid experienced greater anxiety reduction than those on placebo, but no greater decrement in avoidance. Limitations of this study include prior MAO inhibitor treatment in one-third of the patients and no ratings at baseline or termination for panic attacks.

Solyom et al. (1973) compared flooding, phenelzine plus supportive psychotherapy, and placebo plus supportive psychotherapy in a study involving thirty patients with agoraphobia, social phobia, or specific phobia. The study lasted three months, and maximum phenelzine dosage was 45 mg/day. Flooding produced a greater decrement on the Wolpe-Lang Fear Survey, while the phenelzine group had greater amelioration of anxiety. Significant phenelzine-placebo differences were also found in reduction of phobia, neurotic symptoms, and social maladjustment. At two-year follow-up, all patients who had tried to stop phenelzine had relapsed. Limitations of this study include the failure to keep raters blind to psychotherapy status and no ratings for panic attacks.

Mountjoy et al. (1977) contrasted phenelzine plus diazepam and placebo plus diazepam in a study of 36 patients with anxiety neurosis (panic disorder or generalized anxiety disorder) and 22 patients with agoraphobia or social phobia. Maximum phenelzine dose was 75 mg/day, and the study lasted four weeks. Few drug-placebo differences were found; however, for phobic patients phenelzine was superior to placebo on a social phobia scale, while for the patients with anxiety neurosis placebo was superior on the Hamilton Anxiety Scale. Limitations of this study include short duration, small Ns for different treatment groups within diagnosis, heterogeneous patient sample, and lack of ratings for panic attacks.

The most complete trial of MAO inhibitors with panic attacks and agoraphobia, and the only one to contrast a MAO inhibitor and a tricyclic, was the study by Sheehan et al. (1980). Fifty-seven patients with panic attacks and phobic avoidance were assigned to imipramine (up to 150 mg/day), phenelzine (up to 45 mg/day), or placebo for 12 weeks. Both drugs were found superior to placebo on a variety of measures, with a slight edge for phenelzine on two scales. The only limitations of this well-designed trial were its modest dosages and its sample size (big Ns are needed to detect differences between two active drugs) and the fact that all patients received concomitant group psychotherapy.

The most recent MAO inhibitor trial, by Solyom et al. (1981), involved forty patients with agoraphobia or social phobia in a 2 × 2 phenelzine vs. placebo design in which some patients also received exposure therapy. Maximum dosage in this six-week trial was 45 mg/day. Phenelzine was found superior to placebo on anxiety reduction during exposure, but not on avoidance, for which exposure was superior to nonexposure on several measures. No differences between phenelzine and exposure were found in this study, which suffers methodologically from low phenelzine dosage, no separation of outcome by the two phobic types, lack of control for exposure therapy, and no ratings for panic.

None of the MAO inhibitor studies discussed have had all the necessary requisites for an adequate trial: sufficient dosage and duration; sufficient sample size; homogeneous sample, or, if heterogeneous, separate randomization and reporting of different patient types; and adequate ratings of panic attacks. The Sheehan et al. (1980) study comes closest to the mark, in that its only limitations were its modest dosage schedule and sample size. Since the study found distinct phenelzine-placebo differences for phobic patients with panic attacks, it would appear that phenelzine is active with this group. Further well-designed trials are, however, indicated to study MAO inhibitors with all subtypes of anxiety and phobia.

None of the MAO inhibitor trials incorporated a follow-up period in which poststudy treatment was adequately controlled. However, reporting on a large open clinical series, Kelly et al. (1970) found that 30 percent of patients who were well after a year on MAO inhibitors were able to stop medication, while another 36 percent had relapsed after attempting to reduce or stop their MAO inhibitor. The remaining 34 percent were advised, for unstated reasons, not to attempt a reduction in their medication.

Other Antidepressants

Two small open trials found modest efficacy for the specific serotonin-reuptake blocker, zimelidine, in phobic anxiety (Evans and Moore, 1981; Koczkas et al., 1981); however, neither report indicated the type of phobic patients involved. Clinical experience suggests that trazodone may block panic attacks, while a single blind clinical trial found a lack of efficacy for buproprion in patients with panic attacks and phobic avoidance (Sheehan et al., 1983).

Discussion

RELATIONSHIP TO DEPRESSION   Since imipramine and phenelzine are established antidepressants, it is tempting to speculate that their efficacy with patients who have panic and agoraphobia is related to their amelioration of depression. Weighing against this are the following findings.

1. The most adequately designed studies have either found no correlation between baseline depression and outcome (Sheehan et al., 1980) or have found a negative correlation (Zitrin et al., 1980).
2. Buproprion, an effective antidepressant, is ineffective in treating patients with panic (Sheehan et al., 1983).
3. Several cases have been reported in which patients with both panic attacks and depression had their panics blocked with a tricyclic, but required ECT to alleviate their depressions (Nurnberg and Coccaro, 1982).
4. In a series of patients with panic, screened to exclude major depression, a high rate of response was still seen with tricyclics (Liebowitz et al., unpublished data, 1983).
5. Clinical experience indicates ECT is ineffective or noxious for panic attacks.

Nevertheless, panic and depression do not appear entirely independent, as suggested by the recent data showing that patients with histories of both panic attacks and depression have more family histories of depression than do patients with depression only (Leckman et al., 1983). Klein (1981) recently speculated that vulnerability to both panic attacks and depression may be related to defects in normal physiological mechanisms controlling protest and despair reactions to separation.

MECHANISMS OF ACTION   The best current hypothesis for the antipanic effects of imipramine and phenelzine is their ability to suppress central noradrenergic firing via inhibition of the locus coeruleus (Svensson, 1980). The locus coeruleus is the major CNS sympathetic nucleus and has been implicated in the fear responses of primates (Redmond, 1979). It is hypothesized, but not yet proven, that panic blockade is the requisite for the antiphobic effect of tricyclics or MAO inhibitors.

SUMMARY   The efficacy of imipramine has been established for patients with spontaneous panic attacks and for at least some with phobic avoidance. Most patients appear to require 150 to 300 mg/day for several months to become panic free, and some patients require adjunctive exposure therapy to overcome avoidance patterns. Clinical experience, not yet supported by controlled data, also suggests antipanic efficacy for desmethylimipramine, nortriptyline and clomipramine. Optimum length of treatment to minimize relapse remains to be determined. Phenelzine appears similar to imipramine in potency and mechanisms of action with this patient population.

OBSESSIVE-COMPULSIVE DISORDER

The only pharmacologic agent at all systematically tested for patients with obsessive-compulsive disorder has been the tricyclic, clomipramine, which was first shown in the late 1960s to benefit such patients (Reynynghe de Voxrie, 1968). This finding was subsequently affirmed in numerous open studies (Marshall, 1971; Capstick and Seldrup, 1973; Walter, 1978). More recently, a number of controlled trials have been reported. Since these studies have been extensively reviewed elsewhere (Liebowitz, in press), they will be briefly summarized here (see Table 3).

Thoren et al. (1980) assigned 24 obsessive-compulsive patients to clomipramine, nortriptyline, or placebo, and found a significant clomipramine-placebo difference, but found no superiority for nortriptyline over placebo or for clomipramine over nortriptyline. Montgomery (1980) compared clomipramine and placebo in a double-blind crossover design involving 14 obsessive-compulsive patients and noted a significant clomipramine effect on compulsive thoughts but not rituals. Rappaport and colleagues (1980) conducted a 15-week crossover study involving clomipramine, desmethylimipramine, and placebo with 9 obsessive-compulsive adolescents and found no significant differences, although clomipramine effects have been more marked in recently studied cases (Judith Rappaport, personal communication, 1983).

Marks et al. (1981) compared clomipramine and placebo in a study involving forty patients and a complicated eight-month trial, in which patients also received relaxation or exposure in vivo during weeks four to seven and exposure in vivo during weeks seven to ten. With this study, only the first four weeks can be used to ascertain the drug response uncomplicated by psychotherapy. At week four, a significant drug effect appeared on 3 of 15 variables, including time spent on rituals and self-rating on a compulsion checklist. Throughout the study, patients on clomipramine improved more than those on placebo on rituals, mood,

Table 3. Controlled Trials of Antidepressants in Obsessive-Compulsive Disorder

Study (Year)	Sample	Design	Daily Dosage*	Duration	Final Outcome	Limitation
Thoren et al. (1980)	Obsessive-compulsive (RDC criteria) N = 24	Clomipramine vs. nortriptyline vs. placebo	CMI up to 150 mg NORT up to 150 mg	5 weeks	Clomipramine superior to placebo	Small sample. Short duration. Significant effect seen only for scale containing both obsessive-compulsive and depression items
Montgomery (1980)	Obsessive-compulsive (RDC criteria) N = 14	Crossover design: Clomipramine vs. placebo	CMI up to 75 mg	4 weeks of each treatment	Clomipramine effect for compulsive thoughts but not rituals	Concomitant behavior therapy throughout. Carry-over effects of crossover design. Low dosage
Rappaport et al. (1980)	Obsessive-compulsive adolescents N = 9	Crossover design: Clomipramine vs. desmethylimipramine vs. placebo	CMI + DMI up to 150 mg	5 weeks of each treatment	No active drug effects seen	Small N. Carry-over effects of crossover design

Table 3. Continued

Study (Year)	Sample	Design	Daily Dosage*	Duration	Final Outcome	Limitation
Marks et al. (1981)	Obsessive-compulsive N=40	2 × 2 design: Clomipramine vs. placebo; Exposure vs. relaxation	CMI up to 225 mg Mean CMI: 183 mg (week 10); 145 mg (weeks 11–36)	36 weeks	Clomipramine effects on rituals, mood, and social adjustment	Behavior therapy for all patients in weeks 4–10
Ananth et al. (1981)	Obsessive-compulsive N=20	Clomipramine vs. amitriptyline	CMI & AMI up to 300 mg Means: CMI 133.3 mg AMI 197.4 mg	4 weeks	CMI but not AMI effect on obsessive, depressive, and anxiety symptoms CMI superior to AMI on depression, anxiety	Short length of active treatment
Insel et al. (1983)	Obsessive-Compulsive N=12	Crossover design: Clomipramine vs. clorgyline	CMI up to 300 mg Clorgyline 30 mg	6 weeks of each active drug with 4-week placebo period before and after each drug	Clomipramine superior to clorgyline	Small sample, short duration. Lack of simultaneous placebo group. Crossover design

*Note: Final study week; scheduled dosages indicated by "up to"; actually administered doses (if available) denoted by "mean" or "median" and social adjustment, but the investigators did not report proportions of responders versus nonresponders to each treatment.

Summing up, one finds clear or emerging evidence of efficacy in four out of four placebo-controlled trials, suggesting that obsessive-compulsive patients do benefit from clomipramine, but actual response rates cannot be generated from the reported data.

Another trial involving obsessive-compulsive patients compared clomipramine and amitriptyline in a four-week randomized double-blind trial (Ananth et al., 1981). Pre- and posttreatment comparisons showed significant decrement in number and severity of obsessive-compulsive symptoms within clomipramine but not within amitriptyline, but no significant differences between the two drugs for obsessive-compulsive symptoms.

More recently, Insel et al. (1983) have reported a double-blind cross-over trial comparing the response of 13 obsessive-compulsive patients to clomipramine and the selective MAO-A inhibitor clorgyline. Clomipramine, but not clorgyline, appeared effective for obsessive-compulsive symptoms, and clomipramine was superior to clorgyline after six weeks of treatment. The effects of clomipramine on the obsessive-compulsive symptoms did not depend on the presence of depression, but were correlated with plasma concentrations of the drug. While a simultaneous placebo control was not included, patients had failed to respond to four weeks of placebo prior to each active drug phase.

Whether clomipramine is more effective than other antidepressants with obsessive-compulsive patients is still unresolved. In three controlled trials, clomipramine appeared to outperform nortriptyline, amitriptyline, and clorgyline, but significant differences between clomipramine and the other two tricyclics were not demonstrated. Large sample sizes are required to demonstrate differences in active drugs, however, and are difficult to assemble for obsessive-compulsive patients. Case reports suggesting the efficacy of phenelzine and tranylcypromine have also appeared (Annesley, 1969; Jain, 1970; Isberg, 1981; Jenike, 1981), and controlled studies of nonspecific MAO inhibitors and MAO-B inhibitors are indicated.

Should clomipramine prove to be more effective than other tricyclics, a serotonin mechanism may be implicated, since clomipramine is the most potent serotonin-reuptake blocker among the tricyclics. However, as a MAO-A inhibitor, clorgyline should raise serotonin levels as well, and yet was ineffective in doses of 30 mg/day (Insel et al., 1983).

The role that relieving depression plays in the drug response of obsessive-compulsive patients is more complicated than for panic attacks. Many obsessive-compulsive patients also meet the criteria for major depression, and these patients cannot be excluded from drug trials without making it impossible to obtain an adequate sample size. Instead, investigators usually admit the depressed obsessive-compulsive patients if the obsessive-compulsive symptoms came first, dominate the clinical picture, and appear to have led to the depression. Dexamethasone escape was 40 percent in one obsessive-compulsive sample (Insel et al., 1982), which approximates the rate for patients with endogenous depression (Carroll, 1982) and which is also higher than the rate reported for patients with panic disorder (Curtis et al., 1982). Yet Insel et al. (1983) reported that the obsessive-compulsive patients who benefited from clomipramine did not have high pretreatment depression scores.

GENERALIZED ANXIETY DISORDER

Generalized Anxiety Disorder is a residual diagnostic entity left by the removal of Panic Disorder from the DSM-II category of anxiety neurosis. This category per se has received little study, and no antidepressant trials have yet been reported. The older anxiety literature commonly included antidepressant studies of depressed patients with concomitant anxiety, but those of primarily anxious patients (with the exception of studies with doxepin) are relatively rare. These studies have been extensively reviewed elsewhere (Liebowitz, in press). Table 4 outlines those for tricyclics other than doxepin (Rickels et al., 1974; Shammas, 1977; Kleber, 1979; Johnstone et al., 1980; Kahn et al., 1981).

Among these five studies, four show evidence of tricyclic efficacy, two of these in comparison with a benzodiazepine and two in comparison with placebo. The fifth study (Shammas, 1977), which was interpreted as showing benzodiazepine superiority over a tricyclic, was seriously flawed in data-analytic technique. However, all five studies included patients with varying admixtures of depression and anxiety, with only the Kahn et al. (1981) study requiring predominant anxiety. It thus remains unclear whether tricyclics have antianxiety effects separate from their antidepressant effects. The Kahn et al. study suggests that they do, but patients with panic attacks were included, since this study began before the dichotomy between panic and generalized anxiety disorder was widely appreciated. Patients with panic attacks may also have been included in the other four studies, which would predispose the results toward tricyclic superiority. Future studies of patients with generalized anxiety must control carefully for ongoing panic attacks, as well as for depressive symptomatology, even when patients meet DSM-III criteria for Generalized Anxiety Disorder. They should also extend beyond four weeks, since the tricyclic effects in the Kahn et al. (1981) study became more pronounced in weeks six and eight. Whether tricyclic antianxiety effects are distinct from sedative effects also requires careful attention.

In terms of nontricyclic antidepressants, efficacy with primarily anxious patients has been reported for trazodone (Wheatley, 1976) and mianserin (Conti and Pinder, 1979). Since high baseline anxiety seems to be a predictor for phenelzine's efficacy with outpatient nonendogenous depressed patients (Paykel et al., 1982), and MAO inhibitors have been found superior in antianxiety effect to tricyclics with depressed outpatients (Nies et al., 1982), the efficacy of MAO inhibitors in generalized anxiety disorder also merits further study.

OTHER ANXIETY DISORDERS

Posttraumatic Stress Disorder

Although Posttraumatic Stress Disorder is officially listed as a separate DSM-III Anxiety Disorder, patients with this disorder at times experience paniclike reactions. One open trial suggested a MAO inhibitor benefit for five patients who had posttraumatic stress disorder and con-

Table 4. Controlled Studies of Tricyclics in Generalized Anxiety Disorder

Study (Year)	Sample Composition	Design	Daily Dosage*	Duration	Final Outcome	Limitations
Rickels et al. (1974)	Mixed depression and anxiety N=108	Amitriptyline vs. placebo	Mean: AMI 70 mg	4 weeks	AMI>placebo	Significance found in global rating and depressive symptoms only
Shammas (1977)	Mixed anxiety and depression with neither predominant N=72	Amitriptyline vs. bromazepam vs. placebo	Means: AMI 94 mg BROM 24 mg	4 weeks	Bromazepam >AMI	Majority of early dropouts included in end-point analyses Placebo results not provided
Kleber (1979)	Mixed depression and anxiety N=53	Desipramine vs. diazepam	Medians: DMI 150 mg DZPM 20 mg	4 weeks	DMI>diazepam	Greater significance in global and depressive ratings than anxiety rating
Johnstone et al. (1980)	Either anxiety or depression or both in varying combinations N=240	Amitriptyline vs. diazepam	AMI up to 150 mg DZPM up to 20 mg	4 weeks	AMI>diazepam	Differences not sustained when predominantly anxious patients analyzed separately
Kahn et al. (1981)	Greater anxiety than depression N=390	Imipramine vs. chlordiazepoxide vs. doxepin vs. thioridazine vs. placebo	Means: IMI 135 mg CHLORD 56 mg Up to 200 mg IMI, DOX, THIORID Up to 80 mg CHLORD	8 weeks	IMI>placebo DOX>placebo THIORID >placebo	Included patients with panic attacks

*Note: Final study week; dosage scheduled indicated by "up to"; actually administered dose (if available) denoted by "mean" or "median"

comitant panic attacks (Hogben and Cornfield, 1981), but controlled trials of such patients with and without panics are needed. Suggestive of tricyclic efficacy is a report of drug superiority with fifty patients randomized openly to either twice-weekly psychotherapy or a combination of 12 mg perphenazine and 75 mg amitriptyline per day (Thompson, 1977). Open trials of tricyclics alone with this patient group are indicated, to be followed, if warranted, by controlled studies.

Social Phobia

Two studies have reported clomipramine efficacy in social phobia. The first, an open trial involving 765 agoraphobic or social phobic patients treated with clomipramine up to 200 mg/day, found more than 50 percent of patients symptom free at the end of 12 weeks (Beaumont, 1977). Limiting interpretation of these findings, in addition to the noncontrolled design, are the lack of separate results for social phobic versus agoraphobic patients, a greater than one-third dropout rate, the fact that over 50 percent of patients were ill for six months or less, and the lack of specific diagnostic criteria in the report.

More recently, Pecknold et al. (1982) conducted a ten-week double-blind study of 24 agoraphobic and 16 social phobic patients. All patients received clomipramine, and the effects of adding tryptophan or placebo were compared. While no tryptophan-placebo differences were found, patients in both diagnostic groups are reported to have benefited from the treatment regimens. Limitations of this study include the fact that clomipramine administration was not blind or controlled and that diagnostic criteria are not reported for either diagnosis. Also confusing is the report that 80 percent of the patients with social phobia had panic attacks prior to treatment. It is not clear whether the investigators were referring in this instance to spontaneous or situationally induced panics. They do conclude their report, however, by saying that their data support the premise that the main effect of clomipramine, imipramine, and phenelzine is to control spontaneous panic attacks, which suggests that they are referring to spontaneous panic attacks in their social phobic group. DSM-III criteria, on the other hand, do not include spontaneous panic attacks as a feature of social phobia.

The lack of full descriptions or clear criteria for patients with social phobia appears routine in the studies that have included this diagnostic group along with agoraphobic patients in treatment trials (see Table 2). Several studies, including that by Pecknold et al. (1982), appear to have included as social phobic patients those individuals who have spontaneous panic attacks and become socially avoidant because they wish to avoid the embarrassment of having such an attack in the presence of others. This really represents a variant of panic disorder or agoraphobia with panic attacks, rather than a primary form of the social unease, avoidance, or low threshold for shame that characterizes social phobia.

Simple Phobia

No data are available to suggest antidepressant efficacy with patients who have simple phobias and who never have spontaneous panic attacks. The two controlled studies that examined the efficacy of imipramine (Zitrin et al., 1983) or phenelzine (Sheehan et al., 1980) with this population found no drug-placebo differences. These findings are in line with the hypothesis that spontaneous panic attacks are required for a phobic disorder to be amenable to tricyclic or MAO inhibitor therapy.

CONCLUSION

Evidence exists that several classes of antidepressants are extremely effective with patients who have agoraphobia with panic attacks and panic disorder accompanied by limited phobic avoidance. Clomipramine appears effective for obsessive-compulsive patients, but its superiority to other antidepressants remains undemonstrated, and the interrelationship of obsessive-compulsive and depressive symptoms has not been elucidated. Both the tricyclics and the MAO inhibitors may be of benefit in generalized anxiety disorder, but they require further study in this disorder as well as in posttraumatic stress disorder and social phobia. Finally, simple phobias do not appear responsive to antidepressants of any class. The implications of these findings for diagnosis, pathophysiology, and clinical practice are many; they warrant further attention.

Unresolved Questions
by Donald F. Klein, M.D.

INTRODUCTION

Each of the chapters in this part has presented a clear statement concerning recent advances. As we know, current knowledge is a way station toward future, deeper knowledge. Research is always a gamble, given the level of our capabilities and our substantial ignorance of the facts. The unexpected finding is still the greatest generator of scientific advance. Accordingly, although we cannot with any confidence predict future findings, we can at least tabulate some current questions and indicate possible areas where study and experimentation are likely to pay off in the reasonably near future.

As evidence of the rapid scientific growth in the field of anxiety disorders, the Preceptor has prepared a very partial listing of the most apparent and immediately answerable questions raised by these contributions. The length of the list should not be daunting. It is not so much a recitation of the extent of our current ignorance as it is a promise of our future knowledge.

QUESTIONS FOR FUTURE RESEARCH

Diagnostic Issues in the DSM-III Classification of the Anxiety Disorders

Drs. Robert L. Spitzer and Janet B.W. Williams suggest a number of questions related to the nosology of the anxiety disorders. Might generalized anxiety disorder represent the penumbrae of several more discrete conditions? Are there subgroups of generalized anxiety disorders which appear more like panic disorder in remission, others more like compulsive personality disorder, others more like social phobia, and so forth?

Can we reliably identify patients with agoraphobia who do not have panic disorder? What would happen to them if they were given lactate infusions?

Is there any rational way other than convenience and usage whereby preemptive hierarchies can be established? Wouldn't we be better off with fewer hierarchies?

Can generalized anxiety disorder concomitant with major depressive disorder be distinguished from the agitated form of the depressive syndrome? In view of the reports that phenothiazines are helpful for agitated depression but not for anxiety, this may be of some practical consequence.

Are Drs. Spitzer and Williams suggesting that generalized anxiety disorder be given as an additional diagnosis to panic disorder?

Doesn't the suggestion that a patient with panic disorder who avoids eating in public be diagnosed as having a social phobia obscure the notion that a social phobia represents an irrational fear of embarrassment? The patient with panic disorder has more realistic reason to think that he may behave in a socially inappropriate way (as by fleeing a restaurant) than what is usually considered as socially phobic.

Do patients with obsessive-compulsive disorders regularly have generalized anxiety? Aren't there some patients with obsessive-compulsive disorder who have organized their thinking and rituals to a degree that they are relatively calm most of the time?

If the instigating incident in posttraumatic stress disorder is broadened to include stresses within the range of normal experience, how can posttraumatic stress disorder be distinguished from adjustment reactions?

The Role of Genetics in the Etiology of Panic Disorder

Dr. Raymond R. Crowe's chapter prompts the question, Is it clear that neurasthenia, neurocirculatory asthenia, and effort syndrome are actually synonyms for panic disorder? Might they not be overlapping rather than identical conditions? What proportion of patients with panic disorder has easy fatigability? Does this relate to mitral valve prolapse?

Is anxiety beginning after the age of 40 commonly part of a depressive syndrome? How commonly does this occur?

Is an adoption study on anxiety disorders feasible?

What is the relevance of Gray's model for the spontaneous panic attack?

Might the benzodiazepine-receptor system be a component of an anxiogenic circuit?

Anxiety Disorders in Children

Dr. Rachel Gittelman raises many developmental and treatment issues. Is there any objective evidence that separation anxiety is the child's response to unconscious aggressive impulses toward the mother, as Anna Freud has stated? Is such a belief supported by any evidence other than application of the precept that behind every fear lies a wish? Is such a belief consonant with the clinical findings and the benefits of imipramine?

What is the long-term outcome of separation anxiety in children?

Do benzodiazepines have any place in the management of childhood anxiety?

What are the clinical characteristics of overanxious children?

Do social phobic children suffer from marked rejection sensitivity? Might monoamine oxidase (MAO) inhibitors be of benefit?

The Psychotherapy of Anxiety

Dr. Jerome D. Frank suggests that anxiety symptoms alone are not sufficient incentive to bring a person to psychotherapy, but that the patient must also be demoralized. However, a person may feel unable to handle his or her symptoms alone and consequently seek professional help, but this might not damage the person's self-esteem. A person who requires an appendectomy does not necessarily feel demoralized because of not being able to treat the symptoms without assistance. Conceivably, some enlightened patients with anxiety symptoms may recognize their incapacity to deal with these symptoms and apply for appropriate help without undergoing pervasive demoralization. Public education may be useful here, especially with regard to recent pharmacologic advances in developing several different effective anxiolytics, which are frequently confused with addicting drugs.

Can we measure degree of demoralization, and does it affect the course of treatment? One might expect that the severer the demoralization, the more difficulty the patient would have in improving if improvement required goal-directed activity.

Can severe demoralization be distinguished from depression? The Preceptor has suggested elsewhere that severe demoralization is characterized by appetitive inhibition, but not by inhibition of consummatory pleasures (Wender and Klein, 1981).

Can demoralization be treated by pharmacotherapeutic methods? In particular, do stimulants and MAO inhibitors have a role here, since they seem to increase appetitive and pursuit pleasures?

Can it be demonstrated that interaction with anxious family members intensifies the anxiety of the patients? Is this an indication for family treatment?

Does the cathartic method, as with amobarbital injections, have any specific value for the treatment of posttraumatic stress disorders compared with other credible therapies? Is this a function of the recency of the stress?

What abilities, attitudes, or experiences must a patient have to be able to evaluate his or her own recurrent spontaneous panic attacks as harmless and transient? Can this be enhanced?

Can any differences be found between different psychotherapies that cannot be attributed to credibility or persuasiveness (Klein and Rabkin, 1983)?

Dr. Frank finds the professionalism of the therapist to be an important variable in creating a secure attachment and facilitating therapy. However, professionalism is clearly a matter of degree. Can degrees of professionalism be scaled? After a certain minimum degree of professionalism is established in the patient's eyes, does increased professionalism yield further benefits?

Can the minimum degree of professionalism that most patients find credible and useful be determined? Might this differ depending upon the nature of the disorder? What about the expectations of the patient? Do different social strata have different expectations concerning the degree of professional training that the therapist must have to be credible?

Is the therapist's ability to listen important for all patients? Might not some patients benefit from an entirely didactic approach and find self-revelation positively burdensome? Can this be assessed prior to treatment?

Is emotional arousal a crucial variable for therapeutic effect, since in the field of phobia treatment we have seen a shift from abreactive flooding to graded exposure? Can procedures be developed to help patients view medication as enhancing self-efficacy?

Anxiety and Psychodynamic Theory

Dr. John C. Nemiah cites Freud as saying that if you compel an agoraphobic to cross the street alone, the consequence will be an attack of anxiety. In fact, this is not usually the case, as shown by behavioral tests. What are the implications for dynamic theory?

Is there any way of telling in advance, on examinational grounds, which patients are suffering from structural intrapsychic conflicts and which are not?

What information is available regarding the specific diagnosis of alexithymia and its relationship to treatment? What is the operational definition for alexithymia, and has this been shown to be a reliable judgment? Do alexithymics find insight-oriented therapy credible?

Just because a patient is psychologically minded does not indicate that the etiology of that patient's anxiety state is psychogenic. Should one routinely recommend dynamic psychotherapy for psychologically minded people with panic attacks?

What about a study where psychologically minded patients with panic attacks were randomly assigned to medication plus noninsightful behavioral procedures vs. medication plus psychodynamic procedures, assuming that both therapies are found credible by the patients? Wouldn't psychodynamic theory predict a sharp decrease in the eventual relapse rate in the dynamically treated patients, given resolution of underlying conflicts? Can this be demonstrated?

The Relaxation Response and the Treatment of Anxiety

Dr. Herbert Benson reports the interesting, counterintuitive result that while training in the relaxation response causes an increase in plasma norepinephrine levels, this change is not associated with increases in heart rate and blood pressure. His suggestion is that these observations are consistent with reduced norepinephrine end-organ responsivity. In other words, the relaxation response appears to work analogously to pharmacologic β-blockade, which also has been reported to be associated with increased plasma and urinary catecholamines. Is there a neural circuit that induces β-blockade?

Benson cites the work of Peters et al. (1977a; 1977b) which compared the effects on working volunteers of the relaxation response vs. instructions to sit quietly vs. no instructions. Although the relaxation response showed statistical superiority to the no-instruction group, it was not superior to the simple instruction to sit quietly. In a study involving patients with anxiety neuroses, Benson et al. (1978) compared self-hypnosis and a meditational relaxation technique and found no differences.

Therefore, in both studies when the relaxation response was compared with another credible alternative, no superiority was found. Furthermore, substantial clinical improvements were not apparent in either case.

Do these results indicate a specific value for training in the relaxation response in the treatment of anxiety? Aren't these results consonant with the usual finding that credible psychotherapies have indistinguishable effects?

Exposure Treatment of Agoraphobia

Dr. Matig Mavissakalian's report on his study raises the question of how much consequence antidepressant dosage differences have in the comparative studies of antidepressants and nonpharmacologic approaches.

Can it be physiologically demonstrated that flooding actually blockades the recurrence of spontaneous panics?

If exposure stops panics, why do patients with pure panic disorders who have no phobic avoidances continue to have panics? Does a decrease in anticipatory anxiety make the occurrence of spontaneous panics less likely?

Mortality After Thirty to Forty Years: Panic Disorder Compared with Other Psychiatric Illnesses

Dr. William Coryell's follow-up raises several questions regarding the nature of the circulatory system disease reported to be in excess in patients with panic disorder. Does this relate to mitral valve prolapse? What about the relative cardiotoxic importance of tobacco and alcohol as secondary to anxious states? Does panic disorder predispose to hypertension? Does this suggest the utility of chronic β-blockers in the treatment of panic disorder?

Does a successful treatment of panic disorder obviate the increased risk of suicide?

The Biology of Anxiety

Dr. Jack M. Gorman's review leads to the question, Do the differences described for anxious patients in autonomic nervous system physiology differ between anxiety disorder subgroups? What about patients with depression, schizophrenia, or other distressing psychopathology?

Is lessened vagal tone important in anxiety states? How can this be demonstrated? For instance, are there differential effects of cholinergic and anticholinergic agents between anxious patients and normal subjects?

Is the reported increase in platelet MAO levels in agoraphobic patients compensatory for increased circulating catecholamines? Does chronic tricyclic treatment increase circulating catecholamines? Does this cause any change in MAO?

Are carbon dioxide–induced panic attacks prevented by antidepressant treatment?

Do β-agonists such as isoproterenol produce panic attacks or just cardiorespiratory distress?

Will antidepressants block the anxiogenic effects of yohimbine in normal subjects or patients with panic disorder?

What are the merits of chronic β-blockers in the treatment of anxiety?

What role do the various definitions of mitral valve prolapse play in the differences reported in the incidence of mitral valve prolapse?

The Biochemistry of Anxiety: From Pharmacotherapy to Pathophysiology

Drs. Steven M. Paul and Phil Skolnick have given us a fascinating review of a tremendously promising area.

What can we make of the fact that a complete pharmacologic effect is observed if only 25 percent of the benzodiazepine receptors are occupied? Does this indicate some selectivity of action within a mixed class of benzodiazepine receptors?

Is there any evidence for an endogenous ligand that may play a role in anxiogenesis?

Do specific benzodiazepine-receptor antagonists, such as Ro15-1788, have any effect upon states of pathological anxiety?

What role, if any, would GABA'ergic compounds play in the management of anxiety? Might they be useful synergistic agents with benzodiazepines?

β-Adrenergic Blockers and Buspirone

Dr. Jonathan O. Cole highlights two poorly understood but potentially valuable groups of antianxiety agents.

Since buspirone resembles apomorphine in some of its actions, can it cause a significant degree of nausea?

Would β-blockers or buspirone have any role in treating the patient with severe examination anxiety?

Is it possible that the beneficial effects of β-blockers on performance anxiety are due to their disrupting a vicious, positive feedback cycle where initial treatment and tachycardia are overreacted to with yet further autonomic discharge?

Is there any evidence of different clinical effectiveness of β-blockers with regard to their capacity to pass the blood-brain barrier?

Is there any evidence of synergistic effects between benzodiazepines and β-blockers? Similarly, does adding buspirone to a benzodiazepine produce any benefits that could not have been accomplished by simply raising the dose of benzodiazepine?

The Efficacy of Antidepressants in Anxiety Disorders

Dr. Michael R. Liebowitz's review leads to the question of what proportion of agoraphobic patients do not experience a clinical onset consisting of spontaneous panic attacks. Do such patients differ in response to treatment from those whose illness does begin in this way?

Do relapses regularly start with panic attacks? Are relapses heralded by signs of increasing autonomic or respiratory disturbance?

What determines when simple panic disorder progresses to phobic avoidance? Is it the frequency and intensity of the attacks? Is it the presence of obsessional trends antedating the onset of the panic attacks?

Might high-dose benzodiazepines be of use in blockade of panic attacks?

If alprazolam is demonstrated to blockade spontaneous panic attacks, is this different from other high-potency benzodiazepines such as clonazepam?

What are the characteristics of the small group of panic disorder patients who do not respond to imipramine but do respond to MAO inhibitors? Is this related to features of atypical depression?

What is the optimum length of drug treatment of panic disorder to minimize relapse when medication is discontinued?

How fast will panic attacks come under control if medication (as compared with placebo) is started immediately on relapse? Might there be an immediate blockade?

Are antidepressants effective in pure generalized anxiety disorders?

Are antidepressants useful for posttraumatic stress disorder in patients without concomitant panic attacks?

CONCLUSION

Psychiatry has always been plagued by unanswered questions. This chapter presents a sampling of current queries. However, we can take heart from the fact that these questions are not abstract quandaries but are eminently researchable, given currently available techniques. We can look forward to the answers and the new questions.

References for Part V

References for the Introduction

Klein DF: A proposed definition of mental illness, in Critical Issues in Psychiatric Diagnosis. Edited by Spitzer RL, Klein DF. New York, Raven Press, 1978

Klein DF, Davis JM: Diagnosis and Drug Treatment of Psychiatric Disorders, 1st ed. Baltimore, Williams & Wilkins, 1969

Klein DF, Gittelman R, Quitkin FM, Rifkin A: Diagnosis and Drug Treatment of Psychiatric Disorders: Adults and Children, 2nd ed. Baltimore, Williams & Wilkins, 1980

Wender PH, Klein DF: Mind, Mood, and Medicine: A Guide to the New Biopsychiatry. New York, Farrar, Straus & Giroux, 1981

References for Chapter 25

Diagnostic Issues in the DSM-III Classification of the Anxiety Disorders

American Psychiatric Association, Diagnostic and Statistical Manual of Mental Disorders, 3rd ed. Washington DC, American Psychiatric Association, 1980

Amies PL, Gelder MG, Shaw PM: Social phobia: A comparative clinical study. Br J Psychiatry 142:174–179, 1983

Atkinson RM, Henderson RG, Sparr LF, Deale S: Assessment of Viet Nam veterans for posttraumatic stress disorder in Veterans Administration disability claims. Am J Psychiatry 139:1118–1121, 1982

Barlow DH, Beck JG: The psychosocial treatment of anxiety disorders: Current status, future directions, in Psychotherapy Research: Where Are We and Where Should We Go? Edited by Williams JBW, Spitzer RL. New York, Guilford Press, 1984

Boyd JH, Burke JD, Gruenberg E, Holzer CE, George LK, Karno M, Stoltzman R, McEvoy L, Nestadt G: The diagnostic hierarchies of DSM-III. Paper presented at the Annual Meeting of the American Psychiatric Association, New York, May 1983

Celsus AC: Celsus on Medicine (in eight books) (first century A.D.). Translation of L. Targa edition by Lee A. London, E Cox, 1831

Cloninger CR, Martin RL, Clayton P, Guze SB: A blind follow-up and family study of anxiety neurosis: Preliminary analysis of the St. Louis 500, in Anxiety: New Research and Changing Concepts. Edited by Klein DF, Rabkin JG. New York, Raven Press, 1981

DaCosta JM: On irritable heart: A clinical study of a functional cardiac disorder and its consequences. Am J Med Sci 61:17–25, 1871

Di Nardo PA, O'Brien GT, Barlow DH, Waddell MT, Blanchard EB: Reliability of DSM-III anxiety disorder categories using a new structured interview. Arch Gen Psychiatry (in press)

Falloon IRH, Lloyd GG, Harpin RE: The treatment of social phobia: Real-life rehearsal with nonprofessional therapists. J Nerv Ment Dis 169:180–184, 1981

Feighner JP, Robins E, Guze SB, Woodruff RA, Winokur G, Munoz R: Diagnostic criteria for use in psychiatric research. Arch Gen Psychiatry 38:57–63, 1972

Finlay-Jones R, Brown GW: Types of stressful life events and the onset of anxiety and depressive disorders. Psychol Med 11:803–815, 1981

Foa EB, Foa UG: Differentiating depression and anxiety: Is it possible? Is it useful? Psychopharm Bull 18:62–68, 1982

Frances A, Cooper AM: The DSM-III controversy: A psychoanalytic perspective. Am J Psychiatry 138:1198–1202, 1981

Freud S: On the grounds for detaching a particular syndrome from neurasthenia under the description "anxiety neurosis," (1894) in Complete Psychological Works, standard ed, vol 3. London, Hogarth Press, 1962

Frye JS, Stockton RA: Discriminant analysis of posttraumatic stress disorder among a group of Viet Nam veterans. Am J Psychiatry 139:52–56, 1982

Gurney C, Roth M, Garside RF, Kerr TA, Schapira K: Studies in the classification of affective disorders. II. The relationship between anxiety states and depressive illnesses. Br J Psychiatry 121:162–166, 1972

Horowitz MJ, Wilner N, Kaltreider N, Alvarez W: Signs and symptoms of posttraumatic stress disorder. Arch Gen Psychiatry 37:85–92, 1980

Hough RL, Gongla PA: Research problems in relation to post-traumatic stress disorders in Viet Nam veterans. Paper presented at the workshop on anxiety disorders, National Institute of Mental Health, Rockville MD, May 6–7, 1982

Insel TR: Obsessive compulsive disorder—five clinical questions and a suggested approach. Compr Psychiatry 23:241–251, 1982

Keiser L: The Traumatic Neurosis. Philadelphia, JB Lippincott Co, 1968

Klein DF: Delineation of two drug responsive anxiety syndromes. Psychopharmacologia 5:397–408, 1964

Klein DF: Anxiety reconceptualized, in Anxiety: New Research and Changing Concepts. Edited by Klein DF, Rabkin JG. New York, Raven Press, 1981

Klein DF: Medication in the treatment of panic attacks and phobic states. Psychopharm Bull 18:85–90, 1982

Klein DF, Rabkin JG. (eds): Anxiety: New Research and Changing Concepts. New York, Raven Press, 1981

Klerman GL: Anxiety and depression, in Handbook of Studies on Anxiety. Edited by Burrows GD, Davies B. Amsterdam, Elsevier/North Holland Biomedical Press, 1980

Leckman JF, Weissman MM, Merikangas KR, Pauls DL, Prusoff BA: Panic disorder increases risk of depression, alcoholism, panic and phobic disorders in families of depressed probands. Arch Gen Psychiatry, in press

Lewis A: Problem of obsessional illness. Proc R Soc Med 29:325–326, 1936

Lopez-Ibor J Jr, Lopez-Ibor JM: Spanish psychiatry and DSM-III, in International Perspectives on DSM-III. Edited by Spitzer RL, Williams JBW, Skodol AE. Washington DC, American Psychiatric Press, 1983

Mackenzie TB, Popkin MK: Organic anxiety syndrome. Am J Psychiatry 140:342–344, 1983

Marks IM: The classification of phobic disorders. Br J Psychiatry 116:377–386, 1970

Raskin M, Peeke HV, Dickman W, Pinsker H: Panic and generalized anxiety disorders. Developmental antecedents and precipitants. Arch Gen Psychiatry 39:687–689, 1982

Regier DA, Myers JK, Kramer M, Robins LN, Blazer DG, Hough RL, Eaton WW, Locke BZ: The NIMH Epidemiologic Catchment Area (ECA) program: Historical context, major objectives, and study population. Paper presented at the Annual Meeting of the American Public Health Association, Montreal, Canada, November 1982

Shader RI, Greenblatt DJ: Antidepressants: The second harvest and DSM-III. J Clin Psychopharmacol 1:51–52, 1981

Spitzer RL, Williams JBW: Proposed revisions in the DSM-III classification of anxiety disorders based on research and clinical experience. Paper presented at Anxiety and the Anxiety Disorders, National Institute of Mental Health-sponsored Conference. Tuxedo Park NY, September 12–14, 1983a

Spitzer RL, Williams JBW: Structured Clinical Interview for DSM-III (SCID). New York, Biometrics Research Department, New York State Psychiatric Institute, 1983b

World Health Organization: Mental Disorders: Glossary and guide to their classification in accordance with the Ninth Revision of the International Classification of Diseases. Geneva, World Health Organization, 1978

Zitrin CM, Klein DF, Woerner MG: Behavior therapy, supportive psychotherapy, imipramine and phobias. Arch Gen Psychiatry 35:307–316, 1978

References for Chapter 26

The Role of Genetics
in the Etiology of Panic Disorder

Ackerman SH, Sachar EJ: The lactate theory of anxiety: A review and reevaluation. Psychosom Med 36:69–81, 1974

Andreasen NC, Endicott J, Spitzer RL, Winokur G: The family history method using diagnostic criteria. Arch Gen Psychiatry 34:1229–1235, 1977

Appleby IL, Klein DF, Sachar EJ, Morton L: Biochemical indices of lactate-induced panic: A preliminary report, in Anxiety: New Research and Changing Concepts. Edited by Klein DF, Rabkin JG. New York, Raven Press, 1981

Beard GM: Neurasthenia or nervous exhaustion. Boston Med Surg J 3:217–221, 1869

Brown FW: Heredity in the psychoneuroses. Proc Royal Soc Med 35:785–790, 1942

Carey G, Gottesman II, Robins E: Prevalence rates for the neuroses: Pitfalls in the evaluation of familiality. Psychol Med 10:437–443, 1980

Cloninger CR, Martin RL, Clayton PJ, Guze SB: A blind follow-up and family study of anxiety neurosis: Preliminary analysis of the St. Louis 500, in Anxiety: New Research and Changing Concepts. Edited by Klein DF, Rabkin JG. New York, Raven Press, 1981

Cohen ME, White PD: Life situations, emotions and neurocirculatory asthenia (anxiety neurosis, neurasthenia, effort syndrome). Assn Res Nerv Ment Dis Proc 29:832–869, 1950

Cohen ME, Badel DW, Kilpatrick A, Reed EW, White PD: The high familial prevalence of neurocirculatory asthenia (anxiety neurosis, effort syndrome). Am J Hum Genet 3:126–158, 1951

Crowe RR, Pauls DL, Slymen DJ, Noyes R: A family study of anxiety neurosis: Morbidity risk in families of patients with and without mitral valve prolapse. Arch Gen Psychiatry 37:77–79, 1980

Crowe RR, Gaffney G, Kerber R: Panic attacks in families of patients with mitral valve prolapse. J Affective Disord 4:121–125, 1982

Crowe RR, Noyes R, Pauls DL, Slymen D: A family study of panic disorder. Arch Gen Psychiatry 40:1065–1069, 1983

Devereux RB: Mitral valve prolapse. Am J Med 67:729–731, 1979

Devereux RB, Brown T, Kramer-Fox R, Sachs I: Inheritance of mitral valve prolapse: Effect of age and sex on gene expression. Ann Intern Med 97:826–832, 1982

Gershon ES, Hamovit J, Guroff JJ, Dibble GE, Leckman JF, Sceery W, Targum SD, Nurnberger JI, Goldin LR, Bunney WE: A family study of schizoaffective, bipolar I, bipolar II, unipolar, and normal control probands. Arch Gen Psychiatry 39:1157–1167, 1982

Gorman JM, Fyer AF, Glicklich J, King DL, Klein DF: Mitral valve prolapse and panic disorders: Effect of imipramine, in Anxiety: New Research and Changing Concepts. Edited by Klein DF, Rabkin JG. New York, Raven Press, 1981

Gray JA: Anxiety as a paradigm case of emotion. Brit Med Bull 37:193–197, 1981a

Gray JA: The Neuropsychology of Anxiety: An Inquiry Into the Functions of the Septo-Hippocampal System. Oxford, Oxford University Press, 1981b

Grosz HJ, Farmer BB: Blood lactate in the development of anxiety symptoms: A critical examination of Pitts' and McClure's hypothesis and experimental study. Arch Gen Psychiatry 21:611–619, 1969

Grosz HJ, Farmer BB: Pitts' and McClure's lactate-anxiety study revisited. Br J Psychiatry 120:415–418, 1972

Grunhaus L, Gloger S, Rein A, Lewis BS: Mitral valve prolapse and panic attacks. Israel J Med Sci 18:221–223, 1982

Hallam RS: Agoraphobia: A critical review of the concept. Br J Psychiatry 133:314–319, 1978

Hartman N, Kramer R, Brown T, Devereux RB: Panic disorder in patients with mitral valve prolapse. Am J Psychiatry 139:669–670, 1982

Hoehn-Saric R: Neurotransmitters in anxiety. Arch Gen Psychiatry 39:735–742, 1982

Kannel WB, Dawber TR, Cohen ME: The electrocardiogram in neurocirculatory asthenia (anxiety neurosis or neurasthenia): A study of 203 neurocirculatory asthenia patients and 757 healthy controls in the Framingham study. Ann Int Med 49:1351–1360, 1958

Kelly D, Mitchell-Heggs N, Sherman D: Anxiety and the effects of sodium lactate assessed clinically and physiologically. Br J Psychiatry 119:129–141, 1971

Kendler K, Gruenberg AM, Strauss JS: An independent analysis of the Copenhagen sample of the Danish adoption study of schizophrenia: I. The relationship between anxiety disorder and schizophrenia. Arch Gen Psychiatry 38:973–977, 1981

Kidd KK, Cavalli-Sforza LL: An analysis of the genetics of schizophrenia. Soc Biol 3:254–265, 1973

Klein DF: Anxiety reconceptualized, in Anxiety: New Research and Changing Concepts. Edited by Klein DF, Rabkin JG. New York, Raven Press, 1981

McInnes RG: Observations on heredity in neurosis. Proc Roy Soc Med 30:895–904, 1937

Marks I, Lader M: Anxiety states (anxiety neurosis): A review. J Nerv Ment Dis 156:3–18, 1973

Noyes R, Clancy J, Crowe RR, Slymen D: The familial prevalence of anxiety neurosis. Arch Gen Psychiatry 35:1057–1059, 1978

Oppenheimer BS, Rothschild MA: The psychoneurotic factor in the irritable heart of soldiers. JAMA 70:1919–1923, 1918

Pariser SF, Pinta ER, Jones BA: Mitral valve prolapse syndrome and anxiety neurosis/panic disorder. Am J Psychiatry 135:246–247, 1978

Paul SM, Marangos PJ, Skolnick P: The benzodiazepine-GABA-chloride ionophore receptor complex: Common site of minor tranquilizer action. Biol Psychiatry 16:213–229, 1981

Pauls DL, Crowe RR, Noyes R: Distribution of ancestral secondary cases in anxiety neurosis (panic disorder). J Affective Disord 1:287–290, 1979

Pauls DL, Bucher KD, Crowe RR, Noyes R: A genetic study of panic disorder pedigrees. Am J Hum Genet 32:639–644, 1980

Pitts FN, McClure JN: Lactate metabolism in anxiety neurosis. N Engl J Med 277:1329–1336, 1967

Reich T, Cloninger CR, Guze SB: The multifactorial model of disease transmission: I. Description of the model and its use in psychiatry. Br J Psychiatry 127:1–10, 1975

Slater E, Cowie V: The Genetics of Mental Disorders. Oxford, Oxford University Press, 1971

Squires RF, Braestrup C: Benzodiazepine receptors in rat brain. Nature 266:732–734, 1977

Tallman JF, Paul SM, Skolnick P, Gallager DW: Receptors for the age of anxiety: Pharmacology of the benzodiazepines. Science 207:274–281, 1980

Thompson WD, Orvaschel H, Prusoff BA, Kidd KK: An evaluation of the family history method for ascertaining psychiatric disorders. Arch Gen Psychiatry 39:53–58, 1982

Torgersen S: Contribution of twins to psychiatric nosology, in Twin Research: Part A. Psychology and Methodology. Edited by Nance WE. New York, Allen R Liss, 1978

Venkatesh A, Pauls DL, Crowe RR, Noyes R, Van Valkenburg CV, Martins JB, Kerber RE: Mitral valve prolapse in anxiety neurosis (panic disorder). Am Heart J 100:302–305, 1980

Wheeler EO, White PD, Reed EW, Cohen ME: Familial incidence of neurocirculatory asthenia ("anxiety neurosis," "effort syndrome") (abstract). J Clin Invest 27:562, 1948

Wheeler EO, White PD, Reed EW, Cohen ME: Neurocirculatory asthenia (anxiety neurosis, effort syndrome, neurasthenia): A twenty year follow-up study of one-hundred seventy-three patients. JAMA 142:878–889, 1950

Wooley CF: Where are the diseases of yesteryear? DaCosta's syndrome, soldier's heart, the effort syndrome, neurocirculatory asthenia—and the mitral valve prolapse syndrome. Circulation 53:749–750, 1976

References for Chapter 27

Anxiety Disorders in Children

Abe K: Sulpiride in school phobia. Psychiatr Clin 8:95–98, 1975

Ainsworth MDS: Infancy in Uganda: Infant Care and the Growth of Love. Baltimore, Johns Hopkins University Press, 1967

Bauer D: Childhood fears in developmental perspective, in Modern Perspectives in Truancy and School Refusal. Edited by Hersov L, Berg I. New York, John Wiley & Sons, 1980

Berney T, Kolvin I, Bhate SR, Garside RF, Jeans J, Kay B, Scarth L: School phobia: A therapeutic trial with clomipramine and short-term outcome. Br J Psychiatry 138:110–118, 1981

Bowlby J: Attachment and Loss, vol 1: Attachment. New York, Basic Books, 1969

Bowlby J: Attachment and Loss, vol 2: Separation Anxiety and Anger. New York, Basic Books, 1973

D'Amato G: Chlordiazepoxide in management of school phobia. Disease Nerv Syst 23:292–295, 1962

Eisenberg L: School phobia: A study in the communication of anxiety. Am J Psychiatry 114:712–718, 1958

Fish B: Drug therapy in child psychiatry: Pharmacological aspects. Compr Psychiatry 1: 212–227, 1960

Fish B: Drug use in psychiatric disorders of children. Am J Psychiatry 124:31–36, 1968

Freud S: Analysis of a phobia in a five-year-old boy (1909), in Complete Psychological Works, standard ed, vol 10. London, Hogarth Press, 1955

Frommer EA: Treatment of childhood depression with antidepressant drugs. Br Med J 1:729–732, 1967

Frommer EA: Depressive illness in childhood. Br J Psychiatry Special Publ 2:117–136, 1968

Gittelman-Klein R: Pharmacotherapy of pathological separation anxiety, in Recent Advances in Child Psychopharmacology. Edited by Gittelman-Klein R. New York, Human Sciences Press, 1975

Gittelman-Klein R, Klein DF: Controlled imipramine treatment of school phobia. Arch Gen Psychiatry 25:204–207, 1971

Gittelman-Klein R, Klein DF: School phobia: Diagnostic considerations in the light of imipramine effects. J Nerv Ment Dis 156:199–215, 1973

Hayes TA, Panitch ML, Barker E: Imipramine dosage in children: A comment on "Imipramine and electrocardiographic abnormalities in hyperactive children." Am J Psychiatry 132:546–547, 1975

Jones MC: A laboratory study of fear: The case of Peter. Pedag Seminary 31:308–315, 1924

Klein DF: Delineation of two drug-responsive anxiety syndromes. Psychopharmacologia 5:397–408, 1964

Klein DF, Zitrin CM, Woerner MG, Ross DC: Treatment of phobias. II. Behavior therapy and supportive psychotherapy. Arch Gen Psychiatry 40:139–145, 1983

Kraft IA: Treatment of school phobia with chlordiazepoxide. Am J Psychiatry 118:841–842, 1962

Lapouse R, Monk MA: An epidemiologic study of behavior characteristics in children. Am J Pub Health 48:1134–1144, 1958

Lapouse R, Monk MA: Fears and worries in a representative sample of children. Am J Orthopsychiatry 29:803–818, 1959

Miller LC, Barrett CL, Hampe E, Noble H: Comparison of reciprocal inhibition, psychotherapy and waiting list control for phobic children. J Abnorm Psychol 79:269–279, 1972

Ollendich T, Mayer JA: School Phobia in Behavioral Treatment of Anxiety Disorders. Edited by Turner SM. New York, Plenum Press, 1982

Rutter M: Separation, loss, and family relationships, in Child Psychiatry: Modern Approaches. Edited by Rutter M, Hersov L. Oxford, Blackwell Scientific Publications, 1977

Saraf KR, Klein DF, Gittelman-Klein R, Groff S: Imipramine side effects in children. Psychopharmacologia 37:265–274, 1974

Saraf KR, Klein DF, Gittelman-Klein R, Gootman N, Greenhill P: EKG effects of imipramine treatment in children. J Am Acad Child Psychiatry 17:60–69, 1978

Skynner ACR: Effects of chlordiazepoxide (ltr to ed). Lancet 1:110, 1961

Sperling M: School phobias: Classification, dynamics and treatment. Psychoanal Study Child 22:375–401, 1967

Suomi SJ, Seaman SF, Lewis JK, DeLizio RD, McKinney WT: Effects of imipramine treatment of separation-induced social disorders in rhesus monkeys. Arch Gen Psychiatry 35:321–327, 1978

Weinraub M, Lewis M: The determinants of children's responses to separation. Monogr Soc Res Child Dev 42:1–78, 1977

Winsberg BG, Goldstein S, Yepes LE, Perel JM: Imipramine and electrocardiographic abnormalities in hyperactive children. Am J Psychiatry 132:542–545, 1975

Zitrin CM, Klein DF, Woerner MG, Ross DC: Treatment of phobias. Arch Gen Psychiatry 40:125–138, 1983

References for Chapter 28

The Psychotherapy of Anxiety

American Psychiatric Association: Diagnostic and Statistical Manual of Mental Disorders, 3rd ed. Washington DC, American Psychiatric Association, 1980

Asch SE: Effects of group pressure upon the modification and distortion of judgments, in Groups, Leadership and Men. Edited by Guetzkow H. Pittsburgh, Carnegie Press, 1951

Beck AT: Cognitive Therapy and the Emotional Disorders. New York, International Universities Press, 1976

Bowlby J: Attachment theory, separation anxiety and mourning, in American Handbook of Psychiatry, 2nd ed, vol 6. Edited by Hamburg DA, Brodie HKH. New York, Basic Books, 1975

DeFigueiredo JM, Frank JD: Subjective incompetence, the clinical hallmark of demoralization. Compr Psychiatry 23:353–363, 1982

Frank JD: Therapeutic components shared by all psychotherapies, in Psychotherapy Research and Behavior Change (The Master Lecture Series, vol 1). Edited by Harvey JH, Parks MM. Washington DC, American Psychological Association, 1982

Freud S: A General Introduction to Psychoanalysis. New York, Horace Liveright, 1920

Grinker RR, Spiegel JP: War Neuroses. Philadelphia, Blakiston, 1945

Havens LL: The existential use of the self. Am J Psychiatry 131:1–10, 1974

Horney K: The Neurotic Personality of Our Time. New York, WW Norton & Co, 1937

Janov A: The Primal Scream: Primal Therapy, the Cure for Neurosis. New York, GP Putnam's Sons, 1970

Kardiner A: Traumatic neuroses of war, in American Handbook of Psychiatry, vol 1. Edited by Arieti S. New York, Basic Books, 1959

Shader RI, Goodman M, Gever J: Panic disorders: Current perspectives. J Clin Psychopharmacol (Suppl 6) 2:2S–10S, 1982

Shapiro RI, Shapiro D: Meta-analysis of comparative therapy outcome studies: A replication and refinement. Psychol Bull 92:581–604, 1982

Smith NL, Glass GV, Miller TI: Benefits of Psychotherapy. Baltimore, Johns Hopkins University Press, 1980

Stampfl TG, Levis DJ: Essentials of implosive therapy. J Abnorm Psychol 72:496–503, 1967

Sullivan HS: The Interpersonal Theory of Psychiatry. New York, WW Norton & Co, 1953

Weeks C: Agoraphobia. New York, EP Dutton & Co, 1977

Wolpe J: Psychotherapy by Reciprocal Inhibition. Stanford CA, Stanford University Press, 1958

References for Chapter 29

Anxiety and Psychodynamic Theory

Breuer J, Freud S: Studies on Hysteria (1895): Complete Psychological Works, standard ed, vol 2. London, Hogarth Press, 1955

Freud S: The neuro-psychoses of defense (1894), in Complete Psychological Works, standard ed, vol 3. London, Hogarth Press, 1962

Freud S: Obsessions and phobias (1895a), in Complete Psychological Works, standard ed, vol 3. London, Hogarth Press, 1962

Freud S: On the grounds for detaching a particular syndrome from neurasthenia under the description of "anxiety neurosis" (1895b), in Complete Psychological Works, standard ed, vol 3. London, Hogarth Press, 1962

Freud S: The Interpretation of Dreams (1) (1900): Complete Psychological Works, standard ed, vol 4. London, Hogarth Press, 1953

Freud S: A phobia in a five-year-old boy (1909), in Complete Psychological Works, standard ed, vol 10. London, Hogarth Press, 1955

Freud S: Inhibitions, Symptoms and Anxiety (1926): Complete Psychological Works, standard ed, vol 20. London, Hogarth Press, 1959

Group for the Advancement of Psychiatry, Committee on Research: Pharmacotherapy and Psychotherapy: Paradoxes, Problems and Progress, Report No 93. New York, Mental Health Materials Center, 1975

Janet P: L'Automatisme Psychologique. Paris, Félix Alcan, 1889

Janet P: The Major Symptoms of Hysteria. New York, Macmillan, 1907

Janet P, Raymond F: Les Obsessions et la Psychasthénie, 2 vols., Paris, Félix Alcan, 1903

Karush A, Daniels G: The response to psychotherapy in chronic ulcerative colitis. Psychosom Med 31:201–227, 1969

Klein DF, Fink M: Psychiatric reaction patterns to imipramine. Am J Psychiatry 119:432–438, 1962

Klein DF, Rabkin JG (eds): Anxiety: New Research and Changing Concepts. New York, Raven Press, 1981

Marty P, de M'Uzan M: La 'pensée opératoire'. Rev Franc Psychoanal 27:Suppl, 1963

Nemiah J: Alexithymia and psychosomatic illness. J Contin Educ Psychiatry Oct: 25–37, 1978

Nemiah J: The psychodynamic view of anxiety, in Diagnosis and Treatment of Anxiety Disorders. Edited by Pasnau RO. Washington DC, American Psychiatric Press, 1984

Nemiah J, Sifneos P: Affect and fantasy in patients with psychosomatic disorders, in Modern Trends in Psychosomatic Medicine, vol 2. Edited by Hill O. London, Butterworths, 1970

Sheehan D: Panic attacks and phobias. N Engl J Med 307:156–158, 1982

Sifneos P: Short-Term Psychotherapy and Emotional Crisis. Cambridge MA, Harvard University Press, 1972

References for Chapter 30

**The Relaxation Response
and the Treatment of Anxiety**

Anand BW, Chhina GS, Singh B: Studies on Shri Ramananda Yogi during his stay in an air-tight box. Indian J Med Res 49:82–89, 1961

Anonymous: A Benedictine of Stanbrook Abbey, in Mediaeval Mystical Tradition and Saint John of the Cross. London, Burns & Oates, 1954

Bagchi BK, Wenger MA: Electrophysiological correlations of some yoga exercises. Electroencephalogr Clin Neurophysiol (Suppl) 7:132–149, 1957

Barber TX: Physiological effects of hypnosis. Psychol Bull 58:390–419, 1961

Beary JF, Benson H: A simple psychophysiologic technique which elicits the hypometabolic changes of the relaxation response. Psychosom Med 36:115–120, 1974

Benson H: The Relaxation Response. New York, William Morrow & Co, 1975

Benson H: Systemic hypertension and the relaxation response. N Engl J Med 296:1152–1156, 1977

Benson H, Beary JF, Carol MP: The relaxation response. Psychiatry 37:37–46, 1974

Benson H, Alexander S, Feldman CL: Decreased premature ventricular contractions through the use of the relaxation response in patients with stable ischemic heart disease. Lancet 2:380–382, 1975

Benson H, Frankel FH, Apfel R, Daniels MD, Schniewind HE, Nemiah JC, Sifneos PE, Crassweller KD, Greenwood MM, Kotch JB, Arns PA, Rosner B: Treatment of anxiety: A comparison of the usefulness of self-hypnosis and a meditational relaxation technique. Psychother Psychosom 30:229–242, 1978

Benson H, Arns PA, Hoffman JW: The relaxation response and hypnosis. Int J Clin Exp Hypn 29:259–270, 1981

Bokser Rabbi Ben Zion: From the World of the Cabbalah. New York, Philosophical Library, 1954

Borysenko JZ: Behavioral-physiological factors in the development and management of cancer. Gen Hosp Psychiatry 4:69–74, 1982

Cannon WB: The emergency function of the adrenal medulla in pain and the major emotions. Am J Physiol 33:356, 1941

Chang C-Y: Creativity and Taoism. New York, Julian Press, 1963

Dean SR: Is there an ultraconscious beyond the unconscious? Can Psychiatr Assoc J 15:57–61, 1970

French RM (trans): The Way of a Pilgrim. New York, Seabury Press, 1968

Fujisawa C: Zen and Shinto. New York, Philosophical Library, 1959

Gorton BE: Physiology of hypnosis. Psychiatr Q 23:317–343, 457–485, 1949

Herbert J: Shinto: At the Fountain-head of Japan. London, Allen & Unwin, 1967

Hess WR: Functional Organization of the Diencephalon. New York, Grune & Stratton, 1957

Hess WR, Brugger M: Das subkortikale Zentrum der affektiven Abwehrreaktion. Helv Physiol Acta 1:33–52, 1943

Hoenig J: Medical research on yoga. Confin Psychiatr 11:69–89, 1968

Hoffman JW, Benson H, Arns PA, Stainbrook GL,

Landsberg L, Young JB, Gill A: Reduced sympathetic nervous system responsivity associated with the relaxation response. Science 215:190–192, 1982

Jacobson E: Progressive Relaxation. Chicago, University of Chicago Press, 1938

James W: The Varieties of Religious Experience. New York, New American Library, 1958

Johnson RC: Watcher on the Hills. New York, Harper & Row, 1959

Johnston W: Christian Zen. New York, Harper & Row, 1971

Kabat-Zinn J: An outpatient program in behavioral medicine for chronic pain patients based on the practice of mindfulness meditation: Theoretical considerations and preliminary results. Gen Hosp Psychiatry 4:33–47, 1982

Karambelkar PV, Vinekar SL, Bhole MV: Studies on human subjects staying in an air-tight pit. Indian J Med Res 56:1282–1288, 1968

Lang R, Dehof K, Meurer KA, Kaufmann W: Sympathetic activity and transcendental meditation. J Neural Transm 44:117–135, 1979

Lehmann JW, Benson H: Nonpharmacologic treatment of hypertension: A review. Gen Hosp Psychiatry 4:27–32, 1982

Levander VL, Benson H, Wheeler RC, Wallace RK: Increased forearm blood flow during a wakeful hypometabolic state. Fed Proc 31:405, 1972

Lowell P: The Soul of the Far East. Boston, Houghton Mifflin, 1892

Lown B, Verrier RL, Rabinowitz SH: Neural and psychologic mechanisms and the problem of sudden cardiac death. Am J Cardiol 39:890–901, 1977

Luthe W (ed): Autogenic Therapy, vols 1–5. New York, Grune & Stratton, 1969

Luthe W: Autogenic therapy: Excerpts on applications to cardiovascular disorders and hypercholesterolemia, in Biofeedback and Self-Control 1971. Chicago, Aldine-Atherton, 1972

Melzack R, Perry C: Self-regulation of pain: The use of alpha feedback and hypnotic training for the control of chronic pain. Exp Neurol 46:452–469, 1975

Michaels RR, Haber MJ, McCann DS: Evaluation of transcendental meditation as a method of reducing stress. Science 192:1242–1244, 1976

Morgane PJ: Historical and modern concepts of hypothalamic organization and function, in Handbook of the Hypothalamus, vol 1. Anatomy of the Hypothalamus. Edited by Morgane DJ, Panksepp J. New York, Marel Dekker, 1979

Morse DR, Martin JS, Furst ML, Dubin LL: A physiological and subjective evaluation of meditation, hypnosis and relaxation. Psychosom Med 39:304–324, 1977

Norwich JJ, Sitwell R: Mount Athos. New York, Harper & Row, 1966

Onda A: Autogenic training and Zen, in Autogenic Training, internat ed. Edited by Luthe W. New York, Grune & Stratton, 1965

Organ TW: The Hindu Quest for the Perfection of Man. Athens OH, Ohio University Press, 1970

Osuna Fray Francisco de: The Third Spiritual Alphabet. London, Benziger, 1931

Peters RK, Benson H, Porter D: Daily relaxation response breaks in a working population: 1. Health, performance and well-being. Am J Public Health 67:946–953, 1977a

Peters RK, Benson H, Peters JM: Daily relaxation response breaks in a working population: 2. Blood pressure. Am J Public Health 67:954–959, 1977b

Progoff I (ed and trans): The Cloud of Unknowing. New York, Julian Press, 1969

Saint Terese of Avila: The Way of Perfection. Edited by Waller AR. London, JM Dent, 1901

Sanborn FB: Familiar Letters of Henry David Thoreau. Boston, Houghton Mifflin, 1894

Scholem GG: Jewish Mysticism. New York, Schocken Books, 1967

Spurgeon CFE: Mysticism in English Literature. Port Washington NY, Kennikat Press, 1970

Sugi Y, Akutsu K: Studies on respiration and energy-metabolism during sitting in Zazen. Res J Phys Ed 12:190–206, 1968

Trimingham JS: Sufi Orders in Islam. Oxford, Clarendon Press, 1971

Underhill E: Mysticism. London, Methuen, 1957

Wallace RK: Physiological effects of Transcendental Meditation. Science 167:1751–1754, 1970

Wallace RK, Benson H, Wilson AF: A wakeful hypometabolic state. Am J Physiol 221:795–799, 1971

Walrath LC, Hamilton DW: Autonomic correlates of meditation and hypnosis. Am J Clin Hypn 17:190–197, 1975

Warrenburg S, Pagano RR, Woods M, Hlastala M: A comparison of somatic relaxation and EEG activity in classical progressive relaxation and Transcendental Meditation. J Behav Med 3:73–93, 1980

References for Chapter 31

Exposure Treatment of Agoraphobia

Agras WS: Transfer during systematic desensitization therapy. Behav Res Ther 5:193–199, 1967

Agras WS, Leitenberg H, Barlow DH: Social reinforcement in the modification of agoraphobia. Arch Gen Psychiatry 19:423–427, 1968

Agras WS, Leitenberg H, Barlow DH, Thomson LE: Instructions and reinforcement in the modification of neurotic behavior. Am J Psychiatry 125:1435–1439, 1969

Appelby IL, Klein DF, Sachar EJ, Levitt M: Biochemical indices of lactate-induced panic: A preliminary report, in Anxiety: New Research and Changing Concepts. Edited by Klein DF, Rabkin J. New York, Raven Press, 1981

Ascher LM: Employing paradoxical intention in the treatment of agoraphobia. Behav Res Ther, 19:533–542, 1981

Bandura A: Self-efficacy: Towards a unifying theory of behavioral change. Psychol Rev 84:191–215, 1977

Barios BA, Shigetomi CC: Coping skills training in the management of anxiety: A critical review. Unpublished manuscript, University of Utah, 1980

Barlow DH, Leitenberg H, Agras WS, Wincze JP: The transfer gap in systematic desensitization: An analogue study. Behav Res Ther 7:191–196, 1969

Beck AT, Ward CH, Mendelson M, Mock J, Erbaugh J: An inventory for measuring depression. Arch Gen Psychiatry 4:53–63, 1961

Chambless DL, Goldstein AJ (eds): Agoraphobia: Multiple Perspectives on Theory and Treatment. New York, John Wiley & Sons, 1982

Chambless DL, Foa EB, Groves GA, Goldstein AJ: Flooding with brevital in the treatment of agoraphobia: Countereffective? Behav Res Ther 17:243–251, 1979

Crowe MJ, Marks IM, Agras WS, Leitenberg H: Time-limited desensitization, implosion and shaping for phobic patients: A crossover study. Behav Res Ther 10:319–328, 1972

De Silva P, Rachman S: Is exposure a necessary condition for fear reduction? Behav Res Ther 19:227–232, 1981

Dyckman JM, Cowan PA: Imagining vividness and the outcome of in vivo and imagined scene desensitization. J Consult Clin Psychol 48:1155–1156, 1978

Emmelkamp PMG: The behavioral study of clinical phobias, in Progress in Behavior Modification, vol 8. Edited by Hersen M, Eisler RM, Miller PM. New York, Academic Press, 1979

Emmelkamp PMG: In vivo treatment of agoraphobia, in Agoraphobia: Multiple Perspectives on Theory and Treatment. Edited by Chambless DL, Goldstein AJ. New York, John Wiley & Sons, 1982

Emmelkamp PMG, Wessels H: Flooding in imagination versus flooding in vivo: A comparison with agoraphobics. Behav Res Ther 13: 7–16, 1975

Emmelkamp PMG, Kuipers ACM, Eggeraat JB: Cognitive modification versus prolonged exposure in vivo: A comparison with agoraphobics as subjects. Behav Res Ther 16:33–41, 1978

Everaerd WTAM, Rijken HM, Emmelkamp PMG: A comparison of "flooding" and "successive approximation" in the treatment of agoraphobia. Behav Res Ther 11:105–117, 1973

Foa EB: Failure in treating obsessive-compulsives. Behav Res Ther 17:169–176, 1979

Foa EB, Blau JS, Prout M, Latimer P: Is horror a necessary component of flooding (implosion)? Behav Res Ther 15:397–402, 1977

Frankl VE: Paradoxical intention: A logotherapeutic technique. Am J Psychother 14:520–535, 1960

Frankl VE: Paradoxical intention and dereflection. Psychotherapy: Theory, Research and Practice 12:226–237, 1975

Freud S: Turnings in the ways of psychoanalytic therapy (1919), in Collected Papers, vol 2. Translated by Riviere J. London, Hogarth Press, 1950.

Gelder MG, Marks IM: Severe agoraphobia: A controlled prospective trial of behaviour therapy. Br J Psychiatry 112:309–319, 1966

Gelder MG, Marks IM, Wolff HH: Desensitization and psychotherapy in the treatment of phobic states: A controlled enquiry. Br J Psychiatry 113:53–73, 1967

Gelder MG, Bancroft JHJ, Gath DH, Johnston DW, Mathews AM, Shaw PM: Specific and non-specific factors in behaviour therapy. Br J Psychiatry 123:445–462, 1973

Gertz HO: The treatment of the phobic and the obsessive-compulsive using paradoxical intention. Sec. Viktor Frankl. Neuropsychiatry 3:375–387, 1962

Gertz HO: Experience with the logotherapeutic technique of paradoxical intention in the treatment of phobic and obsessive-compulsive patients. Am J Psychiatry 125:548–553, 1967

Greist JH, Marks IM, Berlin F, Gournay K, Noshirvani H: Avoidance versus confrontation of fear. Behavior Therapy 11:1–14, 1980

Hafner RJ, Marks IM: Exposure in vivo of agoraphobics: Contributions of diazepam, group exposure, and anxiety evocation. Psychol Med 6:71–88, 1976

Jannoun L, Munby M, Catala J, Gelder M: A home-based treatment program for agoraphobia: Replication and controlled evaluation. Behavior Therapy 11:294–305, 1980

Jansson L, Ost L: Behavioral treatments for agoraphobia: An evaluative review. Clin Psychol Rev 2:322–336, 1982

Johnston DW, Lancashire M, Mathews AM, Munby M, Shaw PM, Gelder MG: Imaginal flooding and exposure to real phobic situations: Changes during treatment. Br J Psychiatry 129:372–377, 1976

Kelly D, Mitchell-Hegg N, Sherman D: Anxiety in the effects of sodium lactate assessed clinically and physiologically. Br J Psychiatry 119:468–470, 1971

Lader MH, Mathews AM: Physiological model of phobic anxiety and desensitization. Behav Res Ther 6:411–421, 1968

Leitenberg H, Agras WS, Edwards JA, Thomson LE, Wincze JP: Practice as a psychotherapeutic variable: An experimental analysis within single cases. J Psychiatr Res 7:215–225, 1970

Liebowitz MR, Klein DF: Agoraphobia: Clinical features, pathophysiology, and treatment, in Agoraphobia: Multiple Perspectives on Theory and Treatment. Edited by Chambless DL, Goldstein AJ. New York, John Wiley & Sons, 1982

McConaghy N: Results of systematic desensitization with phobias re-examined. Br J Psychiatry 117:89–92, 1970

McCutcheon BA, Adams HE: The physiological basis of implosive therapy. Behav Res Ther 13:93–100, 1975

McDonald R, Sartory G, Grey SJ, Cobb J, Stern R, Marks I: The effects of self-exposure instructions on agoraphobic outpatients. Behav Res Ther 17:83–85, 1979

Marks IM: Flooding (implosion) and allied treatments, in Behavior Modification: Principles and Clinical Applications. Edited by Agras WS. Boston, Little, Brown & Company, 1972

Marks IM: Cure and Care of Neuroses: Theory and Practice of Behavioral Psychotherapy. New York, John Wiley & Sons, 1981

Marks IM: Are there anticompulsive or antiphobic drugs? Review of the evidence. Br J Psychiatry 143:338–347, 1983

Marks IM, Gelder MG: A controlled retrospective study of behaviour therapy in phobic patients. Br J Psychiatry 111:571–573, 1965

Marks IM, Mathews AM: Brief standard self-rating for phobic patients. Behav Res Ther 17:263–267, 1979

Marks IM, Gelder MG, Edwards JG: Hypnosis and desensitization for phobias: A controlled prospective trial. Br J Psychiatry 114:1263–1274, 1968

Marshall WL, Gauthier J, Gordon A: The current status of flooding therapy. Progress in Behavior Modification 7:205–275, 1979

Mathews AM: Psychophysiological approaches to the investigation of desensitization and related procedures. Psychol Bull 76:73–91, 1971

Mathews AM: Recent developments in the treatment of agoraphobia. Behavioral Analysis and Modification 2:64–75, 1977

Mathews AM, Shaw PM: Emotional arousal and persuasion effects in flooding. Behav Res Ther 11:587–598, 1973

Mathews AM, Johnston DW, Shaw PM, Gelder MG: Process variables and the prediction of outcome in behaviour therapy. Br J Psychiatry 125:256–264, 1974

Mathews AM, Johnston DW, Lancashire M, Munby M, Shaw PM, Gelder MG: Imaginal flooding and exposure to real phobic situations: Treatment outcome in behavior therapy. Br J Psychiatry 129:362–371, 1976

Mathews AM, Teasdale J, Munby M, Johnston D, Shaw

P: A home-based treatment program for agoraphobia. Behavior Therapy 8:915–924, 1977

Mathews AM, Gelder MG, Johnston DW: Agoraphobia: Nature and Treatment. New York, Guilford Press, 1981

Mavissakalian M: Pharmacological treatment of anxiety disorders. J Clin Psychiatry 43:487–491, 1982

Mavissakalian M: Antidepressants in the treatment of agoraphobia and obsessive-compulsive disorder. Compr Psychiatry 24:278–284, 1983

Mavissakalian M, Barlow DH: Phobia: An overview, in Phobia: Psychological and Pharmacological Treatment. Edited by Mavissakalian M, Barlow DH. New York, Guilford Press, 1981a

Mavissakalian M, Barlow DH (eds): Phobia: Psychological and Pharmacological Treatment. New York, Guilford Press, 1981b

Mavissakalian M, Michelson L: Agoraphobia: Behavioral and pharmacological treatments. Preliminary outcome and process findings. Psychopharmacol Bull 18:91–103, 1982

Mavissakalian M, Michelson L: Agoraphobia: Behavioral and pharmacological treatment (N=49). Psychopharm Bull 19:116–118, 1983a

Mavissakalian M, Michelson L: Self-directed practice in behavioral and pharmacological treatments of agoraphobia. Behavior Therapy 14:506–519, 1983b

Mavissakalian M, Michelson L, Greenwald D, Kornblith S, Greenwald M: Cognitive behavioral treatment of agoraphobia: Paradoxical intention vs. self-statement training. Behav Res Ther 21:75–86, 1983

Meichenbaum DH: Self-instructional methods, in Helping People Change. Edited by Kanfer FH, Goldstein P. New York, Pergamon Press, 1975

Meichenbaum DH: Cognitive-Behavior Modification: An Integrative Approach. New York, Plenum Press, 1977

Mowrer O: A stimulus-response analysis of anxiety and its role as a reinforcing agent. Psychol Rev 46:553–565, 1939

Rachman S: The passing of the two-stage theory of fear and avoidance: Fresh possibilities. Behav Res Ther 14:125–131, 1976

Rachman S: The conditioning theory of fear-acquisition: A critical examination. Behav Res Ther 15:375–387, 1977

Rachman S: Emotional processing. Behav Res Ther 18:51–60, 1980

Rosenthal TL, Bandura A: Psychological modeling: Theory and practice, in Handbook of Psychotherapy and Behavior Change: An Empirical Analysis, 2nd ed. Edited by Garfield SL, Bergin AE. New York, John Wiley & Sons, 1978

Sherman AR: Real-life exposure as a primary therapeutic factor in the desensitization treatment of fear. J Abnorm Psychol 79:19–28, 1972

Solomon RL, Wynne LC: Traumatic avoidance learning: The principles of anxiety conservation and partial irreversibility. Psychol Rev 61:353–385, 1954

Solyom C, Solyom L, LaPierre Y, Pecknold J, Morton L: Phenelzine and exposure in the treatment of phobias. Biol Psychiatry 16:239–247, 1981

Stampfl TG: Implosive therapy: The theory, the subhuman analogue, the strategy and the techniques—Part I. The theory, in Behavior Modification Techniques in the Treatment of Emotional Disorders. Edited by Armitage SG. Battle Creek MI, VA Publication, 1967

Stampfl TG, Levis DJ: Essentials of implosion therapy: A learning theory-based psychodynamic behavioral therapy. J Abnorm Psychol 72:496–503, 1967

Watson JP, Marks IM: Relevant and irrelevant fear in

flooding—A crossover study of phobic patients. Behavior Therapy 2:275–293, 1971

Williams SL, Rappoport JA: Cognitive treatment in the natural environment for agoraphobics. Behavior Therapy, 14:299–343, 1983

Wolpe J: Psychotherapy by Reciprocal Inhibition. Stanford CA, Stanford University Press, 1958

Wolpe J: Quantitative relationships in the systematic desensitization of phobias. Am J Psychiatry 119:1062–1068, 1963

Yorkston JN, Sergeant HGS, Rachman S: Methohexitone relaxation for desensitising agoraphobic patients. Lancet 2:651–653, 1968

Zitrin CM, Klein DF, Woerner MG: Treatment of agoraphobia with group exposure in vivo and imipramine. Arch Gen Psychiatry 37:63–72, 1980

References for Chapter 32

Mortality After Thirty to Forty Years: Panic Disorder Compared with Other Psychiatric Illnesses

American Psychiatric Association: Diagnostic and Statistical Manual of Mental Disorders, 2nd ed. Washington DC, American Psychiatric Association, 1968

American Psychiatric Association: Diagnostic and Statistical Manual of Mental Disorders, 3rd ed. American Psychiatric Association, Washington DC, 1980

Babigian HM, Odoroff CL: Mortality experience of a population with psychiatric illness. Am J Psychiatry 126:470–480, 1969

Coryell W: Diagnosis-specific mortality: Primary unipolar depression and Briquet's syndrome (somatization disorder). Arch Gen Psychiatry 38:939–942, 1981a

Coryell W: Obsessive-compulsive disorder and primary unipolar depression. J Nerv Ment Dis 169:220–224, 1981b

Coryell W, Noyes R, Clancy J: Excess mortality in panic disorder. Arch Gen Psychiatry 39:701–703, 1982

Coryell W, Noyes R, Clancy J: Panic disorder and primary unipolar depression: A comparison of background and outcome. J Affective Disord, in press

Crowe RR, Gaffney G, Kerber R: Panic attacks in families of patients with mitral valve prolapse. J Affective Disord 4:121–125, 1982

Derby, IM: Manic-depressive "exhaustion" deaths. Psychiatr Q 7:435–449, 1933

Feighner JP, Robins E, Guze SB, Woodruff RA, Winokur G, Munoz R: Diagnostic criteria for use in psychiatric research. Arch Gen Psychiatry 26:57–63, 1972

Guze SB, Robins E: Suicide and primary affective disorders. Br J Psychiatry 117:437–438, 1970

Hartman N, Kramer R, Brown WT, Devereux RB: Panic disorder in patients with mitral valve prolapse. Am J Psychiatry 139:669–670, 1982

Innes G, Millar WM: Mortality among psychiatric patients. Scot Med J 15:143–148, 1970

Lee K: Alcoholism and cerebrovascular thrombosis in the young. Acta Neurol Scand 59:270–274, 1979

Noyes R, Clancy J, Hoenk CR, Slymen DJ: Anxiety neurosis and physical illness. Compr Psychiatry 19:407–413, 1978

Rorsman B: Mortality among psychiatric patients. Acta Psychiatr Scand 50:354–375, 1974

Salmons P, Sims A: Smoking profiles of patients admitted for neurosis. Br J Psychiatry 139:43–46, 1981

Sims A, Prior P: The pattern of mortality in severe neurosis. Br J Psychiatry 133:299–305, 1978

Sims A, Prior P: Arteriosclerosis related deaths in severe neurosis. Compr Psychiatry 23:181–185, 1982

Taylor JR: Alcohol and strokes (ltr to ed). New Engl J Med 18:1111, 1982

Tsuang MT, Woolson RF: Mortality in patients with schizophrenia, mania, depression and surgical conditions. Br J Psychiatry 130:162–166, 1977

Tsuang MT, Woolson RF, Fleming JA: Causes of death in schizophrenia and manic depression. Br J Psychiatry 136:239–242, 1980

Wheeler EO, White PD, Reed EW, Cohen ME: Neurocirculatory asthenia (Anxiety neurosis, effort syndrome, neuro-asthenia): A 20 year follow-up study of 173 patients. JAMA 142:878–888, 1950

Woodruff RA, Guze SB, Clayton PJ: Anxiety neurosis among psychiatric outpatients. Compr Psychiatry 13:165–170, 1972

Woolson RF, Tsuang MT, Fleming JA: A method for analyzing mortality data collected in follow-up studies. Methods Inf Med 17:116–120, 1978

References for Chapter 33

The Biology of Anxiety

Akselrod S, Gordon D, Ubel AF, Shannon DC, Barger AC, Cohen RJ: Power spectrum analysis of heart rate fluctuations: A quantitative probe of beat to beat cardiovascular control. Science 213:220–222, 1981

Basowitz H, Korchin SJ, Oken D, Goldstein MD, Gussack H: Anxiety and performance changes with minimal doses of epinephrine. Arch Neurol Psychiatry 76:98–106, 1956

Beckman H, Goodwin FK: Urinary MHPG in subgroups of depressed patients and normal controls. Neuropsychobiology 6:91–100, 1980

Bloom LJ, Houston BK, Burish JG: An evaluation of finger pulse volume as a measure of anxiety. Psychophysiology 13:40–42, 1976

Bond AJ, James DC, Lader MH: Physiological and psychological measures in anxious patients. Psychol Med 4:364–373, 1974

Boudoulas H, Wooley CF, Reynolds J, Mazzaferri E: Mitral valve prolapse syndrome—evidence for a hyperadrenergic state. Am J Cardiol 43:368, 1979

Boudoulas H, Reynolds JC, Mazzaferri E, Wooley CF: Metabolic studies in mitral valve prolapse syndrome. Circulation 61:1200–1205, 1980

Brown OR, Kloster FE, Demots H: Incidence of mitral valve prolapse in the asymptomatic normal. Circulation (Suppl 2):77, 1975

Chattopadhyay B, Cooke E, Toone B, Lader M: Habituation of physiological responses in anxiety. Biol Psychiatry 15:711–721, 1980

Coghlan HC, Phares P, Cowley M, Copley D, James TN: Dysautonomia in mitral valve prolapse. Am J Med 67:236–244, 1979

Cohen ME, White PD: Neurocirculatory asthenia. Milit Med 137:142–144, 1972

Cohen ME, Consolazio FC, Johnson RE: Blood lactate response during moderate exercise in neurocirculatory asthenia, or effort syndrome. J Clin Invest 26:339, 1947

Connolly JF: Tonic physiological responses to repeated presentations of phobic stimuli. Behav Res Ther 17:189–196, 1979

Crowe RR, Gaffney G, Kerber R: Panic attacks in families of patients with mitral valve prolapse. J Affective Disord 4:121–125, 1982

DaCosta JM: On irritable heart: A clinical study of a form of functional cardiac disorder and its consequences. Am J Med Sci 6:17, 1871

Darsee JR, Mikolich JR, Nicoloff NB, Lesser LE: Prevalence of mitral valve prolapse in presumably healthy young men. Circulation 59:619–622, 1979

Davidson J, Turnbull CP, Miller RD: A comparison of inpatients with primary unipolar depression and depression secondary to anxiety. Acta Psychiatr Scand 61:377–386, 1980

Devereux RB, Perloff JK, Reicheck N, Josephson ME: Mitral valve prolapse. Circulation 54:3–14, 1976

Dimsdale JE, Moss J: Plasma catecholamines in stress and exercise. JAMA 243:340–342, 1980

Dynes JB, Tod H: The emotional and somatic response of schizophrenic patients and normal controls to adrenalin and doryl. J Neurol Psychiatry 3:1–8, 1940

Easton JD, Sherman DG: Somatic anxiety attacks and propranolol. Arch Neurol 33:689–691, 1976

Elam M, Yoat TP, Svensson TH: Hypercapnia and hypoxia: Chemo-receptor-mediated control of locus coeruleus neurons and splanchnic, sympathetic nerves. Brain Res 222:373–381, 1981

Elsworth JD, Redmond DE Jr, Roth RH: Plasma and cerebrospinal fluid 3-methoxy-4-hydroxyphenylethyleneglycol (MHPG) as indices of brain norepinephrine metabolism in primates. Brain Res 235:115–124, 1982

Fink M, Taylor MA, Volavka J: Anxiety precipitated by lactate. New Engl J Med 281:1429, 1970

Frankenhaeuser M: Behavior and circulating catecholamines. Brain Res 31:241–262, 1971

Frankenhaeuser M, Jarpe G: Psychophysiological reactions to infusions of a mixture of adrenalin and noradrenalin. Scand J Psychol 3:21–28, 1962

Frohlich ED, Tarazi RC, Duston HP: Hyperdynamic ß-adrenergic circulatory state. Arch Int Med 123:1–7, 1969

Gaffney FA, Karlsson ES, Campbell W, Schutte JE, Nixon JV, Willerson JT, Blomqvist CG: Autonomic dysfunction in women with mitral valve prolapse syndrome. Circulation 59:894–901, 1979

Garfield SL, Gershon S, Sletten I, Sunland DM, Ballou S: Chemically induced anxiety. Int J Neuropsychiatry 3:426–433, 1967

Gellhorn E, Loofbourrow GN: Emotions and Emotional Disorders. New York, Harper & Row, 1963

Glickstein M: Temporal heart rate patterns in anxious patients. Arch Neurol Psychiatry 78:101–106, 1957

Gold MS, Redmond DE, Kleber HD: Noradrenergic hyperactivity in opiate withdrawal supported by clonidine reversal of opiate withdrawal. Am J Psychiatry 136:100–101, 1979

Goldstein L, Munoz C: Influence of adrenergic stimulant and blocking drugs on cerebral and electrical activity in curarized animals. J Pharm Exp Therap 132:345–353, 1961

Gorman JM, Fyer AF, Gliklich J, King D, Klein DF: Effect of imipramine on prolapsed mitral valves of patients with panic disorder. Am J Psychiatry 138:977–978, 1981a

Gorman JM, Fyer AF, Gliklich J, King D, Klein DF: Effect of sodium lactate on patients with panic disorder and mitral valve prolapse. Am J Psychiatry 138:247–249, 1981b

Gorman JM, Fyer AF, Gliklich J, King D, Klein DF: Mitral valve prolapse and panic disorders: Effect of imipramine, in Anxiety: New Research and Changing Concepts. Edited by Klein DF, Rabkin JG. New York, Raven Press, 1981c

Gorman JM, Levy FR, Liebowitz MR, McGrath P, Abbleby IL, Dillon DJ, Davies SO, Klein DF: Effect of acute beta-adrenergic blockade on lactate-induced panic. Arch Gen Psychiatry 40:1079–1083, 1983a

Gorman JM, Askanazi J, Liebowitz MR, Fyer AF, Stein J, Kinney JM, Klein DF: Hyperventilation and panic attacks, unpublished manuscript, 1983b

Grant SJ, Huang YH, Redmond DE Jr: Benzodiazepines attenuate single unit activity in the locus coeruleus. Life Sci 27:2231–2236, 1980

Grant S, Redmond DE Jr: The neuroanatomy and pharmacology of the nucleus locus coeruleus, in The Psychopharmacology of Clonidine. Edited by Lal A, Fielding S. New York, Alan R Liss, 1981

Grayson JB, Nutter D, Mavissakalian M: Psychophysiological assessment of imagery in obsessive-compulsives: A pilot study. Behav Res Ther 18:590–593, 1980

Grunhaus L, Gloger S, Rein A, Lewis BS: Mitral valve prolapse and panic attacks. Isr J Med Sci 18:221–223, 1982

Hart JD: Physiological responses of anxious and normal subjects to simple signal and non-signal auditory stimuli. Psychophysiology 11:443–451, 1974

Hartman N, Kramer R, Brown WT, Devereux RB: Panic disorder in patients with mitral valve prolapse. Am J Psychiatry 139:669–670, 1982

Hoehn-Saric R: Neurotransmitters in anxiety. Arch Gen Psychiatry 39:735–742, 1982

Holmberg G, Gershon S: Autonomic and psychic effects of yohimbine hydrochloride. Psychopharmacologia 2:93–106, 1961

Iskandar S, Bradshaw CM, Szabadi E: The responsiveness of sweat glands to carbachol in anxiety neurosis. J Clin Pharmacol 10:303–305, 1980

Janowsky D, Risch SC, Huey L, Judd L, Rausch J: Physostigmine-induced cardiovascular changes: Behavioral and neuroendocrine correlations. Presented at the Annual Meeting of The American College of Neuropsychopharmacology, San Juan, Puerto Rico, December 1982

Kane JM, Woerner M, Zeldis S, Kramer R, Saravay S: Panic and phobic disorders in patients with mitral valve prolapse, in Anxiety: New Concepts and Changing Research. Edited by Klein DF, Rabkin JG. New York, Raven Press, 1981

Kelly DHW: Measurement of anxiety by forearm blood flow. Br J Psychiatry 152:789–798, 1966

Kelly DHW, Walter CJS: The relationship between clinical diagnosis and anxiety assessed by forearm blood flow and other measurements. Br J Psychiatry 114:611–626, 1968

Kelly DHW, Mitchell-Heggs N, Sherman J: Anxiety and sodium lactate assessed clinically and physiologically. Br J Psychiatry 119:129–141, 1971

Knight ML, Borden RJ: Autonomic and affective reactions of high and low socially-anxious individuals awaiting public performance. Psychophysiology 16:209–213, 1979

Ko GN, Elsworth JD, Roth RH, Rifkin BG, Leigh H, Redmond DE Jr: Panic-induced elevation of plasma MHPG levels in phobic-anxious patients. Arch Gen Psychiatry 40:425–430, 1983

Lader MH: Palmar skin conductance measures in anxiety and phobic states. J Psychosom Res 11:271–281, 1967

Lader MH, Wing L: Physiological Measures, Sedative Drugs, and Morbid Anxiety. London, Oxford University Press, 1966

Lader MH, Gelder MG, Marks IM: Palmar skin conductance measures as predictors of response to desensitization. J Psychosom Res 11:283–290, 1967

Lewis T: The Soldier's Heart and the Effort Syndrome. New York, Paul B Hoebner, 1919

Liebowitz MR, Fyer AJ, McGrath P, Klein DF: Clonidine treatment of panic disorder. Psychopharmacol Bull 17:122–123, 1981

Lindemann E, Finesinger JE: The effect of adrenaline and mecholyl in states of anxiety in psychoneurotic patients. Am J Psychiatry 95:353–370, 1938

Lindemann E, Finesinger JE: Subjective responses of psychoneurotic patients to adrenaline and mecholyl. Psychosom Med 2:231–248, 1940

Lum LC: Hyperventilation: The tip and the iceberg. J Psychosom Res 19:375–383, 1975

Markiewicz W, Stoner J, Louden E, Hunt SA, Popp RL: Mitral valve prolapse in one hundred presumably healthy young females. Circulation 53:464–473, 1976

Mason ST, Fibiger HC: Anxiety: The locus coeruleus disconnection. Life Sci 25:2141–2147, 1979

Matthew RJ, Ho BT, Kralik P, Taylor D, Semchuk K, Weinman M, Claghorn JL: Catechol-O-methyl transferase and catecholamines in anxiety and relaxation. Psychiatry Res 3:85–91, 1980

Matthew RJ, Ho BT, Kralik P, Weinman M, Claghorn JL: Anxiety and platelet MAO levels after relaxation training. Am J Psychiatry 138:371–373, 1981

Meyer V, Reich B: Anxiety management—the marriage of physiological and cognitive variables. Behav Res Ther 16:177–182, 1978

Mirsky IA: Physiology of anxiety, in Management of Anxiety Neuroses for the General Practitioner. Edited by Rickles K. Springfield IL, Charles C Thomas, 1973

Missri JC, Alexander S: Hyperventilation syndrome. A brief review. JAMA 240:2093–2096, 1978

Montgomery GK: Effects of performance evaluation and anxiety on cardiac response in anticipation of difficult problem solving. Psychophysiology 14:251–257, 1977

Newton JEO, Dykman RA, Chapin JR: The prediction of abnormal behavior from autonomic indices in dogs. J Nerv Ment Dis 166:635–641, 1978

Nyback H, Walters JR, Aghajanian GK, Roth RH: Tricyclic antidepressants: Effects on the firing rate of brain noradrenergic neurons. Eur J Pharmacol 32:302–312, 1975

Odegaard O: The psychogalvanic reactivity in affective disorders. Br J Med Psychol 25:3–12, 1932

Praiser SF, Pinta ER, Jones BA: Mitral valve prolapse syndrome and anxiety neurosis/panic disorder. Am J Psychiatry 135:246–247, 1978

Pasternac A, Tubau JF, Cousineau J, De Champlain J: Increased plasma catecholamines in symptomatic mitral valve prolapse. Circulation 60 (Suppl 2):156, 1979

Pasternac A, Tabau JF, Puddu PE, Krol RB, De Champlain J: Increased plasma catecholamine levels in patients with symptomatic mitral valve prolapse. Am J Med 73:783–790, 1982

Pitts FN: Biochemical factors in anxiety neurosis. Behav Sci 16:82–91, 1971

Pitts FN, Allen RE: Biochemical induction of anxiety, in Phenomenology and Treatment of Anxiety. Edited by Fann WE, Karacan I, Pokorny AD, Williams RL. New York, Spectrum Publications, 1979

Pitts FN, Allen RE: β-adrenergic blockade in the treatment of anxiety, in The Biology of Anxiety. Edited by Matthew RJ. New York, Brunner/Mazel, 1982

Pitts FN, McClure JN: Lactate metabolism in anxiety neurosis. New Engl J Med 277:1326–1328, 1967

Redmond DE: Alterations in the function of the nucleus locus coeruleus: A possible model for studies of anxiety, in Animal Models in Psychiatry and Neurology. Edited by Hanin I. New York, Pergamon Press, 1977

Redmond DE: New and old evidence for the involvement of a brain norepinephrine system in anxiety, in Phenomenology and Treatment of Anxiety. Edited by Fann WE, Karacan I, Pokorny AD, Williams RL. New York, Spectrum Publications, 1979

Reese WG: A dog model for human psychopathology. Am J Psychiatry 136:1168–1172, 1979

Rifkin A, Klein DF, Dillon D, Levitt M: Blockade by imipramine or desipramine of panic induced by sodium lactate. Am J Psychiatry 138:676–677, 1981

Roth WT, Ticklenberg JR, Doyle CM, Horvath TB, Kopell BS: Mood states and 24-hour cardiac monitoring. J Psychosom Res 20:179–186, 1976

Santos AD, Mathew PK, Hilal A, Wallace WA: Orthostatic hypotension: A commonly unrecognized cause of symptoms in mitral valve prolapse. Am J Med 71:746–750, 1981

Schandry R: Heart beat perception and emotional experience. Psychophysiology 19:483–488, 1981

Schmidt HS, Elizabeth JI: Mitral valve prolapse: Relationship to panic attacks/anxiety disorders and β-adrenergic hypersensitivity. Presented at the thirty-seventh Annual Meeting of the Society of Biological Psychiatry, Toronto, May 1982

Solomon AP, Fentress TL: Galvanic skin reflex and blood pressure reactions in the psychoneuroses. J Nerv Ment Dis 80:163–182, 1934

Sweeney DR, Maas JW, Heninger GR: State anxiety, physical anxiety, and urinary 3-methoxy-4-hydroxyphenylethyleneglycol excretion. Arch Gen Psychiatry 35:1418–1423, 1978

Toone BK, Cooke E, Lader MH: Electrodermal activity in the affective disorders and schizophrenia. Psychol Med 11:497–508, 1981

Tyrer P, Lee I, Alexander J: Awareness of cardiac function in anxious, phobic and hypochondriacal patients. Psychol Med 10:171–174, 1980

Tzivoni D, Stern Z, Keren A, Stern S: Electrocardiographic characteristics of neurocirculatory asthenia during everyday activities. Br Heart J 44:426–432, 1980

Van Dis H: Hyperventilation in phobic patients, in Stress and Anxiety. Edited by Spielberger CD, Sarason IG. New York, John Wiley & Sons, 1978

White BV, Gilden EF: "Cold pressor test" in tension and anxiety. A cardiochronographic study. Arch Neurol Psychiatry 38:964–984, 1937

Wood P: Diseases of the Heart and Circulation (1941). Philadelphia, JB Lippincott, 1968

Wooley CF: Where are the diseases of yesteryear? Circulation 53:749–750, 1976

Yu PH, Bowen R, Carlson K, O'Sullivan K, Boulton AA: Comparison of biochemical properties of platelet monoamine oxidase in mentally disordered and healthy individuals. Psychiatry Res 6:107–121, 1982

References for Chapter 34

The Biochemistry of Anxiety: From Pharmacotherapy to Pathophysiology

American Psychiatric Association: Diagnostic and Statistical Manual of Mental Disorders, 3rd ed. Washington DC, American Psychiatric Association, 1980

Bosmann HB, Penney DP, Case KR, DiStefano P, Averill K: Diazepam receptor: Specific binding of [³H]diazepam and [³H]flunitrazepam to rat brain subpopulations. FEBS Lett 87:199–202, 1978

Braestrup C, Nielsen M, Olsen CF: Urinary and brain β-carboline-3-carboxylates as potent inhibitors of brain benzodiazepine receptors. Proc Natl Acad Sci USA 77:2288–2292, 1980

Braestrup C, Schmiechen R, Neef G, Nielsen M, Petersen EN: Interaction of convulsive ligands with benzodiazepine receptors. Science 216:1241–1243, 1982

Carey G, Gottesman II: Twin and family studies of anxiety, phobic, and obsessive disorders in Anxiety: New Research and Changing Concepts. Edited by Klein DF, Rabkin JG. New York, Raven Press, 1981

Chang RSL, Snyder SH: Benzodiazepine receptors: Labelling in intact animals with ³H-flunitrazepam. Eur J Pharmacol 48:213–218, 1978

Costa E, Guidotti A, Mao CC, Suria A: New concepts on the mechanism of action of benzodiazepine. Life Sci 17:167–186, 1975

Cowen PJ, Green AR, Nutt DJ, Martin IL: Ethyl β-carboline carboxylate lowers seizure threshold and antagonizes flurazepam-induced sedation in rats. Nature 290:54–55, 1981

Czernik AJ, Petrack B, Kalinsky HJ, Psychoyos S, Cash WD, Tsai C, Rinehart RK, Granat FR, Lovell RA, Brundish DE, Wade R: CGS 8216: Receptor binding characteristics of a potent benzodiazepine antagonist. Life Sci 30:363–372, 1982

Dorow R, Horowski R, Paschelke G, Amin M: Severe anxiety induced by FG 7142, a β-carboline ligand for benzodiazepine receptors. Lancet 8341:98–99, 1983

Geller I, Seifter J: The effects of meprobamate, barbiturates, D-amphetamine, and promazine on experimentally induced conflict in the rat. Psychopharmacologia 1:382–492, 1960

Greenblatt DJ, Shader RI: Benzodiazepines in Clinical Practice. New York, Raven Press, 1974

Haefely W, Kulcsar R, Möhler H, Pieri L, Polc P, Schaffner R: Possible involvement of GABA in the central actions of benzodiazepines. Adv Biochem Psychopharmacol 14:131–151, 1975

Hunkeler W, Möhler H, Pieri L, Polc P, Bonetti EP, Cumin R, Schaffner R, Haefely W: Selective antagonists of benzodiazepines. Nature 290:514–516, 1981

Insel TR, Ninan PT, Aloi J, Jimerson DJ, Skolnick P, Paul SM: A benzodiazepine receptor mediated model of anxiety: Studies in non-human primates and clinical implications. Arch Gen Psychiatry 1984, in press

Klein DF: Delineation of two drug-responsive anxiety syndromes. Psychopharmacologia 5:397–408, 1964

Koe BK: Biochemical effects of antianxiety drugs on brain monoamines, in Anxiolytics. Edited by Fielding S, Lal H. New York, Futura Publishing Co, 1979

Lippa AS, Nash PA, Greenblatt EN: Pre-clinical neuropsychopharmacological testing procedures for anxiolytic drugs, in Anxiolytics. Edited by Fielding S, Lal H. New York, Futura Publishing Co, 1979

McNamara JO, Byrne MC, Dasheiff RM, Fitz JG: The kindling model of epilepsy: A review. Progr Neurobiol 15:139–159, 1980

Mendelson W, Cain M, Cook J, Paul SM, Skolnick P: A benzodiazepine receptor antagonist decreases sleep and reverses the hypnotic actions of flurazepam. Science 219:414–416, 1983

Möhler H, Okada T: Benzodiazepine receptor: Demonstration in the central nervous system. Science 198:849–851, 1977

Ninan PT, Insel TM, Cohen RM, Cook JM, Skolnick P, Paul SM: Benzodiazepine receptor-mediated experimental "anxiety" in primates. Science 218:1332–1334, 1982

Olsen RW: GABA-benzodiazepine-barbiturate receptor interactions. J Neurochem 37:1–13, 1981

Paul SM, Skolnick P: Benzodiazepine receptors and psychopathological states: Towards a neurobiology of anxiety, in Anxiety: New Research and Changing Concepts. Edited by Klein DF, Rabkin JG. New York, Raven Press, 1981

Paul SM, Skolnick P: Comparative neuropharmacology of antianxiety drugs. Pharmacol Biochem Behav 17:37–41, 1982

Paul SM, Syapin PJ, Paugh BA, Moncada V, Skolnick P: Correlation between benzodiazepine receptor occupation and anticonvulsant effects of diazepam. Nature 281:688–689, 1979

Paul SM, Marangos PJ, Skolnick P: The benzodiazepine-GABA-chloride ionophore receptor complex: Common site of minor tranquilizer action. Biol Psychiatry 16:213–229, 1981

Polc P, Ropert N, Wright DM: Ethyl β-carboline-3-carboxylate antagonizes the action of GABA and benzodiazepines in the hippocampus. Brain Res 217:216–220, 1981

Rickels K: Use of anti-anxiety agents in anxious outpatients. Psychopharmacology 58:1–17, 1978

Robertson HA, Martin IL, Candy JM: Differences in benzodiazepine receptor binding in Maudsley reactive and Maudsley non-reactive rats. Eur J Pharmacol 50:455–457, 1978

Rose RM, Sachar E: Psychoendocrinology, in Textbook of Endocrinology, 6th ed. Edited by Williams RH. Philadelphia, WB Saunders Company, 1981

Scheel-Kruger J, Petersen F: Anticonflict effects of the benzodiazepines mediated by a Gabaergic mechanism in the amygdala. Eur J. Pharmacol 82:115–116, 1982

Schweri M, Cain M, Cook J, Paul SM, Skolnick P: Blockade of 3-carbomethoxy-β-carboline induced seizures by diazepam and the benzodiazepine antagonists, Ro15-1788 and CGS 8216. Pharmacol Biochem Behav 17:457–460, 1982

Schweri M, Martin J, Mendelson W, Barrett J, Paul SM, Skolnick P: Pharmacokinetic and pharmacodynamic factors contributing to the convulsant actions of β-carboline-3-carboxylate esters. Life Sci, 1984, in press

Sheehan DV: Current concepts in psychiatry: Panic attacks and phobias. N Engl J Med 307:156–158, 1982

Skolnick P, Paul SM: Molecular pharmacology of the benzodiazepines. Int Rev Neurobiol 23:103–140, 1982

Skolnick P, Moncada V, Barker J, Paul SM: Pentobarbital has dual actions to increase brain benzodiazepine receptor affinity. Science 211:1448–1450, 1981

Squires RF, Braestrup C: Benzodiazepine receptors in rat brain. Nature 266:732–734, 1977

Stein L, Wise CD, Berger BD: Anti-anxiety action of benzodiazepines: Decrease in activity of serotonin neurons in the punishment system, in The Benzodiazepines. Edited by Garattini S, Mussini E, Randall LO. New York, Raven Press, 1973

Study RE, Barker JL: Cellular mechanisms of benzodiazepine actions. JAMA 247:2147–2151, 1982

Tallman JF, Paul SM, Skolnick P, Gallager DW: Receptors for the age of anxiety: Pharmacology of the benzodiazepines. Science 207:274–281, 1980

Tenen SS, Hirsch JD: β-Carboline-3-carboxylic acid ethyl ester antagonizes diazepam activity. Nature 288:609–610, 1980

Williamson MJ, Paul SM, Skolnick P: Labeling of benzodiazepine receptors in vivo. Nature 275:551–553, 1978

Young WS, Kuhar MJ: Autoradiographic localization of benzodiazepine receptor in the brains of humans and animals. Nature 280:393–395, 1979

References for Chapter 35

β-Adrenergic Blockers and Buspirone

Altesman R, Cole JO: Psychopharmacologic treatment of anxiety. J Clin Psychiatry 44:12–18, 1983

Balster R, Woolverton W: Intravenous buspirone self-administration in rhesus monkeys. J Clin Psychiatry 43:34–37, 1982

Becker A: Oxprenolol and propranolol in anxiety states: A double-blind comparative study. S Afr Med J 50:627–629, 1976

Besterman EMM, Friedlander DH: Clinical experiences with propranolol. Postgrad Med J 41:526–535, 1965

Bonn JA, Turner P: D-propranolol and anxiety. Lancet 1:1355–1356, 1971

Brantigan C, Brantigan T, Joseph N: Effect of β-blockade and beta stimulation on stage fright. Am J Med 72:88–94, 1982

Brewer C: Beneficial effect of β-adrenergic blockade on "exam nerves." Lancet 2:435, 1972

Burrows G, Davies B, Fail L: A placebo-controlled trial of diazepam and oxprenolol for anxiety. Psychopharmacology 50:177–179, 1976

Carlsson C: Haemodynamic effects of adrenergic β-receptor blockade in the withdrawal phase of alcoholism. Int J Clin Pharmacol 3:61–63, 1969

Carlsson C, Johansson T: The psychological effects of propranolol in the abstinence phase of chronic alcoholics. Br J Psychiatry 119:605–606, 1971

Cleghorn JM, Peterfy G, Pinter EJ: Verbal anxiety and the β-adrenergic receptors: A facilitating mechanism? J Nerv Men Dis 151:266–272, 1970

Cole JO, Altesman RI, Weingarten CH: β-blocking drugs in psychiatry. McLean Hos J 4:40–68, 1979

Cole JO, Haskell DS, Orzack MH: Problems with the benzodiazepines: An assessment of the available evidence. McLean Hosp J 6:46–74, 1981

Cole JO, Orzack MH, Beake B, Bird M, Bar-Tal Y: Assessment of the abuse liability of buspirone on recreational sedative users. J Clin Psychiatry 43:69–74, 1982

Easton JD, Sherman DG: Somatic anxiety attacks and propranolol. Arch Neurol 33:689–691, 1976

Eisdorfer C, Nowlin J, Wilkie F: Improvement of learning in the aged by modification of autonomic nervous system activity. Science 170:1327–1329, 1970

Feighner J, Meredith C, Hendrickson G: A double-blind comparison of buspirone and diazepam in outpatients

with generalized anxiety disorder. J Clin Psychiatry 43:103–107, 1982

Frohlich ED, Tarazi RC, Dustan HP: Hyperdynamic β-adrenergic circulatory state. Arch Intern Med 123:1–7, 1969

Gaind R, Suri A, Thompson J: Use of β-blockers as an adjunct in behavioral techniques. Scott Med J 20:284–286, 1975

Goldberg H, Finnerty RJ: The comparative efficacy of buspirone and diazepam in the treatment of anxiety. Am J Psychiatry 136:1184–1187, 1979

Goldberg H, Finnerty RJ: Comparison of buspirone in two separate studies. J Clin Psychiatry 43:87–91, 1982

Gottschalk LA, Stone WN, Gleser GC: Peripheral versus central mechanisms accounting for antianxiety effects of propranolol. Psychosom Med 36:47–56, 1974

Granville-Grossman KL, Turner P: The effect of propranolol on anxiety. Lancet 1:788–790, 1966

Hafner J, Milton F: The influence of propranolol on the exposure in vivo of agoraphobics. Psychol Med 7:419–425, 1977

Hallstrom C, Treasden I, Edwards JG, Lader M: Diazepam, propranolol and their combination in the management of chronic anxiety. Br J Psychiatry 139:417–421, 1981

Hawkings J: Clinical experience with β-blockers in consultant psychiatric practice. Scott Med J 20:294–298, 1975

Hayes PE, Schulz SC: The use of β-adrenergic blocking agents in anxiety disorders and schizophrenia. Pharmacotherapy 3:19–117, 1983

Imhof PR, Blatter K, Fuccella LM, Turri M: β-blockade and emotional tachycardia, radiotelemetric investigations in ski jumpers. J Appl Physiol 27:366–369, 1969

James I, Pearson R, Griffith D, Newbury P, Taylor S: Reducing the somatic manifestations of anxiety by β-blockade—a study of stage fright. J Psychosom Res 22:327–337, 1978

Johnson G, Singh B, Leeman M: Controlled evaluation of the β-adrenoreceptor blocking drug oxprenolol in anxiety. Med J Aust 1:909–912, 1976

Kathol R, Noyes R, Slymen D, Crowe R, Clancy J, Kerber R: Propranolol in chronic anxiety disorders. Arch Gen Psychiatry 37:1361–1367, 1980

Kellner R, Collins AC, Shulman RS: The short-term antianxiety effects of propranolol Hcl. J Clin Pharmacol 14:301–304, 1974

Krishnan G: Oxprenolol in the treatment of examination nerves. Scott Med J 20:288–289, 1975

Krope P, Kohrs A, Ott H, Wagner W, Fichte K: Evaluating mepindolol in a test model of examination anxiety in students. Pharmacopsychiatria 15:41–47, 1982

Lader M: Psychological effects of buspirone. J Clin Psychiatry 43:62–67, 1982

LaPierre YD: Psychophysiological correlates of sodium lactate infusion. Paper presented at New Clinical Drug Evaluation Unit Annual Meeting, Key Biscayne, Florida, June 1983

McMillin WP: Oxprenolol in the treatment of anxiety due to environmental stress. Am J Psychiatry 132:965–966, 1975

Mattila M, Aranko K, Seppala T: Acute effects of buspirone and alcohol on psychomotor skills. J Clin Psychiatry 43:56–60, 1982

Meltzer H, Fleming R: Effect of buspirone on prolactin and growth hormone secretion. J Clin Psychiatry 43:76–79, 1982

Moskowitz H, Smiley A: Effects of chronically administered buspirone and diazepam on driving-related skills performance. J Clin Psychiatry 43:45–55, 1982

Nakano S, Gillespie H, Hollister L: Propranolol in experimentally-induced stress. Psychopharmacology 59:279–284, 1978

Newton R, Casten G, Alms D, Benes C, Marunycz J: The side effect profile of buspirone in comparison to active controls and placebo. J Clin Psychiatry 43:100–102, 1982

Nordenfelt O: Orthostatic ECG changes and the adrenergic β-receptor blocking agent, propranolol (Inderal). Acta Med Scand 178:393–401, 1965

Nordenfelt O, Persson S, Redfors A: Effects of a new β-blocking agent, H56/28, on nervous heart complaints. Acta Med Scand 184:465–471, 1968

Pitts F, Allen R: β-adrenergic blockade in the treatment of anxiety, in The Biology of Anxiety. Edited by Matthew RJ. New York, Brunner/Mazel, 1982

Riblet L, Taylor D, Eison M, Stanton H: Pharmacology and neurochemistry of buspirone. J Clin Psychiatry 43:11–16, 1982

Rickels K, Weisman K, Norstad N, Singer M, Stoltz D, Brown A, Danton J: Buspirone and diazepam in anxiety: A controlled study. J Clin Psychiatry 43:81–86, 1982

Sellers E, Zilm D, Degani H: Comparative efficacy of propranolol and chlordiazepoxide in alcohol withdrawal. J Stud Alcohol 38:2096–2108, 1977

Suzman MM: Propranolol in the treatment of anxiety. Postgrad Med J 52:168–174, 1976

Tanna V, Penningroth R, Woolson R: Propranolol in the treatment of anxiety neurosis. Compr Psychiatry 18:319–326, 1977

Temple D, Yevich J, New J: Buspirone: Chemical profile of a new class of anxioselective agents. J Clin Psychiatry 43:4–9, 1982

Turner P, Granville-Grossman KL, Smart JV: Effect of adrenergic receptor blockade on the tachycardia of thyrotoxicosis and anxiety state. Lancet 2:1316–1318, 1965

Tyrer PJ, Lader MH: Response to propranolol and diazepam in somatic and psychic anxiety. Br Med J 2:14–16, 1974a

Tyrer PJ, Lader MH: Physiological and psychological effects of ± propranolol, + − propranolol and diazepam in induced anxiety. Br J Clin Pharmacol 1:379–385, 1974b

Wheatley D: Comparative effects of propranolol and chlordiazepoxide in anxiety states. Br J Psychiatry 115:1411–1412, 1969

Wheatley D: Buspirone: Multicenter efficacy study. J Clin Psychiatry 43:92–94, 1982

Zilm D, Sellers E, McLeod S: Effect of propranolol on treatment of alcohol withdrawal. N Engl J Med 294:785–788, 1976

References for Chapter 36

The Efficacy of Antidepressants in Anxiety Disorders

Anath J, Pecknold JC, Van Den Steen N, Engelsmann F: Double-blind comparative study of clomipramine and amitriptyline in obsessive neurosis. Prog Neuropsychopharmacol 5:257–262, 1981

Annesley PT: Nardil response in a chronic obsessive compulsive (ltr. to ed). Br J Psychiatry 115:748, 1969

Beaumont G: A large open multicentre trial of clomipramine (Anafranil) in the management of phobic disorders. J Int Med Res 5:116–124, 1977

Capstick N, Seldrup J: The pharmacological aspects of obsessional patients treated with clomipramine. Br J Psychiatry 12:719–720, 1973

Carroll BJ: The dexamethasone test for melancholia. Br J Psychiatry 140:292–304, 1982

Conti L, Pinder RM: A controlled comparative trial of mianserin and diazepam in the treatment of anxiety states in psychiatric out-patients. J Int Med Res 7:285–289, 1979

Curtis GC, Cameron OG, Nesse RM: The dexamethasone suppression test in panic disorder and agoraphobia. Am J Psychiatry 139:1043–1046, 1982

Evans L, Moore G: The treatment of phobic anxiety by zimelidine. Acta Psychiatr Scand (Supp 290) 63:342–345, 1981

Gloger S, Grunhaus L, Birmacher B, Troudart T: Treatment of spontaneous panic attacks with clomipramine. Am J Psychiatry 138:1215–1217, 1981

Hogben GL, Cornfield RB: Treatment of traumatic war neurosis with phenelzine. Arch Gen Psychiatry 38:440–445, 1981

Insel TR, Kalin NH, Guttmacher LB, Cohen RM, Murphy DL: The dexamethasone suppression test in patients with primary obsessive-compulsive disorder. Psychiatry Res 6:153–160, 1982

Insel TR, Murphy DL, Cohen RM, Alterman I, Kilts C, Linnoila M: Obsessive-compulsive disorder. Arch Gen Psychiatry 40:605–612, 1983

Isberg RA: A comparison of phenelzine and imipramine in an obsessive-compulsive patient. Am J Psychiatry 138:1250–1251, 1981

Jain VK: Phenelzine in obsessive neurosis (ltr. to ed). Br J Psychiatry 117:237, 1970

Jenike MA: Rapid response to severe obsessive-compulsive disorder to tranylcypromine. Am J Psychiatry 138:1249–1250, 1981

Johnstone EC, Cunningham-Owens DG, Frith CD, McPherson K, Dowie C, Riley G, Gold A: Neurotic illness and its response to anxiolytic and antidepressant treatment. Psychol Med 10:321–328, 1980

Kahn RJ, McNair DM, Covi L, Downing RW, Fisher S, Lipman RS, Rickels K, Smith V: Effects of psychotropic agents on high anxiety subjects. Psychopharmacol Bull 17:97–100, 1981

Kelly D, Guirguis W, Frommer E, Mitchell-Heggs N, Sargant W: Treatment of phobic states with antidepressants. Br J Psychiatry 116:387–398, 1970

King A: Phenelzine treatment of Roth's calamity syndrome. Med J Aust 1:879–883, 1962

Kleber RJ: A double-blind comparative study of desipramine hydrochloride and diazepam in the control of mixed anxiety/depression symptomatology. J Clin Psychiatry 40:165–170, 1979

Klein DF: Delineation of two drug-responsive anxiety syndromes. Psychopharmacologia 5:397–408, 1964

Klein DF: Importance of psychiatric diagnosis in prediction of clinical drug effects. Arch Gen Psychiatry 16:118–126, 1967

Klein DF: Anxiety reconceptualized, in Anxiety: New Research and Changing Concepts. Edited by Klein DF, Rabkin JG. New York, Raven Press, 1981

Koczkas S, Holmberg G, Wedin L: A pilot study of the effect of the 5-HT-uptake inhibitor, zimelidine, on phobic anxiety. Acta Psychiatr Scand (Suppl 290) 63:328–341, 1981

Leckman JF, Merikangas KR, Pauls DL, Prusoff BA, Weissman MM: Anxiety disorders and depression: Contradictions between family study data and DSM-III conventions. Am J Psychiatry 140: 880–882, 1983

Liebowitz MR: Tricyclic therapy of the DSM-III anxiety disorders: A review with implications for further research. J Clin Psychopharmacol, in press

Lipsedge JS, Hajjoff J, Huggins P, Napier L, Pearce J, Pike DF, Rich M: The management of severe agoraphobia: A comparison of iproniazid and systematic desensitization. Psychopharmacologia 32:67–80, 1973

Marks IM, Stern RS, Mawson D, Cobb J, McDonald R: Clomipramine and exposure for obsessive-compulsive rituals: I. Br J Psychiatry 136:1–25, 1981

Marks IM, Gray S, Cohen SD, Hill R, Mawson D, Ramm L, Stern RS: Imipramine and brief therapist-aided exposure in agoraphobics having self-exposure homework: A controlled trial. Arch Gen Psychiatry 40:153–162, 1983

Marshall W: Treatment of obsessional illness and phobic anxiety states with clomipramine. Br J Psychiatry 119:467–471, 1971

Mathews AM, Gelder MG, Johnston DW: Agoraphobia, Nature and Treatment. New York, Guilford Press, 1981

McNair DM, Kahn RJ: Imipramine compared with a benzodiazepine for agoraphobia, in Anxiety, New Research and Changing Concepts. Edited by Klein DF, Rabkin JG. New York, Raven Press, 1981

Montgomery SA: Clomipramine in obsessional neurosis. A placebo-controlled trial. Pharmaceutical Med 1:189–192, 1980

Mountjoy CQ, Roth M, Garside RF, Leitch IM: A clinical trial of phenelzine in anxiety, depressive and phobic neuroses. Br J Psychiatry 131:486–492, 1977

Muskin PR, Fyer AJ: Treatment of panic disorder. J Clin Psychopharmacol 1:81–90, 1981

Nies A, Howard D, Robinson DS: Antianxiety effects of MAO inhibitors, in The Biology of Anxiety. Edited by Matthew RJ. New York, Brunner/Mazel, 1982

Nurnberg HG, Coccaro EF: Response of panic disorder and resistance of depression to imipramine. Am J Psychiatry 8:1060–1062, 1982

Paykel ES, Rowan PR, Parker RR, Bhat AV: Response to phenelzine and amitriptyline in subtypes of outpatient depression. Arch Gen Psychiatry 39:1041–1049, 1982

Pecknold JC, McClure DJ, Appeltauer L, Allan T, Wrzesinski L: Does tryptophan potentiate clomipramine in the treatment of agoraphobic and social phobic patients? Br J Psychiatry 140:484–490, 1982

Rappaport J, Elkins R, Mikkelsen E: Clinical controlled trial of chlorimipramine in adolescents with obsessive-compulsive disorder. Psychopharmacol Bull 16:61–63, 1980

Redmond DE Jr: New and old evidence for the involvement of a brain norepinephrine system in anxiety, in Phenomenology and Treatment of Anxiety. Edited by Fann WE, Karacan I. New York, Spectrum Publications, 1979

Reynynghe de Voxrie: Anafranil in obsession. Acta Neurol Belg 68:787–792, 1968

Rickels K, Csanalosi I, Chung HR, Case WG, Pereira-Ogan JA, Downing RW: Amitriptyline in anxious-depressed outpatients: A controlled study. Am J Psychiatry 131:25–30, 1974

Sargant W, Dally P: Treatment of anxiety states by anti-depressant drugs. Br Med J 1:6–9, 1962

Shammas E: Controlled comparison of bromazepam, amitriptyline, and placebo in anxiety-depressive neurosis. Dis Nerv Syst 38:201–207, 1977

Sheehan DV: Current views on the treatment of panic and phobic disorders. Drug Ther Hosp 74–93, October 1982

Sheehan DV, Ballenger J, Jacobsen G: Treatment of endogenous anxiety with phobic, hysterical, and hypochondriacal symptoms. Arch Gen Psychiatry 37:51–59, 1980

Sheehan DV, Davidson J, Manschreck T, Van Wyck Fleet J: Lack of efficacy of a new antidepressant (Buproprion) in the treatment of panic disorder with phobias. J Clin Psychopharmacol 3:28–31, 1983

Solyom L, Heseltine GFD, McClure DJ, Solyom C, Ledgwidge B, Steinburg G: Behavior therapy versus drug therapy in the treatment of phobic neurosis. Can Psychiatr Assoc J 18:25–31, 1973

Solyom C, Solyom L, LaPierre Y, Pecknold J, Morton L: Phenelzine and exposure in the treatment of phobias. Biol Psychiatry 16:239–247, 1981

Svensson TH: Effect of chronic treatment with tricyclic antidepressant drugs on identified brain noradrenergic and serotonergic neurons. Acta Psychiatr Scand (Suppl 280):121–131, 1980

Thompson GN: Post-traumatic psychoneurosis: Evaluation of drug therapy. Dis Nerv Syst 38:617–619, 1977

Thoren P, Asberg M, Cronholm B, Jornestedt L, Traskman L: Clomipramine treatment of obsessive-compulsive disorder. Arch Gen Psychiatry 37:1281–1285, 1980

Tyrer P, Candy J, Kelly DA: A study of the clinical effects of phenelzine and placebo in the treatment of phobic anxiety. Psychopharmacologia 32:237–254, 1973

Walter CJS: Clinical impression on the treatment of obsessional states with intravenous clomipramine. J Int Med Res 1:413–416, 1978

West ED, Dally PJ: Effects of iproniazid in depressive syndromes. Br Med J 1:1491, 1959

Wheatley D: Evaluation of trazodone in the treatment of anxiety. Curr Ther Res 20:74–83, 1976

Zitrin CM, Klein DF, Woerner MG: Treatment of agoraphobia with group exposure in vivo and imipramine. Arch Gen Psychiatry 37:63–72, 1980

Zitrin CM, Klein DF, Woerner MG, Ross DC: Treatment of phobias: I. Comparison of imipramine and placebo. Arch Gen Psychiatry 40:125–138, 1983

References for Unresolved Questions

Benson H, Frankel FH, Apfel R, Daniels MD, Schniewind HE, Nemiah JC, Sifneos PE, Crassweller KD, Greenwood MM, Kotch JB, Arns PA, Rosner B: Treatment of anxiety: A comparison of the usefulness of self-hypnosis and a meditational relaxation technique. Psychother Psychosom 30:229–242, 1978

Klein DF, Rabkin JG: Specificity and strategy in psychotherapy research and practice, in Psychotherapy Research (Proceedings of the Annual Meeting of the American Psychopathological Association, 1983). Edited by Spitzer RL, Williams JBW. New York, Raven Press, 1983

Peters RK, Benson H, Porter D: Daily relaxation response breaks in a working population: 1. Health, performance, and well-being. Am J Public Health 67:946–953, 1977a

Peters RK, Benson H, Peters JM: Daily relaxation response breaks in a working population: 2. Blood pressure. Am J Public Health 67:954–959, 1977b

Wender PH, Klein DF: Mind, Mood, and Medicine: A Guide to the New Biopsychiatry. New York, Farrar, Straus & Giroux, 1981

Index

A

AA (Alcoholics Anonymous), **84**:299, 300, 311–19 passim, 343, 344, 346, 361
  and Alateen, **84**:343, 346
  and Al-Anon, **84**:300, 343, 346
Aamark, C., **84**:316
Aarens, M., et al., **84**:369
Aaron, P., **84**:360
AASECT (American Association of Sex Educators, Counselors and Therapists), **82**:7
ABC (alcoholic beverage control) system, **84**:361.
  See also Alcoholism
Abdulla, Y. H., **82**:146
Abe, K., **84**:416
Abell, C. W., et al., **82**:126
Aberfan (Wales) disaster, **84**:111
Aberg, T., **84**:264
Abernethy, V., **84**:139
Ablon, S. L., et al., **83**:250, 456
Abortion: legalized, advent of, **82**:7
Abraham, K., **82**:511, **83**:319, 385, 522
Abram, H. S., **84**:263, 266
Abrams, A., et al., **82**:214
Abrams, D. B., **84**:331
Abrams, R., **82**:152; **83**:273, 279, 440, 443; **84**:208;
  et al., **83**:279
Abulafia, Rabbi, **84**:442
Abuse, *see* Child abuse; Drug abuse/addiction;
  Sexual abuse; Substance abuse; Violence
Accidents: and accident-proneness, **83**:366; **84**:216
  alcohol and, **84**:369
  and mortality rate, **84**:217
  See also Disaster, studies of
Acetaldehyde accumulation, *see* Alcohol (metabolism of)
Acetylcholine, **83**:459, 460; **84**:351, 470, 476
Acetylcholinesterase (AChE) activity: in Alzheimer's disease, **83**:109–10; **84**:233
  drug inhibition of, **84**:476
Achenbach, T. M., **82**:269, 291
Ackerman, Nathan W., **83**:170, 189, 190, 191, 208, 234, 235
Ackerman, S. H., **84**:224, 407
Acquired immunodeficiency syndrome, *see* AIDS
Acromegaly, **82**:37
Acting-out behavior: adolescent, **83**:190, 192, 285
  parents' divorce and, **84**:152
  in borderline disorders, **82**:454, 455, 465, 467, 475, 477, 482
  in narcissistic disorder, **82**:522
  psychotherapeutic management of, **84**:21–22
  separation/divorce and, **82**:44; **84**:152
  of therapist, **83**:330–31
  in time-limited psychotherapy, **84**:43
  transference, **82**:475, 476, 478–79, 485
Active-interpretive technique, **84**:7
Adams, H. E., **84**:450
Adams, J., **84**:109
Adams, P. L., **84**:156

Adams, R. W., **84**:351, 355
Adamson, J. D., **84**:217
ADD (Attentional Deficit Disorder), **82**:457, 468; **83**:443
  drug therapy for, **82**:462–63, 467, 470
  DSM-III criteria for, **82**:442, 463
  residual, **82**:442
  and schizophrenia, **83**:292
Addams, Jane, **83**:169
Addiction, *see* Alcoholism; Drug abuse/addiction;
  Substance abuse
Addiction Research Center Inventory, **84**:501
Addiction Research Foundation (Toronto), **84**:336, 337
Addison's disease, **82**:37
Adebimpe, V. R., **82**:102; **83**:290
Adelstein, A. M., et al., **83**:419
Adenosines, **84**:350
Ader, R., **84**:217, 223, 224
ADH (alcohol dehydrogenase), **84**:324, 349
  and ALDH (aldehyde dehydrogenase), **84**:324, 356
ADIS (Anxiety Disorders Interview Schedule), **84**:402
Adjustment Disorder: with anxious mood, **84**:208, 246, 247, 419
  cancer and, **84**:246, 247
  childhood, **82**:263
  with depressed mood, **83**:367, 410; **84**:63, 206, 246, 247
    childhood depression and, **82**:305
  DSM-III category for, **83**:140, 357, 367, 375, 410; **84**:63, 203, 246, 247, 419
  epidemiology/prevalence rate of, **84**:203, 214
  late-life, **84**:236
  with mixed mood, **84**:246
Adjustment reaction(s): depression as, **83**:361–62, 375
  late-life, **83**:95, 140–41, 146
  See also Grief reaction; Stress
Adler, Alfred, **82**:488, **83**:47, 513; **84**:7, 44
Adler, G., **82**:480
Adler, S. A., et al., **82**:126; **83**:467
Administration on Aging, U.S., **83**:85
Adolescent(s): and age of consent, **82**:352
  and alcoholism, **84**:313, 338
  anorexic, **83**:189
  anxiety disorders in, **84**:410
  and bipolar illness, **83**:270, 280–85 passim, 329, 456
  EE and prediction of risk in, **84**:95
  family therapy and, **82**:279; **83**:171, 188–92 passim, 195, 200, 209–11, 241, 247
  gender dysphoria of, **82**:51–52, 53
  impaired/psychotic parents and, **84**:132, 133
  mentally retarded, **84**:122
  noncompliance with chemotherapy by, **84**:240
  parents' separation/divorce and, **84**:145, 149–53 passim, 157
  pre-schizophrenic, **82**:89, 106, 108; **83**:175; **84**:415
  psychic trauma and, **84**:39

as rape victims, **82:**62, 63
suicide and attempted suicide by, **82:**51–52, 278, 301, 303; **83:**433; **84:**152
See also Adolescent depression; Childhood; Juvenile delinquency; Young adults
Adolescent depression, **82:**278–79, 291, 294; **83:**365
clinical signs of, **82:**297, 300, 301, 303
concept of, **82:**264, 289
criteria for diagnosis of, **82:**289, 298–99
frequency of, **82:**284; **83:**364
and mania, **83:**287
Adoption: of children of mentally ill, **84:**131
of mentally retarded children, **84:**123
Adoption studies: of affective disorders, **83:**435, 444–45; **84:**97
of alcoholism, **84:**320, 321
of anxiety disorders, **84:**405–06
of depressives, need for, **83:**405
development of, and genetic evidence, **84:**391
of mentally retarded children, **84:**123
of schizophrenia, **82:**95–96, 445–48; **84:**405–06
of suicide, **83:**432, 443
See also Genetic factors
Adrenergic response: anxiety and: **84:**471–76
drug therapy and, **84:**490–503
unresolved questions about, **84:**524
See also Epinephrine; Norepinephrine(NE)
Adreno-genital syndrome, **82:**37
Adult depression, *see* Depression
Advertising: alcohol, controversy over, **84:**368
Aesthetic Preference Scale, **83:**336
Affect: defined, **83:**357
Affective Disorders: age and, **83:**456
alcoholism and, **84:**326
atypical, **83:**367
autonomous and nonautonomous, **83:**120–21
borderline personality disorder relation to, **82:**438–44 passim, 452, 454–55
catecholamine hypothesis of, *see* Catecholamines
children at risk for, **84:**96–98
diagnostic criteria for, **82:**432, 436, 440; **83:**285, 362–64
DSM-III, *see* DSM-III categories/criteria
epidemiology/prevalence rate of, **83:**406–28, 435, 438, 447; **84:**97, 203, 235
family approaches to, **83:**249–53
genetic factors in, **83:**274, 282–83, 434–57; **84:**97, 100, 325
in geriatric patient, **83:**118–30, 144
lithium ratio in, **82:**208; **83:**452–53
manifestations of, **83:**356–57
organic, **83:**287, 295; **84:**235
primary and secondary, distinction between, **83:**376–80, 381
as response to physical illness, *see* Physical illness
studies of (international), **83:**293, 294, 407–09, 411; **84:**303
subcategories of, **83:**367, 409–10
and suicide rate, **84:**467 (*see also* Suicide and attempted suicide)

therapy for, **83:**128–30; **84:**97
See also Bipolar (manic-depressive) Disorder; Depressed affect; Depression; Emotions; Schizoaffective Disorder
Affective knowing: in infant, **83:**14
Affect memory, *see* Memory
Affect suppression: and childhood depression, **82:**297
Africa: depression prevalence in, **83:**415
Age: and affective disorders, **83:**456
and alcoholism, **84:**316–17
and anxiety/anxiety disorders, **84:**208, 404
and bipolar illness, **83:**119, 125, 283–85, 296, 304, 306, 329, 424–25, 427, 443
and cancer mortality, **84:**240
of children of divorce, **84:**144–45
and effects on children, **84:**151–52
of consent, **82:**352
demographic statistics regarding, **83:**88–89
and depression, *see* Depression
and drug toxicity, *see* Drug side effect(s)
and emotional impact of uterus removal, **82:**40
and hostility toward/distrust of psychiatry, **83:**40, 129
of infant when individuation occurs, **83:**19
and mental illness, **83:**92; **84:**190, 191, 198, 202, 203, 206, 214, 231
minimum legal drinking, **84:**300, 361, 363, 364–65
of mother, and schizophrenia, **84:**99, 100
and paraphrenia, **82:**149; **83:**133
and political leadership, **83:**84
and postmarital sexuality, **82:**43
and psychotherapy (short-term), **84:**25
and reaction to psychic trauma, **84:**114
and schizophrenia (male vs. female), **82:**108
and self-perception (changes in), **83:**216
and sex therapy, **82:**25
and sleep, *see* Sleep disorders
and suicide, **83:**433
and tardive dyskinesia, **82:**147
See also Aging
Age Discrimination Act in Employment (1967), **83:**106
Aggression: erotized and nonerotized, **82:**30–32
latent indications of, **84:**19
mob manifestation of, **83:**22, 23, 24–25
narcissism and, **82:**511, 513, 514–16
pregenital and oral, **82:**473
primary and secondary, **82:**31
in therapeutic relationship, **84:**227
See also Anger; Hostility
Aging: and adjustment to retirement, **83:**106
biologic changes and theories of, **83:**97–100
cross-linkage or eversion theory, **83:**98–99
and epidemiology of psychiatric disorder, **83:**87–93; **84:**184, 232
physiological changes in, **83:**99, 113, 140–51; **84:**234 (*see also* Metabolism)
psychosocial theories of and approaches to, **83:**105–06
primary and secondary, **83:**96
and sexuality, **82:**7, 8, 42, 45–47; **83:**147–51

societies and agencies concerned with, **83:**84–86

as term, **83:**96

See also Age; Late-life psychiatric disorders

Agnoli, A., et al., **82:**200

Agoraphobia, **82:**440, 457, 468; **83:**443; **84:**403, 413, 437, 472, 473, 479, 482–83

drug therapy for, **82:**465, 467; **83:**483, 488; **84:**414, 454–55, 483, 495, 501, 503–11, 518

DSM-III category for, **84:**394, 396–98, 401, 410, 419, 495, 503

exposure treatment of, **84:**448–60, 507

unresolved questions about, **84:**523

Freud's view of, **84:**431, 437

subtypes (with and without panic attacks), **84:**394, 397, 398, 503

See also Panic disorders; Phobic Disorders

Agranulocytosis, **84:**248. See also Drug side effect(s)

Agras, W. S., **84:**451; et al., **84:**453

Ahlenius, S., et al., **84:**349

Ahlfors, U. G., et al., **83:**310, 311

AIDS (acquired immunodeficiency syndrome), **84:**250

Ainsworth, M. D. S., **84:**128, 412; et al., **84:**142

Ainsworth Strange Situation scale, **84:**142

Akiskal, Hagop S., **82:**436, 437, 442, 443; **83:**270–84 passim, 288–90 passim, 442; et al., **82:**440–41, 444, 453, 454; **83:**271–92 passim, 374, 375

A. K. Rice Group Relations Conferences, **83:**32

Akselrod, S., et al., **84:**469

Akutsu, K., **84:**445

Al-Anon, Alateen, see AA (Alcoholics Anonymous)

Albert, H., **84:**260

Albert, N., **82:**282

Albert, S. N., et al., **84:**354

Albrecht, P., et al., **82:**121

Alcohol: drugs combined with, **83:**127, 491; **84:**253, 358

studies of, **84:**500, 501

metabolism of

acetaldehyde accumulation, **84:**321, 323–24, 327, 349, 356–57

ethanol reaction, **84:**321–28 passim, 348–49, 350

MAOIs and, **84:**358 (see also Drug therapy)

use of (as life style), and mortality rate, **84:**217

See also Alcoholism

Alcohol, Drug Abuse, and Mental Administration, U.S., **83:**406n, 409

Alcohol and Health (1971 report to Congress), **84:**357

Alcohol dehydrogenase, see ADH

Alcoholics Anonymous, see AA

Alcoholics Anonymous (publication), **84:**346

Alcoholism: abstinence vs., **84:**317–18, 319, 332, 344, 361

unacceptability of, **84:**337

(see also AA [Alcoholics Anonymous])

alcohol abuse (as category), **84:**301, 302–03, 307, 308, 340

alcohol amnestic disorder (Korsakoff's syndrome), **83:**115, **84:**301, 347

alcohol dependence (as category), **84:**68, 213, 301–08 passim, 340

alcohol hallucinosis, **84:**301, 347

antipsychotics in treatment of, **84:**355

distinguished from schizophrenia, **83:**289, 290

anxiety and, see Anxiety

and BAC (blood alcohol concentration), **84:**323, 326

behavioral assessment of, **84:**329–31 (see also Behavioral approach)

behavior modification and, **84:**319

in bipolar illness, **83:**279, 281, 282, 286, 320, 442, 453; **84:**314

borderline disorders and, **82:**438, 441, 442, 454; **84:**299

and children at risk, **84:**135, 136, 299, 311–13, 324, 330 (see also of parent, below)

classification of (five types), **84:**315, 339–40

and delirium tremens, **84:**310 (see also and withdrawal, below)

dementia associated with, **84:**301, 307, 347

denial of, **84:**299, 343, 344

and depression, **83:**365, 373–81 passim, 420, 422, 432; **84:**326, 356, 357, 358

diagnosis of

criteria for, **84:**303–10

differential, **84:**61

DSM-III categories for disorders related to, **84:**68, 213, 299, 301–10, 340, 351

as disease, see as "mental illness" or disease, below

drug dependencies or abuse concurrent with, **84:**334–35, 340, 353

and environmental risk (reduction of), **84:**368–69

etiology of

environmental factors and, **84:**313, 320, 339

the family/family history and, **83:**178; **84:**320, 322, 323, 326, 327, 340 (see also of parent, below)

genetic and biochemical factors in, **84:**300, 313, 320–28

illusions about, **84:**311–13

multidimensional theories of, **84:**329

preexisting factors in, **84:**309

social expectancies and, **84:**330–31, 360, 365–66

social learning theory and, **84:**328–38

surgery and, **84:**276

intoxication and idiosyncratic intoxication, **84:**301

and Korsakoff's syndrome, see alcohol amnestic disorder, above

late-life, **83:**94, 109, 115

MAO activity decrease in, **82:**126; **83:**452; **84:**325

medical complications resulting from, **84:**307, 331, 465

as "mental illness" or disease, **82:**337; **83:**286, 442; **84:**299, 313–14, 331, 344, 361

contradictory conceptions of, **84:**315–16

and minimum drinking age, *see* prevention of, *below*

morbidity risk/prevalence rates, **82:**290; **84:**213, 299, 321, 324, 326–27

and mortality rate, **84:**460 (*see also* and suicide, *below*)

of parent, **84:**135, 299, 330
  and adult alcoholism, **84:**312
  biological vs. adoptive, **84:**320
  (*see also* and children at risk; etiology of, *above*)

personality and, **84:**310, 321–22, 325

police and, **82:**385

preoperative, in cancer patients, **84:**276

prevention of, **84:**338
  minimum drinking age and, **84:**300, 361, 363, 364–65
  public policy and, **84:**359–70

and "problem drinker," **84:**315, 316, 329, 336–37, 338

and prognosis, **84:**308, 318

as progressive disease, **84:**314–17, 318

psychiatric disorders concurrent with problems of, **84:**299, 307, 312–13, 321, 358

public policy toward, *see* prevention of, *above*

studies of, **83:**174; **84:**303–05, 315–19, 320–28, 330–31, 348–59 passim
  adoption, **84:**320, 321
  animal research, **84:**320, 323, 329, 349, 350, 355, 359
  behavior change, **84:**335–36
  "problem drinkers," **84:**336–37
  prospective, and need for, **84:**318–19

and suicide, **83:**429, 430, 431, 432; **84:**326, 357, 467

symptoms of, **84:**303–05
  ever present (vs. currently present), **84:**315

and tolerance of alcohol, **84:**303, 305–06, 308, 322

treatment of
  behavioral, *see* Behavioral approach
  chemical aversion, **84:**328, 333–34
  counseling, **84:**186
  detoxification, **84:**299, 342, 353, 355, 356
  drug, *see* Drug therapy
  electrical aversion, **84:**328, 329, 332–33
  family therapy, **83:**189; **84:**300
  goals of, **84:**317–18, 331–32, 337, 343, 344, 345, 361 (*see also* abstinence vs., *above*)
  illusions about futility of, **84:**311, 313–14
  multimodal, **84:**318
  psychotherapy, **84:**299, 338–46
  relapse from, **84:**342, 343, 345

and withdrawal, **84:**301–06 passim, 351–56 passim, 493
  symptoms of, **84:**306, 310, 347, 351–52
  therapy for, *see* Drug therapy
  withdrawal delirium (delirium tremens), **84:**301, 351–56 passim

Aldehyde, aldehyde dehydrogenase (ADH, ALDH), *see* ADH (alcohol dehydrogenase)

Aldosterone: stress and, **84:**222. *See also* Endocrine system

Aldrich, R. F., **82:**332

Alexander, A. A., et al., **83:**139

Alexander, Franz, **83:**55; **84:**7, 30; et al., **84:**216

Alexander, G. J., **82:**351

Alexander, J. F., **83:**190

Alexander, P. E., et al., **82:**210

Alexander, S., **84:**477

Alexanderson, B., **83:**499

Alexithymia concept, **84:**217, 218, 227, 437–39

Alfredsson, G., et al., **82:**200

Alfrey, A. C., et al., **83:**111

Alignment with potential states of being: mother-infant relationships and, **83:**20–21. *See also* Empathy; Mother-child relationship

Alkalosis: panic attacks and, **84:**477, 478

Alkana, R. L., **84:**347, 348, 349, 351; et al., **84:**349, 350

Allen, C., **84:**346

Allen, Edward B., Award, **83:**85

Allen, Frederick, **82:**264

Allen, J. C., et al., **84:**252

Allen, R. E., **84:**474, 478, 491, 492

Allergies: decreased prevalence of, **82:**118
  drug effects on allergic symptoms, **84:**223
  as "psychosomatic" disorders/psychological effects on, **84:**198, 224
  See also Immune system

Altesman, R., **84:**490

Althusser, L., **83:**34

Altman, J. H., **83:**387, 389, 392

ALTRO Health and Rehabilitation services, **84:**11

Altruism, pathological: and sexual dysfunction, **82:**30

Aluminum concentration: and Alzheimer's disease, **83:**101, 111

Alzheimer's disease, *see* Dementia, Primary Degenerative

Amarasingham, L. R., **83:**173

Ambelas, A., **83:**277

American Association of Sex Educators, Counselors and Therapists (AASECT), **82:**7

American Board of Medical Specialties, **83:**86

American Board of Psychiatry and Neurology, **83:**86

American Geriatrics Society, **83:**85

American Law Institute (ALI) Rule, **82:**391, 392

American Law Reports, **82:**328

American Medical Association, **82:**7, 329

American Psychiatric Association (APA), **82:**425, 449; **84:**393
  cited, **82:**143, 209, 339nn16, 18, 450; **83:**84, 89, 90, 106–08 passim, 118–20 passim, 131, 140, 272, 277, 290–94 passim, 357, 367–70 passim, 408, 479, 492, 512, 528; **84:**49, 109, 110, 121, 234, 301, 302, 340, 392–99 passim, 419, 460–61, 482, 488 (*see also* DSM-III)
  and confidentiality issue, **82:**330, 331–32, 334
  Council(s)
    on Aging, **83:**84
    on Government Policy and the Law, **82:**326
    on Research, **83:**85
  and criterion of dangerousness, **82:**339
  and legislation, **82:**323, 330
  Principles of Medical Ethics, **82:**329
  Task Force(s)
    on geriatric psychiatry, aging, dying, **83:**85

on psychiatric participation in sentencing, **82:**395
on Vitamin Therapy, **82:**143
Amies, P. L., et al., **84:**399
Amish population: affective disorders among, **83:**271, 448
Amkraut, A., et al., **82:**115
Amnesia: alcoholism and, *see* Alcoholism
as criterion for incompetence, **82:**388
as drug side effect, **84:**252
infantile, **83:**17–18
late-life, **83:**109
amnestic syndrome, **83:**115
and "pseudodementia," **84:**234
secondary, in manic psychosis, **83:**328
See also Memory
Amphetamine, **82:**131, 132, 462; **83:**127, 480, 483
affective disorders produced by, **83:**365, 374, 379, 461, 484
for cancer patient, **84:**249
as ethanol antagonist, **84:**350
misuse of, **84:**350
and paranoid psychosis, **82:**137, 138, 197; **83:**290
-PEA model of schizophrenia, **82:**137, 148, 152
for school-phobic children, **84:**416
stereotyped behavior induced by, **82:**137, 144
Amputation, *see* Surgery
Amsterdam, J. D., **83:**512; et al., **83:**492
Amyloidosis, **83:**98
Analysis of the Self, The (Kohut), **82:**500; **83:**59
Analyst, the: and "middle game," **83:**51–56, 59
psychoanalytic theory applied by, **83:**65–66
and role reversal, **82:**516 (*see also* Transference)
task of, **82:**497; **83:**55, 59–60, 65–66
technical neutrality of, **82:**476–78
See also Psychoanalysis; Therapeutic relationship; Therapist, the
Anand, B. W., et al., **84:**445
Ananth, J. V., **82:**118; et al., **84:**514, 515
Anatomy, **82:**9–11
child's discovery of distinctions in, **83:**42–43
repudiation of (and gender disturbance), **82:**51, 55, 56
See also Genitalia
Andersen, S. M., **83:**134
Anderson, B., **83:**103
Anderson, C. D., **84:**218
Anderson, C. M., **83:**253; et al., **82:**163, 173; **83:**245–46, 248, 253, 256
Anderson, G. J., **84:**233
Anderson, P., **83:**34
Andreasen, N. C., **83:**279, 280, 285, 289; et al., **82:**290; **84:**404
Andrew, J. M., **84:**257
Androgen: futility of administration of, **82:**11
stress effect on, **84:**222
Andrulonis, P. A., et al., **82:**437, 441–42, 443, 453, 454
Anemia: and dementia, **84:**234. *See also* Physical illness
Anesthesia: fear of, **84:**260–61. *See also* Surgery
Aneuploidy, **83:**110

Anger: depression and, **84:**19
divorce as cause of
in child, **84:**151, 152
in parent, **84:**148, 149, 154, 155
impulsive, borderline patient expression of, **82:**416, 417, 457, 464–65, 467
toward therapist, **84:**43 (*see also* Therapeutic relationship)
of traumatized individual, **84:**118
See also Aggression; EE (expressed emotion); Rage
Angrist, B. M., et al., **82:**133
Angst, J., **83:**269, 272, 305, 313, 315, 423, 439, 440, 447; et al., **82:**208, 210; **83:**285, 305, 306, 438, 439, 440, 447
Anhedonia, **82:**156, 296, 297, 300, 463; **83:**279, 282, 331, 479, 514. *See also* Depression; Dysphoria
Animal research: alcoholism studies, **84:**320, 323, 329, 349, 350, 355, 359
anxiety studies, **84:**409, 412, 416–17, 471–72, 475, 476, 484–88 passim, 498
drug dependence studies, **84:**501
operant conditioning studies; **84:**227, 329
parent-offspring separation studies, **84:**417
relaxation response studies, **84:**444–45
stress studies, **84:**110, 222, 224
Annesley, P. T., **84:**515
Annis, H. M., **84:**337, 338
Anomie: gender disturbance and, **82:**51
Anorexia: as depression symptom, **83:**479; **84:**248
childhood depression, **82:**297, 304
as drug side effect, **84:**233
family therapy for, **83:**189, 191
in geriatric patient, **83:**144
Philadelphia studies of, **84:**225
Anorexia nervosa, **82:**423; **83:**121, 122; **84:**219, 220, 225
in children, family psychotherapy and, **84:**225
circadian rhythms and, **84:**222–23
family history and, **83:**442
therapy for, **83:**169, 171; **84:**229
See also Weight loss
Anorgasmia, primary: therapy for, **82:**21. *See also* Psychosexual dysfunctions
Ansbacher, H. L. and R. R., **84:**44
Anstee, B. A., **84:**231
Anthony, E. J., **82:**266, 273, 278, 288; **83:**25, 27, 190, 192; **84:**106, 132, 141, 143
Anthony, W. A., et al., **82:**110, 176, 177
Anthropology: diagnosis compared to, **83:**178–79
Antibiotics, antidepressants, antipsychotics, etc., *see* Drugs
Antibody levels: in Alzheimer's disease, **83:**111
behavioral conditioning and, **84:**224
in schizophrenia (elevated), **82:**117, 118, 121
See also Immune system
Antigens: human leukocyte (HLA) and bipolar illness, **83:**436, 445, 449–50
response to, in schizophrenic patients, **82:**115, 121, 146
Anti-Saloon League, **84:**360. *See also* Alcoholism

Antisocial features (in borderline and narcissistic disorders): and prognosis, **82:**487, 515–16, 520. *See also* Social isolation; Social skills
Antisocial personality, **84:**460
  alcoholism and, **84:**307, 313, 321, 326
  genetic factors and, **84:**325
Antisocial Personality Disorder, **82:**290, 435, 436
  as risk indicator, **84:**95–96
Anxiety, **83:**443
  and alcoholic relapse during treatment, **84:**345
  alcoholism as result of, **84:**329, 465
  alcohol withdrawal causing, **84:**351, 357, 493
  ascorbic acid (Vitamin C) level and, **82:**144
  benzodiazepine-GABA-receptor model of, **84:**488
  biology and biochemistry of, **84:**409–10, 457, 467–90
    unresolved questions about, **84:**523–24
  cancer and, *see* Cancer
  carbon dioxide and, **84:**474, 477, 478
  cardiovascular illness and, **82:**36; **84:**465–67
  castration, **82:**34, 38, 40, 503; **83:**23, 42
  among children, **84:**98, 410–18
  "contagious," *see* Contagion
  definition of, **84:**418, 482–83
  depression and, **83:**273, 381, 393, 463
    childhood depression distinguished from, **82:**297
    (*see also* panic, *below*)
  DSM-III and, *see* DSM-III categories/criteria
  etiology of, **84:**419–20
  Freud's theories of, *see* Freud, Sigmund
  and heart rate, **84:**418, 468–69
  hospitalization and, **84:**208
  Janet's theory of, **84:**427–29
  lactate and, *see* Drug therapy (for anxiety states)
  late-life states of, **83:**91, 92, 95, 127, 140–42, 146
    postoperative, **84:**275
  neurophysiology of, **84:**408–09, 471–79
  panic, **84:**414, 436–37
    depression and, **84:**511–12
    (*see also* Panic Disorder)
  pharmacological provocation of, *see* Drugs
  posttraumatic, **84:**110–15 passim, 421 (*see also* Trauma, emotional/psychic)
  prevalence of, **84:**84:203, 214
  psychodynamic view of, **84:**417, 426–40
    unresolved questions about, **84:**522
  and psychological defenses, **84:**432–36
  separation, *see* Separation fears
  and sexual dysfunctions, **82:**15, 23, 25, 26, 31, 34, 38
  signal, **84:**433, 436–37
  stress and, **83:**395; **84:**439, 469, 482, 496–97
  and suicide, **83:**429; **84:**467
  surgery and (preoperative, perioperative, postoperative), **84:**222, 229, 256–61
  treatment of, *see* Anxiety Disorders
  See also Dysphoria; Panic Disorder; Stress
Anxiety Disorders, **83:**443; **84:**392
  atypical, **84:**393 (*see also* Anxiety; Obsessive-Compulsive Disorder; Phobic Disorders; Posttraumatic Stress Disorder)

avoidant, **84:**410
cancer and, **84:**254
childhood or adolescent, **84:**410–18
  avoidant, **84:**410
  unresolved questions about, **84:**520–21
  -depression relationship, **84:**511–12
diagnosis of
  criteria for, **84:**392–93 (*see also* DSM-III)
  differential, **84:**61
epidemiology/prevalence rate of, **84:**203, 208, 209, 403–04, 407–08
  among children, **84:**411
etiology of, **84:**184, 402–10, 419–20
generalized anxiety disorder, **84:**395–401 passim, 482, 488, 499–503 passim, 510, 516, 517
  DSM-III and, *see* DSM-III categories/criteria
genetic factors in, **84:**391, 402–10, 479, 520
Interview Schedule (ADIS), **84:**402
and mortality rate, **84:**460–67, 523
overanxious disorder, **84:**410
physical illness and, **84:**184, 407–08
separation anxiety disorder, **84:**410–13 passim, 417, 418
therapy for
  behavior therapy, **83:**483; **84:**401, 417, 421, 424, 439, 440, 448–60
  in childhood, **84:**411–12, 413–18
  drug therapy, *see* Drug therapy
  exposure, **84:**448–60
  group, **84:**424–25
  psychotherapy, **84:**412, 416, 417, 418–26, 439–40, 521–22
  relaxation therapy, **84:**258, 439, 440–48, 522–23
unresolved questions about, **84:**519–25
See also Agoraphobia; Anxiety; Panic Disorder
Anxiety neurosis, **84:**394, 395, 403, 430–31
  alcoholism and, **84:**465
  drug therapy for, **84:**478, 498, 510
  DSM category for, **84:**393, 516
  and hypertension, **84:**465–67
  and lactate metabolism, **84:**407
  prevalence of, **84:**404
  RDC criteria for, **84:**494
  See also Anxiety Disorders
Anxiety-provoking psychotherapy, short-term (STAPP), *see* Psychotherapy(ies), brief
Anzieu, D., **83:**23, 24, 25, 33, 35
Apfel, R. J., **84:**218
Apnea: as drug effect, **84:**353
  sleep, **83:**147; **84:**220–21
Appelbaum, Paul S., **82:**325, 326, 330, 331, 333, 351–56 passim, 361n2, 368, 379–83 passim, 384n8; **84:**260; et al., **82:**357, 359
Appleby, I. L., et al., **84:**407, 457
APUDomas, **84:**250. *See also* Cancer
Arato, M., et al., **82:**202
Aretaeus, **83:**269
Arib, M., **82:**186
Arie, T., **83:**116, 117
Arieti, S., **82:**272, 273; **83:**522; **84:**57, 59
Arlow, J. A., **83:**33
Armor, D. J., et al., **84:**299, 307, 318, 332, 356
Armstrong, S., **82:**363

Arthritis, rheumatoid, **84:**220, 221, 229
  mood of patient and prognosis, **84:**218, 224
  as "psychosomatic" disorder, **84:**202, 216, 437
  schizophrenia and, **82:**117, 118
  and sexual dysfunction, **82:**37
Arthur, R. J., **84:**213
Artiss, L. K., **84:**245
Art-therapeutic work (with children), **84:**112, 113; 120
Asano, N., **83:**441
Asarnow, R. F., et al., **84:**100
Asberg, M., et al., **83:**452, 477
Asch, S. E., **84:**424
Ascher, L. M., **84:**458
Ascorbic acid (Vitamin C), **82:**143–44. *See also* Vitamins
Ashby, W. R., et al., **82:**143
Ashford, W., **83:**127
Ashkenazi, A., et al., **82:**146
Ashley, M., et al., **82:**356
"As if" identity, **82:**56
"As if" personality, **82:**515
"As if" reaction, **84:**475
Asnis, G. M., et al., **82:**204, 294
Assertiveness training, **82:**23; **83:**142, 518; **84:**10
Association of State Mental Health Program Directors, **82:**348
Associations: interpretation of (in psychoanalysis), **83:**63–64. *See also* Free association
Associations for Retarded Citizens, **84:**128
Asthma, **84:**219, 220, 221
  absence of, in psychotic patients, **82:**115
  drug effects on, **84:**223, 502
  family therapy in cases of, **83:**189
  as "psychosomatic" disorder/psychological effects on, **84:**202, 211, 216, 224
  in children, **84:**225
  social support networks and, **84:**229, 230
Astrachan, B. M., **84:**182
Astrup, C., et al., **83:**372
Atkinson, R. M., et al., **84:**401
Atomic bomb, *see* Nuclear disaster threat
Atsmon, A., et al., **82:**205, 206
Attachment bonds, *see* Relationships
Attentional Deficit Disorder, *see* ADD
Atypical disorders, *see* Bipolar (manic-depressive) Disorder; Depression, Psychosexual dysfunctions; Psychosis(es)
Auchincloss, H., **84:**259
Auditory impairment, *see* Hearing loss
Austin, V., et al., **82:**417, 434, 437
Australia: CMI results in, **84:**202
  suicide rate in, **83:**433
Autism: of normal infant, questioned, **83:**10–11
  as schizophrenia symptom, **83:**130, 290
Autonomic nervous system (ANS): dysfunction, **84:**479, 480–81
  physiology, **84:**468–71
  See also CNS (central nervous system)
Averback, P., **82:**120
Avery, D., **83:**366, 431
Avoidant Disorder of Childhood or Adolescence, **84:**410. *See also* Anxiety Disorders
Avoidant Personality Disorder, **82:**15, 18

Axelsson, R., **82:**203
Ayd, F. J., **83:**125, 487
Aylon, O., **84:**109
Azrin, N. H., **84:**334

B

Baastrup, P. C., **83:**304, 326, 327; et al., **83:**307, 308, 309, 315
Babigian, H. M., **84:**460
BAC (blood alcohol concentration), *see* Alcoholism
Bach, G. R., **83:**26
Bachrach, L., **82:**370n1
Baekeland, F., **84:**356
Bagchi, B. K., **84:**445
Bagley, C., **82:**120; **83:**426; **84:**252
Bailey, D. N., **83:**501
Bairitt, J. A., **84:**276
Bakst, J., **84:**263
Baldessarini, R. J., **82:**129, 147; **83:**271, 475, 476; et al., **83:**272
Baldwin, A. L., et al., **84:**101
Baldwin, C. P., et al., **84:**132
Baldwin, J. A., **82:**115
Balint, M., **83:**56
Ballenger, J. C., **83:**303, 311
Balster, R., **84:**501
Balter, M. D., **83:**95
Baltimore City Hospitals, **84:**330, 334
Ban, T. A., **83:**305, 317; et al., **82:**143
Bandura, A., **84:**337, 453
Bane, M. J., **84:**144
Baratham, G., **84:**353
Barber, T. X., **84:**446
Barcai, A., **83:**443
Barchas, J., **83:**102
Bard, M., **84:**270
Barglow, P., **83:**40
Baringer, J. R., et al., **83:**111
Barios, B. A., **84:**458
Barker, D. J. P., **82:**283; **83:**87
Barker, J. L., **84:**485, 486
Barker, M. G., **84:**262
Barlow, D. H., **84:**393, 401, 449, 450, 454; et al., **84:**451
Barnes, M., **84:**106
Barnes, R. F., **83:**106
Barnes, T. R. E., **83:**273
Baron, M., **82:**126; **83:**449; et al., **82:**429, 430, 432, 452; **83:**447, 448
Barraclough, B., **83:**431; et al., **83:**429, 430
Barrett, J., et al., **83:**371
Barrett, J. E., **83:**379, 381, 384, 406, 407, 420, 425
Barry, H., III, **84:**347, 348, 349
Barsky, A. J., **84:**184
Bartko, J. J., **82:**167
Barton, A., **84:**117
Barton, R., **82:**88
Bartrop, R. W., et al., **84:**223

Bartus, R. T., et al., **84**:233
Basch, M. F., **82**:502, 503
Bash, K. W., **83**:416
Bash-Liechti, J., **83**:416
"Basic-assumptions group," *see* Group psychology
Basic Handbook on Psychiatry, The (Noshpitz), **84**:115
BASIC IB, **84**:67
BASIC ID, **84**:10, 67–73 passim, 76
Baskin, D. S., **84**:351
Basowitz, H., et al., **84**:475
Batchelor, I. R. C., **83**:285
Bates, E., **83**:18
Bateson, Gregory, **83**:170, 242
Battered wives/husbands, *see* Violence
Baudry, F., **84**:276, 277
Bauer, D., **84**:412
Bauer, M. L., **83**:95
Bauersfeld, K. H., **82**:282
Bayley scale, **84**:142
Bazelon, David L., **82**:362, 371, 372–73, 377
Bazzoui, W., **83**:271
BDI (Beck Depression Inventory), **82**:270, 282; **83**:336, 362; **84**:50, 52, 54, 189, 203, 206, 208, 455
Bean, M. H., **84**:339, 344
Beard, B. H., **84**:266, 268
Beard, G. M., **84**:404
Beard, J. H., et al., **82**:176
Beardslee, W. R., **84**:107, 116–17; et al., **84**:97, 133
Beary, J. F., **84**:444, 446
Beatty, E. T., **84**:228
Beaubrun, M. H., **84**:364
Beaumont, G., **84**:518
Beaumont, William, **84**:219
Beaver Valley nuclear plant, **83**:403. *See also* Nuclear disaster threat
Bebbington, P. E., **82**:284–85; **83**:406, 417, 421
Bech, P., et al., **83**:386, 387, 388
Beck, Aaron T., **82**:161, 268, 282, 283; **83**:322, 364, 431, 512, 513, 525; **84**:8, 45–48 passim, 421; et al., **83**:513; **84**:47–50 passim, 56, 455
Beck, D. F., **83**:190
Beck, E. C., **83**:441
Beck, J. G., **84**:393, 401
Beck Depression Inventory, *see* BDI
Becker, A., **84**:495
Becker, J., **84**:57
Beckhardt, R. M., **84**:182, 186
Beckman, G., et al., **83**:449
Beckman, H., **83**:461, 467, 468, 473, 474; **84**:472
Beels, C. Christian, **83**:172, 189, 242, 244, 248, 255; **84**:95n
Beg, A. A., et al., **82**:204
Begleiter, H., **84**:327
Behavior: prediction of, *see* Prediction of behavior
Type A and Type B, *see* Personality
Behavioral approach:
to alcoholism, **84**:299
assessment of, **84**:329–31

aversion techniques, **84**:328–29, 332–34
contingency, **84**:332, 334, 337
future trends in, **84**:337–38
goals of, **84**:331–32
history of, **84**:328–29
individualized (IBTA), **84**:335–36
integrated behavior change techniques, **84**:336
to anxiety states, **83**:483; **84**:401, 417, 421, 424, 439, 440, 504, 507
phobia, **84**:448–60
(*see also* flooding technique [implosion], *below*)
in brief psychotherapy, **84**:8
to cancer, **84**:244, 245
in child therapy, **82**:265
in consultation-liaison psychiatry, **84**:186
in couples therapy, **83**:220, 222, 223, 225; **84**:53
to depression, **83**:515–28 passim
in family therapy, **83**:196, 201–02, 246–47
flooding technique (implosion), **84**:222, 424, 439, 450–52, 459, 510
combined with other therapies, **84**:454–56
to medical/psychosomatic disorders, **84**:227, 228–29, 230
to mental retardation, **84**:126, 129
to obesity, **84**:53
to older patients, **83**:114, 146
to psychic trauma, **84**:118
in rape crisis therapy, **82**:63
to schizophrenia, **82**:111; **83**:246–47
in screening police applicants, **82**:385
to sex therapy, **82**:21–26 passim, 35, 40; **84**:53
See also Sensitization
Behavioral immunology, *see* Immune system
Behavioral medicine: defined, **84**:227
Behavior disorders, *see* Externalization
Behrens, M. L., **83**:235
Beigel, A., **83**:295
Beigler, J. S., **82**:330; et al., **84**:181
Beitman, B., **82**:457
Bell, John E., **83**:170
Bell, N. W., **83**:233
Bellack, A. S., **82**:108, 109
Bellak, Leopold, **82**:463; **84**:7, 8–9, 11–21 passim; et al., **84**:17
Bell Jar, The (Plath), **83**:428
Belmaker, R. H., et al., **82**:126, 206; **83**:467
Bemporad, Jules, **82**:264, 279; **83**:522; **84**:57, 59
Bender, L., **82**:58; **84**:99
Bender, M. B., **83**:116
Bender-Gestalt test, **84**:131
Benedek, E. P. and R. S., **84**:157
Benjamin, F., et al., **82**:204
Benjamin, J. D., **83**:9
Benjaminsen, S., **83**:386, 387, 388, 395–99 passim
Bennahum, D. A., **83**:449; et al., **83**:449
Bennett, I., **84**:96
Bennett, J. P., et al., **82**:130, 139
Bennett, M., **84**:299
Benney, Celia, **84**:11
Bennie, E. H., **82**:204

Benson, Herbert, 84:440–47 passim, 522; et al., 84:440–47 passim, 522
Benson, R., 83:328
BEP (brief and emergency psychotherapy), see Psychotherapy(ies), brief
Bereavement, see Grief reaction; Loss; Widowhood
Beresford, T. P., 84:186
Bergen, J. R., et al., 82:119
    and Bergen's plasma fraction, 82:119
Bergener, M., 84:354
Berger, K. S., 83:132, 133
Berger, P. A., et al., 82:129, 141, 212
Bergler, Edmund, 82:494
Bergmann, K., 83:107
Bergner, R. M., 84:53
Bergstrom, S., et al., 82:146
Berkman, P. L., 83:90
Berkowitz, R., 83:246
Berlin, R. M., 84:182
Berman, Ellen M., 83:171, 172, 199, 216; 84:53; et al., 83:216
Berman, M., 84:212
Berner, P., 83:279
Berney, T., et al., 84:414, 416
Bernstein, N., 84:115, 125
Bernstein, S., 84:181
Bernstein, S. M., et al., 82:53
Beroz, E., et al., 84:356
Berrettini, W. H., 82:126; et al., 82:126
Bertelsen, A., 83:444; et al., 83:444
Bertilsson, L., et al., 83:495
Besser, R. S., et al., 84:275
Besses, G. S., et al., 82:200
Besterman, E. M. M., 84:492
Beta blockers: in anxiety disorders, 84:490–503
    unresolved questions about, 84:524
    See also Anxiety Disorders; Drugs, list of
Beta-CCE, see CCE
Beth Israel Hospital (Boston): Department of Psychiatry, 84:34
Beumont, P. J. V., et al., 82:202, 204
Beverly Hills Supper Club disaster, 84:118
Bewell, M. E., 84:275
Bexton, W. H., 83:30
Bialos, D., et al., 83:315
Bibring, E., 82:272, 273, 286, 480; 83:522
Bibring, G. L., 84:180
Bielski, R. J., 83:122, 125, 126
Bierman, J. S., et al., 82:276
Bigelow, G., et al., 84:330, 334
Bigelow, L. B., et al., 82:130, 132, 152
Bigger, J. T., 83:123
Biggs, J. T., 83:506
Bijou, S. W., 84:126
Bille, D. A., 84:273
Billings, Edward G., 84:179
Billings, R. F., et al., 84:233
Biofeedback: defined, 84:227
    use of, 84:10, 70, 73, 76, 227–28, 230, 456, 473
Bion, W. R., 82:471, 477; 83:21, 22, 24, 26–35 passim
Biopsy, see Tumors

Bipolar (manic-depressive) Disorder: age and, 83:119, 125, 283–85, 296, 304, 306, 329, 424–25, 427, 443
    alcoholism and, 83:279, 281, 282, 286, 320, 442, 453; 84:314
    atypical, 83:119, 125, 271, 273, 275, 295, 367, 410, 441
    as autonomous affective disorder, 83:120
    bipolar I, see Manic state (bipolar I)
    bipolar II, see Hypomania
    circular, 83:275, 277
    classification of/criteria for, 83:119, 271–75 passim, 295, 296, 354, 367, 368, 371, 410, 423, 427
    definition of, 83:422–23
    dementia praecox separated from, 82:82; 83:269
    depressive phase, 83:126, 279–80, 328, 332, 367, 386, 420 (see also Depression)
    diagnosis of, 83:122, 271, 278–79, 407, 410; 84:61
        childhood, 83:283
        differential, 83:125, 285, 287–90, 293, 295, 465–66
        DST in, see DST (dexamethasone suppression test)
        and misdiagnosis, 83:280, 281, 284
    drug therapy for, see Bipolar (manic-depressive) Disorder, treatment of, below; Lithium therapy
    epidemiology/prevalence rate of, 83:270–71, 275, 283, 407, 415, 420–27 passim, 435, 439, 447, 455
    etiology of, 83:249, 285, 319, 320
    and the family (impact on), 83:249, 279, 302, 305, 329
    family therapy for, 83:249–52
    genetics/family history and, 82:265; 83:272–78 passim, 282–83, 287, 289, 329, 427, 435–57; 84:97
    Kraepelin's concept of, see Kraepelin, Emil
    late-life, 83:125–26, 285
    manic state, see Manic state (bipolar I)
    MAO activity in, 83:467–68
    mixed states in, 83:280–81, 367
    mood changes and discrimination in, 83:281, 286, 326–30 passim, 334, 374
    and mortality rate, 83:287; 84:217
    parental (and effect on child), 84:133
    personality and, 83:384, 386–92, 426
    prevention of, 83:454–57
    prognosis for, 83:250–51, 282
        recurrence and fears of, 83:285, 304, 305–07, 311–16 passim, 327–35 passim, 425
    psychoanalytic view of (pre-lithium), 83:319
    rapid-cycling, 83:303, 312, 318
    related to borderline disorders, 82:439, 442, 448, 454
    risk factors in, 83:423, 438–45 passim, 454–56 (see also genetics/family history and, above)
    social implications of, 83:285–86, 297, 303, 320, 331, 423
    subgroups of, 83:367, 410, 439

and suicide, **83**:286–87, 320, 329, 330, 334, 429, 430

symptoms of, **83**:280, 281–82, 320

unipolar compared to/distinguished from/related to, *see* Unipolar/nonbipolar depression

urinary MHPG and VMA levels in, **83**:272– 73, 460–66, 468–69

validation of typology of, **83**:282–83

See also Cyclothymic Disorder; Dysthymic Disorder; Major Depression; Schizoaffective Disorder

Bipolar (manic-depressive) Disorder, treatment of:

drug therapy, **83**:250, 276, 303–18, 368

  compliance/noncompliance with, **83**:251, 301, 315–18 passim, 321–37

  conditions requiring, **83**:305–07

  dosage, **83**:126, 316–17

  duration of, **83**:315

  family approach to, **83**:249–52, 305

  imipramine/TCA, **83**:307, 311, 312, 371, 380, 480

  lithium, *see* Lithium therapy

  long-term vs. continuation, **83**:304

  other drugs, **83**:126, 312, 318, 370

  psychotherapy combined with, **83**:316, 320–37

  UCLA-Columbia study of, **83**:322, 332–37 passim

ECT, **83**:126, 302

family or marital therapy, **83**:189, 249–52

hospitalization, **83**:125, 249, 275, 293–97 passim, 303, 306, 318, 320, 326, 330, 334, 423, 424, 438, 439

outpatient, **83**:271, 297–98, 303, 326

psychoanalysis, **83**:319–20, 329

psychotherapeutic issues in, **83**:319–37

psychotherapy (brief) contraindicated for, **84**:44

Bipolar self, *see* Self

Bird, E. D., **82**:138; et al., **82**:132, 133

Birkett, D. P., **83**:114

Birleson, P., **82**:287

Birley, J. L. T., **82**:102, 172; **83**:174, 242; **84**:95

Birnbaum, Morton, **82**:361–62

Birnbom, F., **84**:236

Birren, J. E., **83**:108

Birtchnell, J., **83**:431

Birth control, **82**:7

contraception, **84**:138, 139

  vasectomy as means of, **82**:39

family planning services and, **84**:137, 138–39

for intelligence control (condemned), **84**:126

Birth weight, **83**:229; **84**:131

Bisexuality, **82**:55. *See also* Sexuality

Bishop, M. P., **82**:180, 181, 184

Bizzoco, D. H., **84**:353

Blachly, P. H., **84**:262, 263

Black, A. L., **83**:114

Black, S., et al., **84**:224

Blackburn, I. M., **83**:279, 387, 389; **84**:49

Blackouts: alcoholism and, **84**:304

Blacks: and anxiety at hospitalization, **84**:208

bipolar illness among, **83**:270, 290, 426

and cognitive dysfunction; **84**:203

depressive symptoms among, **83**:413, 420; **84**:208

in elderly population, **83**:88

schizophrenia among, **82**:102; **83**:270, 290

single-parent families among, **84**:144

Blackwell, B., **83**:304; **84**:188, 214

Blanchard, M., **83**:277

Bland, R. C., **82**:100

Blane, H. T., **84**:313, 339, 343, 345

Blath, R. A., et al., **83**:432

Blaufarb, H., **84**:117

Blazer, Dan G., **83**:87, 90–95 passim, 132; **84**:235

Bleuler, Eugen P., **82**:82–88 passim, 112–13, 149, 166, 197, 444; **83**:289, 357–58, 359

Bleuler, Manfred, **82**:88, 161; **84**:94, 99, 134, 137, 138

Blindness, *see* Vision

Bliss, E. L., et al., **84**:262

Bloch, Donald A., **83**:171, 172; **84**:225n; et al., **84**:107, 118

Block, J. H., et al., **84**:153

Block, M. A., **84**:352

Blombery, P. A., et al., **83**:461

Blood alcohol concentration (BAC), *see* Alcoholism

Blood flow, *see* Peripheral blood flow

Blood glucose levels, **82**:293

Blood pressure: antidepressant effect on, **82**:291–92; **83**:469, 477–78, 484–85

β-blocker effect on, **84**:491

biofeedback regulation of, **84**:227, 228

during orgasm, **82**:12

penile, **82**:46

personality type and, **84**:220

relaxation response and, **84**:444, 446, 447

separation from mother (in animal model) and, **84**:225

See also Drug side effect(s); Hypertension

Blood type O, **83**:450

Bloom, B. L., et al., **84**:58, 145

Bloom, F. E., **84**:223, 323, 350

Bloom, L., **83**:20

Bloom, L. J., et al., **84**:469

Blum, H. P., **83**:44, 46, 62

Blum, J. E., **83**:129

Blum, K., et al., **84**:349

Blume, Sheila B., **84**:300, 339, 341, 343, 344; et al., **84**:346

Blumenfield, S., et al., **84**:238

Blumenthal, J. A., et al., **84**:216

Blumenthal, M. D., **83**:123, 412, 413; **84**:235, 236

Body image, *see* Self

Bohannon, P., **83**:227

Bohman, H., et al., **84**:320

Boklage, C., **82**:124

Bokser, Rabbi Ben Zion, **84**:442

Bolen, D. W., **83**:189

Bonaparte, M., **84**:104

Bond, A. J., et al., **84**:470

Bond, P. A., et al., **83**:461

Bondareff, W., et al., **83**:110, 117

Bonfiglio, G., et al., **84:**355
Bonn, J. A., **84:**495
Böök, J. A., et al., **82:**126, 127
Bookhammer, R. S., **82:**158; et al., **82:**217–18
Borden, R. J., **84:**469
Borderline Personality Disorder, **82:**491
  characteristics of, **82:**417, 452–54, 464–66, 468, 512–13
    vs. institutionalization symptoms, **82:**456
    MBD, **82:**441–42, 454
    in psychotherapeutic situation, **82:**472–76
    transference patterns, **82:**489 (*see also* Transference)
  coexistence of, with other disorders, **82:**466; **84:**299
  as definable/discrete syndrome, **82:**416, 417, 424, 425, 433–37 passim, 454, 455, 456
  epidemiology/prevalence rate of, **82:**415, 455
  etiology of, **82:**438, 452–56
  and gender disturbance, **82:**48, 52, 56
  genetic factors in, **82:**437–56
    biologic markers, **82:**452–56
  morbidity in, **82:**416
  prognosis for, **82:**486–87
  and psychosexual dysfunctions, **82:**19
  regression in, **82:**473
  schizophrenia compared to/discriminated from/related to, **82:**416, 436, 439–43 passim, 444–57 passim
  treatment of
    drug therapy, **82:**444, 456–67, 469–70, 484; **83:**480
    and effect on nursing staff, **83:**28–29
    goals of, **82:**482–83, 485
    hospital, **82:**424, 450, 470–74 passim, 482
    problems in, **82:**415
    psychoanalytic, **82:**471
    psychotherapeutic, **82:**425, 467, 470–87; **84:**44, 49
Borderline Personality Disorder, diagnosis of, **82:**465
  in adoptive studies, **82:**446–48
  criteria for, **82:**424–28, 436, 441, 443, 444, 457
    Borderline Personality Scale (BPS) II, **82:**431–34 passim
    Diagnostic Interview for Borderlines (DIB), **82:**417, 423, 424, 428–35 passim, 439–40, 456, 466
    DMS-III, **82:**428–36 passim, 440–43 passim, 448, 449–51, 454–66 passim, 470; **83:**288
    Gund-R scale, **82:**429, 430
    Research Diagnostic Criteria (RDC), **82:**423, 434
    Schedule for Affective Disorders and Schizophrenia (SADS), **82:**432
    Schedule for Interviewing Borderlines (SIB), **82:**429, 430, 432, 433, 452
    Schedule for Schizotypal Personalities (SSP), **82:**432
    Spitzer et al. (17) Item List, **82:**424–25, 429–34 passim
    Structural Interview (Kernberg), **82:**431, 432, 433, 438, 440, 454

Symptom Scale for Borderline Schizophrenia, **82:**448
    and cyclothymic personality, **82:**444; **83:**288
    diagnostic schemes compared, **82:**433–35
    differential, **83:**288
    empirical studies and, **82:**415–37, 448
Borderline Personality Scale, *see* BPS
Borga, O., **83:**495, 497
Borison, R. L., et al., **82:**137
Borkenstein, R. F., et al., **84:**366
Bornstein, M. H., **83:**12
Bornstein, P. H., et al., **84:**129
Borocas, C. and H., **84:**110
Borowski, T., **82:**171
Borton, R. W., **83:**12
Borysenko, J. Z., **84:**447
Boscolo, L., **83:**247
Bosmann, H. B., et al., **84:**485
Bosron, W. F., **84:**324
Boston, L. N., **84:**352
Boston: family planning services in, **84:**139
    STAPP studies in, **84:**32–33
Boston University Center for Law and Health Sciences, **82:**364
Boswell, J., **83:**430
Boszormenyi-Nagy, Ivan, **83:**170, 187, 194, 199, 219, 223, 236
Boucharlat, P. J., et al., **84:**352
Boudoulas, H., et al., **84:**480, 481
Boushey, H. A., **84:**223
Bowden, C., **83:**274
Bowen, D. M., **83:**109; et al., **83:**109, 110
Bowen, Murray, **83:**170, 194, 222, 223, 234, 235, 242
Bower, G., **83:**16, 17
Bowers, M. B., **82:**133, 140; **83:**480
Bowlby, J., **82:**266, 275; **83:**360, 404, 519; **84:**57–58, 106, 128, 412, 418, 420, 423
Boyar, R. M., **84:**223; et al., **84:**223
Boyd, Jeffrey H., **83:**270, 355, 406, 406n, 438; **84:**206, 214; et al., **84:**396
Boyd, W. H., **83:**189
BPRS (Brief Psychiatric Rating Scale), **82:**199
BPS (Borderline Personality Scale): I, **82:**432; II, **82:**432–33, 434
Braden, G., et al., **83:**314
Braden, W., et al., **83:**289
Bradley, C., **82:**263
Bradley, J., **83:**144
Bradley, S. J., **82:**434
Braestrup, C., **84:**409, 485; et al., **84:**483, 487
Brain, the: aging effects on, **83:**99–101
    and brain wave amplitude in alcoholism, **84:**327
    damage to, *see* Encephalopathy
    neurobiology of, **83:**458
    trauma, and borderline disorders, **82:**442
    See also Catecholamines; Neurotransmitters; Protein factors
Brain disorders, *see* Organic Mental Disorders; Stroke
Braithwaite, R., et al., **83:**495, 499
Branchley, M. H., et al., **83:**114, 137

Branconnier, R., et al., **83**:476
Brandeis, L. D., **82**:328
Brant, R., **82**:57
Brantigan, C., et al., **84**:496
Bratfos, O., **83**:286, 372
Braunschweig, D., **83**:33
Braverman, E., **82**:144
Brazelton, T. B., **83**:9; et al., **83**:10
Breast, the: cancer of, *see* Cancer
  and postoperative phantoms, **84**:272
  tumor biopsy, emotional effect of, **84**:222, 223
  See also Surgery (mastectomy)
Breathing exercises, *see* Exercise (as therapy)
Brennan, Justice William, **82**:323n5
Brenner, M. H., **82**:100, 103
Breskin Rigidity Test, **83**:336
Bretherton, I., **83**:19
Brethren, The (Woodward and Armstrong), **82**:363
Breuer, J., **84**:430
Brewer, C., **84**:496
Bridge, T. P., **83**:131, 132, 139; et al., **83**:131
Bridging: defined, **84**:75
Brief Psychiatric Rating Scale (BPRS), **82**:199
Brieter, C., **84**:126
Briley, M. S., et al., **83**:470
Brinkley, J., et al., **82**:457, 460, 464
Brinkman, S. D., et al., **83**:113
Briquet's syndrome, *see* Somatization Disorder
Briscoe, C. W., **84**:59
British Medical Journal, **83**:114
Brockington, I. F., **82**:102
Brockington, L., et al., **82**:209
Brodie, H. K. H., **83**:100, 286, 456
Brody, J. E., **82**:26
Brogden, R., et al., **83**:490
Bromet, E., **83**:401, 403, 404
Bronfenbrunner, U., **84**:126
Bronx Municipal Hospital Center, **82**:423
Brook, Mary Potter, **83**:170
Brooks, A., **82**:391
Brooks, G. W., **82**:88
Brotman, Judge, **82**:383
Brotman, R. K., et al., **82**:188
Broverman, I. K., et al., **83**:38
Brown, B. F., **84**:145
Brown, C., **84**:125
Brown, F. W., **84**:404
Brown, George W., **82**:102, 172; **83**:94, 395, 396,
  400–04 passim, 421–22; **84**:95, 133, 135, 397; et
  al., **82**:88, 109; **83**:94, 174, 242, 244, 385, 394–
  400 passim, 414, 416; **84**:58, 95
Brown, G. M., **82**:293; et al., **82**:200
Brown, H. N., **84**:186
Brown, J., **83**:431, 433, 434
Brown, J. B., **84**:325
Brown, O. R., et al., **84**:479
Brown, R. J., **84**:217
Brown, R. S., et al., **84**:273
Brown, S. L., **83**:230, 236
Brown, W. A., **82**:135, 200, 203
Brown, W. T., **83**:316
Brownell, K., et al., **84**:53
Brownmiller, S., **82**:58

Bruch, H., **84**:219
Bruch, Hilde, **82**:155
Brugger, M., **84**:444
Brunell, L. F., **84**:69
Bruner, J. S., **83**:13
Brunswick, D. J., **83**:501; et al. **83**:500
Bruun, K., et al., **84**:362, 364
Bucher, K. D., **83**:446; et al., **83**:446
Buchsbaum, M. S., **82**:453; et al., **82**:125, 452
Bucht, G., **83**:314
Buckman, M. T., **82**:203
Buffalo Creek (West Virginia) flood, **84**:110, 111–
  12, 117
Buie, D. H., **82**:480, 496
Buikholder, G. U., **84**:275
Bukberg, J., et al., **84**:246
Bulemia, **84**:223
Bumberry, W., et al., **82**:270
Bunney, W. E., **83**:272, 278, 311, 448, 470; et al.,
  83:298, 469
Burger, Chief Justice Warren, **82**:323, 361, 363–
  64, 373
Burgess, A., et al., **84**:116
Burgess, A. W., **82**:61, 62, 63
Burlingham, D., **84**:105, 106
Burnet, F. M., **83**:111
Burnside, I. M., **83**:114
Burrows, G., et al., **84**:358, 495
Burstein, C. L., **84**:353
Burt, R., **82**:387
Burton, N., **82**:266, 267–68
Burton, Richard, **83**:512
Burvill, P. W., **84**:214
Busch, D. A., et al., **82**:200
Busse, Ewald W., **83**:84, 86, 102, 104, 142, 143;
  84:232
Bustamenta, J. P., **84**:231
Butcher, R. W., **84**:350
Butler, Robert N., **83**:84, 86

C

Caddy, G. R., **84**:331
Cade, J. F., **83**:298, 320, 328
Cadoret, R. J., **83**:440; **84**:97, 213
Caffeine: and caffeinism, **83**:146, 280, 296
  as ethanol antagonist, **84**:350
Caffey, E. M., **82**:205, **83**:316; et al., **82**:190, 192,
  226
Cahalan, D., **84**:315, 316, 321, 329; et al., **84**:330
  and Cahalan scale, **84**:315
Cain, A., **84**:115
Caine, E. D., **83**:119
CALGB (Cancer and Leukemia Group B), **84**:242
California: Department of Health, **84**:122
  Department of Mental Health, **82**:350
  divorce studies/Children of Divorce Project,
  84:145, 148–53 passim
  family law, **84**:155
Callaway, E., **84**:228

Camara, K. A., **84**:154
Cambridge-Somerville Study (of alcoholism), **84**:312
Campbell, A., et al., **84**:133
Campbell, J. C., **82**:288–89; **83**:279, 283
Canada: depressive disorders diagnosed in, **83**:108
  lithium therapy used in, **83**:481
  schizophrenia studies in, **82**:98, 145
Canadian Mental Health Association, **82**:143
Cancer: anxiety/distress of patients with, **84**:187, 203, 208, 245–47, 254
  and alcoholism (preoperative), **84**:276
  following cure, **84**:254–55
  (*see also* psychiatric disorders concurrent with, *below*)
  breast, **82**:40, 202; **84**:223, 253
    mood of patient and prognosis for, **84**:218
    treatment of, **84**:218, 252, 254, 255, 270–71
    (*see also* Surgery [mastectomy])
  chromosome damage and, **83**:97
  depressive patients and, **83**:366; **84**:49, 208, 217, 235, 246–47, 248–49
  epidemiology of, **84**:239, 253
  and mortality rate, **84**:217, 240
  psychiatric consultations for patients with, **84**:243–45
  psychiatric disorders concurrent with, **84**:203, 245–54
    anxiety disorders, **84**:254
    delirium and dementia, **84**:249–53
    major depression, **84**:246, 248–49
    prevalence of, **84**:245–47
    reactions to crises, **84**:247
    schizophrenic disorders, **82**:115; **84**:253–54
  psychological problems of surviving patients, **84**:254–55
  radiation therapy for, **82**:39
    combined with drugs, **84**:252
    distress at end of, **84**:255
    side effects of, **84**:248, 250, 252, 255
  risk factors in, **84**:239–42
  surgery for, **82**:39, 40; **84**:273
    disfiguring and reconstructive, **84**:276
    (*see also* Surgery)
  therapeutic approach to, **84**:240–45
    behavioral, **84**:244, 245
    psychopharmalogic, *see* Drug therapy
    psychotherapeutic, **82**:39; **84**:244, 245, 247, 248
  (*see also* radiation therapy for, *above*)
  uterine, dangers of, **83**:149
  See also Leukemia
Cancer and Leukemia Group B (CALGB), **84**:242
Cancro, Robert, **82**:83, 95, 153; **84**:325n
Canetti, E., **83**:25
Canino, I. A., **83**:283
Cannon, W. B., **84**:217, 445
Canter, A., **83**:285
Cantwell, D. P., **82**:266, 268, 282, 297; et al., **83**:442
Capitalism: sexuality repressed by, **83**:34
Caplan, G., **84**:157, 229

Capone, M. A., **84**:274
Capstick, N., **84**:512
Carbon dioxide: and panic attacks, **84**:474, 477, 478
Carcinoid syndrome: as drug side effect, **83**:128
Cardiac disorders: β-blockers and, **84**:492–93, 502
  biofeedback vs. relaxation therapy for, **84**:228, 447
  as drug side effect, *see* Drug side effect(s)
  of elderly patients, **83**:96, 123, 498; **84**:232
  MVP (mitral valve prolapse), **84**:407–08, 465, 479–82
    incidence of, **84**:479
  myocardial infarction and psychiatric morbidity, **84**:214
    social support network and, **84**:229, 230
  and pacemakers, **83**:478
  sleep (REM or NREM), sleep apnea and, **84**:220, 221
  surgery for, **84**:262–65
  TCAs and, **83**:123, 477–78, 509
  See also Heart rate; Physical illness; Vascular disorders
Cardozo, Justice Benjamin, **82**:350
CARE (Comprehensive Assessment and Referral Evaluation), **83**:116
Carey, G., **84**:483; et al., **84**:403
Carey-Trefzer, C., **84**:106
Carlen, P. L., **84**:347
Carlin, J., **84**:115
Carlson, G. A., **82**:266, 268, 282, 289, 291, 294, 297; **83**:279, 284, 289, 302, 434; et al., **83**:250
Carlsson, A., **82**:132, 135, 196
Carlsson, C., **84**:493
Carp, R., **82**:121
Carpenter, G., **83**:10
Carpenter, L., **82**:102; **84**:258
Carpenter, William T., Jr., **82**:85–89 passim, 108, 109, 154–61 passim, 167, 416; **83**:130; et al., **82**:157, 170, 416, 418; **83**:279, 289
Carrier Clinic, **84**:313
Carroll, Bernard J., **83**:283, 289, 355, 452; **84**:515; et al., **82**:290, 436, 452–53; **83**:121, 273, 460, 463
Carroll, P. J., **83**:114
Carskodan, M., et al., **83**:147
Carter, E. A., **83**:216
Casacchia, M., et al., **82**:200
Casey, D. E., et al., **82**:141
Casey, J. F., et al., **82**:209
Casper, R. C., et al., **83**:461; **84**:219
Cassano, G. B., et al., **82**:201
Cassel Hospital (England), **84**:139
Cassem, E. H., **84**:183
Castelden, C. M., **83**:114
Castelnuovo-Tedesco, P., **84**:219, 268
Castration anxiety, *see* Anxiety
CAT (choline acetyltransferase): in Alzheimer's disease, **83**:109–10, 113
Cataracts, *see* Vision
Catastrophic events, *see* Disaster; Stress
Catatonic stupor or excitement: bipolar illness misdiagnosed as, **83**:280
  and competency, **82**:354

Catecholamines, **82:**127, 129, 139, 144, 146, 147
and catecholamine-derived products, **84:**323
and catecholamine hypothesis of affective disorders, **82:**265; **83:**380, 458–59
Catechol-O-methyltransferase (COMT), **82:**128, 131; **83:**451, 454
heightened levels of
anxiety and, **84:**472–73
β-CCE and, **84:**488
and ethanol effects, **84:**349–50
MVP and, **84:**480–81
in older males, **83:**133
in postoperative patients, **84:**258
stress and, **84:**222
urinary, **83:**464–67; **84:**258 (*see also* Urinary MHPG levels)
CATEGO (computer diagnosis), *see* Diagnosis
Catholic Church, **84:**208, 442, 447. *See also* Religion
Cation transport parameters, **83:**451, 452–53. *See also* Genetic factors
Catley, D. M., et al., **84:**351
Caudill, B. D., **84:**330
Cause-effect, *see* Relationships
Cautela, J. R., **84:**333
Cavalli-Sforza, L. L., **84:**406
Cavanaugh, Stephanie, **84:**177–78, 188, 189, 201, 203, 206, 207, 208
Cawley, R. H., **84:**214
β-CCE, **84:**487–88, 489–90
CDI (Children's Depression Inventory), **82:**270–71
Cebiroglu, R., **82:**291; et al., **82:**282
Cecchin, G., **83:**247
Celiac disease, **82:**145, 146. *See also* Physical illness
Celsus, A. C., **84:**392
Census, U.S. Bureau of the, **83:**88; **84:**144, 156
Center for Epidemiological Studies Depression Scale, *see* CES-D
Center for Science in the Public Interest, **84:**362
Central nervous system, *see* CNS
Cerebral atrophy: schizophrenia and, **82:**117, 120, 122, 148
Cerebrospinal fluid, *see* CSF
Cervulli, M., et al., **84:**228
Cesarec-Marke Personality Scale, **83:**386–87
CES-D (Center for Epidemiological Studies Depression Scale), **84:**189, 203, 208
Chalmers, R. J., **82:**204
Chambers, W., et al., **82:**270
Chambless, D. L., **84:**460; et al., **84:**450
Chandler, M. J., **83:**229, 230; **84:**88, 125
Chang, C-Y., **84:**443
Chang, R. S. L., **84:**485
Chang, S. S., **83:**452; et al., **83:**299
Changing the Body: Psychological Effects of Plastic Surgery (Goin and Goin), **84:**276
Chapanis, Natalia, **82:**49n2
Chapman, C. J., **83:**424, 438, 446
Chapman, R. M., et al., **84:**255
Charalampous, K. D., et al., **82:**180, 182, 184

Charatan, F. B., **83:**114
Charcot, Jean Martin, **84:**93, 427, 429
Charles, E., **82:**423
Charney, D. S., et al., **83:**459, 460, 469
Chasin, R., **83:**186, 230, 238
Chasseguet-Smirgel, J., **83:**23, 24, 25, 35, 36
Chatham, M. A., **84:**262
Chattopadhyay, B., et al., **84:**470
Chazan, M., **84:**124
Cheadle, J., **82:**193
Cheah, K. C., et al., **84:**201, 207
Cheek, D. S., **84:**260
Cheetham, R. W. S., **82:**102
Chell, B., **82:**350
Chemotherapy, *see* Drug therapy
Cherlin, A. J., **84:**145, 148
Chester, W. J., **84:**218
Chevron, Eve S., **83:**519; **84:**8, 10
Chien, C. P., et al., **82:**204
Child abuse, **83:**188, 196, 229; **84:**105, 108
and child psychosis, **83:**206 (*see also* Psychosis[es])
mandatory reporting of, **82:**332
posttraumatic effects of, **84:**115, 116
sexual, **82:**58
and sexual dysfunction, **82:**28, 31, 32
See also Children at risk
Childhood: "adjustment disorder" in, **82:**263
adoption in, **84:**123, 131 (*see also* Adoption; Adoption studies)
"adultomorphic" approach to, **84:**104, 105
alcohol education in, **84:**367–68
anxiety disorders of, **84:**410–18, 520–21
behavior disorders of, **84:**96 (*see also* Externalization; Juvenile Delinquency)
bipolar illness in, **83:**283, 284
and child participation in couples therapy, **83:**225
CT scan use for ailments of, **83:**184
deprivation during, effects of, **82:**32, 273; **83:**229; **84:**125, 143
development during, **82:**276; **83:**42
latent stages of, **82:**277–78
and "pandevelopmental retardation," **84:**130, 131
possible outcomes, **84:**87
prediction of, **83:**229
of retarded child, **84:**121–22 (*see also* Mental retardation)
separation/divorce effect on, **84:**151–52, 153–54
Western belief in continuity of, **84:**130
(*see also* Children at risk; Environmental factors)
drug therapy in, **83:**283, 498, 505, 509
encopresis in, **83:**176–77
family therapy for disorders of, **82:**265, 307; **83:**171, 188–201 passim, 209, 228–41
gender differentiation in, **83:**42–43
gender dysphoria in, **82:**49–51, 53, 55
and infant mortality, **82:**274
leukemia in, **84:**242, 252
memories of, Freud's view of, **83:**63; **84:**105

object relations in, **83**:218
psychoanalysis in, **83**:55, 192
psychosomatic disorders of, **84**:225
punishment for sexual behavior in, **82**:32
radiation effects in, **84**:252
rheumatic fever in, later surgery for, **84**:264
and scapegoating of child, **83**:233–34, 239, 240
schizophrenia in, **82**:89, 108, 263, 306
seduction in, **82**:57–58 (*see also* Incest)
selfobject in structure building in, **82**:501
studies of disorders of, **83**:174, 176–77
superego in, **82**:272
surgery during, *see* Children at risk
withdrawal during, and later schizophrenia, **82**:89
See also Adolescent(s); Age; Child abuse; Family, the; Infancy; Mother-child relationship; Parent(s); Parent-child relationship; School, attitude toward or performance in; Separation fears
Childhood depression: adult model for, **82**:26, 269, 270, 289–90
vs. developmental, **82**:271–72
definition of, **82**:267–69
denial of existence of, **84**:98
diagnosis of
biological correlates, **82**:290, 292–95
as clinical entity, **82**:263–72 passim, 283, 288–90; **84**:98
criteria (and RDC) for, **82**:270, 288, 289–90, 293, 296–99, 304
depressed affect and, **82**:269, 297, 305, 306
differential, **82**:305–07
failure in, **82**:287
measurement techniques in, **82**:269–71
epidemiology/prevalence rate, **82**:267, 281–88, 289
high risk factors in, **82**:285–88, 290–91
sociodemographic variables in, **82**:283–85
etiology of, **82**:274, 275, 280, 285–86, 288
prevention of, **82**:287–88
psychobiological correlates of, **84**:98
separation and divorce and, **84**:145, 154
and suicide, **82**:278, 301, 303
symptoms of, **82**:274–78, 287
clinical characteristics, **82**:296–305
cluster of, **82**:268, 296
as developmental phenomena, **82**:267, 268, 269
at developmental stages, **82**:280
masking (depressive equivalents), **82**:268, 272, 297
and symptom-oriented methods for assessing, **82**:270–71
treatment of, **82**:278, 287–88, 302, 307
family therapy, **82**:265, 307
imipramine/TCA, **82**:290, 291–92, 307; **83**:505, 509; **84**:414
Child psychiatry, **82**:263–65, 289, 305
diagnostic principles in, **84**:410–11
drug therapy in, **83**:509
family therapy in, **82**:265, 307; **83**:228–41
and mental retardation, **84**:127, 128–29

multimodal therapy in, **84**:69
new categories in, **84**:410
psychic trauma as viewed by, **84**:107 (*see also* Children at risk)
Children at risk: adaptivity of, *see* as "superkids," *below*
for affective disorders, **84**:96–98
alcoholism and, *see* Alcoholism
antisocial personality disorders in, **84**:95–96
definitions of, **84**:87, 129
disasters and, **84**:107, 110–14
divorce and, *see* Separation and divorce
education programs for, **84**:123, 125–26
genetic factors and, **84**:96, 97, 126
the law and, **84**:115–16
mentally retarded, *see* Mental retardation
parental attitudes and, **84**:102–03, 105–06, 107, 110, 118–19 (*see also* Contagion)
parental impairment/stress and, **84**:87, 94, 97, 98, 100, 129–38, 143 (*see also* Mother-child relationship; Parent[s])
perinatal complications or injury, **84**:101, 103
pessimism of, toward future, **84**:114, 117
and prediction of adult behavior, **84**:95–96
and prediction of children's problems
divorce and, **84**:145
EE and, **84**:95
preventive intervention for, **84**:90–91, 125–29, 136–43, 157
and protective factors, **84**:88, 91, 93, 94, 95
search for, **84**:102–03
psychic trauma and, **84**:104–20
vicarious, **84**:107, 116–17
research on, *see* Research
for schizophrenia, **84**:98, 99–101
separation from parents and, **84**:106 (*see also* Separation fears)
stress and, **84**:103, 109–10, 130, 150, 225
age of child and, **84**:151–52
as "superkids," **84**:103, 134, 135, 137–38, 149, 152 (*see also* Role[s])
surgery and, **84**:258, 263
amputation, **84**:115, 272
orthopedic, **84**:275
and postoperative delirium, **84**:263
and psychic trauma, **84**:106–07, 115
treatment of, **84**:111–12, 117–20
wartime effects on, **84**:105–06, 107, 110–11, 115
See also Child abuse; Childhood
Children at Risk for Schizophrenia: A Longitudinal Perspective (Watt et al.), **84**:99, 131
Children's Depression Inventory (CDI), **82**:270–71
Children's Rights Report, **82**:352
Childs, B., **83**:450
China: age of leaders of, **83**:84
Chisholm, S. E., et al., **84**:232
Cho, J. T., et al., **83**:303
Chodoff, P., **82**:89; **83**:364, 365, 383, 385–86, 407, 421; **84**:57, 110
Chodorow, N., **83**:40, 41
Cholecystectomy, *see* Surgery
Cholecystokinin, **84**:223

Choline acetyltransferase, *see* CAT
Cholinergic agents: in anxiety, **84:**476
in dementia, **83:**113
Cholinergic system: Alzheimer's disease and, **83:**110, 111
and depressive disorders, **83:**463
drugs and, *see* Drug side effect(s)
Cholinesterase: aging and, **83:**96
Chouinard, G., et al., **83:**488
Chowchilla (California) kidnapping, **84:**110, 112–14, 119
Christianity, **84:**442. *See also* Religion
Christiansen, J., **83:**495
Christie, A. B., **83:**107
Christie, J. E., et al., **83:**113
Christopherson, L. K., **84:**268, 269
Chromatography, *see* GC (gas chromatography); HPLC (high performance liquid chromatography)
Chromosome loss or damage, **83:**97, 110. *See also* Genetic factors
Chu, H. M., et al., **83,**139
Ciompi, L., **82:**88, 161; **83:**132
Ciraulo, D. A., et al., **83:**508
Circadian rhythm: and disease, **84:**220, 222–23, 230
Circumcision, **82:**10
Cirrhosis of the liver, **84:**310, 322
and mortality rate, **84:**217, 360
See also Physical illness
Civil commitment: constitutional rights and, **82:**321–22, 363
distinguished from criminal, **82:**334–35
least restrictive alternative in, **82:**322, 348–49, 364, 370–79; **84:**123
legal criteria for, **82:**334–50, 378, 380, 384, 390
legal objections to, **82:**362
police and, **82:**385
without treatment, **82:**381
See also Law and psychiatry
Civil rights movement, **82:**323, 334, 339, 371
CJD, *see* Creutzfeldt-Jakob disease
Claghorn, J. L., et al., **82:**171, 219
Clarenback, P., et al., **82:**204
Clark, E. R., et al., **84:**349
Clark, M. L., et al., **82:**180, 181, 184, 188
Clark, R., et al., **83:**147
Clark, W. B., **84:**315, 316, 355, 362
Clarkin, J. F., et al., **83:**187
Class action suits, **82:**324. *See also* Law and psychiatry
Clausen, J. A., **82:**107, 109
Clayson, D., **84:**275
Clayton, Paula J., **83:**269, 271, 272, 279, 287, 290, 355, 430, 438, 443, 446; **84:**217, 235; et al., **83:**279, 289, 291, 431, 434, 440; **84:**187
Cleghorn, J. M., et al., **84:**496
Clemens, J. A., et al., **82:**200
Clements, C. B., **83:**114
Cleveland, Ohio: postoperative studies in, **84:**263
State Law Review: "Comment," **82:**364n9
Clingembeel, W. G., **84:**156
Clinics, *see* Outpatient treatment

Clitoris, **82:**18
stimulation of, **82:**10–11, 12; **83:**41
Cloninger, C. R., **84:**320; et al., **84:**96, 401, 404
Cloud of Unknowing, The (Anon.), **84:**441
Clough, L., et al., **84:**139
CMI (Cornell Medical Index), **84:**189, 190, 202
CNS (central nervous system), **82:**144, 146; **83:**127, 358
in anxiety attack, **84:**477
cancer and, **84:**249–50
degeneration of, **82:**120; **83:**121
drug effect on, **82:**215; **83:**126; **84:**233, 347, 350, 352, 475, 485, 512
chemotherapy, **84:**250, 252–53
(*see also* Drug side effect[s]; Lithium therapy)
hormone regulation by, **84:**221, 223
and immunity, **82:**114
metabolites, in CSF, **83:**452 (*see also* DBH [dopamine]; Serotonin)
neurobiology of, **83:**457–58
psychosis and, **82:**129; **84:**123
Cobb, S., **84:**229
Cobbin, D. M., et al., **83:**468, 469
Coble, P., et al., **82:**290, 295
Coblentz, J. M., et al., **83:**109
Coccaro, E. F., **84:**511
Cochran, S. D., **83:**322
Cochrane, C., **83:**381
Cocozza, J., **82:**361n2
Coddington, R. D., **84:**94
Code of Federal Regulations, **82:**330
Cofer, D. H., **83:**387, 389
Coghlan, H. C., et al., **84:**481
Cognition, **83:**106
and body image, **84:**218–19 (*see also* Self)
and cognitive knowing in infant, **83:**14
defined, **83:**513; **84:**46
Cognitive dysfunction: alcohol consumption and, **84:**347, 358
as drug side effect, **84:**499, 501
in elderly patient, **84:**236
physical illness and, **84:**203
psychosocial factors and, **84:**202, 203
radiation therapy and, **84:**252
Cognitive therapy, **83:**513–17; **84:**65, 421
in brief psychotherapy, **84:**8, 9, 44–56
cognitive schemata in, **83:**513; **84:**9, 46–47
couples, **84:**52–56 (*see also* Marital therapy)
for depression, **83:**513–16, 524–27 passim
childhood depression, **82:**307
drug therapy vs. or combined with, **83:**525; **84:**49, 50–52
and exposure, **84:**457–59
fundamental characteristics of, **83:**516
indications for, **84:**48–50
and contraindications, **84:**49
and lithium compliance, **83:**322
for pain, **84:**229
theoretical background of, **84:**44–45
therapeutic relationship in, **83:**514–15; **84:**46, 47–48
therapeutic technique in, **84:**46–48
Cohen, B., et al., **83:**487

Cohen, Donna, 83:87
Cohen, F., 84:213, 257
Cohen, G. D., 83:85
Cohen, K. L., et al., 82:202
Cohen, L. B., 83:10
Cohen, M., et al., 84:330
Cohen, Mabel Blake, et al., 83:375, 386, 426; 84:57, 66
Cohen, M. E., 84:407, 479; et al., 84:403, 404, 477
Cohen, M. S., 83:183
Cohen, N., 84:224
Cohen, R., 84:349
Cohen, R. M., et al., 83:469
Cohen, S. M., et al., 83:441
Cohen, W. J. and N. H., 83:301
Cohler, B. J., 84:133, 135, 138, 140; et al., 84:100, 131
Cohn, J. V., 84:352
Cole, Jonathan O., 82:169, 188–94 passim, 413, 436, 463; 83:292, 321, 356, 475, 480, 481, 486–90 passim, 512; 84:358n, 490, 524; et al., 82:178, 198; 83:483, 488; 84:491, 501, 502
Cole, R. E., et al., 84:133
Coleman, J. H., 84:358
Coleman, R., et al., 83:147
Colitis, ulcerative, see Gastrointestinal disorders
Coll, M., et al., 84:219
Collagen: aging effects on, 83:98–99
Collins, G. S., 83:452
Collu, R., et al., 82:204
Colman, A. D., 83:30
Colombia: schizophrenia in, 82:101
Color(s): infant "knowledge" of, 83:12
Colorado General Hospital (Denver), 84:179
Color blindness, see Vision
Colostomy, see Surgery (ostomies)
Columbia University, 84:263
  Department of Psychiatry, 84:98
  Medical Center, 84:179
  in UCLA-Columbia study, 83:334–36
Coma: ethanol-induced, reversal of, 84:350
Comfort, A., 83:84, 129
Comings, D. E., 83:453
Communication: couples therapy and, 83:223
  defined, 83:19
  discontinuity of, within group, 83:22–23
  family/marital therapy and, 83:190, 198, 220, 223, 521
    nonverbal, 83:231
  with infant, 83:19–20
  lack of, see Sensory deficits; Social isolation; Withdrawal, social
  patient-staff, in therapeutic community, 83:29; 84:181
  in psychotherapy, 83:521, 527; 84:18
  of suicide intent, 83:430–31 (see also Suicide and attempted suicide)
  See also Relationships
Communication deviance (in schizophrenia), 83:155; 83:242, 247, 280; 84:101, 132
  and communication therapies, 83:247–49, 255–56 (see also Family therapy)
Community, therapeutic, see Health care sys-

tem; Nursing staff; Therapeutic relationship
Community care, see Therapy
Community Mental Health Centers Act (PL 88–164), 82:371
Competency/incompetency: and consent to or refusal of treatment, 82:335n3, 348, 350–60, 384 (see also Therapy)
  criteria for, 82:353–55, 387–88
  as crucial legal issue, 82:324, 339, 350
  de jure and de facto, 82:351–53, 359, 360, 380
  examination for, 82:387–89
  and release of information, 82:333, 334
  to stand trial, 82:386–89
  See also Coping capacities; Diminished capacity/responsibility; Grave disability; Law and psychiatry
"Complementary identification," 82:474. See also Identification
Comprehensive Assessment and Referral Evaluation (CARE), 83:116
Compulsive Personality Disorder, 82:18. See also Obsessive-Compulsive Disorder; Personality disorders
Computed tomography, see CT (computed tomography) findings
Comstock, G. W., 83:412, 413
COMT, see Catecholamines
Comte, Auguste, 84:391
Conditioning: of immune system, 84:224
  learning by, 84:18 (see also Learning)
  operant
    in animal studies; 84:227, 329
    and conditoned aversion (in alcoholism therapy), 84:328, 329, 332–34
    seizure reduction by, 84:228
    in treatment of psychosomatic disorders, 84:228–29, 230
  phobic anxiety as conditioned response, 84:449
Confidentiality: in dyadic therapy, 84:423
  ethical principle of, 82:327–28, 333–34
  in family therapy, 83:202–03, 210
  legal support for, impediments to, status of, 82:328–34
  in marital/couples therapy, 83:221–22, 227
  in police work, 82:385
  third-party payment or protection and, 82:325, 331–32
  See also Ethical considerations
Conflict: definition of, 82:503
  psychological, Freud's concept of, 84:430
Conger, J. J., 84:96, 329
Conjoint therapy, see Psychotherapy(ies)
Connell, H. M., 82:291
Connell, P. H., 82:137
Conners, C. K., et al., 82:286
Connolly, J. F., 84:470
Connolly, P. B., 82:37
Consanguinity method, see Genetic factors
Consent decrees, 82:365–70, 375
Consent to treatment, see Informed consent; Therapy
"Conspicuous psychiatric morbidity" (CPM), see Epidemiology

Constantinidis, J., **83**:111

Constitution, *see* U.S. *Constitution*

Consultation-liaison psychiatry: clinical setting for, **84**:184–85

  definition and use of terms, **84**:179, 183, 185

  development and growth of, **84**:179–83

  dichotomy in, **84**:183

  drug therapy and, **84**:186

  for geriatric patient, **84**:184, 231–38

  journals devoted to, **84**:182

  need for leadership by, **84**:215

  and oncology, **84**:239–56

  role of consultant in, **84**:127–28, 185, 236–38, 243–45, 266

  and surgery, **84**:256, 258, 265, 275, 276–77

  therapy in, **84**:185–86

  training for, **84**:179, 180, 186

Contagion: of psychic trauma or anxiety, **84**:105–06, 110, 113, 119, 145, 420

  of symptoms (among children in group), **84**:142

Conti, L., **84**:516

Contraception, *see* Birth control

Conversion Disorder: DSM-III category for, **84**:211

Convulsions, *see* Epileptic disorders

Coogler, O. J., **84**:155

Cook, P. J., **84**:363, 364, 365

Cooper, A. E., **82**:328

Cooper, A. F., **83**:133–34; et al., **83**:133, 136

Cooper, Arnold M., **82**:414; **83**:55; **84**:393

Cooper, D. G., **82**:217

Cooper, J. E., et al., **82**:86; **83**:299

Cooper, P., **84**:274

Cooper, T. B., **83**:500; et al., **83**:293

Coping capacities: anxiety and, **84**:419, 420

  assessment and aid of (in consultation-liaison psychiatry), **84**:180, 185–86

  childhood

    and alcohol/drug use, **84**:368

    separation and divorce and, **84**:152, 154

    stress and, **84**:94, 109

    of "superkids," *see* Children at risk

  depression and, **83**:387, 520; **84**:217

  and hormone response, **84**:222

  medication and, **84**:425

  of older patient, **83**:136, 212

  and pain management, **84**:229, 230

  and sexual dysfunctions, **82**:32–33

    treatment of, **82**:35

  and social competence/adjustment of schizophrenics, **82**:88, 107–10, 111–12

  social support networks and, **82**:106–07

  of surgical patient, **84**:257, 259, 260, 261

  See also Diminished capacity/responsibility

Coping with Depression (Beck and Greenberg), **84**:48

Coppen, A., et al., **83**:307, 308, 312, 314, 468, 470, 506; **84**:274

Corbett, J., **84**:124

Cornblatt, B., **84**:132

Corneal deposit: as drug side effect, **82**:169

Cornell Medical Index, *see* CMI

Cornfield, R. B., **84**:518

Coronary disease: etiologic factors in, **84**:216–17, 220. *See also* Vascular disorders

Corse, C. D., et al., **84**:216, 220

Corsini, G. U., et al., **82**:135, 196

Cortical atrophy: in diagnosis, **84**:234

Cortisol: in aging process, **83**:99

  alcohol effects on, **84**:326

  CNS regulation of, **84**:222

  drug effects on, **83**:460, 463, 469; **84**:488

  hypersecretion, and depression, **82**:293–94, 295, 452; **83**:121, 460, 463; **84**:236

    in children, **84**:98

  stress effects on, **84**:222

  urinary free (UFC) levels, **83**:462–63

Coryell, William, **83**:282, 283, 285; **84**:461, 464, 523; et al., **83**:430, 438; **84**:461, 464

Costa, E., et al., **84**:486

Costello, C. G., **82**:267; **83**:401, 403, 404

Costello, R. M., **84**:318, 319

Cotes, P. J., et al., **82**:200

Co-therapy, *see* Psychotherapy(ies); Sex therapy

Cotton, N. S., **84**:320

Cotzias, G. C., et al., **82**:133

Countertransference, *see* Transference

Couples therapy, *see* Marital therapy; Sex therapy

Coursey, R. D., **82**:453; et al., **82**:452; **84**:325

Covert sensitization, *see* Sensitization

Covi Anxiety Scale, **84**:498

Cowan, P. A., **84**:451

Cowdry, R. W., **83**:280; et al., **82**:454

Cowen, P. J., et al., **84**:487

Cowie, V., **84**:97, 405

Cox, M., **83**:314

Coyne, J. C., **84**:59

CPK (creatinine phosphokinase): in schizophrenia, **82**:128–29

CPM ("conspicuous psychiatric morbidity"), *see* Epidemiology

Crabtree, R. E., **82**:203

Crammond, W. A., **84**:266, 267

Crane, G. E., **83**:482

Crapper, D. R., et al., **83**:110, 111

Creese, I., et al., **82**:131, 134, 196

Creutzfeldt-Jakob disease (CJD), **82**:120; **83**:111, 117. *See also* Physical illness

Crews, F. T., **83**:474, 489

Crime: and criminal parents, children of, **84**:99, 136, 141

  homicide, personality type and, **84**:216, 460

  MAO activity and, **82**:126

  and role of psychiatrist, **82**:384–96

  in U.S. (annual arrests), **84**:367

  vandalism, **83**:190

  See also Juvenile delinquency; Prison(s); Violence

Crisis intervention: in borderline disorders, **82**:472, 482

  in cancer cases, **84**:247

  in consultation-liaison psychiatry, **84**:185

  and crisis management in bipolar and unipolar disorders, **83**:250, 252

and crisis theory, **84:**157, 180
in divorce process, **84:**157
and emergency psychotherapy, **84:**8
in family therapy, **83:**239, 245
in late-life psychiatric disorders; **83:**129, 141
in psychic trauma, **84:**117–18
See also Intervention
Crisis reaction, *see* Stress
Crisp, A. H., **84:**219; et al., **84:**225
Critcher, E. C., **84:**323
Criteria: difficulty in writing, **84:**308. *See also* DSM-III categories/criteria
Croatia: schizophrenia in, **82:**120
Crocetti, G. M., et al., **83:**417
Crohn, H., et al., **84:**149
Crook, T., **83:**404
Crosignani, P. G., et al., **82:**201
Cross, A. J., et al., **82:**127, 128
Cross, Christine K., **83:**355, 385, 406, 413, 414; **84:**58n, 97, 226n
Crow, T. J., **82:**148; et al., **82:**115, 132, 134
Crowder, M. K., **84:**233
Crowe, M. J., et al., **84:**453
Crowe, Raymond R., **83:**372; **84:**520; et al., **83:**446, 450; **84:**403–08 passim, 465, 480
Crowley, T. J., **82:**200
Crown, S., et al., **84:**224
Crumley, F., **82:**301
Cruz, R., **82:**144
Crying, *see* Weeping
CSF (cerebrospinal fluid): in Alzheimer's disease, **83:**109
and DBH activity, **82:**127; **83:**452
GABA concentrations, **82:**139
hydroxy metabolites of tricyclics in, **83:**494
PEA and, **82:**152
and schizophrenia, **82:**121, 129, 132, 133, 139, 141, 144–45; 146
serotonin metabolite (5-HIAA) in, **83:**431, 446, 452
CT (computed tomography) findings, **82:**120, 122–25, 130, 148–49, 150
and overuse of CT scan for children, **83:**184
position emission tomography (PET), **82:**125; **83:**117
in senile dementia, **83:**117; **84:**234
Cuber, J. F., **82:**42, 45; **83:**233
Cuche, H., **82:**208
Cuculic, Z., **82:**185
Cudeck, R., et al., **84:**131
Culpan, M. B., **84:**193; et al., **84:**193
Cults, **82:**279
Cultural factors: alcohol problems, **84:**362, 365
and cultural expectations (male vs. female), **83:**334
cultural shock, **83:**139
indigenous family culture, **83:**179–83
in schizophrenia, **82:**100–102, 120
and traumatized children, **84:**115
See also Alcoholism; Environmental factors; Ethnicity; Values
Culver, C. M., et al., **82:**359
Cumming, E., **83:**105

Cundall, R. L., et al., **83:**307, 308
Curran, W. J., **82:**332
Curry, A. R., **83:**133
Curry, S. H., et al., **82:**183
Curtis, G. C., et al., **84:**515
Cushing's syndrome, **82:**37, 140; **83:**121
Cutler, M., **84:**270
Cutler, Neal R., et al., **82:**135
Cutter, H. S. G., et al., **84:**332
Cyclic adenosine monophosphate (cAMP), **84:**350
Cyclothymic Disorder, **82:**455; **83:**119, 195, 392–93
as bipolar variant, **83:**271, 275, 278, 285, 374–75, 439, 442–43
and borderline disorders, **82:**444; **83:**288
course and manifestations of, **83:**281, 282, 374
diagnosis of, **83:**288–89, 373
drug or substance abuse in, **83:**285, 286
DSM-III category for, **83:**292, 354, 367, 410
dysthymic kinship with/distinction from, **83:**276–77, 373
epidemiology/prevalence rate of, **84:**206
etiology of, **83:**375
See also Bipolar (manic-depressive) Disorder
Cytryn, L., **82:**266, 269, 287, 303; **84:**124; et al., **82:**267, 284, 289, 297, 303
Czechoslovakia: CJD and dementias in, **83:**111
Czernik, A. J., et al., **84:**487, 489

D

Dabbagh, F., **83:**432
DaCosta, J. M., **84:**394, 479
and Da Costa's syndrome, **84:**394, 479, 492
Dahl, G., **83:**112
Dally, P. J., **83:**119, 126; **84:**225, 507
D'Amato, G., **84:**416
Damgaard, S., et al., **84:**349
Dangerousness: and commitment, **82:**337–38, 348, 349, 380–81, 384, 390
and competency/incompetency, **82:**386, 387
criterion of, **82:**339–47
and involuntary treatment, **82:**383
prediction of, **82:**393, 394, 395, 396
and right to treatment, **82:**364
to self, **82:**345 (*see also* Self-destructiveness)
See also Violence
Daniels, G., **84:**439
Danilowicz, D., **84:**258
Dann, S., **84:**105
Darondel, A., **82:**196
Darsee, J. R., et al., **84:**479
Dartmouth College, **84:**247
Darwin, Charles, **83:**359–60; **84:**57
Datan, N., **83:**216
Davanloo, H., **84:**8, 12
Davenport, Y. B., et al., **83:**250, 251, 316, 322, 324
David, D. J., **84:**276
Davidson, J. R. T., et al., **82:**452; **83:**467; **84:**473

Davie, J. W., **83:**121
Davies, B., **83:**314; **84:**193
Davies, P., **83:**109, 110; **84:**362, 363
Davis, C. E., **84:**258
Davis, G. C., **83:**147, 148; et al., **82:**212
Davis, John M., **82:**133, 147, 169, 178, 179, 183, 188–91 passim, 199, 214; **83:**459, 463, 481; **84:**390; et al., **82:**154, 168, 183, 187
Davis, K. L., **83:**132; et al., **83:**113, 463
Davis, R. E., **83:**283
Davis, R. H., **83:**150
Davison, A. N., **83:**109
Davison, R., **82:**120
Dawling, S., et al., **83:**498
DBH (dopamine), **82:**144; **83:**454, 459
  aging and, **83:**96–97, 110
  alcoholism and, **84:**325
  antidepressants and, **83:**487, 490
  antipsychotics and, **82:**178, 182, 196, 200, 203
  anxiolytics and, **84:**497–98, 501, 503
  CNS metabolites of, **83:**452
  heritability of, **83:**451
  in Parkinson's disease, **83:**101
  and schizophrenia, **82:**123, 126–36 passim, 147, 178–79, 196–97, 200–201
  and TRH/TSH response, **83:**122
  See also Catecholamines
Deafness, see Hearing loss
Dean, S. R., **84:**441
De Aravjo, G., et al., **84:**229
Death: children's awareness of, **84:**111
  children's dreams of, **84:**113, 114 (see also Dreams)
  fears of, surgery and, **84:**260, 267, 268, 270
  vs. immortality/rejuvenation, **83:**83–84
  and morbid ideation of child, **82:**300
  of parent, reaction to, **83:**212, 216, 400, 403, 404, 421; **84:**145 (see also Grief reaction; Loss)
De Board, R., **83:**30
DeConti, R. C., **84:**253
Defense mechanism(s): of alcoholic patient, **84:**344
  anxiety and, **84:**430, 432–36
  in borderline disorders, **82:**433, 473, 474, 477, 478, 482, 483–85
  brief psychotherapies and, **84:**36
  denial as, **84:**20, 222 (see also Denial)
  internalization and externalization, **83:**237
  of organ transplant donor, **84:**266
  primitive (dissociation or splitting), **82:**54, 472–73, 477–85 passim, 494, 511–18 passim
    as group reaction, **83:**22, 29
  and sexual dysfunctions, **82:**32–34, 56, 58
  treatment of, **82:**35
deFigueiredo, J. M., **84:**419
DeFrancis, V., **82:**58
de Haan, S., **83:**452
Dekirmenjian, H., **82:**187
DeLeon-Jones, F. D., et al., **83:**461
del Guidice, J., et al., **82:**195
Delirium: dementia and, **83:**106, 107, 108, 115
  diagnosis of, **83:**108
  and nonrecognition of, **84:**232

as drug side effect, **83:**108, 475; **84:**232–34, 248–52
  among elderly, **83:**107, 108; **84:**232–34, 275
  etiology and treatment of, **83:**108, 137; **84:**232
    alcoholism and, **84:**351–52, 354–55, 356
    cancer and, **84:**249–53
    hormone-induced, **84:**250
    postoperative, **84:**261, 262, 271, 275
    of children, **84:**263
    postcardiotomy, **84:**261, 262–64
  See also Hallucinations
Delirium tremens (withdrawal delirium), see Alcoholism
DeLisi, Lynn E., et al., **82:**115, 121, 125–30 passim
Dellelis, R., **84:**250
DeLoache, J. S., et al., **83:**13
DeLuca, J., **84:**347
Delusions: and delusional states of geriatric patients, **83:**132, 134, 137, 138, 285; **84:**236
  depression and, **83:**362, 370, 371, 373, 381, 527
  of grandeur or persecution, **82:**139; **83:**134
    antipsychotics and, **82:**197
    in bipolar illness, **83:**275, 281, 285, 297, 302, 312, 423
    childhood, **82:**306
    schizophrenia and, **82:**85–87 passim, 149, 167, 197; **83:**130, 131, 138
  and mania, **83:**278, 285
  and plasma levels, **83:**509
  therapy for, **84:**61
  of worthlessness, guilt, or illness, **83:**134
    as predictor of nonresponse to TCAs, **83:**122, 125
  (see also Self-esteem)
Delves, H. T., **82:**144
de Mare, P. B., **83:**25
Dembrowski, T. M., et al., **84:**220
Dement, W. C., et al., **83:**91, 147
Dementia: alcoholism and, **84:**301, 307, 347
  defined, **84:**234
  as drug or radiation side effect, **84:**234, 252, 253
  See also Dementia, Primary Degenerative
Dementia, Primary Degenerative, **83:**130
  Alzheimer's disease, **83:**98, 107, 113, 115, 476; **84:**233, 234
    infection theory regarding, **83:**111
    neurochemical pathology of, **83:**100, 101, 109–11
    and delirium, **83:**106, 107, 108, 115
  depression/depressive pseudodementia and, **83:**90, 107, 109, 119, 127, 279, 280, 366, 476; **84:**234, 236
  diagnosis of, **83:**107, 108–09, 119, 366; **84:**235, 236
  DSM-III category for, **83:**108, 109; **84:**234
  epidemiology/prevalence rate, **83:**107
  etiology of, **83:**111
  genetic factors in, **83:**110
  manic, **83:**285
  multiinfarct, **83:**109, 113, 114–15
  and paranoia, **83:**132, 137

senile dementia, **83:**92, 97, 100, 101, 107–15 passim, 476
sleep disorders in, **83:**145, 146–47
treatment of, **83:**111–12, 113–14, 115, 137, 476, 480
Dementia praecox, **82:**84, 113
bipolar (manic-depressive) disorder separated from, **82:**82; **83:**269
children at risk of, **84:**93
See also Schizophrenia
Dementia Praecox and Paraphrenia (Kraepelin), **84:**93
Dementia Praecox or the Group of Schizophrenias (Bleuler), **82:**113
Demography, *see* Age
de Montigny, C., et al., **83:**481
Demoralization, **84:**419, 420, 421. *See also* Anxiety; Anxiety Disorders; Coping capacities
Dempsey, G. M., et al., **84:**273
deM'Uzan, M., **84:**218, 437
Denber, H., **82:**185
Dencker, S. J., **83:**112
Denial:
of illness
alcoholism, **84:**299, 343, 344
in bipolar disorder, **83:**317, 320, 322, 328, 330, 331, 335
and competency, **82:**354, 355, 356
as defense mechanism, **84:**20
by depressed mothers, **84:**142
in late-life dementia, **83:**108
by parent, of child, **84:**142
of loss, **83:**277
of reality
under stress, **84:**109, 114
surgery and, **84:**257, 259, 269, 272
of responsibility for illness, **83:**190
of treatment termination date, **84:**42 (*see also* Therapy)
De Nicola, P., **83:**148
Deniker, P., **82:**208
Denmark: schizophrenia studies in, **82:**95, 98, 101, 103, 121, 445, 447; **84:**405
suicide studies in, **83:**432, 445
twin studies in, **83:**432, 443, 444
Denner, L. J., **84:**353
Denney, D., et al., **84:**200, 202, 236
Dennis, W., **82:**274
Denson, R., **82:**143
DePalma, R. G., et al., **82:**46
Department of Health, Education, and Welfare, U.S., **83:**85
Department of Health and Human Services, **83:**304
DePaulo, R. J., et al., **83:**313, 314
Dependency: alcohol or drug, *see* Alcoholism; Drug abuse/addiction; Substance abuse
of child on parent substitute, **84:**106
of depressive/manic-depressive, **83:**251; **84:**61
on family, **83:**195, 241, 251–52
as "female quality," **83:**38–44 passim
within group, **83:**21–22, 26
invalidism and, **84:**267

on medication, **84:**425 (*see also* Drug abuse/addiction)
narcissistic lack of, **82:**513, 518, 520
oral-dependent traits
and alcoholism, **84:**314
and depression, **84:**20
of parent on child, **83:**231–32; **84:**138, 149, 152
pathological, **84:**155
and sexual dysfunctions, **82:**28, 29
Dependent Personality Disorder, **82:**17
Depressed affect: in borderline patients, **82:**417
and childhood depression, **82:**269, 297, 305, 306
symptom cluster of, **82:**296
Depression: as adjustment reaction/disorder, **83:**361–62, 367, 375, 410
childhood, **82:**305
age of onset of, **82:**295; **83:**287, 296, 364, 365–66, 372, 412, 420, 422, 443; **84:**206, 208, 231, 404 (*see also* late-onset, *below*)
alcoholism and, *see* Alcoholism
atypical, **82:**466, **83:**119, 120, 126–28, 281, 359, 367, 370, 410, 479
in elderly patient, **83:**119, 121
in borderline patients, **82:**417, 436, 465–66, 467
catecholamine hypothesis of, **82:**265
cognitive theory of, **84:**46–47
components (three) of, **84:**59
concepts of, **83:**514, 517–23 passim
cortisol hypersecretion in, **82:**140, 293–94, 295; **83:**121, 460, 463
definition of, **83:**265–66, 272–73; **83:**411
dementia coexisting with, **83:**107, 366; **84:**234
developmental perspective of, **82:**272–81
diagnosis of, **83:**359, 362–64, 410, 428, 460
in cancer patient, **84:**246–47
clinical data and, **83:**462, 471, 510
differential, **82:**457; **83:**108–09, 366, 374, 466; **84:**61, 236, 248
difficulties in, **82:**266; **83:**118, 291–92, 366, 406–07; **84:**236
of donor, in organ transplant case, **84:**267
"double," **83:**276
dread of future in, **82:**278
as drug side effect, **83:**369, 374, 379; **84:**233, 235, 242, 252, 499, 500, 502
DSM-III criteria for, *see* DSM-III categories/criteria
endogenous, **82:**293–94, 452–53; **83:**272, 273, 276, 287, 288, 292, 354, 371, 395, 414, 479, 482, 488, 503, 526–27; **84:**20, 49
age and, **84:**235
and TCA response, **83:**359, 381
term reevaluated, **83:**369
epidemiology/prevalence rate of, **82:**281–85 passim, 290; **83:**271, 392, 406, 411–22; **84:**203–08, 214, 235, 246–47
terms defined, **83:**410
ethanol-induced, **84:**349
etiology of, **83:**364–65, 371, 383, 400, 404, 463, 519, 522; **84:**19, 184, 235
family history of/genetic factors in, **82:**290; **83:**273, 276, 364–65, 368, 392–93, 404, 420–21, 422, 449–50, 458, 519; **84:**511

among females, *see* Females(s)
and GH response, **82:**293; **83:**460
group therapy contraindicated for, **82:**25
and habituation process, **84:**457
historical descriptions of, **83:**354, 357
and immunosuppression, **84:**208
late-onset, **83:**90–91, 92, 107, 118, 119–30, 132, 136, 141, 142, 144, 275, 285, 355, 366, 373, 443, 476, 477; **84:**235–36
MAO activity in, **82:**452; **83:**467
and marital problems, **83:**195, 252n, 364, 365–66; **84:**53, 58–59, 132
masked, **82:**304; **83:**373; **84:**98
MHPG levels during, **83:**272–73, 461–65 passim, 468–69
and mortality rate, **84:**462, 463, 464
narcissism and, **82:**491
neurotic, **83:**281, 370, 371, 380, 381, 399, 414, 503
nonendogenous, **82:**295, 457, 465–66; **83:**273, 467, 479, 482
as normal emotion, **83:**359–60, 362, 411
nosology of depressive disorders, **83:**356–82
-panic relationship, **84:**511–12
of parent, and children at risk, **82:**285, 286; **84:**97, 98, 100, 129, 133 (*see also* Mother-child relationship)
personality related to, *see* Personality
among police officers, **82:**385
postmarital, **82:**43, 44
-postoperative, **82:**38–41 passim; **84:**267 68, 272, 274, 275
and prognosis, **84:**264, 269
postpartum, **83:**277, 287, 414, 422
posttraumatic, **84:**110
of prison inmates, **82:**396
psychiatric chemistry and, **83:**457–71 (*see also* treatment of, *below*)
psychosocial factors and, **83:**364, 365, 371, 382–405, 411–14, 420–22; **84:**57, 97, 208
deterioration, pathoplasty, predisposition, subclinical approaches to, **83:**383, 385–94, 399–400, 404–05
(*see also* Alcoholism; Social class; Stress)
psychotic, **83:**399, 414, 420
defined, and prevalence rate, **83:**415
-neurotic distinction, **83:**371, 380
psychotherapy (brief) contraindicated for, **84:**44
and risk of mania, **83:**287–88
RDC in, **82:**289, 296, 305
reactive, **83:**354, 370, 371, 395, 414, 482, 503
and alcoholism, **84:**312
retarded (in bipolar illness), **83:**279–80
role transition and, **83:**512; **84:**63
schizophrenia-related, **82:**88; **83:**291
secondary to medical or other psychiatric illness, **83:**118–19, 288, 369, 374–81 passim, 430; **84:**49, 184, 206, 208, 217–18, 230, 235, 246–27, 248
separation and divorce and, *see* Separation and divorce
sex differentiation in, **82:**284, **84:**206

and sexual dysfunctions, **82:**16–17; **83:**150, 366, 373
and spouse of depressed patient, **84:**53–56
stress and, *see* Stress
subtypes of, **82:**288, 289, 293; **83:**384, 414; **84:**234
and suicide, **83:**287, 362–70 passim, 429–34, 527; **84:**326, 460, 467
of survivors of diaster, **84:**110
as symptom, **83:**360–61
symptoms of, **83:**411–14, 479
tardive dyskinesia and, **82:**204
treatment of, **83:**370
drug, *see* Drugs; Drug therapy
ECT, **83:**121, 125, 366, 369, 370, 381, 382, 480; **84:**49, 511
hospitalization, **83:**271, 274, 294, 295, 364–70 passim, 415, 420, 438, 439; **84:**142
psychotherapy, **83:**252, 319, 369, 511–28; **84:**10, 20, 44, 46–52, 56–67
See also Adolescent depression; BDI (Beck Depression Inventory); Bipolar (manic-depressive) Disorder; Childhood depression; Depressed affect; Major Depression; Mood disorders; TCA (tricyclic antidepressant) response; Unipolar/nonbipolar depression
Deprivation: in childhood, *see* Childhood
sensory (psychic trauma and), **84:**109 (*see also* Sensory deficits)
sexual, **82:**30
Depue, R. A., **83:**272; et al., **83:**281
Derby, I. M., **84:**460
Derdeyn, A. P., **84:**155
DeRivera, J. L., et al., **82:**202
Derogatis, L. R., et al., **82:**8; **84:**203, 246, 247
Descartes, René, **84:**177
Descriptive-normative role of theory, **83:**39
Desensitization, *see* Sensitization
De Silva, P., **84:**453
Desire disorders, **82:**32, 33. *See also* Psychosexual dysfunctions
Despert, J. L., **82:**263; **84:**106
Detre, T., et al., **83:**279
Deutsch, F., **83:**44
Deutsch, H., **84:**260, 276
Deutsch, M., **82:**143
DeVane, C. L., **83:**492, 504, 510; et al., **83:**494
Developmentally Disabled Assistance Act, **82:**375, 376
Devereux, R. B., **84:**407, 408; et al., **84:**407, 479
Deviant Children Grown Up (Robins), **84:**96
Devine, V., **84:**136
de Wind, E., **84:**110
Dexamethasone suppression test, *see* DST
Dexter, J. D., **84:**221
Dhadphale, M., et al., **84:**197, 198, 203, 205, 206, 209, 211
Diabetes mellitus, **83:**121
drug therapy and, **84:**502
maturity-onset, **83:**96, 98, 99
as "psychosomatic" disorder, **84:**198
in children, **84:**225

and sexual inhibition, **82**:17–18, 37; **83**:151
Diagnosis: of alcoholism, **84**:61
  computer (CATEGO), **82**:100; **83**:408, 409, 427
  defined (assessment distinguished from), **83**:363
  and diagnostic labels, **82**:265; **84**:75, 142
  and doctor as anthropologist, **83**:178–79
  and legal considerations of misdiagnosis, **83**:272
  psychiatric screening instruments used in, **84**:187, 188–89 (*see also individual tests*)
  psychopathological vs. physical symptoms in, **84**:184
  standardized procedures in, **83**:408
  See also individual disorders
Diagnostic and Statistical Manual of Mental Disorders, see DSM
Diagnostic Interview Schedule, *see* DIS
Dialysis, **84**:265–66, 271
  ethanol eliminated by, **84**:348
  as schizophrenia treatment, **82**:141
Diaphoresis: in alcohol withdrawal, **84**:351
  as anxiety symptom, **84**:474, 492
DIB (Diagnostic Interview for Borderlines), *see* Borderline Personality Disorder, diagnosis of
DIC (disseminated intravascular coagulation), *see* Vascular disorders
DiChiara, G., et al., **82**:135
Dickes, Robert, **82**:8, 436
Dicks, H. V., **83**:218, 236
Didactic techniques, *see* Psychotherapy(ies)
Diet: cereal grain- and milk-free (CMF), **82**:145–46
  and eating disorders, *see* Anorexia; Anorexia nervosa; Obesity
  in prevention of mental deficiency, **84**:127
  restrictions on (in MAOI therapy), **83**:127, 484, 490–91, **84**:249, 358
  in treatment of dementia, **83**:113
  and schizophrenia, **82**:142, 145–46
  See also Malnutrition; TPN (total parenteral nutrition); Vitamins
Digit symbol substitution test (DSST), **84**:500
Dillon, H., **84**:117
Dimension: defined, **82**:113n1
Diminished capacity/responsibility, **82**:389–90, 392. *See also* Competency/incompetency; Coping capacities; Grave disability; Law and psychiatry
Dimsdale, J. E., **84**:472; et al., **84**:216
Di Nardo, P. A. et al., **84**:398, 402
Dinerstein, D., **84**:135
Dirksen, R., et al., **84**:351
DIS (Diagnostic Interview Schedule), **83**:90, 408; **84**:61, 309
Disability, *see* Grave disability; Learning disorders; Physical handicap
Disability benefits: as rehabilitation disincentives, **82**:109–10
Disaster: studies of, **84**:107, 110–14, 117–18
  therapeutic management of, **84**:24
"Disaster at Buffalo Creek," **84**:111
Disease, *see* Physical illness

Disease-entity approach, **82**:82–83
Dissociation: Freud's theory of, **84**:429–30
  Janet's theory of, **84**:430
Dissociative Disorders: DSM-III category for, **84**:393
Divorce, *see* Separation and divorce
Divorce Mediation Research Project (Denver, Colorado), **84**:145
Dix, G. E., **82**:394
Dizziness: anxiety and, **84**:492
  as drug side effect, **84**:500
Djenderedjian, A. H., **83**:442
DNA: in aging process, **83**:97, 98
  clinical use of technology of, **83**:436, 449, 453–54
Doane, J. A., et al., **83**:175, 176, 247
Docherty, J. P., et al., **82**:88
Doctor-patient relationship, *see* Therapeutic relationship
Dohan, F. C., **82**:145; et al., **82**:145
Dohrenwend, B. S. and B. P. **84**:94
Dois, L. C. W., **82**:195
Dole, V. P., et al., **84**:351
Domino, E. F., et al., **82**:115
Don Juan syndrome, **82**:34
Donlon, P. T., et al., **82**:171, 187, 195; **83**:291
Donnelly, C. H., **83**:452
Donnelly, E. F., et al., **83**:250, 387, 389
Donovan, D. M., **84**:329, 330
Dopamine and dopamine hypothesis, *see* DBH
Dorian, B., et al., **84**:223
Dorow, R., et al., **84**:488, 489
Dorpat, T. L., **83**:429, 430
Dorus, E., et al., **83**:452, 453, 454
Douduin, T., **84**:261
Douglass, R. L., **84**:365
Doust, J. W. L., **82**:115
Dovenmuehle, R. H., **84**:235
Down's syndrome (mongolism), **83**:100, 101, 110; **84**:121, 126. *See also* Mental retardation
Dowson, J. H., **83**:112
Dreams: childhood trauma inferred from, **84**:104
  importance of, **84**:15
  and memory, **83**:18
  postoperative, **84**:260
  posttraumatic, **84**:113, 114, 115
  in psychotherapy, **84**:64
  and transference relationship, **84**:14
  See also Sleep
Drive: infant research implications concerning, **83**:13, 15
Drug abuse/addiction: adolescent, **83**:190, 270, 284, 285
  alcoholism/alcohol withdrawal and, **84**:334–35, 340, 353
  and amnestic syndrome, **83**:115
  bipolar illness and, **83**:279, 281, 282, 286
  by borderline patients, **82**:416–17, 441, 454; **84**:299
  children at risk for, **84**:136, 143
  criterion for, **84**:309
  and depression, **83**:365, 374, 375
  as "mental illness," **82**:337

preexisting factors and, **84:**309
and suicide, **83:**429
studies of (buspirone), **84:**501
treatment of, **84:**343
Drugs: adrenergic, **84:**223
alcohol-sensitizing, **84:**356–57
amethystic, **84:**347–51
analgesic, *see* sedative or tranquilizing, *below*
antibiotic, overuse of, **83:**184
anticoagulant, **83:**112, 115
anticonvulsant, **82:**454, 455, 465; **83:**303, 311,
497; **84:**487
in alcohol withdrawal treatment, **84:**355
antidepressant, **82:**436, 453; **83:**112, 269, 278,
311, 312, 458, 472–91; **84:**49, 357–58
for anxiety/panic disorders, *see* Drug therapy
avoidance of, **83:**303, 476, 478, 479–80;
84:233, 237, 238
for borderline disorders, **82:**461–66 passim
for cancer patients, **84:**244, 247, 248–49
for children, **84:**414–17
combined with psychotherapy, **83:**321
criteria for clinical studies of, **83:**504
dosage, **83:**112, 128, 317, 487
for elderly patients, **83:**107, 112, 142, 146,
150; **84:**235, 236
nontricyclic, **83:**485, 487–88
plasma level measurement of, **83:**470–71
and polysomnographic patterns, **82:**294
stress and, **83:**400
(*see also* antipsychotic/neuroleptic, *below*; tricyclics [TCAs], *below*; Lithium therapy; MAO
[monoamine oxidase])
antiepileptic, **83:**312
antiparkinsonian, **82:**204–05; **83:**302
antipsychotic/neuroleptic, **82:**117–18, 127, 152,
180–96; **83:**269, 359, 472, 487; **84:**248
for alcohol-related disorders, **84:**354–55
and anxiety, **84:**484, 498
antidepressants/TCAs combined with,
82:208, 209; **83:**125, 382, 479, 480, 484
for bipolar illness, **83:**287, 298–99, 311, 312
for borderline disorders, **82:**461–67 passim
for dementia, **83:**113, 115, 137
for geriatric disorders, **83:**126, 139, 145
and growth hormone (GH) levels, **82:**135,
136, 203–04
high-dosage, **82:**183, 187–90
and immunological abnormalities, **82:**117–18,
121
for paraphrenia, **83:**139
and PG (prostaglandin) absorption, **82:**146
and psychotherapy vs. or combined with,
82:156, 157, 160, 168–69, 178, 215, 219–
25
(*see also* Lithium therapy; Schizophrenia,
treatment of)
anxiety-producing, **84:**474–79
anxiolytic, **84:**409, 426, 471–72, 491–503
and GABA, **84:**409–10, 481–90 passim
cardioglycosides, **84:**232, 233
CL (total body clearance) of, **83:**113, 492, 499–
500

depressant, **84:**346–47
half-life of, **83:**113, 115–16, 476, 492–500 passim, 504, 511
hallucinogens, **82:**130, 139–41; **83:**295
hypnotics, **83:**113, 116, 150, 485; **84:**250, 352,
354
judicial view of use of, **82:**381–82, 383
MAO inhibitors, *see* MAO (monoamine oxidase)
new, **82:**180–96; **83:**485–90
prolactin (PRL) response to, **82:**135–36, 200–
203; **83:**487; **84:**253, 498
psychotropic, **82:**175, 215, 359–60, 455; **83:**95,
121, 436, 497; **84:**186, 237, 247, 484
rauwolfias, **83:**369, 379
reaction to, and child psychosis, **82:**306
and REM sleep, **83:**115
restrictions on, in MAOI therapy, **83:**127, 484,
490–91
sedative or tranquilizing, **83:**121, 476, 480–88
passim, 526
for alcohol withdrawal treatment, **84:**352,
353–54, 355
benzodiazepines as, **84:**483, 484–85, 487
chronic or overuse of, **83:**365, 374
contraindicated, **84:**299
and delirium, **84:**250
for elderly, **83:**95, 115–16, 126, 141, 146, 150
for manic illness, **83:**281, 301
for schizophrenics, **82:**217
and suicide, **83:**430, 433
sensitivity to, of elderly patients, **83:**96–97, 113,
126, 498; **84:**232, 233
side effects of, *see* Drug side effect(s)
steroids and corticosteroids, **82:**140; **83:**121, 123,
369, 374, 379, 478; **84:**250, 253
with supportive therapy, **82:**484, 485
tricyclics (TCAs), **82:**464–67 passim; **83:**321,
359, 361, 458, 472–97, 503; **84:**233, 237, 357–
58 (*see also* TCA [tricyclic antidepressant]
response)
volume of distribution of, **83:**492
See also Drug abuse/addiction; Drugs, list of;
Drug therapy; Hormone(s)
Drugs, list of: acebutol, **83:**492
alprazolam, **83:**472, 474, 485, 488; **84:**485n, 504,
507
alprenolol, **84:**492
aminophylline, **84:**350
amitriptyline, **82:**466; **83:**123, 124, 127, 312, 371,
462, 468–96 passim, 524–25; **84:**49, 50, 248–
49, 515, 518
-alcohol combintions, **84:**358
dangers of (in cardiac disease), **84:**358
and plasma levels, **83:**500, 505–06, 507
amobarbital, **82:**462, 464; **84:**119, 420
amoxapine, **83:**124–25, 312, 472, 474, 480, 485,
487, 495
amphetamines, *see* Amphetamine
apomorphine, **82:**134–35, 136, 196, 203, 204;
84:498
arecoline, **83:**113
asparaginase, **84:**252
atenolol, **84:**491

atropine, **84:**223, 248
baclofen, **84:**235
benzodiazepines, **82:**139, 461, 464, 465; **83:**121, 141, 479, 481; **84:**352–55 passim
  for anxiety/panic, **83:**146, 480, 488; **84:**254, 260, 409–10, 437, 472, 483–90, 491–502 passim, 516
  failure/disadvantages of, **84:**493, 500, 501, 504
  receptors of, **84:**483, 485–90, 497
  (*see also individual forms*)
bethanecol, **83:**476
bleomycin, **84:**252
bromocriptine, **82:**135, 197
buproprion, **83:**312, 474, 485, 490; **84:**511
buspirone, **84:**497–503, 524
butaperazine, **82:**189
butyrophenones, **83:**323; **84:**354
caffeine, **84:**350 (*see also* Caffeine)
calcium carbamide (citrated), **84:**356
carbachol, **84:**470
carbamazepine, **83:**303, 307, 311–12, 318
carbidopa, **82:**200; **83:**461
carmustine (BCNU), **84:**252
centrophenoxine, **83:**112
chloral hydrate, **83:**115; **84:**352, 353
chlorazepate, **84:**499, 500, 501
chlordiazepoxide, **82:**465; **83:**381, 479, 480; **84:**353, 416, 493, 495, 504
chlorimipramine (clomipramine), **83:**480, 500
chlormethiazole (clomethiazole), **84:**352, 354, 493
chlorpromazine (CPZ), **83:**271, 484, 497; **84:**503–04
  in acute mania, **83:**298, 300–301, 302
  in borderline disorders, **82:**462, 463, 464
  in delirium, **84:**353
  in schizophrenia, **82:**118, 143, 178, 180, 189, 199–200, 201, 208
cimetidine, **83:**123, 475; **84:**232–33
cis-platinum (cis-platin, DDP), **84:**249, 252, 254
clomipramine, **84:**416, 512, 515–16, 518, 519
clonidine, **84:**235, 471, 472
clorgyline, **84:**515
clozapine, **82:**182, 201
cocaine, **82:**197; **84:**501
cyclandelate, **83:**112
cyclophosphamide, **84:**252
dacarbazine, **84:**252
deprenyl, **83:**485
desipramine, **82:**466; **83:**123, 124, 472–80 passim, 486, 487
  and plasma levels, **83:**477, 498, 506, 507
  prediction of response to, **83:**468, 473, 499–500
desmethylimipramine, **84:**512
dexamethasone, **83:**121, 469; **84:**250, 253, 515 (*see also* DST [dexamethasone suppression test])
diazepam, **82:**461; **83:**115–16, 488; **84:**353, 356, 471–72, 485, 488, 493–503 passim, 510
digitalis, **84:**233
dihydroergotoxine, **83:**112
diphenhydramine, **84:**416

diphenylhydantoin, **82:**465, 467; **83:**121, 122, 497; **84:**355
disulfiram, **84:**318–24 passim, 334–35, 343, 346, 347, 356–57
domperidone, **82:**200
dopamine, **82:**144; **83:**122 (*see also* DBH)
doryl, **84:**476
doxepin, **82:**461; **83:**123, 125, 146, 472–80 passim, 493, 496; **84:**248, 358, 516
  and plasma levels, **83:**124, 498, 500, 506, 507
doxorubicin hydrochloride, **84:**254
EDTA, **84:**478
emetine, **84:**333, 334
ephedrine, **84:**333, 350
epinepherine, *see* Epinephrine
ethanol, *see* Ethanol
fludrocortisone, **83:**478
fluorouracil, **84:**252
fluoxetine, **83:**474, 489–90
flupenthixol decanoate, **83:**307, 311, 318
fluphenazine, **82:**463; **83:**139
  in schizophrenia, **82:**178, 182, 187–88, 195–96, 204–05, 219
flurazepam, **83:**115–16
haloperidol, **83:**487
  in delirium, **84:**234, 253, 354, 355
  and GH response, **82:**203, 204
  in mania, **83:**113, 126, 298, 300, 301
  in schizophrenia, **83:**183, 195–96, 199
hydralazine, **83:**123
5-hydroxytryptophan (5-HTP), **83:**113, 312
hydroxyurea, **84:**252
imipramine, *see* Imipramine
iproniazid, **83:**482; **84:**507
isocarboxazid, **83:**472, 482, 483
isoproterenol, **83:**470; **84:**474, 475, 491, 493, 496
L-dopa (levodopa), **82:**131, 132, 136; **83:**113, 123, 368; **84:**235, 349–50
L-tryptophan, **83:**312, 483
legatrile, **82:**197
levorphanol, **84:**250
limbitrol, **83:**480
lisuride, **82:**197
lithium (carbonate), *see* Lithium therapy
lorazepam, **83:**116; **84:**500
lormetazepam, **84:**488
loxapine, **82:**180, 182, 184–86; **83:**487
LSD (lysergic acid diethylamide), **82:**130, 139, 140
magnesium sulphate, **84:**356
maprotiline, **83:**146, 312, 468–74 passim, 478, 485–90 passim, 495; **84:**248
marijuana, **82:**140; **84:**254
mecholyl, **84:**474, 476
melperone, **82:**201
meperidine, **84:**250
meprobamate, **82:**461; **83:**121
mescaline, **82:**139, 140
methadone, **84:**334–35
methamphetamine, **82:**462 (*see also* Amphetamine)
methaqualone, **84:**501
methohexitone, **84:**507
methotrexate, **84:**250–52

methscopolamine, 84:476
methyldopa, 83:123; 84:235
methylphenidate, 82:197, 462; 83:480
metoclopramide, 84:254
mianserin, 83:312, 469, 489, 495, 500; 84:358
molindone, 82:180, 181
morphine, 84:471
muscimol, 82:139
mustargen, 84:255
nadolol, 84:491
naftidrofuryl, 83:112
naloxone, 82:141, 209, 212–14; 83:113; 84:323, 350–51
nomifensine, 83:474, 490
nortriptyline, 83:123, 124, 312, 468, 472–80 passim, 493–500 passim; 84:248, 512, 515
  -alcohol antagonism, 84:358
  and plasma levels, 83:499–500, 505–11 passim
nylidrin hydrochloride, 83:112
oxaprotiline, 83:462, 469, 485, 490
oxazepam, 83:116; 84:501
oxprenolol, 84:491–97 passim, 501, 502
p-chlorophenylalenine (PCPA), 82:130
papaverine, 83:112
paraldehyde, 84:352, 353
pargyline, 83:482
pemoline, 82:462–63
penfluridol, 82:182, 195
pentobarbital, 84:501
perphenazine, 82:183, 461; 83:125; 84:518
phencyclidine (PCP), 82:139–40
phenelzine, 82:464, 466; 83:127–28, 471, 472, 479, 482–84, 485; 84:416, 459, 507–18 passim
phenobarbital, 84:501
phenothiazine, 82:131, 198, 218, 220, 461, 463; 83:139, 323, 370; 84:234, 253, 354 (see also individual forms)
phentolamine, 83:484
physostigmine, 83:113, 463, 476; 84:233–34, 474, 476
pilocarpine, 84:333
pimozide, 82:182, 204; 83:122
pindolol, 84:491, 492
piperoxane, 84:472
pipotiazine, 82:195
piracetam, 83:112
piribedil, 84:498
practolol, 84:492
prazosin, 84:476
prednisone, 84:250, 253, 255, 269
primidone, 82:465
probenecid, 82:133
procaine hydrochloride, 83:112
procarbazine, 84:248, 252–53, 255
prochlorperazine, 84:254
propanediol carbamates, 84:483, 484
propanolol, 82:131–32, 152, 205, 208; 83:123, 478; 84:118, 235, 349, 472, 475, 478, 491, 492, 493, 501, 502, 503
  vs. placebo, studies of, 84:494–95, 496–97
  and stage fright, 84:496–97, 502

protriptyline, 83:124, 147, 472–80 passim, 493–500 passim, 506, 507
  dangers of (in cardiac disease), 84:358
quanethadine, 83:123
quinidine, 83:123, 478
reserpine, 82:131, 196; 83:123, 459, 488; 84:235, 253, 349
scopolamine, 84:248
sodium lactate, 84:407, 457, 474–81 passim
sodium valproate (n-dipropylacetate), 84:355
sulpiride, 82:201; 84:416
synaptamine, 83:489
tetrahydrocannabinol, 84:254
theophylline, 84:350
thioridazine, 82:200–201, 203, 218, 461, 463; 83:113, 301; 84:234, 253
thiothixene, 82:182, 188, 200–201, 461; 83:113, 125, 301
tranylcypromine, 82:462; 83:127, 472, 482–85 passim; 84:515
trazodone, 83:312, 472, 474, 475, 485, 487–88; 84:248, 511, 516
triazolam, 84:485n
trifluoperazine, 83:125, 484; 84:253
  in borderline disorders, 82:461–64 passim
  in schizophrenia, 82:178, 180, 183, 188
triiodothyronine, 83:481
trimipramine, 83:472–76 passim, 480 (see also Imipramine)
tyrosine, 83:113
valproic acid, 83:312
vinblastine, 84:252
vincamine, 83:112
vincristine, 84:242, 252, 255
yohimbine, 84:472, 474, 475–76
zimelidine, 83:489–90, 495; 84:511
Drug side effect(s), 83:142, 147, 323, 512
  of adrenergics, 84:223
  affective disorders, 83:287, 369, 379; 84:184, 235
  age and, 83:96–97, 113, 123, 126, 128, 301, 321n, 477, 497–98, 509–10; 84:232–34, 254
  agitation, 84:233, 234, 253, 353
  on allergic symptoms, 84:223
  anticholinergic, 83:113, 123, 124, 127, 302, 313, 315, 317, 332, 336, 459–60, 463, 474–80 passim, 484–88 passim, 498; 84:232, 233, 248
  of antidepressants, 83:142, 459–60, 463, 469
  of antipsychotics, 82:182, 183, 196, 205, 208, 382, 464, 465; 83:125, 126, 130, 291, 301, 302; 84:248 (see also tardive dyskinesia, below)
  apnea, 84:353
  brain damage, 83:301; 84:252
  cardiac/cardiovascular, 83:114, 126, 128, 314, 475, 477–78, 484–86 passim, 491, 494, 498, 505, 509–10; 84:233, 255, 358, 415
  of chemotherapy, 82:39; 84:242, 244, 248, 250, 252–53, 254, 255
  cognitive dysfunction, 84:499, 501
  cross-dependence with ethanol, 84:347
  delirium/hallucinations, 83:108, 475; 84:232–34, 248–53
  dementia, 84:249–53 passim

depression, **83:**369, 374, 379; **84:**233, 235, 242, 252, 499, 500, 502
epileptic disorders, **83:**478, 486; **84:**357, 358
fatigue, **84:**494, 499
gastrointestinal symptoms, **84:**233, 248
headache, **83:**484, 488, 491; **84:**233, 252, 358, 499, 500
hepatic necrosis, **83:**482
hepatitis, **84:**232, 357
hypertension, **83:**482, 484
hypomania, **82:**464; **83:**273–77 passim, 280, 369, 375, 479–80, 488
hypotension, **83:**113–14, 123, 302, 475, 477–78, 485–88 passim, 498, 509; **84:**237, 491
infertility/sterility, **84:**255
as legal issue, **82:**382
lethargy/drowsiness, **84:**233, 252, 253, 254, 499, 500
mania/manic episode, **83:**126, 277, 278, 287, 311; **84:**235, 253
of MAO inhibitors, **83:**127–28, 475, 484–85; **84:**253
on memory, **83:**113, 336, 475–76
myoclonic twitching, **84:**233
nervousness, **84:**499–500
parkinsonian, **82:**196, 205; **83:**128, 302, 478, 487
peripheral neuropathy, **84:**252
plasma-level monitoring for, **83:**507 (*see also* Plasma factors/levels)
and "psychological toxicity," **84:**242
psychosis, **82:**137, 138, 139–40, 197; **83:**290; **84:**253
renal damage, **83:**126, 301, 314, 316; **84:**232, 255
on sex life, **82:**8, 39; **83:**150, 475, 485
tardive dyskinesia, **82:**147–48, 152–53, 169, 193, 195; **83:**125, 480, 487; **84:**498, 501
on vision, **82:**169; **83:**475, 484; **84:**233
weight gain, **83:**313, 332, 336, 475, 478, 485
See also Extrapyramidal symptoms; Imipramine; Lithium therapy; TCA (tricyclic antidepressant) response
Drug therapy, **83:**172, 358–59
for alcoholism, **84:**346–59
chemical aversion, **84:**328, 333–34
contraindicated, **84:**299, 354, 356–57
ethanol antagonists (amethystic agents, **84:**347–48
and withdrawal reactions, **84:**351–56, 493
(*see also* placebo, *below*)
for anxiety states, **83:**142, 479, 483, 488; **84:**439, 440, 472, 483–90
antidepressant, **84:**392, 414–17, 437, 439, 454–60 passim, 472, 484, 493, 503–19, 524–25
β-blockers, **84:**490–503, 524
in children, **84:**413–18
differential, **84:**483
lactate infusion, **84:**407, 457, 474–82 passim, 493
(*see also* Agoraphobia)
for bipolar illness, *see* Bipolar (manic-depressive) Disorder, treatment of; Lithium therapy

for borderline disorders, **82:**444, 456–67,469–70, 484
in cancer treatment
antidepressant, analgesic, etc., **84:**244–50 passim, 253, 254
chemotherapy, **82:**39; **84:**239–44 passim, 247–55 passim, 270
MOPP regimen (for Hodgkin's disease), **84:**255
for women with breast cancer, **84:**254
for children, **83:**283, 498, 505
in anxiety disorders, **84:**413–16, 418
compliance/noncompliance with, **82:**170, 467, 470; **83:**124, 127, 139, 251, 301, 312, 315–18 passim, 321–37, 504, 508, 509, 512
by alcoholic patient (and detection of), **84:**357
by cancer patient, **84:**239–40, 249, 254
contraindicated, **83:**123, 126, 479–80, 512; **84:**119, 233, 237, 248, 299, 354, 356–57, 502
for dementia, **83:**111–12, 113–14, 137
for depressive disorders, **82:**466; **83:**122–28, 195, 366, 370, 371, 381, 457–71, 472–91, 512; **84:**495
psychotherapy vs., **83:**252, 369, 524–28 passim; **84:**49
(*see also* Lithium therapy; MAO [monoamine oxidase]; TCA [tricyclic antidepressant] response)
dosage, **83:**317, 472, 479, 482–83, 487, 488
for alcoholic, **84:**353, 357
of anxiolytics, **84:**414, 415–16, 455, 485, 493–94, 498, 502–12 passim, 518
for cancer patient, **84:**248, 253, 254
for children, **84:**414, 415–16
for elderly, **83:**112, 123–28 passim, 141, 150
high vs. normal, **82:**112, 183, 187–190
and overdose, **83:**478, 486, 487, 488
plasma-level monitoring of, **83:**492, 498–501, 508, 511
(*see also* Lithium therapy; TCA [tricyclic antidepressant] response)
for geriatric patients, **83:**95, 112, 113, 123–28, 137–50 passim, 497–98, 499; **84:**237–38
for hostility, **83:**487
lithium, *see* Lithium therapy
for manic episode, **83:**293–303
for MBD (minimal brain dysfunction), **82:**463, 467, 470
in mental retardation, **84:**129
for paranoia or paraphrenia, **83:**137, 138, 139
placebo
in alcoholism/withdrawal, **84:**331, 353, 356, 493
in anxiety disorders, **84:**459, 490–502 passim, 503–04, 507–18 passim
in cardiac symptoms, **84:**492–93
in hypochondriasis, **83:**143
lithium therapy vs., **83:**298, 307, 318, 481
in school-phobic children, **84:**414–16
and polypharmacy, **83:**490, 498, 508–09
psychiatry/psychotherapy combined with (dual

mechanism theory), **82:**215, 224; **83:**128, 137, 146–47, 173, 183–84, 316, 320–37
in alcohol withdrawal treatment, **84:**357
in anxiety disorders, **84:**416, 418, 425, 440, 454–55, 459–60, 504, 512
in depression, **83:**512; **84:**50–52, 59
effect of, on psychiatric theory and practice, **83:**269
in family/marital therapy, **83:**195, 243, 252
studies of, **83:**321
psychotherapy vs., **82:**156–57, 160, 168–69, 178, 215, 219–25; **83:**252, 369, 524–28 passim; **84:**49
for schizoaffective disorder, **82:**152
for schizophrenia, **82:**102–11 passim, 117–18, 121, 123, 130–48 passim, 156–76 passim, 178–228, 462, 464; **83:**130, 243, 248, 271, 479–80, 487, 526; **84:**95, 498
for stage fright, **84:**496–97, 502 (see also for anxiety states, above)
stress and, **83:**400
for suicidal patient, **83:**527
"therapeutic window" in, **82:**183, 187, 203; **83:**477, 505, 509
urinary MHPG levels as predictors of response to, **83:**468–69, 473–74, 486, 490
and withdrawal effects, **83:**481
See also Drugs; Drugs, list of; Drug side effect(s); Hormone(s)
Druss, R. G., et al., **84:**273
Drye, R., **82:**416
DSM (*Diagnostic and Statistical Manual of Mental Disorders*, American Psychiatric Association)
DSM-I (1st ed.), **84:**198, 208, 395
DSM-II (2d ed.), **82:**14; **83:**118, 290, 293, 380, 381, 410; **84:**206, 393, 394, 395, 516
DSM-III (3d ed.), **82:**339n16; **83:**137, 408, 427; **84:**178, 188, 301, 302, 390
DSM-III-R, **84:**393
DSM-IV (4th ed.), **84:**504
DSM-III categories/criteria, **83:**90, 92, 106, 367–68; **84:**246
ADD (attentional deficit disorder), **82:**442, 463
adjustment disorder, **83:**140, 357, 367, 375, 410; **84:**63, 203, 246, 247, 419
affective disorders, **82:**269, 271, 465; **83:**118, 119, 271–72, 282, 291, 295, 354, 357, 367–75 passim, 380–81, 410, 479; **84:**61, 203, 246, 393, 396, 397
agoraphobia, **84:**394, 396–98, 401, 410, 419, 495, 503
alcohol-related diagnoses, **84:**68, 213, 299, 301–10, 315, 340, 351
history of, **84:**307–08
anxiety disorders, **84:**203, 246, 392–402, 419, 482, 495, 503, 519–20
with childhood onset, **84:**410
generalized, **84:**394, 395, 397, 400–401, 419, 499, 516
unresolved questions about, **84:**519–20
bereavement (uncomplicated), **83:**375
bipolar disorder, **83:**119, 274, 275, 295, 296, 354, 367, 369, 410

borderline disorders, **82:**413, 428–36 passim, 440–43 passim, 448, 449–51, 454–66 passim, 470; **83:**288
cyclothymic disorder, **83:**292, 354, 367, 410
dementia, **83:**108, 109; **84:**234
depression, **82:**269, 282, 287, 288, 289, 294–99 passim, 466; **83:**90, 279, 362, 375, 381, 411, 492; **84:**61
atypical, **82:**466; **83:**119, 127, 367, 410
major, **83:**119–20, 367–75 passim, 410, 479, 506; **84:**63, 246, 396
dissociative disorders, **84:**393
dysthymic disorder, **82:**465, 466; **83:**120, 275, 354, 368, 372, 410, 479; **84:**393
geriatric disorders, **83:**90
histrionic personality disorder, **82:**470
hypochondriasis, **83:**142
mania, **83:**278–79, 293–95, 296
melancholia, **83:**369–70
mental retardation, **84:**120–21
narcissistic personality disorder, **82:**414, 435, 470, 490, 516
obsessive-compulsive disorder, **84:**393–97 passim, 401, 419
organic mental disorders, **84:**49, 203, 246, 301
panic disorder, **84:**394–97 passim, 400, 404, 410, 460, 461, 493, 495, 504
paranoid personality disorder, **82:**470; **83:**135
phobic disorders, **84:**393–400 passim, 419, 518
posttraumatic stress disorder, **84:**109–10, 393–402 passim, 419, 516
primary degenerative dementia, **83:**108, 109
psychogenic pain disorder, **84:**211
psychological factors affecting physical condition, **84:**211
psychosexual dysfunctions, **82:**8, 9, 12–21 passim
schizoaffective disorder, **83:**290–91, 302
schizophrenia, **82:**83–91 passim, 98, 101–02, 113, 149, 167, 448; **83:**131, 271, 282, 291, 293; **84:**101, 102, 396
schizotypal/schizoid personality disorder, **82:**432, 449, 451, 454, 465, 471
sexual response cycle, **82:**12, 13–14
somatoform disorders, **84:**211, 393
substance use disorders, **84:**301, 302
transsexualism, **82:**53
DSST (digit symbol substitution test), **84:**500
DST (dexamethasone suppression test), **83:**355
of bipolar disorder, **83:**121, 273, 280, 281, 283, 289
of borderline disorders, **82:**452–53
of depressive disorders, **82:**294; **83:**121, 122, 273, 291, 460, 463
vs. dementia, **84:**236
of late-life psychiatric disorders, **83:**89, 117, 121
of schizoaffective states, **83:**291, 292
Dual mechanism theory (drugs combined with psychotherapy), see Drug therapy
Dual-sex therapy, see Sex therapy
Dube, K. C., **82:**185; **83:**417
Duby, J., **84:**323
Duckworth, G. S., **83:**108

Duff, R. S., **83**:184
Duffin, H. M., **83**:114
Duke University Medical Center, **83**:86
  Center for Study of Aging and Human Development, **83**:103, 134
Dunbar, Helen Flanders, **84**:179, 186, 216
Duncan, G. W., **84**:235
Duncan-Jones, P., **83**:409, 416
Dunea, G., et al., **83**:111
Dunham, H. W., **83**:424, 425, 426
Dunitz-Johnson, E., **84**:126
Dunner, David L., **83**:250, 270–75 passim, 287, 299, 303, 312; et al., **83**:281, 286, 287, 294–304 passim, 313, 442, 452
Durkin, H. E., **83**:26
Dustman, R. E., **83**:441
Dwarfism, psychosocial, **82**:293; **84**:225
Dweck, C. S., et al., **82**:271
Dwight, R., **83**:281
Dyckman, J. M., **84**:451
Dynes, J. B., **84**:476
Dyrud, J. E., **82**:461
"Dyscontrol syndrome," **82**:455
Dysken, M. W., **82**:214
Dyson, W. L., **83**:443
Dyspareunia, **82**:14, 16, 20. See also Psychosexual dysfunctions
Dysphoria, **82**:273; **83**:337, 377, 514
  as drug side effect, **84**:254
  gender, see Gender identity
  of infant or child, **82**:274–79 passim, 289, 296, 306
  mania and, **83**:279
  rejection-sensitive or hysteroid, **82**:457, 463–64, 467, 468, 470
  See also Depression; Grief reaction
Dysthymic Disorder, **82**:441; **84**:61
  as bipolar variant, **83**:275–77, 278, 281–82, 285
  course and manifestations of, **83**:276–77, 281–82, 289, 365, 366, 372–73
  and depression, **83**:365, 371–74
  DSM-III category for, see DSM-III categories/criteria
  late-life, **83**:91, 92, 95, 119, 128
  thymoleptic-responsive, **83**:275–76, 281
  variants of, **83**:373–74

E

Earle, E., **84**:115
Easton, J. D., **84**:475, 493
Eastwood, M. R., **84**:213; et al., **84**:217
Eastwood, P. R., **83**:320
Eastwood, R., et al., **83**:138
Eating disorders, **84**:230. See also Anorexia; Anorexia nervosa; Obesity
Eaton, J. S., et al., **84**:182
Eaton, W. W., **82**:100, et al., **83**:90, 408

Ebaugh, F. G., **84**:179
Ebstein's anomaly, **83**:314
ECA, see Epidemiologic Catchment Area Program
Eckert, E. D., et al., **84**:229
Eckman, T., **83**:434
Eckstein, R., **82**:475
ECT (electroconvulsive therapy): in alcoholism, **84**:328, 329, 332–33
  consent to, **82**:357–58, 359
  for depression, **83**:121, 125, 366, 369, 370, 381, 382, 480; **84**:49, 511
    in elderly (unilateral vs. bilateral), **83**:126; **84**:238
  legislation regarding, **82**:332–33, 353
  for manic patient, **83**:281, 302
  for panic attacks, **84**:511
  and schizophrenia, **82**:142, 143, 209, 220
  and suicide, **83**:431
Edgerton, M. T., **84**:262, 263
Edgerton, R. B., **82**:100
Education/educational intervention: about alcohol, **84**:367–68
  for children at risk, **84**:123, 125–26
  in family, see Family therapy
  See also Childhood; Learning disorders; Teaching (of medical psychiatry); Therapist, the
Education for All Handicapped Children Act, see P.L. 94–142
Edward B. Allen Award, **83**:85
Edwards, D. J., **83**:452; et al., **83**:452, 461, 467
Edwards, Griffith, **84**:299, 303, 315, 316
EE (expressed emotion): and family at risk, **84**:101
  and prediction of risk in adolescents, **84**:95
  and schizophrenia relapse, **82**:103–105, 110, 111, 172–74; **83**:175, 242–49 passim, 256; **84**:95
  See also Anger; Hostility; Rage
EEG (electroencephalogram), **82**:124
  abnormal, **82**:118, 148, 453–54, 455, 465
  alcoholism and, **84**:326, 349, 355
  biofeedback regulation of, **84**:227–28
  delirium and, **83**:107
  of elderly patient, **83**:102, 126, 145
  ethanol's depressant effects on, **84**:328, 350
  of infant, **83**:10
  relaxation response and, **84**:444, 446
  of schizoaffective, **83**:291
  sleep studies, **83**:122, 145, 291; **84**:221
"Effort syndrome," **84**:403, 479, 492. See also Cardiac disorders
Egbert, L. D., et al., **84**:258
Egeland, J. A., **83**:270, 271, 448
Eger, C. L., **82**:328
Ego, **82**:497, 500, 502
  anxiety and, **84**:428–29, 433, 436, 437
  and dissociation, **84**:429–30
  development of, **82**:493, 494, 501; **83**:49
  and ego identity/identity diffusion, **83**:24 (see also Identity)
  and ego states of borderline patients, **82**:472–81 passim, 486

functions, **83:**31, 370
  adaptive, **82:**515
  appraisal of twelve, **84:**17
  autonomous, **83:**15
  deficiencies of, **82:**29–30, 35, 286
  development of, **82:**501
  reduction of (in mob), **83:**21, 34
  therapeutic relationship and, **84:**16
  impairment of, in gender dysphoria, **82:**54, 56
  -libido conflict, **84:**432, 433
  primitive (preoedipal) ideal, in group, **83:**23
  -self distinction, Freud and, **82:**488, 489
  strength, and success of therapy, **82:**33, 56,
    478; **84:**26, 30, 44
  -superego conflict, **82:**272; **84:**19
  See also Narcissism; Self
Ego boundaries, **83:**31
Ego-dystonic behavior, **82:**31, 416; **84:**19, 21
Ego psychology, **82:**500, 503, 516
  depression as viewed by, **82:**272
  development of, **82:**488; **83:**21; **84:**13
  and narcissism, **82:**488, 490, 519
  and psychoanalysis, **83:**7
  psychotherapeutic use of, **84:**13
  See also Self psychology
Ego-syntonic behavior, **82:**29; **83:**190, 217, 280,
  374; **84:**19, 21
Eighteenth Amendment, *see* Prohibition
Eimas, P. D., **83:**12; et al., **83:**12
Eisdorfer, Carl, **83:**87, 133, 134, 135, 136, 150; et
  al., **83:**132, 136, 138; **84:**496
Eisen, H. J., **84:**357
Eisenberg, L., **84:**418
Eisenberg, T., **82:**324n8
Eisendrath, R. M., **84:**265, 266, 267, 268
Eissler, Kurt, **82:**476; **83:**42, 54, 60
Ejaculation, **82:**10
  aging and, **82:**46
  impairment of, in cancer therapy, **84:**255
  and postejaculation difficulties, **82:**16
  premature, **82:**10, 15, 16, 19, 32
    therapy for, **82:**22, 24, 25, 32
  retarded, therapy for, **82:**21
  retrograde (prostatectomy and), **82:**39
  as separate from male orgasm, **82:**15
  urethral surgery and, **82:**38
  See also Orgasm
Ekdahl, M. C., et al., **84:**138
EKG (electrocardiogram), **82:**291–92; **83:**122, 126,
  299; **84:**233, 468
  in monitoring TCA therapy, **83:**478, 498
Ekstein, R., **82:**444
Elam, M., et al., **84:**477
Elderly, the, *see* Aging; Geriatric psychiatry; Late-
  life psychiatric disorders
Electrocardiogram, *see* EKG
Electroconvulsive therapy, *see* ECT
Electrodermal response: anxiety and, **84:**469–71
  of child of schizophrenic, **84:**131
Electroencephalogram, *see* EEG
Electrolyte imbalance, **84:**250, 352, 355. *See also*
  Hypercalcemia
Electromyogram, *see* EMG

Eliot, J., **83:**404
Elizabeth, J. I., **84:**475
Elizur, A., et al., **82:**207
Elkins, R. L., **84:**333
Ellenberg, M., **82:**37
Ellerbook, R. C., **82:**143
Ellis, Havelock, **82:**8
Ellsworth, R. B., **82:**174; et al., **82:**175
Elmasian, R., et al., **84:**327
Elmhurst, New York, City Hospital, **84:**11
Elston, R. C., **83:**445, 446, 450; et al., **83:**451
Elsworth, J. D., et al., **84:**472
Emde, R. N., **83:**229, 230; **84:**125; et al., **83:**10
Emerson, Ralph Waldo, **83:**37
Emery, R. E., **84:**153, 154
EMG (electromyogram): biofeedback regulation
  of, **84:**227–28
  relaxation response and, **84:**446
Emler, N. T., **83:**37
Emmelkamp, P. M. G., **84:**449, 451, 454, 457; et
  al., **84:**457
Emmeneger, H., **83:**112
Emotionally Unstable Character Disorder, **82:**457,
  463, 467, 468, 470; **83:**288
Emotions: and emotional disorders, *see* Affec-
  tive disorders; Depression; Mental retarda-
  tion; Mood disorders
  hierarchy of, **82:**273
  role of, in health and disease, **84:**177, 187, 191,
    217–18, 224
Empathy: during infancy, **83:**19–20
  narcissism and, **82:**490–91, 495, 496–97, 513
  parental or caretaker, failure of, **82:**492, 494 (*see
    also* Parent-child relationship)
  of patient, with projected aggression, **82:**474
  of therapist, *see* Therapist, the
Emphysema, **83:**98
Employment, *see* Work
Emrich, H. M., et al., **82:**213
Encephalitis, **82:**121; **84:**127
  and borderline disorders, **82:**442
  CMV (cytomegalovirus), **84:**250
  herpes, lethargica, Vilyuisk, **82:**120
  See also Viruses
Encephalopathy: alcoholism and, **84:**322
  cancer and, **84:**250
  drug therapy and, **83:**301; **84:**252
  hyperbilirubinemia and bilirubin, **84:**127
  lead, **84:**127
  radiation therapy and, **84:**252
  See also Brain, the
Encopresis: childhood, studies of, **83:**176–77. *See
  also* Incontinence
Endicott, Jean, **82:**424; **83:**408; **84:**303
Endocrine system: aging and, **83:**99
  antipsychotic effects on, **82:**200–204
  disorders of
    and mood dysfunction, **83:**379, 422, 460
    and psychosexual dysfunctions, **82:**37
    and reversible dementia, **84:**234
    and TSH response, **83:**122
  hypothalamic-pituitary-adrenocortical (HPA)
    axis, **83:**460, 463; **84:**488

lithium effects on, **83:**126, 303
neuroendocrine correlates with depression, **83:**512
childhood depression, **82:**290, 292–94
and sexual development, **82:**11
stress and, **84:**221–23, 225
See also Hormone(s)
Endorphins, **82:**146; **84:**249, 351, 410
and schizophrenia, **82:**141–42
stress and, **84:**222, 223
Engel, B. T., **84:**220; et al., **84:**228
Engel, G. L., **82:**161, 274; **83:**107, 204; **84:**216, 217, 220, 225, 268; et al., **84:**181, 219
Engelmann, S., **84:**126
England, *see* Great Britain
English, O. S., **83:**319, 329
Enna, S. J., **83:**469
Ennis, B. J., **82:**339
Enuresis, *see* Incontinence
Environmental factors: in aging process (and in treatment of older patient), **83:**105, 114, 139
in antisocial personality, **84:**96
in child development, **83:**229, 230; **84:**102
and mental retardation, **84:**125–26, 127
and psychosis, **84:**134
in consanguinity method studies, **82:**93
and culture shock, **83:**139
and depression, **82:**284, **83:**413, 421, 458, 518, 520, 526, 528
and manic states, **83:**278
in paranoia, **83:**137, 138, 139
physical, and health (cancer), **84:**239
in schizophrenia, **82:**88–89, 96–97, 99, 106, 155; **83:**138
See also Diet; Nurture-nature debate; Psychosocial factors; Social support networks
Enzymatic alterations, **82:**125–29, 130–31, 138–39, 144. *See also* DBH (dopamine); MAO (monoamine oxidase)
EPI (Eysenck Personality Inventory), **83:**336, 386; **84:**325
Epidemiologic Catchment Area Program (ECA), **83:**406n, 408, 410, 428; **84:**92, 396
Epidemiology: and "conspicuous psychiatric morbidity" (CPM), **84:**190, 191
defined, **82:**281; **83:**406
among elderly, **83:**87–95
of psychiatric illness among medical populations, **84:**184, 187–215, 467
reduced by intervention, **84:**213
of psychiatric illness among mentally retarded, **84:**123–25
research/studies of, **84:**97, 214, 217
of risk and protective factors, **84:**91, 92
terms (point prevalence, morbid risk, incidence, risk factor) defined, **83:**410
See also individual disorders
Epileptic disorders, **83:**296
as alcohol withdrawal reaction, **84:**351, 355
and borderline disorders, **82:**442, 455
as drug reaction, **83:**478, 486; **84:**357, 358
as "mental illness," **82:**337
operant conditioning and, **84:**228

temporal lobe epilepsy, drug therapy for, **83:**311
Epinephrine, **84:**472, 475, 476, 480, 488. *See also* Norepinephrine (NE)
Episodic dyscontrol, **82:**465, 467, 468
EPS (extrapyramidal symptoms), **82:**182, 195, 196, 201, 205, 208; **83:**113, 125, 487. *See also* Drug side effect(s)
Epstein, H., **84:**110
Epstein, N. B., **83:**215
Equilibrium (in family systems approach), **83:**205–06, 213. *See also* Family therapy
Equus-Laingian view of madness, **83:**331
Erection: of nipples, **82:**12
penile, **82:**9, 10, 12, 23, 39, 43
age and, **82:**46; **83:**149, 151
failure of, **82:**17, 37, 39; **83:**151
Ericksen, S. E., **82:**187; et al., **83:**183, 188, 189
Erikson, Erik H., **82:**278, 490; **83:**15, 51, 83
Erikson, K., **84:**111, 118
Erlenmeyer-Kimling, L., **84:**132; et al., **84:**132, 138
Ervin, C. W., **84:**270
Ervin Act, **82:**373, 374
Escalona, S., **84:**116
Eskelson, E. S., et al., **84:**348
Esman, A. H., **83:**9; **84:**108
Essen-Möller, E., **82:**451; **83:**415, 416, 418, 420, 441; **84:**316
Essman, W. B., **83:**512
Esterson, A., et al., **82:**217
Estroff, N., **83:**248
Estrogen: CNS regulation of, **84:**222
post-menopausal levels of, **82:**10, 11; **83:**149
risk in use of, **82:**11; **83:**149
and TSH response, **83:**122
E.T. (film), **84:**146
Eth, S., **84:**112, 116
Ethanol: drug antagonism to, **84:**347–51, 353–54, 359
reaction to, **84:**326, 346–47 (*see also* Alcohol [metabolism of])
as therapeutic agent, **84:**352, 354, 483, 484
Ethical considerations: in cancer treatment, **84:**242, 245
in consultation-liaison psychiatry, **84:**182
in criminal cases, **82:**386, 393–96
and refusal of treatment, **84:**182, 259–60 (*see also* Therapy)
See also Confidentiality; Values
Ethnicity: and coronary artery disease, **84:**216
and depression or bipolar illness, **82:**284; **83:**361, 413, 420, 426
and schizophrenia, **82:**101, 102
See also Blacks
Ettig, P., et al., **82:**203
Eule, E. M., **84:**272
Euphoria: in bipolar illness, **83:**279, 423. *See also* Bipolar (manic-depressive) Disorder
Evans, L., **84:**511
Evans, M., **82:**26
Evans, N. J. R., et al., **84:**217
Evans, W. E., **84:**358
Everaerd, W. T. A. M., et al., **84:**453

Everett, H. C., 83:476
Ewatt, J. R., et al., 84:272
Ewing, J. A., 84:351
Exercise (as therapy), 83:142, 146
  autogenic training, 84:445
  breathing exercises, 84:10, 70
Existential therapy, see Psychotherapy(ies)
Exner, J., 82:209
Expectations: cultural, see Cultural factors
  of family members, 82:279; 83:196–97, 198–99,
    217, 218, 426 (see also Family, the; Family
    therapy; Marital therapy)
  of organ transplant recipient, 84:266, 268, 269
  parental, of treatment effects on child, 84:417
  by patient, of outcome of treatment, 84:26, 36,
    52
  social, and alcoholism, 84:330–31, 360, 365–66
  staff, of patients, 83:30
  See also Relationships; Role(s)
Exposure treatment (of phobia), 84:448–60, 507,
  510
  cognitive therapy and, 84:457–59
  combined with other therapies, 84:454–56, 459,
    512
  habituation in, 84:450, 453, 456–57, 459
  practical implications of, 84:459–60
  self-directed, 84:452–54, 459, 507
  unresolved questions about, 84:523
  See also Behavioral approach
Expressed emotion, see EE
Expressive psychotherapy, see Psychother-
  apy(ies)
Extein, I., et al., 83:289, 470
Externalization, 83:237; 84:136, 142. See also De-
  fense mechanism(s)
Extrapyramidal symptoms, see EPS
Eye movement, see REM (rapid eye movement);
  SPEM (smooth pursuit eye movement)
Eysenck, H. J., 83:387
Eysenck Personality Inventory, see EPI
Ezriel, H., 83:27, 28

F

Face-Hand Test (FHT), 83:116
Faerman, I., et al., 82:37
Fagan, J. F., 83:15
Faguet, R. A., et al., 84:182
Faiman, M. D., 84:347
Fain, J. H., 83:470
Fain, M., 83:33
Fairbairn, W. R. D., 82:470, 490; 83:26, 218
Fairburn, C. G., 82:212
Faithorn, E. P., 84:12
Falloon, I. R. H., 82:111; 83:245–48 passim, 253,
  256; et al., 82:109, 110–111; 84:399
Falret, Jean Pierre, 83:269
Family, the: adolescent dependence on, 82:279;
  83:241

and alcoholism, see Alcoholism (etiology of)
bipolar illness and, 83:249, 279, 297–98, 302,
  305, 329, 374, 426, 435
child as scapegoat of, 83:233–34, 239, 240
and childhood phobias, 84:411, 416
and childhood psychosomatic disorders, 84:225
and children at risk, 84:138–42, 225 (see also
  Children at risk)
in consultation-liaison psychiatry, 84:181, 186,
  237–43 passim, 258, 266
critical events/stress and, 83:188, 197–98, 214–
  15, 216, 239
of depressive patient, 83:364, 372, 380, 405, 414
and elderly members of, 83:88, 114, 129, 138,
  150
and family identity, 83:177–78
and family law and policy, 84:146–47, 155–57
and family planning services, see Birth control
and gender development, 82:55
genogram of, 83:199, 207, 209, 215
importance of, 83:169–70, 364
  for children at risk, 84:103, 134
and indigenous family culture, 83:179–83
intergenerational family-of-origin problems in,
  83:199, 212, 222, 223, 231, 236–37, 241
lack of moral guidance by, 83:35
life cycles of, 83:209–12, 216; 84:63, 156 (see also
  Adolescent[s]; Aging; Childhood; Infancy;
  Young adults)
loyalties to, 83:199, 219, 234
of mentally retarded child, 84:121, 125–26 (see
  also Mental retardation)
in organ transplant cases, 84:266, 268–69
patriarchal, and capitalism, 83:34
and physical illness, 83:169, 193, 195, 213–14
  cancer, 84:255, 273
  and TPN, 84:271–72
  at risk, 84:101, 110, 111, 121, 126, 128, 132, 275
  "psychosomatogenic,"84:225
and schizophrenia (etiology and relapse),
  82:103–06, 107, 110, 112, 163, 172–74; 83:171,
  175–76, 242–49
See also Children at risk; Marriage; Mother-
  child relationship; Parent(s); Parent-child
  relationship; Separation and divorce; Sib-
  ling(s)
Family Crucible, The (Napier and Whitaker),
  83:215
Family history: of affective disorders, 83:274,
  282–83, 288, 295, 380, 420–21, 434–57 (see also
  Depression)
  in alcoholism studies, 83:178; 84:320–27 pas-
    sim
  of anxiety disorders, 84:403–08 passim, 511
  "living" (initial interview and), 83:208
  and mania/manic episode, 83:288, 295
  of mitral valve prolapse, 84:407, 408, 480
  -negative and -positive (FHN, FHP), 84:322–
    27 passim
  of schizophrenic states, 83:132, 283
  See also Genetic factors; History-taking
Family Planning Project, 84:143. See also Birth
  control

Family Support Project, **84:**141
Family therapy: for alcoholism, **83:**189,; **84:**300
  for bipolar or unipolar disorder, **82:**265, 307;
  83:249–53
  for childhood disorders, **82:**265, 307; **83:**171,
    188–201 passim, 209, 228–41
    anxiety, **84:**416
    psychosomatic, **84:**225
  choice of, **83:**187–92
  combined with drug therapy, **83:**195, 243, 252
  consultation-liaison work and, **84:**186
  defined, **83:**185
  education of family in, **82:**173; **83:**201, 243–50
    passim, 253–56; **84:**95
  family or marital evaluation, **83:**188–91, 193–
    95, 197, 222
  "family systems theory" in, **83:** 186, 194, 203–
    15, 217, 229, 239–40
  geriatric patients and, **83:**129
  group process theories and, **83:**33
  importance and advantages of, **83:**169–70, 185,
    234–35
  vs. individual, **83:**188, 189–92, 203, 204, 239–
    41; **84:**119
  and multiple family group (MFG), **83:**242, 244,
    246, 247, 256
  for psychic trauma, **84:**118–19
  psychosocial studies of, **84:**225
  in schizophrenia, **83:**189, 252
    behavioral, **83:**246–47
    psychoeducational, **82:**163, 173; **83:**245–46,
      253–56
    and relapse, **82:**106, 110–11, 172–74; **83:**242–
      49 passim
    studies of, **82:**217, 219, 225; **83:**170, 175, 242
  strategic and systemic, **83:**247–48, 256
  the therapist and, **83:**179–80, 182–85, 186
    empathy of, **83:**171, 173, 194, 200, 201, 206–
      07, 244, 246
    intervention by, **83:**187, 196–203, 211, 238–
      39, 241
    interviews by, **83:**207–09, 231, 232, 238, 239
    role assumption by, **83:**201, 223–24, 226, 238
    training for, **83:**183
  See also Marital therapy
Fang, V. S., **82:**135
Fann, W. E., **83:**150
Fantasies: absence of, see Alexithymia
Farberow, N., **84:**117
Faris, R. E. L., **83:**424, 425, 426
Farkas, T., et al., **83:**117
Farley, I. J., et al., **82:**132
Farley, J., et al., **84:**212
Farmer, B. B., **84:**407
Farmer, P. M., et al., **83:**110
Farr, S. P., **84:**347
Farrington, D. P., **84:**96
Fascism, **83:**35
Fasman, J., et al., **84:**138
Fast, I., **84:**115
Father, the: absence/rejection of, **83:**35
  depressive, **84:**132, 133
  in divorce, **84:**150, 152, 156

oedipal, Freud's view of, **83:**34–35, 36
participation of, in family therapy, **83:**194, 233n
schizophrenic, see Parent(s)
stresses on, **84:**133, 135
See also Male(s); Parent-child relationship
Father image: "contamination" of (by aggres-
  sion), **82:**473
Fatigue: depression and, **83:**127, 328, 480, 514;
  84:248
  childhood depression, **82:**303–04
  as drug side effect, **84:**494, 499
  in panic or anxiety disorder, **84:**407, 429, 492,
    493
Fauman, B. J., **82:**140
Fauman, M. A., **82:**140, **84:**223
Fava, G. A., et al., **83:**395, 396; **84:**207, 208
Favazza, A. R., **84:**353
Fawcett, J., et al., **83:**480
Fay, A., **84:**75
Fazekas, J. F., et al., **84:**354
Fazio, M., et al., **84:**252
FDA, see Food and Drug Administration
Fear, see Anxiety; Phobias; Separation fears
Fear Questionnaire, **84:**455
Federal Bureau of Investigation, **84:**367
Federal Organizations for Professional Women,
  82:57
Federal Trade Commission, **82:**325
Federn, P., **82:**444
Feedback, see Biofeedback
Feer, H., et al., **82:**141
Feighner, J. P., et al., **82:**289, 422; **83:**272, 278,
  286, 293, 294, 376, 408, 409, 512; **84:**303, 395,
  460, 461, 499
  and Feighner criteria, **84:**191, 206, 303–06
    passim, 309, 395, 460
Feinberg, I., **83:**145; et al., **83:**145
Feinberg, M. P., **83:**452
Feldberg, W., **82:**146
Felder, W., **83:**440
Feldman, M., **84:**231
Fellner, C. H., **84:**266, 267
Felner, R. D., et al., **84:**145
Female(s): anatomy of, **82:**10–11 (see also Genitalia)
  antipsychotic prolactin levels of, **82:**202–03
  bipolar illness of, **83:**304, 424, 426
  depressive, **83:**373, 387, 393, 400–04, 411–14
    passim, 420–22, 433, 524; **84:**58, 62, 133, 206,
    208, 472
    impact of, on offspring, see Mother-child
      relationship
    "involutional," **83:**92, 412
  in divorce studies, **84:**153
  dysthymic disorders among, **83:**373
  elderly
    and late-life psychiatric disorders, **83:**94, 107,
      110, 132, 133, 142, 420; **84:**238
    sexual functions of, **83:**149, 151
    U.S. population figures, **83:**88
  as heart transplant donor, reaction to, **84:**269
  infertility of (as chemotherapy effect), **84:**255
  life expectancy for, **83:**89

lithium reactions of/compliance by, **83:**333, 334, 335

masturbation by, **82:**10, 11, 18, 21

pre- and postmarital sexuality of, **82:**43, 44

psychiatric morbidity rate among, **84:**190, 192, 198, 206, 208, 214

role concepts, impairments, disputes, **83:**38; **84:**58, 62, 133, 135

schizophrenia in, **82:**108 (*see also* Parent[s])

stress and, **83:**94

surgery on, **82:**39–41 (*see also* Cancer)

in therapeutic relationship, **83:**38–40

treatment goals of, **83:**39–40

See also Female psychology; Feminist movement; Menopause; Orgasm; Rape; Sex differentiation

Female psychology, **83:**36–50

Freud and, **83:**38, 40–50 passim

psychoanalysis and, **83:**39–50

Feminist movement, **83:**39, 47–48, 215

attacks double standard, **82:**7

and decline in depression among women, **83:**92

Fengler, B., **82:**196

Fenichel, O., **83:**370; **84:**108

Fenton, F. R., **82:**227

Fentress, T. L., **84:**470

Ferenczi, S., **82:**57–58; **83:**55; **84:**7, 29

Ferguson, R. M., et al., **82:**118

Ferris, R., **83:**490

Ferris, S. H., **83:**112; **84:**234; et al., **83:**117

Ferster, C. B., **83:**516

Fessel, W. J., **82:**115, 117

Fetishism, **82:**33, 34, 58. *See also* Psychosexual dysfunctions

Fetus: external genitalia of, **82:**11

infections of, **82:**120

FHN, FHP (family-history-negative, family-history-positive), *see* Family history

FHT (Face-Hand Test), **83:**116

Fibiger, H. C., **84:**472

"Fibrositis" syndrome, **84:**221

Field, T., **83:**13

Fieve, R. R., **83:**272, 274, 275, 312, 326–35 passim, 449; **84:**61; et al., **82:**117; **83:**467

"Fight-flight" behavior: within group, **83:**22, 26 vs. relaxation response, **84:**445, 448

Filho, V. V., et al., **82:**180

Finch, S. M., **82:**301

Fine, B. D., **82:**489

Finesinger, J. E., **82:**276; **84:**474, 476

Fink, G. B., **84:**354

Fink, M., **83:**126; **84:**437, 504; et al., **84:**478

Finland: schizophrenia studies in, **82:**98, 145

Finlay-Jones, R., **83:**395, 396; **84:**214, 397

Finn, R., **84:**191, 194, 203–12 passim

Finnerty, R. J., **84:**498, 499

Fischer, A. K., **83:**92

Fischer, E., et al., **82:**137, 138

Fischer, M., **82:**94, 451; **83:**291; et al., **83:**441

Fischman, A. M., **82:**62

Fish, Barbara, **84:**87, 99, 101, 130, 131, 416

Fish, F. J., **83:**132

Fisher, C., et al., **82:**46

Fisher, L., et al., **84:**133

Fisher's Exact Probability Test, **83:**307

Fishman, George, **84:**34

Fishman, S. H., **84:**135

Fisman, M., **82:**120; et al., **83:**113

Fitz, G., et al., **82:**62, 63

Fitzgerald, R. G., **83:**249, 324, 331

Fleck, S., **83:**189; **84:**208, 210

Fleiss, J. F., **82:**182

Fleiss, J. L., **83:**448

Fleming, R., **84:**498

Fleminger, J. J., **83:**107

Flink, E. B., **84:**355, 356; et al., **84:**355

Flooding, *see* Behavioral approach

Flor-Henry, P., **82:**124

Flugel, J., **82:**58

Foa, E. B., **84:**402, 457; et al., **84:**450

Foa, U. G., **84:**402

Folks, D. G., **84:**231, 232

Follow Through program, **84:**125

Folstein, M. F., **83:**107, 108; **84:**234; et al., **84:**237

Food, *see* Diet

Food and Drug Administration (FDA), **82:**325; **83:**124, 307, 477, 482, 483, 490; **84:**355

Ford, Charles V., **83:**117, 127; **84:**178, 184, 231–35 passim

Ford, M. D., **82:**382n5

Fordyce, W. E., et al., **84:**229

Forensic psychiatry, *see* Psychiatry

Forney, R. B., **84:**350, 358; et al., **84:**349

Forssman, H., **82:**211

Forster, B., **82:**200, 203

Fosdick, R., **84:**361

Fossum, A., **83:**372

Foster, H. H., **84:**155

Foster, J. R., et al., **83:**126; **84:**238

Foster care: of children at risk, **84:**99, 138

costs of, **84:**139

in schizophrenia, **82:**225, 227

Foucault, M., **83:**34

Foulkes, S. H., **83:**25, 27–28

Foundations Fund Research in Psychiatry, **82:**350n; **83:**491n

Fountain House, **82:**176, 177

Foust, L. L., **82:**349

Fox, B. H., **84:**240

Fox, H.M., et al., **84:**262, 263

Fox, J. H., et al., **83:**117

Fox, R. C., **83:**173

Fraiberg, S., **83:**15, 16; **84:**115; et al., **84:**128

Framingham, Massachusetts; panic disorder study in, **84:**403

Framo, J. L., **83:**218, 222, 223

France: fascism and "new left" in, **83:**35

Frances, A., **84:**393

Frank, E., et al., **82:**46

Frank, Jerome D., **84:**57,63, 319, 419, 420, 521

Frank, J. L., **84:**272

Frank, K. A., et al., **84:**216, 263, 264

Frank, S., **82:**120

Frankenhaeuser, M., **84:**472, 475

Frankfurter, Justice Felix, **82:**361, 362, 371

Frankl, V. E., **84**:458
Frantz, A. G., **82**:204
Frazer, A., **83**:452
Frazier, S. H., **84**:272
Frederick, A. N., **82**:180, 181
Frederickson-Overøo, K., **83**:495
Free association: childhood trauma inferred from, **84**:104
   in group therapy, **83**:26, 27
   interpretation of, **83**:63
Freed, D. J., **84**:155
Freed, W. J., et al., **82**:140
Freedman, A. M., et al., **84**:355
Freedman, B., **82**:351, 355, 356
Freedman, D. X., **82**:139, 461; **83**:363; **84**:353, 354; et al., **82**:130
Freeman, C. P. L., **82**:212
Freeman, H., **82**:180, 181
Freeman, R., **84**:129
Freemon, F. R., **83**:109
Free radical theory (in aging), **83**:97–98
French, R. M., **84**:442
French, T. M., **84**:7, 30
Freud, Anna, **83**:229; **84**:105–06, 108
Freud, Sigmund, **82**:8, 9, 35, 305; **83**:65, 370, 522; **84**:11, 13, 18, 66, 427
   and "analysis as chess game," **83**:51
   anxiety theories of, **84**:394, 395, 418, 421, 429–33, 437, 438
   "Little Hans," **84**:411, 417, 432
   cause-effect framework used by, **83**:66
   and childhood memories, **83**:63; **84**:105
   clitoral-vaginal transfer theory of, **82**:11; **83**:41
   and the family as "interference," **83**:169
   and female psychology, **83**:38, 40–50 passim
   group processes explained by, **83**:21–22, 24, 25, 34, 35
   Guilty Man of, **82**:493
   and ICH, **82**:488, 489
   ideas of, challenged, **83**:7, 404; **84**:66, 105
   on infancy, **83**:9
   influence of, on intellectual tradition, **83**:37
   "interpretation" first used as term by, **83**:63
   libido theory of, **83**:15, 41
   narcissism concept of, **82**:487, 488–89, 493, 494, 497, 512
   patriarchal bias of, **83**:45
   penis envy theory of, **83**:40–48 passim
   on phobia, **84**:448
   psychotherapeutic techniques of, **84**:7
   and sexual trauma, **84**:93
   "traumatic" defined by, **84**:107–08
Freyberger, H., **84**:273
Fridovich, I., **83**:98
Friedel, Robert O., **82**:457; **83**:87, 122–26 passim, 146, 506; et al., **83**:506
Friedlander, D. H., **84**:492
Friedlander, Steven, **82**:264; et al., **82**:266, 271, 272
Friedman, A. S., **83**:252
Friedman, D., et al., **84**:100
Friedman, L., **83**:20, 61
Friedman, M., **84**:216; et al., **84**:216

Friedman, P. R., **82**:358
Friedman, S. B., et al., **82**:115
Friedmann, L. W., **84**:272
Friend, W. C., et al., **82**:203
Friesen, H. G., **82**:204
Frigidity, **82**:14, 58; **83**:41. See also Psychosexual dysfunctions
Frohman, C. E., et al., **82**:118–19
Frohman factor, **82**:118, 119
Frolich, E. D., et al., **84**:475, 493
Frommer, E. A., **82**:267, 291; **84**:416
Fromm-Reichmann, Frieda, **82**:161, 172; **83**:242, 319, 330; **84**:57, 66
Frosch, John, **82**:428, 444, 477
Fructose: as ethanol eliminator, **84**:349
Fruensgaard, K., et al., **82**:186
Frye, J. S., **84**:401
Fuchs, C. Z., **83**:524
Fujisawa, C., **84**:443
Fujita, K., et al., **82**:127
Fuller, R. K., **84**:356
Functional disorder: term defined, **84**:390
Funding, T., **83**:132
Funkenstein, D. H., **82**:115
Funkenstein, H. H., **83**:112
Furer, M., **82**:511; **83**:14
Furnan, E., **84**:119
Furstenberg, F. F., Jr., **84**:146, 150
Future: child's pessimism toward (posttraumatic), **84**:114, 117
   dread of (in depression), **82**:278
Fyer, A. J., **84**:504

G

GABA (L-γ-aminobutyric acid): in Alzheimer's disease, **83**:110, 112
   as amethystic agent, **84**:351
   anxiolytic drug effect on, **84**:409–10, 482–90 passim, 497
   and schizophrenia, **82**:138–39
   sodium valproate and brain levels, **84**:355
Gabriel, H. P., **84**:258
Gadpaille, W., **82**:48
Gaensbauer, T. J., **82**:283, 285
Gaertner, H. J., et al., **83**:468
Gaffney, F. Andrew, **84**:481; et al., **84**:481
Gagnon, J. H., **82**:58
Gagrat, D. D., **83**:286
Gaind, R., et al., **84**:497
Galactosemia, **84**:127
Galadburda, A., et al., **82**:124
Galante, R., **84**:112, 118
Galanter, M., **84**:344
Galdston, R., **84**:115
Galenberg, A. J., **83**:314
Galenson, E., **82**:55; et al., **82**:55
Gallant, D. M., **82**:180, 181, 184, 201, 213; **84**:140, 351

Gallemore, J., **83**:144
Galton, Francis, **83**:435
Gambling: family therapy for, **83**:189
Gamer, E., et al., **84**:131, 132
Gandhi, Mohandas K., **83**:83–84
Ganz, V. H., et al., **83**:287
GAP (Group for the Advancement of Psychiatry), **83**:85, 189, 190, 191; **84**:156, 437
   Committees on Aging, Hospitals, **83**:85
Gapen, P., **84**:250
Garber, H., **84**:126
Garcia-Sainz, J. A., **83**:470
Garcia-Sevilla, J. A., et al., **83**:470
Gardiner, B. M., **84**:224
Gardner, E. A., **84**:191, 194, 213, 215
Gardner, R. A., **84**:120, 145, 156, 157
Gardos, G., **82**:169; **83**:443; et al., **82**:188, 206
Garfield, S. L., et al., **84**:476
Garfinkel, P. E., **84**:219, 223, 225; et al., **83**:461; **84**:219, 229
Garland, F. N., **84**:220
Garmezy, Norman, **82**:106; **84**:87, 88, 90, 99–102 passim, 136
Garner, D. M., **84**:219, 223, 225; et al., **84**:219
Garrard, S. D., **84**:126
Garside, R., **83**:381
Garver, D. L., **82**:136, 208; **83**:459, 463; et al., **82**:183
Gas chromatography, *see* GC
Gastrointestinal disorders, **84**:191
   cancer, **84**:248
   and depressive symptomatology, **84**:208
      childhood depression, **82**:288
   as drug side effect, **84**:233, 244, 254
   drug side effects increased by, **84**:248
   ileitis, **84**:202
   psychological effects on, **84**:216
   as "psychosomatic" disorder, **84**:198, 202, 211, 216, 437, 439, 493
   ulcerative colitis, **84**:198, 202, 211, 216, 273, 437, 439
   ulcers, peptic, **84**:198, 202, 211, 216, 220, 221, 232, 437
Gath, D., **84**:274
Gattaz, W. F., **83**:467
Gaultieri, C. T., **84**:237
Gaussian system, **83**:447
Gauthier, J., **84**:450
Gaylin, W., **83**:522
GC (gas chromatography), **83**:501, 503
Gebhard, P. H., **82**:42, 43, 44
Gediman, H., **83**:9
Gee, W. F., **83**:151
Gelder, M. G., **84**:450; et al., **84**:450, 451
Gelenberg, A. J., **83**:127, 128, 142, 478, 481
Geller, B., et al., **83**:498, 505
Geller, I., **84**:484
Gellhorn, E., **84**:476
Gelman, D., **84**:105
Gender identity, **82**:48–49
   changing theories of, **83**:42–44
   child's recognition of, **83**:42–43
   family therapy in problems of, **83**:189

and gender dysphoria, **82**:48, 49–56
   adolescent, **82**:51–52, 53
   adult, **82**:52–53
   childhood, **82**:49–51, 53, 55
and sex-reassignment surgery, **82**:7, 48, 53–56 passim
See also Transsexualism
Gender Identity Disorder, **82**:8
General Health Questionnaire, *see* GHQ
General Hospital Psychiatry (journal), **84**:182
Generalized Anxiety Disorder, *see* Anxiety Disorders
Genetic factors: in affective disorders, **83**:434–57; **84**:97, 100, 325, 391
   bipolar, **82**:265; **83**:272–78 passim, 282–83, 287, 289, 329, 427, 435–57 passim; **84**:97 (*see also* Depression)
   in aging, **83**:97, 110
   in alcoholism, **84**:300, 313, 320–28
   in Alzheimer's disease, **83**:110
   in antisocial personality, **84**:96, 325
   in anxiety disorders, **84**:391, 479
      panic disorder, **84**:402–10, 482, 520
   in borderline personality disorder, **82**:437–56
   and children at risk, **84**:96, 97, 126
   consanguinity method in study of, **82**:92–93
   contraindicated, **83**:93
   environmental effects on, **83**:458
   and genetic counseling, **83**:436, 443, 454, 456–57; **84**:126
   Genetic Data Sheet showing, **82**:438, 439
   genetic markers, **83**:436, 445, 448–54
   and genetic vulnerability, **83**:140, 437–50 passim, 454
   and modes of transmission, **83**:445–54
      multifactorial, **83**:447; **84**:406
      single-autosomal-locus, **83**:436, 445–46, 450, 451; **84**:406
      X-chromosome, **83**:436, 445–49 passim
   and nervous energy, **84**:429
   in schizophrenia, **82**:92–97, 121, 438, 444–48; **84**:100, 130, 325, 391 (*see also* Schizophrenia, etiology of)
   in suicide, **83**:432
   and theory of genetic redundancy, **83**:97
   See also Adoption studies; Family history; Nurture-nature debate; Twins
Genitalia: female, **82**:10–11, 12, 13, 18, 34
   masculinization of (endocrine disorder), **82**:37
   fetal external, hormone susceptibility of, **82**:11
   male, **82**:9–10, 12, 13 (*see also* Penis)
Genogram, *see* Family, the
George, J. M., et al., **84**:258
Gerard, D. L., et al., **84**:317
Gerber, L. A., **84**:275
Geriatric medicine, **82**:47. *See also* Aging
Geriatric Mental Health Academic Award, **83**:85
Geriatric psychiatry, **83**:84–87, 129, 130
   consultation-liaison, **84**:184, 231–38
   fellowship programs, **83**:86
   See also Late-life psychiatric disorders
German, G. A., **83**:290

Gerner, R., **83:**117; **84:**236
Gerocomy, **83:**83–84
Gerontological Society of America, **83:**85
Gerontology, **83:**86
Gerontophobia, **83:**84
Gershenson, J., **83:**183
Gershon, Elliot S., **83:**270–73 passim, 355, 368, 375, 434n, 435n, 442, 448–51 passim, 455–57 passim, 488; **84:**97, 476; et al., **82:**135, 440, 444; **83:**273, 283, 286, 390, 392, 435n, 437–54 passim, 483, 488; **84:**97, 403
Gerson, S. C., **82:**129
Gerstein, Dean R., **84:**300, 360–69 passim
Gertz, H. O., **84:**458
Gessner, P. K., **84:**347, 352, 354, 356
Geyer, S., **84:**133
GH (growth hormone), *see* Hormone(s)
Gherke, S., **83:**233
Ghose, K., **83:**315
GHQ (General Health Questionnaire), **84:**187, 188–89, 191, 198, 202, 203
Giardana, E. G., et al., **83:**505, 510
Giardana, R., et al., **83:**478
Gibbon, M., **82:**424
Gibson, R. W., **83:**426
GI disorders, *see* Gastrointestinal disorders
Gilden, E. F., **84:**468
Giles, D. E., **84:**46
Gilgamesh, Epic of, **83:**83
Gill, M. M., **82:**476; **83:**65
Giller, E. L., **83:**483; et al., **83:**317
Gilligan, C., **83:**41
Gillin, J. C., **83:**463; et al., **82:**140, 145, 290
Gilman, A. G., et al., **84:**358
Ginsberg, A. L., **84:**357
Giovacchini, P., **82:**472
Gitlin, M., **82:**213
Gittelman, Rachel, **84:**98
Gittelman-Klein, R., **82:**108; **84:**414
Glaser, K., **82:**266, 268, 289
Glass, B., et al., **83:**476
Glass, D. C., et al., **84:**220
Glass, E., **84:**253
Glass, R. M., et al., **84:**189, 191, 196, 203, 204, 206, 209
Glassman, Alexander H., **83:**123, 478, 492; et al., **83:**123, 477, 480, 495, 504, 505
Glatt, M. M., et al., **84:**354
Glaucoma, *see* Vision
Glazer, W. M., **84:**182
Glen, A. I. M., et al., **83:**113
Glenner, G. G., **83:**117
Gleser, G., et al., **84:**117
Gleser, G. C., **82:**144
Glick, Ira D., **82:**225, 226; **83:**171, 172, 183, 188, 193, 215, 217; et al., **82:**225
Glickman, L. S., **84:**182, 183
Glickstein, M., **84:**468
Global illness score, **82:**466
Gloger, S., et al., **84:**504
Glover, B. H., **83:**150
Glover, E., **82:**58; **83:**65; **84:**108
Glueck, B. C., **82:**453

Glueck, S. and E., **84:**96, 311, 313
Gluten hypothesis' (in schizophrenia), **82:**145–46
Godin, Y., et al., **84:**355
Goedde, H. W., et al., **84:**324
Goetzl, V., et al., **83:**438, 446
Goin, J. M. and M. K., **84:**276
Golbert, T. M., et al., **84:**353, 354
Gold, B., **84:**350
Gold, M. S., et al., **83:**122, 460; **84:**472
Goldberg, A., **82:**511; **83:**55–56
Goldberg, D. P., **84:**188, 189, 191, 195, 214; et al., **84:**198, 202
Goldberg, H., **84:**498, 499
Goldberg, R. L., **84:**182
Goldberg, S. C., **82:**178, 179, 190, 192, 193, 195; et al., **82:**175, 178, 188; **84:**219
Golden, C., et al., **82:**125
Goldfarb, Alvin I., **83:**86–87
Goldhand, S., **84:**220
Goldiamond, I., **84:**186
Goldin, L. R., et al., **83:**446, 450, 451
Goldman, R., **84:**38
Goldsmith, G. N., **83:**112
Goldsmith, L., **82:**423
Goldstein, A. A., **82:**111
Goldstein, A. J., **84:**460
Goldstein, H. S., **84:**149
Goldstein, J., **82:**351; **84:**106, 156
Goldstein, L., **84:**475
Goldstein, Michael J., **82:**155; **83:**174, 175, 243, 245, 250, 253, 256; **84:**95, 99; et al., **82:**160, 172, 219, 220; **83:**189
Goldstein, S. E., **84:**236
Goldzband, M. G., **84:**157
Gomberg, E. S., **84:**310
Gongla, P. A., **84:**401
Gonzdilov, A. V., et al., **84:**258
Good, M. I., **83:**107
Good, R. S., **84:**274
Goode, D. J., et al., **82:**203
Goodin, D. S., et al., **83:**117
Goodman, S., **84:**143
Goodwin, D. W., **83:**89; **84:**313, 320, 329; et al., **84:**316, 320
Goodwin, E., **83:**272
Goodwin, Frederick K., **83:**270, 279–81 passim, 289, 302, 306, 316, 317, 319n, 461, 468, 473, 474; **84:**472; et al., **83:**298, 481
Gorczynski, R. M., et al., **84:**224
Gordis, E., **84:**357
Gordon, A., **84:**450
Gordon, J., **83:**25
Gordon, N., **84:**117
Gorham, D. R., **82:**198
Gorman, Jack M., **84:**523; et al., **84:**407, 408, 477–80 passim
Gornick, J., **82:**62
Gorton, B. E., **84:**446
Götestam, K. G., **83:**114, 128, 129
Gottesman, I. I., **82:**94, 95, 451; **83:**291; **84:**483
Gottfries, C. G., **83:**113; et al., **83:**467
Gottheil, E., et al., **84:**332
Gottman, J., et al., **83:**223

Gottschalk, L. A., **82:**144; et al., **84:**496
Goudsmit, J., et al., **83:**111
Gould, E., **83:**490
Governor's Alcohol and Highway Safety Task Force, **84:**367
Gowdy, J. M., **82:**115, 118
Grad, J. D., **84:**124
grad de Alarcón, J., et al., **83:**417, 420
Graduate Medical Education National Advisory Committee, **84:**215
Graf, O., **84:**350
Graham, Garth, **83:**320
Grahame-Smith, D. G., **82:**129
Gralla, R., et al., **84:**254
Gram, L. F., **83:**495, 505; et al., **83:**492
Granacher, R. P., **83:**476
Grant, G. M., **82:**364n9
Grant, M., et al., **84:**368
Grant, S. J., **84:**471; et al., **84:**472
Granville-Grossman, K. L., **84:**494
Grave disability, **82:**345–47, 350. *See also* Competency/incompetency; Diminished capability/responsibility; Law and psychiatry
Graves' disease, **84:**216, 220, 222. *See also* Physical illness
Gray, J. A., **84:**408, 409, 410, 520
Grayson, J. B., et al., **84:**469
Great Britain: affective disorders studied in, **83:**293, 294, 407, 411, 479; **84:**58, 303
    behavior disorders studied in, **84:**96, 136
    diagnosis systems in, **83:**108, 407, 408–09
    drug studies and therapy in, **83:**482, 483, 485, 489
    epidemiology studies in, **84:**92, 190, 202, 206
    geriatrics in, **83:**86, 114, 116
    group-relations conferences in, **83:**32
    Hampstead Nurseries (wartime), **84:**105–06
    lithium use in (UK), **83:**320
    psychiatric morbidity in, **84:**190
    psychoanalytic approach in, **83:**26
    psychosomatic diseases studied in, **83:**174; **84:**211, 217
    schizophrenia studies in, **82:**94, 98–107 passim, 173, 217; **83:**174–75; **84:**95, 303
    suicide rate in, **83:**433
Greco, M. A., **82:**110
Greden, J. F., et al., **83:**291
Green, A., **82:**471; **84:**108, 115
Green, E. J., **83:**516
Green, J., **82:**291
Green, L. W., **84:**229
Green, M. A., **83:**116
Green, R. A., **82:**129
Greenacre, P., **83:**63; **84:**104, 105
Greenberg, I., et al., **83:**188, 189
Greenberg, I. M., **84:**181
Greenberg, R. L., **84:**48
Greenblatt, D. J., **83:**142, 493; **84:**233, 397, 483, 484, 489
Greenblatt, G. D., et al., **83:**115
Greenblatt, M., et al., **82:**218, 219
Greene, B. L., et al., **83:**189, 249
Greene, J. G., et al., **83:**114

Greene, S. M., et al., **84:**217
Greenfield, M. J., **84:**324
Greenhill, M. H., **84:**179, 180, 182, 185
Greenson, R. R., **83:**61, 330
Greenspan, K., et al., **83:**461
Greenspan, S. I., **84:**340
Greenwald, E. S., **84:**252
Greer, S., et al., **84:**218
Gregg, D., **82:**117
Gregoire, F., et al., **82:**290
Gregory, D. W., **84:**233
Gregory, J. G., **84:**275
Greist, J. H., et al., **84:**452
Gridlock couples, **82:**28. *See also* Marital problems
Grief reaction: abnormal, treatment of, **83:**520–21; **84:**62
    of amputee, **84:**272
    bereavement and, **83:**359, 361, 362, 365, 520–21; **84:**62, 157, 230, 235
        DSM-III category for (uncomplicated), **83:**375
        and immunosuppression, **84:**187, 223
        as "psychiatric syndrome," **84:**187, 217, 226
        studies of, **84:**217
    childhood, **84:**106, 111
        in separation or divorce, **84:**151, 152
    depression following, **83:**362, 365; **84:**235
        childhood depression, **82:**285, 300, 305
    of family of schizophrenic, **83:**244n
    and late-life psychiatric disorders, **83:**90–91; **84:**235
    maniacal, **83:**277
    role transition distinguished from, **84:**63
    total parenteral nutrition (TPN) and, **84:**271–72
    See also Loss
Griest, J. and T., **83:**378
Griffith, J. D., et al., **82:**137
Griffiths, J. A., **82:**102
Griffiths, R. R., et al., **84:**330
Grinker, R. R., **82:**266, 268, 416, 417, 425, 433, 437, 472, 480; **84:**107, 117, 119, 420; et al., **82:**415–18 passim, 423, 424, 426, 434, 449, 450
Grinspoon, Lester, et al., **82:**158, 218; **84:**232
Grisso, T., **82:**352
Grof, P., **83:**305, 313, 315; et al., **83:**285, 306
Groom, G. V., **82:**200
Groshong, R., et al., **82:**128; **83:**451
Gross, A., **83:**191
Gross, M., **83:**37
Gross, Milton M., **84:**303; et al., **84:**347, 354
Grosser, G. H., **83:**235; et al., **84:**117
Grossman, L., **82:**357
Grossman, M., **82:**331
Grossman, S., **84:**182, 183
Grossman, W. I., **83:**46
Grosz, H. J., **84:**407
Group for the Advancement of Psychiatry, *see* GAP
Group psychology: and "basic assumptions group," **83:**21, 25–31 passim
    Freud's explanation of, **83:**21–22, 24, 25, 34, 35

hospital staff and therapeutic community models of, **83:**28–30
and the mob/crowds, **83:**21, 22, 24, 34, 36
object-relations approach to, **83:**24–25, 31
psychoanalytic studies of, **83:**7–8, 33
Group-relations conferences (England and U.S.), **83:**32–33
Group therapy: advantages (and disadvantage) of, **84:**424–25
for alcoholism, **84:**318 (*see also* AA [Alcoholics Anonymous])
for anxiety, **84:**424–25
in childhood depression, **82:**307
couples therapy combined with, **83:**195
dangers of (with children), **84:**142
development of, **83:**26–28
family therapy difference from, **83:**184
for geriatric patient, **83:**130
for psychic trauma, **84:**118, 119
in schizophrenia, **82:**170–72, 217, 219
in sex therapy, **82:**21, 24–25, 26
for stress, **84:**229
for vascular amputee, **84:**273
See also Family therapy
Grove, O., **83:**434
Growe, G., et al., **82:**209, 211
Growth hormone (GH), *see* Hormone(s)
Gruen, P. H., et al., **82:**200, 201, 203, 290
Gruenberg, E. M., **82:**281, 283, 287; **84:**91, 93, 94
Grugett, A., **82:**58
Gruman, G. W., **83:**83
Grunberger, B., **82:**519
Grunebaum, Henry, **83:**182, 186, 195, 215, 217, 230, 238; **84:**90, 135, 139, 140, 142; et al., **83:**190, 244n; **84:**130, 131, 133, 138, 139, 140
Grunebaum, J., **84:**143
Grunhaus, L., et al., **84:**408, 479
Gruzelier, J., et al., **82:**208
Guam: neurofibrillary degeneration in, **83:**100
Gudeman, J. E., et al., **83:**467
el-Guebaly, N., **84:**135
Guerra, F., **84:**260
Gugl, **84:**352
Guilleminault, C., et al., **84:**220–21
Guilt feelings: of alcoholic, **84:**344
of bipolar patient, **83:**329
of child of divorce, **84:**151
of child of mentally ill parent, **84:**132
as depression symptom, **83:**479
childhood depression, **82:**302
incestuous experiences and, **82:**59
of rape victims, **82:**62, 63
and sexual dysfunction, **82:**31, 38, 62
of spouse of ill patient, **82:**36
surgery as cause of, **82:**38
of survivors of disaster or illness, **84:**110–11, 255
of therapist, **83:**331
Gulledge, A. D., et al., **84:**271–72
Gulliver's Travels (Swift), **83:**83
Gunderson, John G., **82:**88, 159, 413–19 passim, 423–30 passim, 433–56 passim, 466, 467, 468,

470; et al., **82:**416, 418, 419, 428, 430, 434, 436, 466
Gund-R scale, **82:**429, 430
Gunne, L. M., et al., **82:**141, 212, 214
Gunnels, J. C., **84:**266
Gurevitz, H., **82:**331
Gurland, B. J., **83:**116; et al., **83:**116
Gurman, A. S., **83:**171, 185, 190, 191
Gurney, C., et al., **84:**402
Gusfield, J., **84:**360
Gustafson, J. I., et al., **83:**112
Gutheil, Thomas G., **82:**323, 326, 327, 330, 333, 351, 353, 361n2, 368, 379–83 passim, 384n8; **84:**259n
Gutman, D., **84:**135
Guttman-type scale, **84:**309
Guttstein, S. E., **84:**182
Guze, S. B., **82:**8, 415; **83:**89, 287, 376, 379, 381, 429; **84:**96, 320, 329, 467

H

Haase, A. T., et al., **82:**122
Habituation: in skin conductance response, **84:**470
in therapy (exposure principle), *see* Exposure treatment (of phobia)
Habot, B., **83:**108
Hachinski, V. C., et al., **83:**114
Hackett, T. P., **84:**180, 186, 232, 260, 262
Haefely, W. E., **82:**139; **84:**486
Hafner, J., **84:**497
Hafner, R. J., **84:**450
Hagens, J. H., **84:**261, 263
Haglund, R. M., **83:**116; **84:**323
Hagnell, O., **83:**415, 416, 418, 420
Haier, R. J., et al., **82:**126
Hakstian, A. R., **83:**524, 525
Haley, Jay, **83:**170, 192, 220, 244, 247, 248–49
Halfway houses, *see* Rehabilitation
Hall, K., **83:**250
Hall, R. C. W., **84:**184; et al., **84:**233, 235, 253, 271
Hallam, R. S., **84:**403
Halleck, Seymour L., **82:**58, 326, 327, 361, 366n12, 392; **84:**76
Haller, L., **84:**116
Hallstrom, C., et al., **84:**494
Hällström, T., **83:**412, 413, 416–20 passim
Hallucinations, **82:**139
antipsychotics and, **82:**197, 200, 209
bipolar illness and, **83:**278, 281, 312
childhood, **82:**306
depressive disorders and, **83:**125, 362, 370, 371, 373, 381, 527
paranoid, in geriatric patients, **83:**132, 136, 137
and plasma levels, **83:**509
postoperative, **84:**263

schizophrenia and, **82**:85, 86, 87, 126, 141, 148, 149, 167, 197, 200, 209; **83**:130, 131, 138
during trauma, **84**:112, 114
See also Alcoholism; Delirium; Drug side effect(s)
Hallucinogens, *see* Drugs
Halmi, K. A., et al., **84**:219
Halonen, P., et al., **82**:121
Halpern, C. R., **82**:387
Hamadah, K., **82**:146
Hamburg, D., **84**:109, 110; et al., **84**:247
Hamilton, D. W., **84**:446
Hamilton Anxiety Scale, **84**:494–95, 498–99, 510
Hamilton Depression Rating Scale, **82**:466; **83**:362, 400, 467
Hammen, C. L., **82**:270
Hammer, M., **84**:200, 202
Hamovit, J. R., **83**:435n, 455
Hampson, J. L. and J. G., **82**:55
Hampstead Nurseries, *see* Great Britain
Handicap, *see* Learning disorders; Mental retardation; Physical handicap
Hankin, J. R., **84**:187, 189–90, 203, 205, 213; et al., **84**:213, 214
Hanlon, T. E., et al., **82**:204, 209
Hansen, J. C., **83**:222
Hanson, L. B., et al., **82**:209
Hanssen, T., et al., **82**:207
Harada, S., et al., **84**:324
Harding, C. M., **82**:88
Harding, T. W., et al., **84**:197, 205, 206, 209, 211
Hare, M., **83**:116
Hargreaves, W. A., **82**:225, 226
Harms, I., **84**:123
Harris, J. E., **84**:364
Harris, R., **83**:189
Harris, T., **83**:94, 421–22; **84**:133, 135
Harrison, M. J. G., **83**:109
Harroff, P. B., **83**:233
Harrow, M., et al., **82**:88
Hart, J. D., **84**:468
Hart, R. W., **83**:98
Hartford, J. T., **83**:99, 115
Hartford, M. E., **83**:129
Hartigan, C., **83**:304
Hartman, N., et al., **84**:408, 465, 479
Hartmann, E., **82**:128
Hartmann, Heinz, **82**:489
Hartocollis, P., **84**:35
Harvard University, **84**:360
    Department of Psychiatry, **84**:98
    Harvard Law Review, **82**:323n6, 348n66, 365, 366–67, 368, 381
Hasazi, J., **84**:137, 142, 143
Hastings, D., **82**:55
Haug, J. O., **83**:286, 372
Hauger, M., et al., **83**:444
Hauser, S. T., **83**:184
Havens, L. L., **84**:421
Havighurst, R., **83**:105
Hawkings, J., **84**:494
Hayes, C. P., **84**:266
Hayes, P., **84**:491

Hayes, T. A., et al., **84**:415
Hayes-Roth, F., et al., **84**:68
Hayflick, L., **83**:97
Haynes, J., **84**:155
Haynes, S. N., **84**:228
Hays, S. E., **82**:200, 203, 204
Headache: biofeedback vs. relaxation therapy for, **84**:228, 230, 447
    as drug/food reaction, **83**:484, 488, 491; **84**:233, 252, 358, 499, 500
    nocturnal migraine, **84**:221
    as panic or anxiety attack symptom, **84**:493
Head Start program, **84**:125–26
Health and Human Services, U.S. Department of, **82**:325
Health care system: "aftercare" (post-hospitalization) programs, **84**:140–41
    for cancer patients, **84**:243–44, 245, 255
    and children at risk, **84**:118, 138–42
    challenges to, **84**:142–43
    and consultation-liaison psychiatry, **84**:182
    dysthymic patients' use of, **83**:372, 373
    family as component of, **83**:213
    late-life use of, **83**:94–95, 117
    and mediation in divorce, **84**:155
    and mental retardation, **82**:375; **84**:122–29 passim
    somatizing patient use/overuse of, **84**:184, 213
    See also Consultation-liaison psychiatry; Family, the; Hospitalization; Nursing homes; Nursing staff; Outpatient treatment; Social support networks; Therapy; Third-party payment
Hearing loss: age-related (presbycusis), **83**:103–04, 133–34
    conductive, **83**:104, 133
    family therapy in cases of, **83**:189
    and paranoia, **83**:133–38 passim
    See also Sensory deficits
Heart, "irritable" (DaCosta's syndrome), *see* Da Costa, J. M.
Heart rate: anxiety and (tachycardia), **84**:418, 468–69, 474, 496, 502
    biofeedback regulation of, **84**:227, 228
    drug effect on, **83**:478; **84**:233, 475, 491, 492, 496, 497
    orgasm and, **82**:12
    personality type and, **84**:220
    relaxation response and, **84**:444, 445, 446
    See also Cardiac disorders
Heart transplant/surgery, *see* Surgery
Heath, D. S., **84**:274
Heath, R. G., **82**:115, 118; et al., **82**:118–19
Heber, R., **84**:125–26
Hedberg, D. L., et al., **82**:459, 462
Heermans, H. W., **84**:331
Heimann, P. A., **82**:473, 474
Heinicke and Westheimer study (of child separation from mother), **82**:275
Heinrichs, Douglas W., **82**:154, 158, 160, 161
Helgason, Larus, **83**:419n5, 425n5
Helgason, Tomas, **83**:416, 418, 419, 423, 424, 425
Heller, S. S., et al., **84**:263, 264

Hellon, C., **83**:433
Helsing, K. J., **83**:412, 413
Helzer, J. E., **83**:438, 442, 446; et al., **83**:278; **84**:309
Hematoma, subdural: in delirium, **83**:108
   and mental retardation, **84**:127
Hemmingsen, R., et al., **84**:353
Henderson, S., **83**:409, 416; et al., **84**:58
Hendrickson, E., et al., **83**:117
Hendrie, H. C., **83**:395
Henry, George W., **84**:179
Henry, J. P., **84**:221; et al., **84**:225
Henry, W., **83**:105
Henschke, P. J., et al., **83**:111
Hepatic disease/hepatitis, **84**:232, 357
Herbert, J., **84**:443
Herbert, M. E., **83**:132, 139
Heredity, *see* Family history; Genetic factors
Herjanic, M., **83**:372
Herman, C. P., **84**:219
Herpes virus(es), **82**:120, 121; **83**:109. *See also* Virus(es)
Herrington, B. S., **82**:160
Hersen, M., **82**:108, 109
Hersov, L. A., et al., **84**:96
Hertz, A., et al., **82**:213
Herz, M. I., **82**:88, 226; et al., **82**:226
Hess, R. D., **84**:154
Hess, W. R., **84**:444–45
Hestbech, J., et al., **83**:314
Heston, L. L., **82**:89, 95; **83**:101, 110; et al., **83**:110
Hetherington, E. M., **84**:152; et al., **83**:234; **84**:149, 152, 153
Hetzel, B., **83**:433
Hexter, George, **84**:114
Hicks, R., **83**:112; et al., **83**:113, 498; **84**:237
Hier, D., **82**:124; et al., **82**:124
Higgins, R. L., **84**:330
Higginson, J., **84**:239
High performance liquid chromatography (HPLC), **83**:501
Hilberman, E., **82**:63
Hilgenberg, J. C., **84**:260
Hill, A. B., et al., **83**:115
Hillbom, M. E., **84**:355
Himmelhoch, J. M., et al., **83**:279, 281
Hingson, R. M., et al., **84**:365
Hippocrates, **82**:10, 327; **83**:269; **84**:177
Hird, F., **82**:227
Hiroshima bombing, **84**:111, 116
Hirsch, J. D., **84**:487
Hirsch, S. R., **82**:172; **83**:291; et al., **82**:207
Hirschfeld, Robert M. A., **83**:286, 355, 379, 385, 387, 388, 397, 399, 406, 413, 414, 421; **84**:58n, 97, 226n; et al., **83**:384, 394
Hirschowitz, J., **82**:136; et al., **82**:211
Hispanics: in elderly population, **83**:88
History-taking: in assessment and diagnosis, **83**:116–17, 363, 384–85; **84**:236, 237
   in brief psychotherapy, **84**:13, 14–15, 27, 70
   and note-taking, **84**:31
   from elderly patient, **84**:236, 237

   in family therapy, **83**:188, 208, 231
   in genetic counseling, **83**:456
   See also Family history
Histrionic Personality Disorder, **82**:18, 436
   DSM-III criteria for, **82**:470
HLA (human leukocyte antigen), *see* Antigens
Ho, A. K. S. and C. C., **84**:359
Hoch, P., **82**:444, 462
Hocking, F., **84**:109
Hodge, S. E., **83**:111
Hodgkin's disease, **84**:240, 252, 253, 255. *See also* Cancer
Hoehn-Saric, R., **84**:409, 472
Hoenig, J., **84**:445
Hoeper, E. W., et al., **84**:196, 198, 203–09 passim, 213
Hofer, M., **83**:18; **84**:225
Hoff, L. A., **82**:61
Hoffer, A., **82**:143; et al., **82**:142
Hoffman, B., **82**:361n2
Hoffman, B. B., et al., **83**:470
Hoffman, J. W., et al., **84**:441, 444
Hoffman, P. B., **82**:349
Hogan, R. T., **83**:37
Hogarty, G. E., **82**:173, 190, 191, 193, 195; **83**:245; et al., **82**:88, 160, 173, 176, 177, 195, 219
Hogben, G. L., **84**:518
Hokin-Neaverson, M., et al., **83**:452
Holcomb, G. W., Jr., **84**:275
Holistic medicine, **84**:177, 179. *See also* Orthomolecular psychiatry
Holland, J. F., **84**:239, 243; et al., **84**:252
Holland, Jimmie C., **84**:178, 239, 246, 254, 255; et al., **84**:248, 255
Holland: drug therapy in, **83**:489
Hollender, M. H., **83**:305
Hollingshead, A. B., **83**:93, 184
Hollister, L. E., **84**:358; et al., **83**:462, 468, 473
Hollister, L. F., **83**:111, 113, 116
Holmberg, G., **84**:476
Holmboe, R., **83**:372
Holmes, T. H., **83**:394; **84**:94, 226
Holmstrom, L. L., **82**:61, 62
Holocaust, the: effects of, on surviving children/children of survivors, **84**:105, 110–11
Holroyd, J. C., **84**:228
Holter, F., **84**:115
Holzman, P., **82**:188, 189, 199, 475; **84**:92; et al., **82**:453
Holzman Thought Disorder Index, **82**:199
Homeostasis: aging and, **83**:99
Homesickness, **84**:413. *See also* Separation fears
Homophilia: gender disturbance and, **82**:51
Homosexuality, **82**:33–34
   defensive, **82**:32–33
      treatment of, **82**:34
   family therapy for (tendency), **83**:189
   narcissism and, **82**:488, 512, 519
   and sexual identity, **82**:49
Honecker, H., et al., **83**:467
Hopkins, S. M., **83**:112
Hopkins Symptoms Checklist, *see* HSCL

Hormone(s): adrenocorticotrophic (ACTH), **83**:113; **84**:225, 488
in aging, **83**:99, 102
CNS regulation of, **84**:221
cross-sexual, gender disturbance and, **82**:53
definition of, **83**:102
delirium/psychosis induced by, **84**:250
growth (GH), **84**:221
depression and, **83**:460
drug therapy and, **82**:135, 136, 203–04; **83**:469; **84**:252, 498
response of, to insulin-induced hypoglycemia, **82**:290, 292–93, 295; **84**:98
stress effect on, **84**:222, 223, 225
luteinizing (LH), secretion of, **84**:223
and memory, **83**:113
and neurohomones, **83**:102
postmenopausal use of, **82**:11, 46; **83**:149; **84**:255
and sexual development, **82**:11
thyroid, **83**:102, 303, 503; **84**:222, 223
thyroid-stimulating (TSH) response to stress, **84**:222
thyrotropin-releasing (TRH), **83**:113
thyrotropin-releasing/thyroid-stimulating (TRH/TSH) response test, **83**:121–22, 273, 289, 314
tumors (APUDomas) producing, **84**:250
See also Endocrine system
Horn, A. S., **82**:196
Horn, J. L., **83**:119
Horney, Karen, **82**:490; **83**:42–43, 45, 47, 513; **84**:418
Hornstra, R. K., **83**:365
Horowitz, M., **84**:109; et al., **84**:401
Horrobin, D., **82**:146
Horwitz, W. A., et al., **82**:217
Hosobuchi, Y., **84**:351
Hospitalization: for alcoholism, **84**:213, 299
anxiety of patient at, **84**:208
for bipolar illness, *see* Bipolar (manic-depressive) Disorder, treatment of
of borderline patients, **82**:424, 450, 470–74 passim, 483
children's reactions to, **84**:106–07
for depression, *see* Depression
distinguished (by courts) from treatment, **82**:381
economic conditions and, **82**:103
of elderly, **83**:94, 125, 145, 150; **84**:184, 231, 232, 235
for hip fracture (women), **84**:238
family evaluation preceding, **83**:188
family therapy vs., **83**:191
in forensic hospital, **82**:387, 395, 396
for gender dysphoria, **82**:54
and hospital staff group reactions, **83**:28–29
and intensive care (ICUs), **84**:232, 261–62, 263
joint, of mother and child, **84**:139–40
as least restrictive alternative, **82**:348–49 (*see also* Civil commitment)
length of, as factor, **82**:121, 138, 177, 222, 225–27, 228

and paranoia statistics, **83**:133, 137
of parent, and effect on family, **84**:133, 138
psychiatric disorder as response to, **84**:184, 208, 232, 235
psychiatric morbidity among patients under, **84**:198–203
as rejection or punishment, **83**:326
for schizophrenia, *see* Schizophrenia, treatment of
for transference psychosis, **82**:475
See also Nursing homes; Surgery; Therapy
Hospitalization Anxiety Scale, **84**:208
Hospitalization of the Mentally Ill Act, **82**:373
Hostages: released, treatment of, **84**:116, 118. *See also* Trauma, emotional/psychic
Hostility: drug therapy for, **83**:487
illness viewed as act of, **82**:36
mania and, **83**:279
postmarital, **82**:43, 44
and sexual dysfunctions, **82**:28–31 passim
and scapegoating, **83**:233–34
toward psychiatry, **83**:40, 129
toward therapist, **82**:156–57, 474 (*see also* Therapeutic relationship)
See also EE (expressed emotion)
Hotson, J. R., **84**:357
Houben, M. E., **84**:219
Hough, R. L., **84**:401
Hounsfield Units (HU): in senile dementia, **83**:117
Houpt, J. L., **83**:90, 91
Houston, B. K., **84**:220
Howell, E., **83**:42
HPLC (high performance liquid chromatography), **83**:501
Hrdina, P. D., **83**:500, 506; et al., **83**:492, 498
HSCL (Hopkins Symptoms Checklist), **84**:189, 191, 198, 499
Hsu, L. K. G., et al., **84**:221, 225
HU, *see* Hounsfield Units
Huber, G., et al., **82**:88
Hudgens, R. W., et al., **83**:385
Huessey, H., et al., **82**:463
Huey, L., **84**:359
Huffine, C. L., **82**:109
Hughes, F. W., **84**:350, 358
Hughes, J., **82**:141; et al., **83**:112
Hullin, R. P., **83**:316
Human rights, *see* Right(s)
Human rights committees, **82**:358
Human Sexuality (American Medical Association), **82**:8
Hunkeler, W., et al., **84**:487, 489
Hunt, G. M., **84**:334
Huntington, D. S., **84**:155
Huntington's chorea, **82**:121, 138; **83**:109, 366
Hurt, S. W., **82**:188, 189, 199
Hurvitz, N., **83**:190, 191
Husaini, B. A., et al., **83**:412
Huston, P. E., **83**:372; **84**:191, 194, 203–12 passim
Hutchings, B., **84**:96
Hutchinson, J. L., **84**:253

Huws, D., **82**:200
Hydinger-MacDonald, M., **82**:200
Hydrocephalus, normal-pressure, **83**:109; **84**:127, 234
Hymnowitz, P., **82**:383n6
Hyperactivity, **82**:303; **83**:283, 423, 443; **84**:100
  as symptom, **83**:283, 423, 443; **84**:98
  treatment of, **84**:414
Hypercalcemia, **84**:235, 250
  idiopathic, and mental retardation, **84**:127
Hyperkinetic syndrome, **82**:462; **84**:124, 127. *See also* ADD (Attentional Deficit Disorder)
Hypersexuality: in bipolar illness/manic episode; **82**:15; **83**:281
Hypersomnia, *see* Sleep disorders
Hypertension, **84**:219, 220
  anxiety neurosis and, **84**:465–67
  as drug/food side effect, **83**:482, 484; **84**:358
  drug therapy for, **83**:482
  intercranial, and mental retardation, **84**:127
  as "psychosomatic" disorder, **84**:198, 202, 216, 219
  relaxation therapy for, **84**:228, 230, 447
  and sleep apnea, **84**:220
  and stroke, **83**:114
Hyperventilation: and anxiety attacks, **84**:476–77, 493
  as drug side effect, **84**:233
  psychologically induced, **84**:220, 254
Hypnosis: in "abreactive" therapy, **84**:107
  in alcoholism therapy, **84**:333
  in brief psychotherapy, **84**:8, 10
  in consultation-liaison psychiatry, **84**:186
  contraindicated (for children), **84**:119
  immune response following, **84**:224
  pre- and postoperative, **84**:258, 260
  in relaxation therapy, **84**:446
  self- (in brief psychotherapy), **84**:10
  in sexual dysfunction therapy, **82**:21, 22–23
Hypoactivity: in childhood depression, **82**:297, 303
Hypocalcemia: and panic or anxiety attacks, **84**:407, 478
Hypochondriasis, **82**:491
  depression and, **83**:372, 373
  drug therapy and, **83**:143, 480
  DSM-III category for, **83**:142; **84**:211
  and prognosis for surgery, **84**:274
  See also Somatoform Disorders
  late-life, **83**:91, 142–44; **84**:236
Hypoglycemia: of alcoholic, **84**:352
  β-blockers and, **84**:491
  insulin-induced, **82**:290, 292–93, 295; **84**:98
  and mental retardation, **84**:127
  and panic disorder, **84**:482
Hypomania: as bipolar (II) disorder, **83**:278, 279, 292–98 passim, 304, 423, 424, 466
    and appeal or fear of hypomanic state, **83**:280, 285, 328, 331, 334, 335
    biologic/genetic factors in, **83**:272–73, 439–446 passim, 453
    and compliance in therapy, **83**:330, 332, 335, 337

in cyclothymic/dysthymic variants, **83**:275–77, 281
in borderline disorders, **82**:463, 464, 467
in childhood, **83**:283
depression and, **83**:288, 465
drug-induced, *see* Drug side effect(s)
as drug withdrawal effect, **83**:481
in narcissistic disorder, **82**:514
Hypotension: as drug side effect, *see* Drug side effect(s)
and mitral valve prolapse, **84**:481
Hypothalamus: and aging, **83**:99
and immune system, **84**:223
Hypothyroidism, **84**:127, 234, 235
Hysterectomy, *see* Surgery
Hysteria, **83**:376; **84**:211, 274
  "defense," **84**:429–30
  Janet's studies of, **84**:427–29, 430
  trauma and (Freud's view of), **84**:93, 430–31, 437
  See also Affective Disorders; Somatization Disorder

I

Iacono, W. C., **82**:453
Iacovides, A., et al., **84**:274
Iatrogenic disorders: drug-induced, *see* Drug side effect(s)
Iber, F. L., **84**:355
Ibsen, Henrik, **83**:40
IBTA (individualized behavior therapy for alcoholics) study, **84**:335, 336. *See also* Alcoholism
ICD (*Manual of the International Classification of Diseases, Injuries, and Causes of Death*, World Health Organization)
  ICD-6 (6th rev.), **84**:190–91
  ICD-8 (8th rev.), **84**:198, 206
  ICD-9 (9th rev.), **82**:14; **83**:380, 409, 410; **84**:302, 394
ICH, Freud's use of, **82**:488, 489
Id, **82**:497, 500, 502; **83**:23; **84**:433
ID (Index of Definition), **83**:409, 427
Idealization: of leader by group, **83**:21–22, 24, 25
  narcissistic, *see* Narcissistic Personality Disorder
  of parent(s) by child, **82**:491
Idealizing (selfobject) transference, *see* Transference
Identification: of adolescent with divorced parent, **84**:152
  "complementary," **82**:474
  in family therapy, **83**:200, 201
  of mob with leader, **83**:21, 34
  projective, *see* Projective identification
Identity: family, **83**:177–78
  individual loss of, in group, **83**:21–24 passim
Ideology: defined, **83**:34
  group, **83**: 23, 24, 25, 30, 33
  "preoedipal," **83**: 36

Ileitis, *see* Gastrointestinal disease
Ilfeld, F. W., **83:**413; **84:**58; et al., **84:**157
Illness, *see* Mental illness; Physical illness; Psychosomatic disorders; Somatic symptoms; Surgery
Imhof, P. R., et al., **84:**496
Imipramine, **83:**124, 312, 486, 487, 493–94, 496
 age, and effects of, **83:**498, 499, 509
 in anxiety disorders, **84:**395, 416, 472, 474
  agoraphobia, **84:**454–55, 459
  childhood, **84:**414–16, 418
  combined with other therapies, **84:**454–55, 504
  panic states, **83:**483–84; **84:**395, 408, 476, 480, 503–12 passim, 518
 in borderline disorders, **82:** 462, 463
 dangers of (in cardiac disease), **84:**358
 for depression, **83:**311, 361, 371, 468–69, 473–74, 479, 525
  in cancer patient, **84:**248
  childhood depression, **82:**290, 291–92, 295, 307
 vs. cognitive therapy, **83:**525
 ³H-, **83:**470
 introduction of, **83:**458, 472, 503
 lithium combined with or vs., **83:**307, 311, 318, 481
 and plasma levels, **82:**292, 295; **83:**477, 480, 497–500 passim, 504–11 passim
 sedative vs. energizing effects of, **83:**123, 476, 480
 side effects of, **83:**368, 475–78 passim, 485, 488, 509
 See also Drugs, list of
Immune system: and aging, **83:**98
 and AIDS (acquired immunodeficiency syndrome), **84:**250
 Alzheimer's disease and, **83:**111
 autoimmune disease and depression, **84:**208
 and behavioral immunology (psychoimmunology), **84:**223–24
 emotional stress (bereavement, depression, sleep deprivation) effects on, **84:**187, 222
 and mental retardation, **84:**126
 and organ transplantation, **84:**265, 266 (*see also* Surgery)
 relaxation response and, **84:**447
 and schizophrenia, **82:**114–22
Immunoassay techniques, **83:**501
Implosion, **84:**450. *See also* Behavioral approach
Impotence, **82:**14, 15, 32
 age and, **82:**46, 151
 as drug side effect, **83:**150, 475, 485
 organic dysfunctions and **83:**37–38, 46; **84:**221
 surgery and, **82:**39, 46; **84:**260, 273
 therapy for, **82:**21
  and failure rate in dual-sex therapy, **82:**25
  prosthetics, **84:**275
 See also Psychosexual dysfunctions
Impulse disorders, **82:**33. *See also* Psychosexual dysfunctions
Impulsivity: in borderline patients, **82:**423, 424 450–57 passim, 462
Imura, H., et al., **84:**225

INAC (Intensive Nursing Aftercare Project), **84:**140–41, 143
Incest, **82:**34, 56; **84:**116
 aftermath of, **82:**32, 57–61
 defined, **82:**57
 group prohibition against, **83:**25, 34
Incontinence: depression with psychomotor retardation and, **84:**236
 enuresis, **84:**299
  childhood, **82:**51; **84:**411
 fecal, biofeedback control of, **84:**228, 230 (*see also* Encopresis)
Index of Definition, *see* ID
India: schizophrenia studies in, **82:**98–104 passim, 137–38
Individuation, *see* Self
Industrial revolution, **83:**35
Infancy: "autism" in (normal), **83:**10–11
 depression in, **82:**274–75, 293; **83:**360 (*see also* Childhood depression)
 empathy during, **83:**19–20; **84:**121
 implications of research on, for psychoanalysis, **83:**7, 8–21
 individuation (sense of self) during, **83:**14–15, 19
 infant-object interaction in, **82:**495
 intersubjectivity in, **82:**18–19
 learning and "knowledge" in, **83:**11–15
 memory during, **83:**15–18
 psychosocial risks in, **84:**87
 selfobject in structure building in, **82:**501
 "stimulus barrier," in, **83:**9–11; **84:**108
 symbiotic phase of, **82:**48, 55, 56; **83:**13, 14, 35
 See also Childhood; Children at risk
Infantile personality, **82:**433
Infant mortality, **82:**274. *See also* Mortality rate
Infections(s): Alzheimer's disease as, **83:**111
 and delirium, **84:**232, 250
 and dementia (reversible), **84:**234
 fetal, **82:**120
 resistance to, **82:**115, **83:**98
 schizophrenia and, **84:**460
 See also Immune system; Physical illness; Viruses
Infertility: drug and/or radiation therapy as cause of, **84:**255. *See also* Psychosexual dysfunctions
Informed consent: difficulties of, **84:**242–43, 259–60
 law of, *see* Law and psychiatry
Inglis, J., et al., **84:**228
Inhibited sexual response, *see* Impotence; Orgasm; Sexual response
Inhibitions, Symptoms and Anxiety (Freud), **84:**432
Injury, *see* Physical harm; Physical illness
Innes, G., **84:**460
Inness, I., **84:**350
Inouye, E., **82:**451
Inpatients, *see* Hospitalization; Nursing homes; Surgery
Insanity defense, **82:**387, 389–92. *See also* Law and psychiatry
Insel, T. R., **84:**401; et al., **84:**488, 490, 514, 515–16
Insight: in borderline patients, **82:**475–76

defined, **84:**17
-oriented therapy, *see* Therapy
and success of therapy, **84:**26, 31, 344
Insomnia: as alcohol withdrawal symptom, **84:**356
bipolar illness and, **83:**277, 279, 281
as cancer symptom, **84:**248
depression and, **83:**373, 375
childhood depression, **82:**304
as drug side effect, **83:**485
drug therapy for, **83:**480; **84:**248
dysthymia and, **83:**277, 373
late-life, **83:**145–46
distinguished from sleep needs, **83:**115, 145–46
psychosocial dwarfism and, **82:**293
See also Sleep disorders
Institute of Medicine, **83:**146; **84:**301, 362
Institute of Psychiatry (London), **82:**103
Institutionalization: of elderly, **83:**128
and mortality rate (schizophrenia), **84:**460
See also Civil commitment; Health care system; Hospitalization; Mental retardation
Insulin: hypoglycemia induced by, **82:**290, 292–93, 295; **84:**98
stress and, **84:**222
See also Endocrine system
Insurance companies, *see* Third-party payment
Intelligence quotient, *see* IQ
Intensive care, *see* Hospitalization
Intensive Nursing Aftercare Project, *see* INAC
Internal-External Locus of Control (test), **83:**336
Internalization: as defense mechanism, **83:**237
of object relations, *see* Object relations
of superego, **83:**34
International Congress of Psychotherapy (London, 1964), **84:**25
International Journal of Psychiatry in Medicine, **84:**182
Interpersonal relationships, *see* Relationships
Interpersonal therapy, *see* Psychotherapy(ies), brief
Interpretation: in psychoanalysis and psychoanalytic psychotherapy, *see* Psychoanalysis; Psychotherapy(ies); Transference
Interpretation of Dreams, The (Freud), **84:**432
Intersubjectivity; in infancy, **83:**18–19
Intervention; and medical morbidity/mortality rate, **84:**213
preoperative, **84:**261–62
preventive (with children at risk), **84:**90–91, 125–29, 136–43, 157
psychotherapeutic (active), **84:**29
See also Crisis intervention; Education/educational intervention
Interviews: with elderly, **84:**237
family system, **83:**207–09, 231, 232, 238, 239
See also Borderline Personality Disorder, diagnosis of; History-taking; Note-taking; SCID (Structured Clinical Interview)
Invalidism: and self-esteem, **84:**267
Involuntary treatment, *see* Therapy
"Involutional" melancholia, *see* Melancholia
Iowa: "500" study, **83:**421, 426

psychiatric disorder survey in, **84:**191
IPT (interpersonal therapy), *see* Psychotherapy(ies), brief
IQ (intelligence quotient): and alcoholism, **84:**311
of children at risk, **84:**131, 133
leukemia treatment effect on, **84:**252
of mentally retarded, **84:**121, 123
Iraq: bipolar illness in, **83:**271
Ireland: schizophrenia in, **82:**120
Irritability: depression or mania and, **82:**304; **83:**274, 279, 295, 296, 330, 380, 393, 479
Irwin, H., **83:**476, 477, 478
Isbell, H., **84:**352, 353; et al., **84:**351, 355
Isberg, R. A., **84:**515
Iskander, S., et al., **84:**470–71
Islam, **84:**442. *See also* Religion
Isle of Wight study of mental retardation, **84:**124
Isolation, *see* Social isolation; Withdrawal, social
Israel: alcholism studies in, **83:**442
bipolar illness in, **83:**271, 442
children under stress studied, **84:**109
schizophrenia studies in, **82:**205
Italy: alcoholism studies in, **84:**355
Itil, T. M., et al., **82:**188
Iversen, L., **84:**350

●

J

Jaaskelainen, J., **84:**217
Jackson, Don D., **83:**170, 242
Jackson, Hughlings, **82:**167, 172
Jacob, T., **83:**174
Jacobs, D. R., **84:**216
Jacobs, J., **84:**156
Jacobs, S. C., **82:**103; et al., **83:**395
Jacobs, T. J., et al., **83:**373
Jacobsen, B., **82:**121
Jacobson, D. S., **84:**149, 154
Jacobson, E., **84:**445
Jacobson, Edith, **82:**489, 493, 511; **83:**375; **84:**19, 21
Jacobson, M., et al., **84:**362
Jacobson, N. S., **83:**220, 223
Jacobson, R., **83:**176–77
Jacobson, S., **83:**132, 139
Jain, V. K., **84:**515
James, Henry, **84:**104
James, I., et al., **84:**497
James, N. M., **83:**424, 438, 446
James, William, **84:**441
Jamieson, P. A., **84:**252
Jamison, Kay R., **83:**270, 316, 317, 319n; et al., **83:**280, 315, 317, 323, 326, 328, 333–36 passim; **84:**256, 270, 272
Jandhyala, B. S., et al., **83:**494
Janet, Pierre, **84:**426–30, 438
Janis, I., **84:**109, 257
Jankovic, B. D., et al., **82:**117
Jannoun, L., et al., **84:**452
Janov, A., **84:**425

Janowsky, D. S., **82:**133, 187; **84:**234; et al., **82:**197, 213, 214; **83:**302, 319, 330, 459, 463; **84:**476
Jansen, G., **84:**350
Jansson, L., **84:**449, 454
Japan: alcoholism studies in, **84:**324, 355
  ALDH isoenzyme patterns in, **84:**324
Japelli, G., **82:**146
Jaques, E., **83:**30
Jarpe, G., **84:**475
Jarvik, L. F., **83:**97, 112; et al., **84:**236
Jaspers, K., **82:**162
Jatlow, P. I., **83:**125, 501
Javaid, J. L., et al., **83:**494
Jefferson, J. W., **84:**233
Jeffreys, D. B., et al., **84:**350
Jellinek, E. M., **84:**315, 316, 317, 339, 360, 361
Jenike, M. A., **84:**515
Jenkins, C. D., et al., **84:**216
Jenkins, W. J., **84:**324
Jenkins Activity Survey, **83:**336
Jenner, F. A., **83:**320
Jeremiah, Book of, **84:**129
Jerram, T. C., **83:**316
Jessner, L., et al., **84:**107
Jeste, D. V., **82:**147, 148; et al., **82:**131, 137, 147, 204
Job, Book of, **83:**511
Joffee, W. G., **82:**272–73
Johansson, T., **84:**493
Johns, M. W., **84:**200, 202
Johns Hopkins University, **82:**55, 465
  Johns Hopkins Hospital, **84:**180, 246
Johnson, D. A. W., **83:**291
Johnson, F. N., **83:**320
Johnson, Judge Frank, **82:**363, 371–72, 374
Johnson, G., et al., **83:**300; **84:**495
Johnson, G. F. S., **83:**438
Johnson, J. E., et al., **84:**258
Johnson, K. M., **82:**140
Johnson, Raynor Carey, **84:**443
Johnson, R. M., **84:**354
Johnson, Virginia E., **82:**7–13 passim, 20–22 passim, 25–26, 35, 46, 63; **83:**41, 148, 149, 151; **84:**53
Johnston, D. W., et al., **84:**451
Johnston, E. C., **83:**483
Johnston, J., **84:**155
Johnston, M., **84:**256, 258
Johnston, M. H., **82:**199
Johnston, W., **84:**443
Johnstone, A., **84:**188, 191, 195
Johnstone, E. C., **82:**117; et al., **82:**123, 135, 196; **84:**516, 517
Joint Commission on Accreditation of Hospitals, **82:**325
Jonas, W., **83:**451
Jones, E., **82:**511; **83:**42, 43, 47
Jones, J. E., et al., **84:**132
Jones, J. R., **84:**260
Jones, K. R., **84:**213, 362
Jones, M., **83:**29
Jones, M. C., **84:**411

Joscelyn, K. B., **84:**362
Judaism, **84:**442, 447. *See also* Religion
Judd, L., et al., **82:**203; **84:**358, 359
Judd, Orrin, **82:**324n10
Juel-Nielsen, N., **83:**431; et al., **83:**418, 420
Jung, Carl G., **82:**488
Juvenile delinquency: family therapy for, **83:**190, 191
  mental retardation and, **84:**122
  as prediction of adult behavior, **84:**96
  See also Crime

K

Kabat-Zinn, J., **84:**447
Kaes, R., **83:**33
Kafka, M. S., et al., **82:**131; **83:**470
Kagan, J., **83:**230; **84:**130
Kagle, A., **82:**26, 28, 29, 35
Kahana, R. J., **84:**180
Kahlbaum, Karl Ludwig, **83:**269, 374
Kahn, E., **83:**365
Kahn, J. P., et al., **84:**216
Kahn, R. J., **84:**504, 506; et al., **83:**479; **84:**516, 517
Kahn, R. L., **83:**33; et al., **83:**109, 116
Kaij, L., **84:**101, 131
Kaim, S. C., et al., **84:**353, 355
Kalant, H., **84:**348, 353
Kaldor, J., **82:**128
Kales, A., et al., **83:**145
Kalin, N. H., **82:**127
Kalinowsky, L. B., **84:**352
Kalla, V. A., **82:**186
Kallmann, F. J., **82:**93, 94
Kalter, N., **84:**145, 149
Kaltreiden, M. B., et al., **84:**274
Kalucy, R. S., **84:**219
Kammeier, M. L., et al., **84:**312
Kamp, Van H., **82:**115
Kanas, N., et al., **82:**217
Kane, J., et al., **82:**195, 294; **83:**309, 311; **84:**479
Kannel, W. B., et al., **84:**403, 404
Kansas City community survey (of depression), **83:**365
Kantorovich, N. V., **84:**328, 332–33
Kaplan, B., **83:**14
Kaplan, H. S., **83:**222n1; **84:**53
Kaplan, L., **82:**471
Kaplan, S., **83:**189
Kaplan-DeNour, A., **84:**265
Kapp, F. T., **82:**61
Karacan, I., et al., **82:**46; **83:**151; **84:**221
Karambelkar, P. V., et al., **84:**445
Karasawa, T., **83:**467
Karasu, T. B., **82:**87; **83:**109; et al., **84:**231
Kardiner, A., **84:**421; et al., **82:**495
Karlsson, J. L., **84:**134
Karno, M., **82:**100
Karon, B. P., **82:**158, 217
Karoum, F., et al., **82:**137, 138
Karpel, M. A., **83:**227

Karpinski, E., **82**:57
Karush, A., **84**:439
Kasanin, J., **82**:108, 152; **83**:358
Kashani, Javad, **82**:264, 282, 284; et al., **82**:284–88 passim; **84**:97
Kaslow, F., **83**:227
Kasper, S., et al., **83**:460
Kastin, A. J., et al., **83**:113
Katan, A., **84**:104, 119
Katan, M., **84**:104
Kathol, R. G., **84**:188; et al., **84**:495
Katkin, S., et al., **82**:177
Katsrup, M., et al., **83**:417
Katz, A., **84**:261
Katz, D., **83**:33
Katz, J. L., **84**:223; et al., **84**:222
Katz, S., **82**:58, 61
Katzman, R., **83**:109
Kauai: children of, studied, **84**:88, 134
Kauffman, C., et al., **84**:103, 134, 137
Kaufman, R. M., **84**:181; et al., **84**:198, 199, 203, 207–13 passim
Kaufmann, C. L., **82**:358; et al., **82**:358
Kawecky, C. A., **83**:86
Kay, D. W. K., **83**:107, 109, 132, 133, 137; et al., **83**:91, 110
Kay, J. H., **84**:263
Kay, S. R., **82**:145
Kayed, K., et al., **84**:221
Kazdin, A. E., **82**:269, 270; **83**:516
Keat, D. B., **84**:69
Keeffe, E. B., **84**:357
Keiser, L., **84**:395
Keistein, M. D., **84**:273
Keith, D., **83**:249
Keith, Samuel J., **82**:110, 154, 170, 177; **83**:242n
Kellam, S. G., et al., **82**:174
Keller, M., **83**:276, 512; **84**:316
Keller, S. E., et al., **84**:225
Keller-Teschke, M., **82**:128
Kellner, R., et al., **84**:494
Kelly, D., et al., **84**:407, 457, 507, 511
Kelly, D. H. W., **84**:468, 469; et al., **84**:469, 478
Kelly, George A., **83**:513, 526
Kelly, J. B., **84**:145, 148–54 passim
Kemph, J. P., **84**:268; et al., **84**:266, 267
Kendall, D. A., **83**:469
Kendell, R. E., **84**:357, 358
Kendler, K. S., **83**:132; et al., **82**:89; **84**:406
Kennedy, Hansi, **84**:105
Kennedy, J., **84**:263
Kennedy, John F., effects of assassination, **84**:109
Kennedy, P., **82**:227
Kenya: psychiatric morbidity studies in, **84**:198, 206
Kerbikov, O. V., **82**:118
Kerenyi, C., **83**:83
Kernberg, Otto F., **82**:413, 415, 423–43 passim, 454, 461, 470–74 passim, 480, 486, 490–97 passim, 499n1, 511–23 passim; **83**:7–8, 24–33 passim, 51; et al., **82**:421, 426–36 passim, 471, 486
Kernberg, Paulina, **82**:437

Kernberg's Structural Interview, see Borderline Personality Disorder, diagnosis of
Kerns, R. D., et al., **84**:229
Kerr, R. A., et al., **84**:217
Kerry, R. J., **83**:331
Kessel, W. I. N., **84**:190, 192, 212
Kessler, C., **82**:201
Kessler, D. R., **83**:188, 193
Kessler, L. G., et al., **84**:213, 214
Kessler, R., et al., **84**:135
Kestenbaum, C. J., **83**:283
Kety, S. S., **82**:445n; **83**:432, 445; et al., **82**:95, 444–55 passim
Khan, M. K., **82**:471; **83**:442; **84**:108
Khantzian, E. J., **84**:339, 343, 345
Khatami, M., **84**:53
Khin-Maung-Zaw, **83**:432
Khouri, P. J., et al., **82**:448, 450, 451
Kidd, K. K., **83**:421, 427; **84**:406
Kiddie-SADS, **82**:270. See also Childhood depression; SADS (Schedule for Affective Disorders and Schizophrenia)
Kidney transplant, see Surgery
Kielholz, T., **83**:373; et al., **83**:311
Kiloh, L. G., **83**:107, 108, 381; et al., **82**:186; **83**:479
Kilpatrick, D. M., et al., **82**:61, 63
Kiltie, H., **82**:180, 184
Kimball, C. D., et al., **84**:351
Kimball, C. P., **84**:213
Kincaid-Smith, P., **83**:314
Kindon, D., **84**:273
King, A., **84**:507
King, J. A., **82**:175
King, S., **83**:276, 449
Kingstone, E., **84**:357
Kinney, D., **82**:121
Kinsey, A. C., et al., **82**:7, 20, 43, 58, 62; **83**:151
Kinsman, R. A., et al., **84**:219
Kirk, S. A., **82**:177
Kirkegaard, C., **83**:460; et al., **82**:290
Kirschenbaum, J., **83**:233
Kisimoto, A., **83**:312
Kissin, B., **84**:356, 358
Kitanaka, I., et al., **83**:498
Kjellman, B. F., et al., **83**:315
Klassen, D., **83**:365
Kleber, R. J., **84**:516, 517
Klee, W. A., et al., **82**:146
Klein, Donald F., **82**:108, 413, 436, 443, 458–65 passim; **83**:288; **84**:390–98 passim, 403, 414, 437, 459, 503, 504, 505, 511; et al., **82**:463, 464; **83**:126, 479; **84**:390, 412
Klein, Joel I., **82**:321, 322, 326, 348n, 364
Klein, Melanie, **82**:474, 516; **83**:26, 218
Klein, R. H., **84**:132
Kleinberg, D. L., **82**:204
Kleinman, Joel E., et al., **82**:132–36 passim, 142
Klerman, Gerald L., **82**:281, 283, 284, 415–28 passim, 436, 456; **83**:47, 50, 92, 273, 277, 278, 287, 294, 296, 304, 321, 365, 372, 379–88 passim, 406, 407, 411, 412, 419–26 passim, 519; **84**:8, 10, 58, 99, 184, 187, 402; et al., **82**:161; **83**:381, 481, 519, 524; **84**:8, 10, 63

Klett, C. J., **82:**205
Kline, N. S., **83:**482; et al., **82:**141; **83:**506; **84:**358
Kline, S. A., **84:**357
Knapp, P. H., et al., **84:**219
Knapp, S., **83:**20
Knee, S. T., **84:**357
Knight, A., **83:**291; et al., **82:**227
Knight, M. L., **84:**469
Knight, R. P., **82:**423, 434, 444, 471, 480; **84:**339, 340
Kniskern, D. P., **83:**171, 185, 190, 191
Knorr, N. J., **84:**273
Knowledge: abstract, of infant, **83:**12–14. *See also* Cognition; Memory
Knupfer, G., **84:**315
Ko, G. N., et al., **84:**472
Kobele, S., et al., **82:**422, 423
Koch, C., **84:**219
Koch, Robert, **82:**82
Koch-Weser, J., **83:**493
Kocsis, J. R., **83:**300
Koczkas, S., et al., **84:**511
Koe, B. K., **84:**485
Koenigsberg, H., **82:**422, 424, 428, 433
Kohn, M. L., **82:**98, 107
Kohut, Heinz, **82:**414, 437, 487, 490–505 passim, 510, 511, 512, 523; **83:**20, 51, 55, 59; **84:**339
Kokes, R. F., et al., **82:**108; **84:**131, 133
Kolakowska, T., et al., **82:**200, 202, 203
Kolb, J. E., **82:**417, 419, 423–34 passim, 438–43 passim, 448–57 passim, 467, 468
Kolb, L. C., **84:**272
Koliaskina, G., et al., **82:**117, 119
Koob, G. E., **84:**223
Kopeikin, H. S., **83:**245, 250, 253; et al., **83:**243, 256
Koppanyi, T., et al., **84:**348
Korff, J., **83:**452
Kornblith, S. J., **83:**516, 517, 524
Kornfeld, Donald S., **84:**178, 186, 231, 238, 260, 261, 275; et al., **84:**232, 262, 263, 264, 265
Kornhauser, L., **84:**155
Korsakoff's syndrome (alcohol amnestic disorder), *see* Alcoholism
Korsten, M. A., et al., **84:**323
Koster, F., **84:**263
Kotin, J., **83:**281
Kotz, J., et al., **84:**353
Koutsky, C. D., **84:**353
Kovacs, Maria, **82:**268, 269, 270, 283; **83:**356, 513, 516, 524; et al., **83:**525; **84:**49
Kraepelin, Emil, **83:**372; **84:**57, 93
    and concept of manic-depressive insanity, **83:**272–79 passim, 285, 292, 357–59, 407, 423, 512
    and Kraepelinian tradition, **82:**108, 166, 197; **83:**184, 323, 360, 374, 407, 444
    and nosology, **82:**82–88 passim, 112–13, 149; **83:**269, 270, 282, 392, 487
    on "paraphrenia," **83:**131, 137; **84:**93
Krafft-Ebing, Richard von, **82:**8; **83:**269
Kraft, I. A., **84:**269, 416
Kragh-Sorensen, P., **83:**492, 497, 503, 507, 510

Kraines, S. H., **83:**279
Krakauer, H., et al., **84:**266
Kral, V. A., **83:**107
Kramer, C. H., **83:**236
Kramer, M., **83:**130, 407
Kraml, M., **84:**357
Kramp, P., **84:**353
Krasner, B., **83:**187, 199
Krauthammer, C., **83:**277, 287, 294, 296, 381, 406, 419, 423–26 passim
Kreitman, N., **83:**434
Kretschmer, E., **83:**392
Kringlen, E., **82:**94, 95, 451; **83:**441
Kris, A. O., **83:**64
Kris, Ernst, **84:**11, 108
Kris, M., **84:**110
Krishnan, G., **84:**496
Kroll, J., et al., **82:**415, 420–29 passim, 433–34, 436, 437
Krope, P., et al., **84:**496
Krout, J. A., **84:**360
Krueger, J. C., et al., **84:**274
Krupp, I. M., **82:**115, 118
Kryso, J., **82:**58
Kryspin-Exner, V. K., **84:**354
Krystal, H., **84:**110
Kubanis, P., **83:**110
Kugel, R. B., **84:**128
Kugler, J., et al., **83:**112
Kuhar, M. J., **84:**486
Kuhn, B. and R., **82:**291
Kuhn, R., **83:**472, 503
Kuhn, T. S., **83:**37
Kuiper, N. A., **84:**229
Kuipers, L., **83:**246
Kukopulos, A., et al., **83:**313
Kulcar, Z., et al., **83:**417
Kumar, N., **82:**186; **83:**417
Kuperman, S., **82:**282, 284, 289
Kupfer, D. J., **82:**290, 453; et al., **82:**290, 294; **83:**121, 273, 274, 279, 283, 289, 291, 355, 439, 506; **84:**275
Kuriansky, J. B., et al., **82:**86
Kurland, A. A., **82:**198; et al., **82:**212
Kurland, H. D., **84:**200, 202
Kuro disorder, **82:**120
Kurucz, J., et al., **83:**110

L

L-γ-aminobutyric aid, *see* GABA
L-dopa, L-tryptophan, *see* Drugs, list of
Laakman, G., **82:**290
La Barre, W., **83:**136
L'Abate, L., **83:**223
Labeling: diagnostic, **82:**265; **84:**75, 142
Labor, U.S. Department of, **84:**143
Lacey, G., **84:**111
Lachmann, F., **82:**511

Lactate infusions, *see* Drug therapy (for anxiety states)
Lader, M., **84:**220, 403, 404, 450, 457, 468, 470, 494–501 passim; et al., **84:**470
Laing, R. D., **82:**217
Lake, R. C., et al., **82:**132
Lal, S., **82:**201
Lamb, H. R., **84:**137
Lamb, M. E., **83:**10
Lamendola, N. F., **84:**264
Lampl-de Groot, J., **82:**499n1
Landauer, A. A., et al., **84:**358
Landis, D. H., **83:**460
Landis, J. T., **82:**58
Landowski, J., et al., **83:**467
Lang, R., et al., **84:**444
Langer, E. J., et al., **84:**259
Langer, G., **82:**200; et al., **82:**200, 290
Langer, S. Z., et al., **83:**470
Langer, T. S., **83:**93
Langfeldt, G., **82:**85
Langley, G. E., **83:**125, 137
Langley Porter Psychiatric Institute, **82:**215, 226, 271
Langsley, D. G., et al., **82:**172, 225; **83:**188, 189
Langston, J. W., **84:**357
Language: and memory, **83:**16, 17–18, 70. *See also* Cultural factors; Speech
Lansky, D., **84:**331
LaPierre, Y. D., **83:**500, 506; **84:**493
Laplanche, J., **82:**488, 489
Lapolla, A., **82:**205
Lapouse, R., **84:**411
Larry, J. C., **82:**100
Larsen, N. E., **83:**497
Larsson, T., et al., **83:**110
Lasch, C., **83:**34, 35–36
Last, U., et al., **82:**461
Late-life psychiatric disorders: affective, **83:**118–130
  assessment of, **83:**116–17
  bipolar illness, **83:**125–26, 285
  delirium, **83:**107, 108; **84:**232–34, 275
  depressive, *see* Depression
  epidemiology/prevalence rate of, **83:**87–92, 95
    historical trends in, **83:**92–93
  etiology of, **83:**90–91, 93–94, 140–51
  late-onset schizophrenia, **83:**91–92, 94–95, 130–132, 138
  manic episode, **83:**125, 285; **84:**235, 236
  paranoia ("suspiciousness"), **83:**92, 95, 131–37
  physiological changes and, **83:**140–51
  postoperative, **84:**275
  prognosis for, **83:**116
  somatoform, **83:**119, 127, 140–45 passim; **84:**231, 236
  therapy for, **83:**113, 128–30, 141–44 passim; **84:**25, 232–35, 236–38 (*see also* Drug therapy; Psychotherapy[ies])
  See also Aging; Anxiety; Dementia, Primary Degenerative; Drug side effect(s); Geriatric psychiatry
Latent stages of development, *see* Childhood

Laties, V. G., et al., **84:**354
Laughren, T. P., **82:**135, 203; et al., **82:**135
Law: and alcohol/drunken driving, **84:**366–67
  family (divorce, custody, etc.), *see* Family, the
  and retarded children, **84:**123, 126
  and traumatized children, **84:**115–16
Law and psychiatry, **82:**321–96
  and drug therapy, **82:**382
  and insanity defense, **82:**387, 389–92
  and law of informed consent, **82:**350–55, 396; **84:**259–60 (*see also* Competency/incompetency)
  and least restrictive alternative, *see* Civil commitment
  malpractice claims, **82:**326, 329
  and misdiagnosis, **83:**272
Lawrence, W. G., **83:**30
Lawson, D. M., **84:**331
Layne, O. Z., **84:**263
Lazare-Klerman-Amor Personality Inventory (LKA), **83:**387, 393
Lazarus, Arnold A., **84:**8, 10, 67, 68, 70, 74, 75
Lazarus, H. R., **84:**261, 263
Lazarus, R. S., **84:**257; et al., **84:**109
Leach, K. A., **82:**429
Lead poisoning, **84:**127
Learned helplessness: and depression, **82:**286; **83:**412
Learning: by conditioning, **84:**18
  in infancy, **83:**11–14
  psychotherapy as form of, **84:**19
  of social skills, **83:**517–18, 521, 524
  See also Cognition; Conditioning
Learning disorders: and borderline personality disorders, **82:**441, 454
  and childhood depression, **82:**277, 286, 287, 302, 306
  hemispheric assymetry and, **82:**124
  See also School, attitude toward or performance in
Least restrictive alternative, *see* Civil commitment
Leavy, S. A., **83:**63
LeBlanc, H., et al., **82:**200
Le Bon, G., **83:**22
Leckman, J. F., et al., **83:**448, 467; **84:**396, 511
Lecrubier, Y., et al., **83:**470
Lee, K., **84:**465
Leeman, M. M., **83:**438
Lefave, W. R., **82:**342n31
Leff, Julian P., **82:**88, 102, 104, 105, 172, 173; **83:**174, 175; **84:**95; et al., **82:**102; **83:**245, 246
Leff, M. J., **83:**286, 456
Lefkowitz, M. M., **82:**266, 267–68
Lefkowitz, R. F., **83:**470
Left-handedness: and schizophrenia, **82:**124
Lehmann, H. E., **82:**143; **83:**271, 420; et al., **82:**212
Lehmann, J. W., **84:**447
Lehmann, S., **82:**107
Leifer, R., **84:**181
Leigh, H., **84:**216
Leighton, A. H., **84:**12
Leighton, D. C., et al., **83:**91, 93, 412

Leitenberg, H., et al., **84**:453
LeLord, G., et al., **82**:291
LeMay, M., **82**:124
Lemberger, L., **82**:203
Lemere, F., **84**:328, 333
Lentz, R. J., **82**:110, 175
Leon, G. R., et al., **82**:267, 269, 272
Leonhard, K., **83**:269, 272, 275, 368, 423, 441
Leopold, R., **84**:117
Lepeshinskaya, O. B., **83**:84
Lepsitt, L. P., **83**:16
Lereboullet, J., et al., **84**:354
Lerner, A., **84**:120
Lerner, H., **83**:44
Lerner, P., et al., **82**:127
Lesse, S., **83**:373
Lesser, I. M., **84**:218
Leukemia: Down's syndrome and, **83**:110
    drug (and combined) therapy for, **84**:252
    maintenance (and ending) of, **84**:255
    improved survival from, **84**:240, 242
    See also Cancer
Levander, V. L., et al., **84**:444
Levay, Alexander N., **82**:8, 26, 28, 29, 35
Levenson, A. J., **84**:232, 235
Levine, A. S., **84**:245
Levine, D. B., **84**:275
Levine, H. G., **84**:360, 361
Levine, J., **82**:108, 188, 195; **84**:117; et al., **82**:191, 195
Levine, P. M., et al., **84**:247
Levine, R. S., **82**:364n9, 367n14
Levine, T. M., **83**:283
Levinson, D., et al., **83**:216
Levinson, H., **83**:33
Levis, D. J., **84**:421, 450
Levitan, S. J., **84**:186, 238, 275
Levitt, M., **83**:451; et al., **83**:451
Levy, David, **84**:106–07, 115, 119
Levy, P., et al., **84**:366
Levy, R., et al., **84**:349
Lewin, Kurt, **83**:26
Lewine, R. R. J., **84**:134; et al., **84**:101, 134
Lewinsohn, P. M., **83**:383, 516–19 passim, 524; et al., **83**:516, 517
Lewinsohn, R., **83**:364
Lewis, Sir Aubrey, **84**:401
Lewis, J. L., **83**:278, 311
Lewis, J. M., **83**:184, 230, 233; et al., **84**:95
Lewis, M., **84**:412
Lewis, M. J., et al., **84**:357
Lewis, T., **84**:479
Lewis, W. C., **84**:212
LH (luteinizing hormone), *see* Hormone(s)
Li, T. K., **84**:324
Liaison psychiatry, *see* Consultation-liaison psychiatry
Libb, J. W., **83**:114
Liberman, Robert Paul, **82**:92; **83**:174n, 242n, 245–47 passim, 253, 256, 434; **84**:95n; et al., **82**:107, 110–11
Libido theory, **82**:488–89, 490, 511, 512; **83**:15, 41, 49; **84**:432, 433, 437

Libiková, H., et al., **82**:121
Libow, L. S., **83**:108, 119; **84**:234
Lichtenberg, J., **83**:11
Lichtenstein, H., **82**:499n1; **83**:42, 49
Lidz, Theodore, **83**:170, 242; et al., **82**:172
Lieb, J., **83**:483
Lieber, C. S., **84**:324
Lieberman, M. A., **84**:58
Liebman, R., et al., **83**:189
Liebowitz, J. H., **83**:271, 442
Liebowitz, Michael R., **82**:415, 443, 457, 459, 463; **83**:288; **84**:459, 478, 512, 516, 524; et al., **83**:384, 387, 388; **84**:472, 511
Liebson, I., **84**:330, 356; et al., **84**:334
Liedeman, R. R., **82**:117
Lief, H. I., **83**:173, 216; **84**:53
Liem, J. H., **82**:155; **83**:174
Life cycles, *see* Family, the
Life events, *see* Stress
Life expectancy, **83**:89. *See also* Mortality rate
Life style: and mortality rate, **84**:217, 239. *See also* Alcoholism
Lifton, R. J., **84**:107, 111, 247
Lindberg, D., **82**:216; **83**:112
Lindelius, R., **82**:93
Lindemann, C. A., **84**:261
Lindemann, E., **84**:157, 247, 474, 476
Lindros, K. O., **84**:323; et al., **84**:323, 349
Lindstrom, L. H., **82**:207
Lindy, J., et al., **84**:118
Ling, W., et al., **82**:282, 289, 291
Linkowski, P., **83**:449
Linn, L., **82**:174; **84**:203, 204
Linn, M. W., et al., **82**:175, 177, 227
Linnoila, M., et al., **82**:203; **83**:461; **84**:358
Lipinski, J. F., Jr., **83**:279, 424
Lipinski, T., et al., **82**:212
Lipofusin: in aging process, **83**:97, 100, 112
Lipowski, Z. J., **83**:107; **84**:177–86 passim, 187, 213, 231–38 passim, 250, 253
Lippa, A. S., et al., **84**:484
Lipsedge, J. S., et al., **84**:507, 508
Lipsedge, M., **82**:102
Lipsitt, D. R., **83**:373
Lipsitt, I. R. and M. P., **84**:186
Lipton, F. R., et al., **82**:107
Lipton, G., **84**:115
Lipton, R. B., et al., **82**:453
Lipton, R. C., **84**:128
Lishman, W. A., **82**:124
Lisman, S. A., **84**:326, 330
Liston, E. J., Jr., **83**:107; **84**:232, 236
Lithium Clinic (New York State Psychiatric Institute), **83**:296
Lithium therapy, **82**:465; **83**:269, 271, 320
    in bipolar disorder, **82**:444; **83**:126, 249–51 passim, 272–76 passim, 281–89 passim, 299–304, 307–18, 320–37, 369, 375, 380, 439, 466, 481
    (*see also* in manic states, *below*)
    in borderline disorders, **82**:444, 463–67 passim
    for cancer patient, **84**:249

for children, **83:**283
combined with antipsychotics, **82:**152, 208; **83:**126, 300–301, 302–03
combined with psychotherapy, **83:**320–37
clinical reports on, **83:**324–25
combined with or vs. TCAs, **83:**126, 281, 307, 311–12, 318, 481–82
compliance/noncompliance with, **83:**301, 312–18 passim, 321–37
for depressed alcoholics, **84:**358–59
dosage, **83:**126, 299–300, 303, 316–17, 318
duration of, **83:**315, 318
and genetic studies of affective disorders, **83:**446, 452–53
for geriatric patient, **83:**126, 285, 321n
and high lithium ratio, **83:**452–53
in manic states, **82:**208, 209; **83:**295–303 passim, 359, 453, 454–55
monitoring of, **83:**470; **84:**249
vs. placebo, **83:**298, 307, 318, 481
in schizophrenia/schizoaffective disorders, **82:**136, 152, 208–09, 210–11; **83:**439
side effects of, **83:**126, 299, 301–02, 313–15, 321, 326–27, 331–33, 336
studies of (U.S.), **83:**307, 311, 316–317, 322, 332–37 passim, 371
in unipolar depression, **83:**274
See also Drug therapy
Litin, E. M., **84:**262
Little, M., **82:**471, 472, 475
Littlewood, R., **82:**102
Litwack, T. R., **82:**339n17
Liver disease: drug therapy and, **83:**128
LKA, *see* Lazare-Klerman-Armor Personality Inventory
Lloyd, C., **82:**285; **83:**385, 404; et al., **83:**398, 399, 400
Lloyd, G. G., **84:**214
Locher, L. M., **83:**372
Locke, B. Z., **84:**191, 194, 203, 205, 213
Loevinger, Jane, **82:**279, 280
Loew, C. A., **83:**114
Loewald, H., **83:**60
Logan, J., **83:**327–28
London, W. P., **83:**288
Loo, H., et al., **83:**317
Loofbourrow, G. N., **84:**476
Loosen, P. T., **83:**121; **84:**97
Lopez-Ibor, J., Jr. and J. M., **84:**393
LoPiccolo, J. and L., **83:**222n1
Loranger, A. W., **83:**283
Lorge, I., **83:**128
Los Angeles Police Department, **84:**116
Loss: and childhood depression, **82:**272, 286, 287
denial of, **83:**277
and depressive disorders, **83:**395, 399, 400, 514, 521, 522; **84:**19–20, 217
and geriatric paranoia/anxiety, **83:**135–41 passim
role transition as, **84:**63
See also Drug side effect(s); Grief reaction; Sensory deficits; Separation and divorce; Stress

Lottman, M. S., **82:**363, 365, 366, 367nn14, 15
Lourie, R., **84:**124
Lovett, L. C., et al., **82:**118
Low achievement: in borderline patients, **82:**425, 457
Lowell, P., **84:**443
Lowell, R., **83:**327
Lowenstein, L. M., et al., **84:**349
Lowenthal, M. F., **83:**90, 132
Lown, B., **84:**219; et al., **84:**447
Lucas, A. R., **82:**286
Lucente, F. E., **84:**208, 210
Luchins, Daniel J., et al., **82:**124, 145
Luchterhand, E., **84:**117
Ludwig, A., **82:**109
Luisada, P. V., **82:**140
Lum, L. C., **84:**477
Lunde, D. T., **84:**268, 269
Lundquist, G., **83:**372; **84:**354
Lundwall, L., **84:**356
Luparello, T., et al., **84:**224
Lupus erythematosus, systemic: chlorpromazine and, **82:**118
resemblance of, to bipolar illness, **83:**287
schizophrenia and, **82:**117
Luteinizing hormone (LH), *see* Hormone(s)
Luthe, W., **84:**445
Lutkins, S. G., **84:**217
Luton, F. H., **83:**416
Lydiard, R. B., **83:**487
Lying: as contraindication for supportive psychotherapy, **82:**481
Lykken, D. T., **82:**453
Lymphocytes: and immune response, **82:**114, 115, 117–18; **84:**223
MAO activity in, **82:**147
Lymphoma, *see* Tumors
Lynge, J., **83:**434
Lyons-Ruth, K., et al., **84:**136, 141, 142, 143
Lysenko, T. D., **83:**84
Lyskowski, J., **82:**461

M

Maas, J. W., **83:**459, 460, 461, 474; et al., **82:**144; **83:**459, 461, 468, 473
McAlister, A., **84:**368; et al., **84:**368
McAllister, T. W., **83:**107, 109; **84:**236; et al., **84:**236
McAndrew Score, **84:**325
McCabe, B., **83:**484, 491n
McCabe, L. J., **83:**422
McCabe, M. S., **83:**295, 302, 440, 441
McCahill, T. W., **82:**62
McCarty, D., **84:**351
McClure, J. N., **84:**407, 477
McCollam, J. B., et al., **84:**331
McCombie, S. L., **82:**61
McConaghy, N., **84:**450
McConville, B. J., et al., **82:**276, 277, 282

McCord, W. and J., **84:**96, 312
McCoy, R. T., **84:**330
McCranie, E. W., **82:**177
McCutcheon, B. A., **84:**450
McDaniel, S. M., **84:**224
McDermott, J. R., et al., **83:**111
McDermott, J., Jr., **83:**239
Macdonald, J. M., **82:**58
MacDonald, M. R., **84:**229
MacDonald, N. E., **84:**261
McDonald, R., et al., **84:**452
McDonald, R. J., **83:**112, 316–17
McEvoy, J. P., **84:**237
McFarland, D. D., **84:**231
McFarlane, William R., **83:**172, 220, 244, 248, 253, 255; **84:**95n
McGarry, A. L., et al., **82:**355, 387
McGee, T. E., **83:**115
McGeer, E. G. and P. L., **82:**139
McGhie, A., **83:**90
McGlashan, T. H., **82:**88
McGoldrick, M., **83:**216
McGrath, S. D., **84:**354; et al., **82:**143
McGuffin, P., **82:**121
McHugh, P. R., **83:**107, 289; **84:**234
McInnes, R. G., **84:**404
McIntosh, I. D., **84:**213
Mack, J. E., **82:**415, 437; **84:**107, 116–17, 339, 343
MacKain, K., et al., **83:**13
Mackay, A. V., et al., **82:**134
McKegney, F. P., **84:**182, 186
Mackenzie, A. I., **84:**350
McKenzie, J. M., **84:**222
Mackenzie, T. B., **84:**402
McKinney, W. T., Jr., **83:**272
Macklin, R., **83:**37, 38, 50
McKnew, D. H., **82:**266, 269, 287, 303; et al., **82:**285; **83:**283; **84:**97
McLaughlin, A. I. G., et al., **83:**111
McLean, C. S., **83:**244n
MacLean, G., **84:**120
McLean, P. D., **83:**516, 517, 524, 525
McLean Hospital, **82:**226, 417, 456, 461, 466
MacMahon, B., **83:**87, 89, 94, 406
McMeekan, E. R. L., **82:**124
McMillan, W. P., **84:**495
McNair, D. M., **84:**504, 506
McNamara, J. O., et al., **84:**485
McNamee, H. B., et al., **84:**348
McNaughten Rule, **82:**391, 392
McNeil, T. F., **84:**101, 131
MacRitchie, K. L., **84:**271
MacVane, J. R., Jr., et al., **83:**250
Madanes, C., **83:**223, 244, 247, 248–49
Madden, J. S., et al., **84:**354
Maddox, G. L., **83:**95, 144, 150
Maddrey, W. L., **84:**353
Mader, R., **84:**354
Maggi, A., et al., **83:**469
Maggs, R., **83:**298
Magnes, L. J., **84:**324
Magnesium levels: in alcohol withdrawal reactions, **84:**355–56

Maguire, G. P., et al., **84:**201, 202, 207, 208, 210, 270, 271, 274
Mahler, Margaret S., **82:**275, 471, 493, 511; **83:**14, 51; et al., **82:**49, 55, 511; **83:**10, 14
Mahoney, J. J., **83:**516
Mahoney, M. J., **84:**337
Main, T. F., **83:**28, 29; **84:**139
Majchrowicz, E., et al., **84:**349
Majerus, P. W., et al., **84:**212
Major Depression, **83:**275, 292, 365, 375
alcoholism and, **84:**314
bereavement and, **84:**187
cancer and, **84:**246, 248–49
DSM-III category for, **83:**119–20, 367–75 passim, 410, 479, 506; **84:**61, 63, 246, 396, 397
and supplemental classifications, **83:**375, 379–80
epidemiology/prevalence rate of, **84:**206, 214
late-life, **84:**236
with melancholia/psychotic features, **83:**120, 121, 125, 126, 367, 370; **84:**49, 396
with melancholia and without psychotic features, **83:**122–25, 369–70, 506
without melancholia, **83:**120, 128, 367
neurotic forms of, **83:**371
nonbipolar, **83:**287–88, 410
obsessive-compulsive patients and, **84:**515–16
personality and, **83:**392
prepubertal, **84:**98 (*see also* Childhood depression)
and suicide, **83:**429
treatment of, **83:**369, 370; **84:**49
TCA response in, **83:**122–25, 289, 359, 369, 370, 371, 505
See also Depression; Melancholia; Unipolar/nonbipolar depression
Malan, D. H., **83:**523; **84:**7, 8, 9, 12, 25, 27; et al., **83:**27
Malcolm, M. T., et al., **84:**357
Malcolm, R. M., et al., **84:**271
Male(s): anatomy of, **82:**9–10 (*see also* Genitalia)
catecholamine levels in, **83:**133
dementia (repeated or multiinfarct) in, **83:**115
elderly, U.S. population figures, **83:**88
life expectancy for, **83:**89
lithium compliance by, **83:**333
masturbation by, as therapy, **82:**24
pre- and postmarital sexuality of, **82:**43
schizophrenia in, **82:**108; **84:**101
sterility of (as drug or radiation effect), **84:**255
and suicide, **83:**431, 433
surgery on, **82:**38–39
See also Father, the; Orgasm; Sex differentiation
Malignancy, *see* Cancer
Malih, S. C., **82:**186
Malmquist, C., **82:**58, 266, 274
Malnutrition: of alcoholic, **84:**352, 460
of cancer patients, **84:**250
and geriatric disorders, **83:**93–94
and infant depression, **82:**274
during pregnancy, **84:**126
See also Diet

Malone, Charles A., **83**:171, 172, 192, 220, 229–40 passim; **84**:225n; et al., **83**:229
Maloney, A. J. F., **83**:109
Malpractice claims, *see* Law and psychiatry
Mancini, A. M., et al., **82**:201
Mandel, N., **83**:480
Maneker, J. S., **84**:145
Manganese poisoning, **82**:144
Mania: and competency, **82**:354
defined, **83**:269, 274–75
drug-induced, **83**:323; **84**:235 (*see also* Drug therapy)
DSM-III concept of, **83**:278–79, 293–95, 296, 357
dysphoric mood in, **83**:279
in elderly, **83**:125–26, 285; **84**:235, 236
lithium treatment of, *see* Lithium therapy
morbidity risk of, **82**:290; **83**:287–88
postpartum, **83**:277
precipitants of, **83**:277, 287, 311 (*see also* Drug side effect[s])
reactive, **83**:277 (*see also* Grief reaction)
secondary, **83**:277–78, 279, 287, 294, 296, 297, 376, 381
See also Hypomania; Manic Episode; Manic state (bipolar I)
Manic-depressive illness, *see* Bipolar (manic-depressive) Disorder; Major Depression
Manic-Depressive Scale, **83**:336
Manic Episode: childhood, **83**:283
defined, **83**:423
diagnosis of, **83**:293–97
drug therapy for, **83**:293–303, 337
hypersexuality and, **82**:15
late-life, **83**:125
prediction of (D-type scores), **83**:465–66
See also Bipolar (manic-depressive) Disorder; Mania; Manic state (bipolar I)
Manic state (bipolar I): classification of, **83**:304, 367, 423, 466
course of, **83**:282, 295–96, 297
distinguished from other manias, **83**:274, 279
and drug compliance, **83**:332, 335
drug-induced, **83**:323, 479–80
the family and, **83**:250
lithium treatment of, *see* Lithium therapy
morbidity risk for, **83**:439–46 passim
See also Bipolar (manic-depressive) Disorder; Mania; Manic Episode
Manipulation: as supportive technique, **82**:484; **83**:182
Manipulativeness: in borderline disorders, **82**:457, 464, 465, 467
Mann, A. M., **84**:253
Mann, D. M. A., **83**:110, 112
Mann, James, **83**:467; **84**:7, 8, 9, 12, 35
Manschreck, T. C., **83**:131
Manton, K. G., **83**:88, 89
Manual of the International Classification of Diseases, Injuries, and Causes of Death, see ICD
Manuck, S. B., **84**:220
MAO (monoamine oxidase), **82**:128, 129; **83**:458
in affective (bipolar/unipolar) disorders, **83**:127, 272, 281, 446, 451–54 passim, 466–68

aging and, **83**:96–97, 127; **84**:235
alcoholism and, **82**:126; **83**:452; **84**:325
anxiety and, **84**:473–74
in borderline disorders, **82**:452, 463–67 passim
inhibitors (MAOIs)
alcohol and, **84**:358
and anxiety/panic states, **84**:457, 483, 503, 507–19 passim
in borderline disorders, **82**:463–67 passim
in depression, **83**:127–28, 281, 359, 361, 458, 467–72 passim, 479, 482–85; **84**:249
dosage, **83**:482–83, 485
for phobic children, **84**:416
precautions for people taking, **83**:127, 484–85, 490–91; **84**:249, 358
side effects of, **83**:127–28, 475, 484–85; **84**:253
tricyclics vs. or combined with, **83**:479, 481, 483, 485; **84**:248
(*see also* Drugs, list of)
in schizophrenia, **82**:125–27, 131, 147–52 passim, 452; **83**:467
two forms of (MAO-A, MAO-B), **83**:451–52
Marc-Aurele, J., **84**:348
Marcer, D., **83**:112
March, V., **83**:442
Marchbanks, R. M., **83**:113
Marcus, J., **84**:101; et al., **84**:101, 131
Marcus, S., **83**:48
Marcuse, H., **83**:34
Marder, S. R., **83**:460
Mardh, G., et al., **83**:461
Margolin, G., **83**:220, 223
Marital problems (disillusionment, mismatch, conflict): bipolar illness and, **83**:250–51
and children at risk, **84**:132, 136, 148–49
impact of, on children (boys vs. girls), **84**:153
contracts and, **83**:199, 217–19
depression and, **83**:195, 252n, 364, 365–66; **84**:53, 58–59, 132
detouring of (scapegoating), **83**:233–34, 239, 240, 241
evaluation of (in family or marital therapy), **83**:188, 190, 222, 232
and extramarital involvements, **82**:41
life-cycle stages and, **83**:212
obesity and, **84**:219
presenting styles of, **83**:220–21, 222–23
role disputes and, **84**:58, 62–63
and schizophrenia, **82**:171; **83**:242
and sex therapy failure, **82**:26–29, 32
See also Marriage; Separation and divorce
Marital therapy: combined with other therapies, **83**:195, 252
couples, **83**:192–93, 215–17, 521
for bipolar illness, **83**:189, 250, 251
children and, **83**:216, 225
classes of intervention in, **83**:222–26
in cognitive therapy, **84**:52–56
common problems in, **83**:226–27
vs. individual therapy, **83**:171, 190, 191, 212, 226–27
in IPT, **84**:63

and marital contracts, **83**:199, 217–19
  need for, before sex therapy, **82**:28
  techniques of, **83**:220–27
the disturbed child and, **83**:196–97, 240
indications for, **82**:28; **83**:189–91, 192–93
postparental, **83**:212
See also Family therapy; Separation and divorce; Sex therapy
Marke-Nyman Temperament Scale (MNTS), **83**:386–87
Markianos, E. S., et al., **82**:127, 128
Markiewicz, W., et al., **84**:479
Marks, I. M., **84**:394, 403, 404, 450–57 passim; et al., **84**:450, 506, 507, 512, 514
Marks, J., et al., **82**:159
Marks, J. N., et al., **84**:196
Marlatt, G. A., **84**:329, 330, 332, 337; et al., **84**:330, 331, 332
Marmor, J., **83**:40
Marriage: affective disorders and, **83**:456–57
  bipolar, **83**:249, 250–51, 286, 456–57
  courtship and (sex roles in), **84**:133
  protective role of, **83**:414
  and remarriage, **82**:42–45; **83**:216; **84**:148–49, 156
  See also Marital problems; Marital therapy; Separation and divorce
Marsden, C. D., **83**:109, 115
Marsella, A. J., **82**:98, 285
Marsh, W., **83**:483
Marshall, J. R., **84**:266, 267
Marshall, V., **83**:243
Marshall, W., **84**:512
Marshall, W. L., et al., **84**:450
Martin, F. M., et al., **83**:412
Martin, P., **84**:353
Martin-DuPan, R., **82**:202
Marty, P., **84**:218, 437
Marx, J. L., **83**:99
Marxism, **83**:34
Masala, A., et al., **82**:204
Masochism: as "female" quality, **83**:42, 43
  and masochistic personality (in depression), **83**:374
Mason, J. W., **84**:222
Mason, S. T., **84**:472
Massachusetts Acts of 1979, **82**:330
Massachusetts Department of Mental Health, **82**:367n16
  Memoranda, **82**:366, 368n18
Massachusetts General Hospital (Boston), **84**:180, 393
Massachusetts Mental Health Center, **82**:218; **84**:139, 140
Massie, H. N., **83**:242
Massie, Mary Jane, **84**:178; et al., **84**:245, 247
Mass production and "mass person," **82**:35
Mastectomy, *see* Surgery
Masters, William H., **82**:7–13 passim, 20–22 passim, 25–26, 35, 46, 63; **83**:41, 148, 149, 151; **84**:53
Masterson, J., **82**:470, 480, 486–87
Mastri, A. R., **83**:101, 110

Masturbation: fantasies, narcissism and, **82**:520
  female, **82**:10, 11, 18
    as therapy, **82**:21
  male, as therapy, **82**:24
Masuda, M., **84**:226
Mathé, A. A., et al., **82**:146
Mathew, R., et al., **82**:125; **84**:236
Mathews, A. M., **84**:450–57 passim; et al., **84**:449–54 passim, 459, 507
Matthew, R. J., et al., **84**:473
Matthews, Susan M., **82**:154; **83**:242n
Matthysse, S., **82**:131; et al., **82**:128
Mattila, M. J., et al., **84**:351, 500
Mattisson, K., **84**:350
Mattussek, P., **83**:397, 399
Maudsley Personality Inventory, *see* MPI
Maudsley reactive rat, **84**:485. *See also* Animal research
Maurice, W., **82**:8
Mavissakalian, Matig, **84**:449, 450, 454, 457, 459, 523; et al., **84**:458
May, P. R. A., **82**:158, 174, 175, 209, 216, 217, 220, 221; et al., **82**:158, 220–25 passim
Mayer, J. A., **84**:417
Mayer, V., et al., **83**:111
Mayer-Gross, W., **83**:415, 417
Mayo, J., **83**:251; et al., **83**:329
Mazur, M. A., **82**:58, 61
MBD (minimal brain dysfunction): and borderline disorders, **82**:441–42, 454
  drug therapy for, **82**:463, 467, 470
Meadow, A., et al., **82**:383n6
Meco, G., et al., **82**:196
Medicaid and Medicare, **82**:325n13, 332; **83**:105; **84**:334
Medical psychiatry (psychiatric medicine), **83**:172, 183–84
  and medicine-psychiatry interface, **84**:177, 179–83
  See also Consultation-liaison psychiatry; Drug therapy
Medical World News, **82**:352
Medication, *see* Drugs; Drugs, list of; Drug side effect(s); Drug therapy
Medicine in the Public Interest, Inc., **84**:361
Mednick, B. R., **84**:134
Mednick, S. A., **82**:108; **84**:96, 130; et al., **84**:99, 100, 101, 131, 132
Medvedev (Russian geneticist), **83**:84
Meerloo, J. A. M., **84**:276
Megavitamin therapy, *see* Vitamins
Meichenbaum, D. H., **84**:337, 457
Meierhofer, M., **82**:282
Meier-Ruge, W., **83**:96, 112
Meikle, S., et al., **84**:274
Meisch, R. A., **84**:320
Meisel, A., **82**:331, 350–53 passim, 357, 359; et al., **82**:350, 351
Meissner, W. W., **82**:415, 436
Melancholia, **82**:272, 278, 279; **83**:269, 272, 354, 357, 512
  DSM-III use of term, **83**:369
  DST for, **83**:121, 280

involutional, **83:**367
  among women, **83:**92, 412
  therapy for, **84:**61
  See also Depression; Major Depression
Melick, M. E., **82:**361n2
Melin, L., **83:**114
Mellinger, G. D., et al., **83:**95, 412, 413
Mello, N. K., **84:**329, 330
Mellor, C. S., **83:**289; et al., **83:**289
Mellstrom, B., et al., **83:**500
Mellstrom, D., et al., **84:**217
Meltzer, H. Y., **82:**128–35 passim, 147; **84:**498; et al., **82:**126, 127, 135, 143, 201; **83:**451, 470
Meltzoff, A. N., **83:**12, 13
Melzack, R., **84:**446
Memory, **83:**110; **84:**35
  affect, **83:**16–18
  of childhood, Freud's view of, **83:**63; **84:**431
  drug side effects on (impairment or improvement), **83:**113, 336, 475–76
  of geriatric patients, **83:**116, 139
  infant, **83:**15–18
  language and, **83:**16, 17–18, 70
  motor, **83:**16–18
  recall or evocative, **83:**15–16, 17
  recognition, **83:**15, 16, 17
  sleep and, **83:**18
Memory loss, *see* Amnesia
Mendelian theory, **83:**446; **84:**406. *See also* Genetic factors
Mendels, J., **83:**381, 442, 452, 501, 512
Mendelson, J. H., **84:**330
Mendelson, M., **84:**181
Mendelson, W., et al., **84:**489
Mendlewicz J., **83:**277, 438, 444–51 passim; et al., **83:**440, 441, 448
Mendota State Hospital, **82:**216
Menger, D., et al., **84:**261
Meningitides, bacterial, **84:**127
Menke's syndrome, **82:**144
Menn, A., **82:**175; **83:**248
Menninger, Karl, **83:**269
Menninger Foundation: Psychotherapy Research Project, **82:**471, 480, 486
Menninger Health-Sickness Scale, **82:**220
Menolascino, F., **84:**124
Menopause: and depression, **83:**420
  effect of, on vagina, **82:**10
  and hormone replacement therapy, **82:**11, 46; **83:**149
  treatment-related, **84:**255
Mental Disability Law Reporter **82:**332, 348n69
  "Comment," **82:**364n9
Mental element (legal concept), **82:**390, 392. *See also* Law and psychiatry
Mental Health Clinical Research Center for the Study of Schizophrenia (Camarillo State Hospital), **82:**104
Mental Health Law Project, **82:**372–73
Mental health policies: the courts and, **82:**321–27, 355–36, 349. *See also* Law and psychiatry
Mental health professionals, *see* Health care system

Mental Health Systems Act, **82:**377
Mental illness: age and, **83:**92
  classification of, **83:**357, 358
  criteria of, **82:**337–39, 348, 349, 370
  denial of, *see* Denial
  developmental, *see* Children at risk
  difference or deviation distinguished from, **83:**38
  the family and, **83:**173–85 (*see also* Family, the)
  as functional disorder, **84:**390
  insanity differentiated from, **82:**390–91
  and mortality rate, *see* Mortality rate
  among older females, *see* Female(s)
  prevalence of, *see* Epidemiology
  social factors and, **83:**407 (*see also* Stress)
Mental Patients' Liberation Movement, **83:**248
Mental retardation: behavioral approach to, **84:**126, 129
  and bipolar illness, **83:**289
  children with, **84:**120–29
    misconceptions regarding, **84:**122
  DSM-III definition of, **84:**120–21
  and emotional/psychiatric disorders, **84:**122, 128
    epidemiology of, **84:**123–25
  etiologies of (psychosocial and organic), **84:**121, 122, 124, 126–27
  incidence of, **84:**120–21, 126
  institutionalization, **84:**122–23, 127, 128
    vs. mainstreaming, **84:**122, 123
    vs. mass deinstitutionalization, **82:**375; **84:**122
  as "mental illness," **82:**337
  prevention of, **84:**125–29
  psychosocial factors in, **84:**122, 124, 125, 127
  treatment of, **83:**527; **84:**128–29
  and treatment facilities, **82:**378
Mental status examination: for elderly patient, **84:**234, 237
  and Mental Status Questionnaire, **83:**116
Mental Status Schedule (MSS), **84:**202
Menzies, I. E. P., **83:**30
Mercier, M., **84:**106
Merry, J., **84:**332; et al., **84:**358
Messer, S. B., **84:**68
Messier, M., et al. **82:**218
Metabolic diseases: in infancy, and mental retardation, **84:**127
  and psychosexual dysfunctions, **82:**37
  See also Physical illness
Metabolic screening test, *see* SMAC
Metabolism: aging and, **83:**96, 97, 100, 117, 128, 498
  of alcohol, *see* Alcohol
  cerebral, drug treatment of (in dementia), **83:**111–12
  depression studies of, **83:**380
  and free radicals, **83:**97–98
  neuropeptide influence on, **84:**223
  tricyclics and, **83:**125, 474, 493–506, 508–10
Metals, *see* Aluminum concentration; Lead poisoning; Manganese poisoning; Zinc concentration

Methionine, **82**:140
  -enkephalin concentrations, **82**:142
Meyer, Adolf, **82**:85; **83**:170, 360, 519; **84**:57, 94, 177
Meyer, B. C., **84**:276; et al., **84**:262, 264
Meyer, E., **84**:181; et al., **84**:195
Meyer, Jon K., **82**:8, 48, 52–55 passim; **83**:43n
Meyer, L. C., **82**:62
Meyer, R. E., **82**:140
Meyer, V., **84**:468
MFG (multiple family group), see Family therapy
MHPG, see Urinary MHPG levels
Michael, S. T., **83**:93
Michaels, R. R., et al., **84**:444
Michaux, M. H., et al., **82**:209
Michels, Robert, **82**:351, 355, 483; **83**:7, 8, 65, 68; **84**:35n
Michelson, L., **84**:454
Michigan Alcohol Screening Test, **84**:213
Midanik, L., **84**:362
"Middle game," see Psychoanalysis
Midtown Manhattan Study, **83**:92
Mielke, D. H., **82**:213; et al., **82**:201, 204
Milano, Michael R., **84**:178
Miles, A., **83**:94
Miles, C. P., **83**:286–87
Mill, John Stuart, **82**:279
Millar, W. M., **84**:460
Miller, A. E., et al., **83**:111
Miller, Albert, **83**:457
Miller, D. C., **83**:434
Miller, E., **83**:117
Miller, E. J., **83**:30
Miller, G., **84**:112
Miller, L. C., et al., **84**:412, 417
Miller, N. E., **84**:227
Miller, W. C., **84**:96
Miller, W. R., **84**:331
Millett, K., **83**:45
Mills, Mark J., **82**:323, 324, 326, 361nn2, 3, 382n5; et al., **82**:351
Milne, J. F., **83**:112
Milner, G., **82**:144
Milofsky, E. S., **84**:311, 317, 319, 329
Milton, F., **84**:497
Milwaukee study of deprived children, **84**:125–26
Mims, R. B., et al., **82**:204
Mindus, P., et al., **83**:112
Minerals (diet supplements), **82**:144–45. See also Diet
Minimal brain dysfunction, see MBD
Mini Mental Status Examination, see MMSE
Minkoff, K., et al., **83**:431
Minn, K., **82**:118
Minneapolis study of behavior disorders, **84**:136
Minnesota Multiphasic Personality Inventory, see MMPI
Minors: rights of, **82**:352. See also Adolescent(s); Childhood
Minter, R. D., **83**:480
Minuchin, Salvador, **83**:179, 187, 194; et al., **83**:174, 179, 189; **84**:225

Mirabile, C. S., **82**:453
Mirin, S. M., et al., **83**:481
Mirror (selfobject) transference, see Transference
Mirsky, I. A., **84**:468
Mishler, E. G., **83**:184, 242
Miskimins, R. W., **82**:171
Misogyny: of Freud, **83**:47, 48, 50
Misra, P. S., et al., **84**:354
Missri, J. C., **84**:477
Mitral valve prolapse, see Cardiac disorders
Mitscherlich, A., **83**:35
Mizell, T. A., **82**:177
MMPI (Minnesota Multiphasic Personality Inventory), **84**:202, 274, 312–13, 325
  borderline disorder profile in, **82**:429
  depressive profiles in, **83**:387
  elderly patient scores on, **83**:91
  MAO activity decrease and, **82**:126
MMSE (Mini Mental Status Examination), **84**:189, 203
MMT (Multimodal Therapy), see Psychotherapy(ies), brief
Mnookin, R. H., **84**:155
MNTS (Marke-Nyman Temperament Scale), **83**:386–87
Mob psychology, see Group psychology
Modai, I., et al., **83**:468, 474
Modell, A. H., **82**:480, 519; **83**:46, 56, 59
Moffic, H. S., **84**:206, 207, 208, 235, 247
Mohl, P. C., **84**:182
Mohler, H., **84**:485
Mohr, J., et al., **82**:57
Moja, E. A., et al., **82**:137
Moldofsky, Harvey, **84**:178, 218, 221; et al., **84**:221 **84**:221
Molholm, H. B., **82**:115
Monahan, J., **82**:393
Money, J., et al., **82**:293; **83**:43
Money-Kryle, R. E., **82**:474
Mongolism, see Down's syndrome
Monk, M. A., **84**:411
Monnelly, E. P., et al., **83**:426
Monoamine oxidase, see MAO
Monroe, R. B., **82**:465
Monroe, S. M., **83**:272
Montgomery, D. B., **83**:434
Montgomery, G. K., **84**:469
Montgomery, S. A., **83**:434; **84**:512, 513; et al., **83**:500, 506
Mood disorders, **83**:357
  drug therapy for, **82**:463; **83**:480
  endocrine disorders and, **83**:379, 422
  and mood swings in bipolar illness, **83**:281, 286, 326–30 passim, 334, 374
  See also Affective Disorders; Bipolar (manic-depressive) Disorder; Depression; Emotions; Hypomania; Irritability
Moodswings (Fieve), **84**:61
Mooney, John J., **83**:356
Moore, B. E., **82**:489, 499n1
Moore, D. F., **82**:185
Moore, G., **84**:511

Moore, M. H., **84:**362, 363, 366, 368, 369
Moore, M. K., **83:**13
Moore, N. C., **83:**134
Moorhead, P. S., **83:**97
Moos, R. H., et al., **82:**175
MOPP regimen (for Hodgkin's disease), **84:**255.
    See also Drug therapy
Morbid ideation: in childhood depression, **82:**300
Morbidity, *see* Epidemiology; Mental illness
Morel, Benedict Augustin, **82:**82; **83:**269
Morgan, H. G., **84:**225
Morgan, R., **82:**193
Morgane, P. J., **84:**445
Morgenthau, H., **83:**37
Moriarty, A., **84:**109
Morrell, C., **84:**254
Morris, J. B., **83:**512
Morris, J. N., **83:**88, 90
Morris, N., **82:**387
Morrison, A. L., **84:**148
Morrison, C., **84:**325
Morrison, H. L., **84:**135
Morrison, J. R., **83:**286, 421, 442; **84:**314; et al.,
    83:372
Morrissey, E. R., **84:**340
Morrissey, J. D., **83:**107
Morrow, G. R., **84:**254
Morse, D. R., et al., **84:**446
Morse, R. M., **84:**262
Morse, Robert, **84:**303
Morstyn, R., et al., **84:**100
Mortality rate: alcohol use and, **84:**217, 360
    in alcohol withdrawal reactions, **84:**352, 353
    bereavement and, **84:**217
    in bipolar illness, **83:**287; **84:**217
    cancer, **84:**217, 240
    cardiovascular, **84:**465–67
    decline in, **83:**88–89
    depression and, **83:**366; **84:**217
    infant mortality, **82:**274
    among older females, **83:**89
    psychiatric disorders and, **83:**92; **84:**460
        panic disorders compared to other, **84:**460–
        67, 523
    psychological intervention and, **84:**213
    See also Suicide and attempted suicide
Mortimer, J. A., **83:**107
Moser, J., **84:**362
Mosher, J. F., **84:**363, 369
Mosher, L. R., **82:**110, 159, 170, 175, 177; et al.,
    82:175; **83:**248
Moskowitz, H., **84:**500
Moss, J., **84:**472
Mother, the: preoedipal, and crowd psychol-
    ogy, **83:**23, 35, 36
    schizophrenic, *see* Parent(s)
    See also Female(s); Mother-child relationship;
        Parent-child relationship; Pregnancy
Mother-child relationship: and alcoholism, **84:**312
    attachment bonds in, **84:**57–58, 100, 127
    and children at risk, **84:**99–101, 121, 127, 138
    (*see also* psychotic mother and; separation in,
        below)

depressed mother and, *see* psychotic mother
    and, *below*
    difficulties in, as program entry criteria, **84:**141
    empathic/unempathic, **82:**491–92, 494; **84:**121
    and gender disturbance, **82:**50–51, 52, 55
    hatred (of mother by child) in, **82:**473
    and infant development, **83:**20–21
    in joint hospitalization, **84:**139–40
    and narcissism, **82:**522
    psychotic mother and, **84:**103, 106, 130–31, 133,
        138, 143
        depressive, **84:**58, 100, 131–36 passim, 142,
        144
        INAC and, **84:**140–41
        schizophrenic, *see* Parent(s)
    separation in
        and childhood depression or anxiety,
            82:274–75, 306; **84:**418
        and later pathology (animal models of),
            84:224–25, 412, 417
        traumatic effect of, **84:**106, 412
        (*see also* Separation fears)
    and sexual dysfunction, **82:**28, 32, 34
    See also Mother, the; Parent-child relationship
Mothers Against Drunk Driving (MADD), **84:**362
Motion sickness, **82:**453
Motivation: for change (and success of ther-
    apy), **84:**26–27, 29
    unconscious, inferences regarding, **84:**45
Mottl, J. R., **84:**369
Moulton, R., **83:**47
Mountjoy, C. Q., et al., **84:**509, 510
Mount Sinai Hospital (New York), **84:**180, 198
Mowrer, O., **84:**449
Moyano, C., **82:**184
MPI (Maudsley Personality Inventory), **83:**387,
    393
MSS (Mental Status Schedule), **84:**202
Muchmore, E., **82:**118
Mueller, C. W., **84:**146
Muir, C. S., **84:**239
Muller, D. J., **84:**353
Muller, E. E., et al., **82:**201
Multimodal Life History Questionnaire, **84:**70
Multimodal Therapy (MMT), *see* Psychother-
    apy(ies), brief
Multiple sclerosis: viral etiology suspected,
    82:121; **83:**453
Mumford, E., et al., **84:**213, 258
Munetz, M. R., et al., **82:**357
Munkvad, I., **82:**137
Munoz, C., **84:**475
Murillo, L., **82:**209
Murphy, D. L., **82:**125, 127, 452, 453; **83:**295, 452,
    467, 470; et al., **83:**452, 470
Murphy, E., **84:**236
Murphy, G. E., **83:**430, 431, 433; et al., **83:**372,
    431, 433; **84:**212
Murphy, H. B. M., **82:**120
Murphy, Lois, **84:**109
Murray, H. A., **83:**386
Murray, L. G., **83:**387, 389
Musaph, H., **84:**227

Musick, J., **84:**135, 138; et al., **84:**133, 140
Muskin, P. R., **84:**504
Muslin, H. C., **84:**268
Musto, D., **84:**360
MVP (mitral valve prolapse), *see* Cardiac disorders
Myers, J. K., **82:**103, 281, 283; **83:**91, 271, 275, 374, 408–26 passim; **84:**133, 135; et al., **83:**394
Myers, R. D., **84:**323; et al., **84:**323
Myerson, P., **83:**56
Myoclonic twitching: as drug side effect, **84:**233
   sleep-related, **84:**221
Myopathy, **84:**307. *See also* Physical illness
Myotonia: as sexual response, **82:**12

N

Naber, D., et al., **82:**131, 202
Nachman, P., **83:**16
NAD (nicotinamide-adenine-dinucleotide), **84:**349
   and reoxidation of NADH, **84:**349
Nadelson, Carol, **82:**9, 57, 61, 62, 63
Nadelson, T., **84:**261
Naeser, M., et al., **82:**124
Naipaul, V. S., **84:**104
Nair, N. P. V., **82:**144, 201
Najarian, J., **82:**274
Nakamura, M. M., et al., **84:**358
Nakano, S., et al., **84:**496
Nammalvar, N., **83:**287
Nandy, K., **83:**112
Napier, C. A., **83:**200, 215
Napier, G. G., **84:**272
Narcissism: "as if" personality in, **82:**515
   classification of, **82:**512, 520
   concept of, **82:**487, 488–90
   as "female quality" (Freud), **83:**42, 43
   group ideology and, **83:**23, 24, 25, 30, 35
   healthy/normal, **82:**489, 511–12, 518
      and child's self-esteem, **82:**301
   history-taking as gratification of, **84:**15
   and narcissistic injury in divorce, **84:**148, 155
   pathological, **82:**511–12, 518; **83:**55, 59; **84:**21
      and sexual dysfunction, **82:**30, 54
   (*see also* Narcissistic Personality Disorder)
   relationship of, to current society, **83:**35
Narcissistic Personality Disorder, **82:**436
   characteristics of, **82:**490–91, 512–23
   diagnosis of, **82:**488–89, 491, 512–15
   as discrete syndrome, **82:**437, 490
   DSM-III criteria for, **82:**414, 435, 470, 490, 516
   idealization in, **82:**513, 517–23 passim
      and self-idealization, **82:**514, 516, 518
   and narcissistic rage, **82:**494, 495, 514, 517–21 passim
   prognosis for, **82:**514, 515–16, 520, 523
   treatment of
      psychoanalytic, **82:**487–98, 499, 505–10, 513, 514, 516–20

      psychotherapeutic, **82:**514, 516, 520–23; **84:**44
   See also Primary self pathology
Nash, H., **84:**350
Nash, L. R., **82:**205
Nasrallah, H., et al., **82:**135
Nathan, Peter E., **84:**300, 326, 329–32 passim, 338; et al., **84:**330
National Cancer Institute, **84:**240
National Commission for the Protection of Human Subjects of Biomedical and Behavioral Research, **82:**353
National Commission on Confidentiality of Health Records, **82:**332
National Conference of Commissioners on Uniform State Laws, **82:**354
National Council on Alcoholism (NCA), **84:**307, 361, 362
National Highway Traffic Safety Administration, **84:**362
National Institute of Mental Health (NIMH), **82:**84n, 159, 288n, 416, 452; **83:**491n, 511n; **84:**92, 396
   bipolar illness studies by, **83:**250–51, 446, 454, 456
   borderline patient study by, **82:**416, 417
   Center for Studies of the Mental Health of the Aging of, **83:**85
   Collaborative Studies
      of Lithium Therapy, **83:**307, 311, 316–17, 371, 481
      of Maintenance Drug Therapy in Affective Disorder, **83:**311
      on the Psychobiology of Depression, **83:**286, 394; **84:**303
      of TCA therapy, **83:**479
   conference (1982) on anxiety disorders, **84:**393
   and consultation-liaison psychiatry, **84:**182
   Diagnosis of Depression in Children, Subcommittee for, **82:**271
   Diagnostic Interview Schedule, *see* DIS
   disaster study by, **84:**107, 117
   Division of Biometry and Epidemiology, **84:**92
   ECA program, **83:**406n, 408, 410, 428
   geriatric studies by and programs of, **83:**85, 86
   Intramural Research Program, **84:**98
   neuroleptic drug therapy study by, **82:**123, 178, 179, 198
National Institute on Aging (NIA), **83:**85, 86
National Institute on Alcohol Abuse and Alcoholism, **84:**356
National Institutes of Health, **83:**86
   Consensus Development Conference Statement, **84:**264
National Nursing Home Survey, **83:**94
National Reporter System (West Publishing Company), **82:**349
Nausea: anxiety and, **84:**476
   as drug side effect, **84:**453
   See also Gastrointestinal disorders
Neal, R. A., **84:**357
Neale, J., **83:**143; **84:**99, 131, 132
Neborsky, R., et al., **82:**187

Nebraska study of mental retardation, **84**:124
Negri, F., et al., **83**:443, 456
Neiderhiser, D. H., et al., **84**:357
Neil, J. F., et al., **83**:280
Neill, J. R., et al., **84**:219
Nelson, J. C., **83**:125, 480; et al., **83**:121, 122, 506
Nemiah, John C., **84**:227, 437, 438, 522
Neonates, **83**:9–11. *See also* Infancy
Nervous energy: Janet's theory of, **84**:428–29
Nesse, R. M., et al., **84**:222
Neubuerger, O. W., et al., **84**:334
Neuchterlein, K. H., **84**:100, 228
Neugarten, B., **83**:216
Neuner, R., **83**:397, 399
Neurasthenia, **84**:394, 403. *See also* Panic Disorder
Neurocirculatory asthenia, **84**:403, 468, 477, 479. *See also* Cardiac disorders; Panic Disorder
Neurodermatitis, *see* Skin disease
Neuroendocrine correlates, *see* Endocrine system
Neuroleptics/antipsychotics, *see* Drugs
Neuropeptides, **83**:113; **84**:223
Neurotic, as term, **83**:371
Neurotransmitters, **83**:101–02, 380, 454, 458, 512; **84**:223, 323
  in anxiety, **84**:409, 470, 471–73, 486, 489
  drug effect on, **83**:460, 469, 486
  treatment with, **83**:113
  See also GABA
Newberger, E. H., **82**:332
Newcastle group, **83**:381
New Guinea: schizophrenia in, **82**:120
Newman, C. J., **84**:111–12
Newman, H. W. and E. J., **84**:350
Newman, L., **83**:189
Newman-Keuls analysis, **84**:455
New Mexico, State of, Department of Hospitals and Institutions, **82**:340n21, 344
Newson, J., **83**:19
Newsweek magazine, **84**:104, 105
Newton, J. E. O., et al., **84**:475
Newton, R. E., **83**:488; et al., **84**:499
New York Hospital-Westchester Division, **82**:442
New York State: psychiatric disorder study in, **84**:191
  Psychiatric Institute, Lithium Clinic of, **83**:296
New Zealand: bipolar illness in, **83**:423
Niacin (nicotinic acid, vitamin B₃) and niacinamide, **82**:142–43
Niaura, R. S., **84**:332
Nicholas, P. L., **84**:100
Nickerson, M., **84**:350
Nicotinamide-adenine-dinucleotide, *see* NAD
Niederland, W., **84**:104, 110
Nielsen, A. C., **82**:287; **84**:188, 204, 206
Nielsen, J., **83**:91, 416, 417, 418, 419, 425
Nielsen, J. A., **83**:416, 418
Niemi, T., **84**:217
Nies, A., **83**:97; et al., **82**:126; **83**:452, 467,495; **84**:516
Nietzsche, Friedrich, **83**:47

Nigeria: schizophrenia in, **82**:101
Nikitopoulou, G., et al., **82**:203
Ninan, P. T., et al., **84**:483, 488, 489
Nissen, G., **82**:282
Noble, D., **82**:444
Noble, Ernest P., **84**:300, 347, 348, 349, 357, 358; et al., **84**:347, 349, 351, 355
Nocturnal Penile Tumescence (NPT), **82**:37–38, 46; **84**:221
Noll, J. O., **82**:333
Noone, R. B., et al., **84**:271
Noradrenaline receptors, **83**:474, 482, 483
Norepinephrine (NE), **82**:140, 142, 143, 180, 196; **83**:101, 273, 460
  aging and, **83**:96–97, 110, 112, 127
  antidepressants and, **83**:458–59, 489–90, 494, 508
  anxiety and, **84**:480
  β-CCE and, **84**:488
  metabolite (MHPG), *see* Urinary MHPG levels
  as possible amethystic agent, **84**:350
  relaxation response and, **84**:444, 447
  and schizophrenia, **82**:130–32, 152; **83**:132
  in unipolar depression subtypes, **83**:463, 464–65
Norris, B., **83**:302
North America: ADH isoenzyme patterns in, **84**:324. *See also* Canada; United States
Norton, Arthur J., **84**:144
Norton, N. M., **84**:192, 209, 211, 213
Norway, *see* Scandinavia
Norwich, J. J., **84**:442
Noshpitz, J., **84**:115
Note-taking (advantages of), **84**:31
Notman, M. T., **82**:61, 62, 63
Nott, P. N., **83**:107
Noyes, R., et al., **84**:403, 404, 465
NPT, *see* Nocturnal Penile Tumescence
Nuckolls, K. B., et al., **84**:229
Nuclear disaster threat, **83**:403; **84**:111, 116–17
Nurnberg, H. G., **84**:511
Nurnberger, J. I., Jr., **83**:435n; **84**:97; et al., **83**:453
Nursing homes: consultation-liaison psychiatry in, **84**:184
  National Survey of, **83**:94
  population percentage living in, **83**:88
  schizophrenics in, **83**:130
  See also Hospitalization
Nursing staff: on consultation-liaison team, **84**:215, 245, 259, 261–62
  group reactions of, **83**:28–29, 30
  -patient relations, **83**:29–30, 139
  postoperative intervention by, **84**:261–62, 273, 274
  and staff burnout, **84**:245
  See also Health care system
Nurture-nature debate, **82**:155; **83**:435; **84**:320. *See also* Environmental factors; Genetic factors
Nutrition, *see* Diet; Malnutrition; TPN (total parenteral nutrition)
Nyback, H., et al., **84**:472

Nyland, H., et al., **82:**117
Nystrom, S., **83:**304

O

Oates, J. R., **84:**330
Oberndorf, C. P., **84:**17
Obesity, **84:**219, 220
  therapy for, **84:**53, 229
  See also Weight gain
Obholzer, A. M., **84:**357
Object loss, see Loss
Object relations: absence of, **82:**481, 488
  British theory of, **82:**487, 493
  and group psychology, **83:**24–25, 31
  of individual, **83:**31
  integration of part to total, **82:**476, 478, 479
  internalized, **82:**472–75 passim, 479–80, 512, 513, 520; **83:**24, 49
  and marriage problems, **82:**32; **83:**218–19, 251
  narcissism and, **82:**48, 494, 495, 512–20 passim; **84:**21
  and object loss, see Loss
  pathological vs. normal, **82:**511
  present and past, inability to differentiate, **82:**478
  and prognosis, **82:**486, 487
  splitting of "good" from "bad," **82:**479
  theory of, **83:**7, 49
  therapy and, **84:**21, 66
Object representation: in borderline disorders, **82:**473, 474–75, 479–80
  and ego identity, **83:**24
  in narcissistic disorder, **82:**493, 511–12, 516, 517, 518
O'Brien, C., et al., **82:**171, 218
O'Brien, J. S., **84:**329, 330, 332
O'Brien, P. M., **84:**357
Obsessions and Psychasthenia (Janet), **84:**426
Obsessive-Compulsive Disorder, **84:**469
  drug therapy for, **84:**457, 512–16
  DSM-III category for, **84:**393–97 passim, 401, 419
  and mortality rate, **84:**460–61, 463–64
  See also Anxiety Disorders
Odegaard, O., **84:**470
Odoroff, C. L., **84:**460
Oedipal conflictual disorders, **82:**491
Oedipal issues: and narcissistic disorders, **82:**489, 492, 494, 511–19 passim
  and normal oedipal stage, **82:**48, 501, 503, 504
  oedipal father, **83:**34–35
  and selfobject transferences, **82:**501–08 passim
  and sexual dysfunction, **82:**32
Offer, D., **83:**191
Offit, Avodah K., **82:**8
Ogata, M., **84:**355
O'Grady, P., **82:**217
Ohman, R., **82:**203; et al., **82:**203
Ojesjo, L., **84:**316

Okada, T., **84:**485
Oktay, J. S., **84:**187, 189–90, 213
Okulitch, P. V., **84:**329
Okuma, T., **83:**312; et al., **83:**310, 311–12
O'Leary, K. D., **84:**153
Olin, G. B. and H. S., **82:**357
Oliver, R., **83:**433
Olivier-Martin, R., et al., **83:**505
Ollendich, T., **84:**417
Olsen, E. J., et al., **83:**112
Olsen, R. W., **84:**487
Olson, E., **84:**111
Oltmanns, T. F., **84:**99
Olweus, D., **84:**96
Omens: posttraumatic discovery of, **84:**113, 114, 115. See also Trauma, emotional/psychic
Oncology: psychiatry and, **84:**239–56. See also Cancer
Onda, A., **84:**445
Onset concept, **82:**103
Op Den Velde, W., **83:**110
Operant conditioning, see Conditioning
Oppenheimer, B. S., **84:**404
Oppenheimer, C., **82:**214
Oral (pregenital) aggression, **82:**473. See also Aggression
Oral-dependent traits, see Dependency
Orchidectomy, **82:**39
Oregon: psychiatric morbidity study in, **84:**202
Orford, L., **84:**299, 315, 316
Organ, T. W., **84:**443
Organic Affective Syndrome, **84:**235. See also Affective Disorders
Organic Anxiety Syndrome, **84:**402
Organic Mental Disorders: alcohol-related diagnoses associated with (DSM-III), **84:**301, 307, 347
  cancer and, **84:**246
  DSM-III categories for, **84:**49, 203, 246, 301
  epidemiology/prevalence rate of, **84:**203
  late-life, **83:**91, 94–95, 96, 106–18; **84:**231, 232–36
  postcardiotomy, **84:**262–64
  and sleep patterns, **83:**145
  treatment of, **84:**49
Organization(s): psychoanalytic approach to, **83:**33
  systems theory of, **83:**30–32
  See also Group psychology; Therapeutic community
Organ transplantation, see Surgery
Orgasm: decline in frequency of, **83:**151
  effect of childhood sexual assault on capacity for, **82:**58
  female, **82:**12, 13, 14, 63
    clitoral vs. vaginal, **82:**11; **83:**41
    coital, **82:**11, 44, 58; **83:**41
    inhibited, **82:**16, 18, 44, 62; **83:**41, 485
    multiple, **82:**15, 43
  male, **82:**12, 13, 14, 15, 43
    inhibited, **82:**16, 18–19
  (see also Ejaculation)
  treatment of dysfunction in, **82:**16, 25, 32

Orley, J., et al., **83:**408, 409, 416
Orlov, P., et al., **82:**205
Orn, H., **82:**100
Orne, M. T., et al., **84:**227, 228
Ornstein, A., **82:**498, 502, 503
Ornstein, Paul H., **82:**414, 498, 503
Orr, M., **82:**214
Orr, W. C., **84:**263
Orsulak, Paul J., **83:**356; et al., **83:**467
Ortega, S. T., **82:**100
Ortega y Gasset, J., **83:**36
Orthomolecular psychiatry, **82:**142–46
Orvaschel, H., et al., **82:**284, 285, 286; **83:**283, 404, 421
Orvis, B. R., **84:**362
Osherson, S. E., **83:**173
Osmond, H., **82:**140, 143
Ost, L. G., **84:**449, 454; et al., **84:**76
Ostfeld, A., **84:**263; et al., **83:**112; **84:**187
Ostomies, *see* Surgery
Ostow, M., **82:**461; **83:**285
Osuna, Fray Francisco de, **84:**441–42
Ouellette, D. L., **84:**276
Ouslander, J. G., **84:**235
Outpatient(s): psychiatric morbidity among, **84:**189–98
Outpatient treatment: of bipolar illness, **83:**271, 297–98, 303, 326
   consultation-liaison psychiatry in, **84:**184
   of depression, **83:**524–25; **84:**19
   and diagnosis, **83:**409
   of late-life psychiatric disorders, **83:**94–95
   of schizophrenia, **82:**159, 162, 171, 219, 228
   termination of, *see* Therapy
   See also Social support networks
Ovaries: failure of (chemotherapy and), **84:**255
   surgery on, **82:**41 (*see also* Surgery)
   See also Female(s)
Overanxious Disorder, **84:**410. *See also* Anxiety Disorders
Ovesey, L., **82:**34; **83:**47

P

P300 amplitude: ethanol administration and, **84:**327
   in schizophrenia, **84:**100
Pacha, W., **83:**112
Paffenbarger, R. S., **83:**422
Pain: chronic, short-term management of, **84:**229, 230
   phantom, after amputation, **84:**272
   reaction to, and prognosis, **84:**218
   relaxation therapy and, **84:**447
   See also Psychogenic Pain Disorder
Pair-bonding, **82:**30; **83:**39
Pairing: as basic assumption of group, **83:**22, 25, 26
Palmblad, J., et al., **84:**223
Palmer, A. B., **82:**357
Pallis, D. J., **83:**431

Palmore, E., **83:**103, 105
Palmour, R. M., et al., **82:**141
Pancreatitis, **84:**307. *See also* Physical illness
Pandey, G. N., et al., **82:**136; **83:**452, 470
Panic Anxiety, *see* Anxiety
Panic Disorder, **83:**430; **84:**427, 482
   atypical depression differentiated from, **83:**127
   drug-induced, **84:**493
   drug therapy for, **83:**142, 488; **84:**472, 493, 501, 503–12
      imipramine, **83:**483–84; **84:**395, 408, 476, 480, 503–12 passim
   DSM-III category for, **84:**394–97 passim, 400, 404, 410, 460, 461, 493, 495, 504, 516
   epidemiology of, **84:**403–04, 407–08
   genetic factors in, **84:**402–10, 482
   late-life, **83:**127, 140–41, 142
   and mortality rate, **84:**460–67, 523
      suicide, **84:**467
   MVP and, *see* Cardiac disorders
   as psychosomatic symptom, **84:**438
   psychotherapeutic management of, **84:**22, 421, 457
   subtypes of, **84:**397
   unresolved questions about, **84:**520
   See also Agoraphobia; Anxiety; Anxiety Disorders
Papastamou, P. A., **84:**231
Paprocki, J., **82:**185
Papua: schizophrenia in, **82:**120
Parad, H., et al., **84:**117
Paradoxical Intention (PI), **84:**458, 459
Paranoid Personality Disorder, **84:**397, 399
   DSM-III criteria for, **82:**470; **83:**135
Paranoid reactions, **84:**48
   culture shock and, **83:**139
   depression and, **83:**330
   depression distinguished from, **83:**374
   drug-induced, **82:**137, 138, 197; **84:**253
   in geriatric patients, **83:**92, 95, 131–40
      etiology and characteristics of, **83:**132–37, 140; **84:**233
   in narcissistic personality disorder, **82:**514, 515, 517, 521
   paranoid hallucinosis, **83:**136
   postcardiotomy, **84:**263
   posttraumatic, **84:**421
   sensory deficits/social withdrawal and, **83:**130, 133–39 passim
   suspiciousness, **83:**91, 131–39 passim; **84:**421
   therapy for, **83:**137, 138–39, 480
Paranoid schizophrenia, *see* Schizophrenia
Paraphilia, **82:**52, 54. *See also* Perversion(s)
Paraphrenia, **84:**93
   differentiated from paranoid schizophrenia, **83:**137
   late-life, **82:**149; **83:**107, 131, 133, 137–38
   See also Schizophrenia
Parent(s): abusing, *see* Child abuse
   of adult children, **83:**199, 211; **84:**132
   aging, **83:**212
   alcoholic, **84:**135, 299, 312, 320, 330
   alliance vs. splitting of, **83:**232–33

as auxiliary therapists (for traumatized children), **84**:119
criminal, *see* Crime
death of, *see* Death
depression of, **84**:135
  and children at risk, **82**:285, 286; **84**:97, 98, 100, 129, 133, 135
expectations by, of child's treatment outcome, **84**:417
and parental imagos, **82**:501
possible outcomes for, **84**:88
schizophrenic, **84**:94, 99, 129–37 passim
  father, **84**:101, 130n, 132
  mother, **82**:172; **84**:99–101, 130–31, 132
of schizophrenics, **83**:175–76, 243, 247
single, **84**:141, 144, 145, 146, 148
  and custody, **84**:156
  father, **84**:156
  mother, **84**:156
  (*see also* Separation and divorce)
and social status of parenting, **84**:136, 143
under stress, **84**:58, 135–36, 143
as teachers of handicapped children, **84**:128
-therapist relationship (in child therapy), **82**:264
  (*see also* Therapeutic relationship)
transference links to, **82**:27, 32; **84**:30–31, 39
See also Family, the; Family therapy; Father, the; Mother, the; Mother-child relationship; Oedipal issues; Parent-child relationship
Parent-child relationship: and anorexia nervosa, **84**:225
  and children at risk, **84**:102–03, 107, 110, 132, 158
    deprivation dwarfism, **84**:225
    mentally retarded child, **84**:121, 128
    in reaction to traumatic event, **84**:105–06, 118–19
    in separation and divorce, **84**:148–58 passim
    (*see also* and schizophrenia, *below*)
  conflict in, **83**:218; **84**:62
  empathy in, **83**:19–20
  family therapy and, **83**:192, 210, 211–12, 241
  loyalty and loyalty conflict in, **83**:219; **84**:116
  and prediction of child development, **83**:229–30
  role reversal in, **83**:231–32; **84**:138, 149, 152
  and schizophrenia, **82**:155; **83**:175, 247; **84**:94
  therapist's observation of, **84**:140
  visiting, *see* Separation and divorce
  See also Child abuse; Children at risk; Family, the; Mother-child relationship; Object relations
Paris, J. J., **82**:325
Pariser, S. F., et al., **84**:408, 479
Parisi, A. F., **84**:355
Parker, E. S., **84**:347; et al., **84**:347
Parker, J. C., et al., **84**:331
Parkes, C. M., **84**:217, 272; et al., **84**:217
Parkinson's disease, **83**:101, 109, 128; **84**:235, 349
  parkinsonian symptoms, **82**:204–05; **83**:100; **84**:252, 498

See also Drug side effect(s)
Parloff, M. B., **83**:512
Parsons, H. V., **83**:190
Parsons, O. A., **84**:347
Parsons, P. L., **83**:424
Parsons, Talcott, **83**:142
Pasamanick, B., et al., **82**:225
Pasnau, R. O., **84**:182
Passive-aggressive type: and sexual dysfunction, **82**:15
Passivity: as "female" quality, **83**:42, 43
Pasternac, A., et al., **84**:481
Pasteur, Louis, **84**:177
Pate, J. K., **84**:233
Patient: compliance/noncompliance with drug therapy by, *see* Drug therapy
  consent to or refusal of treatment by, *see* Therapy
  interviewing, *see* Interviews
  responsibility of, in therapy, *see* Responsibility
  role of, **82**:327 (*see also* Therapeutic relationship)
  selection of
    for psychoanalysis, **83**:51–52, 60
    for psychotherapy, **84**:25–27, 44, 440
  somatizing, *see* Somatic symptoms
  -staff relations, **83**:29–30, 139; **84**:181
  See also Hospitalization; Nursing homes; Outpatient(s); Relationships; Surgery
Patrick, V., et al., **83**:395
Patterson, G. R., **83**:174; **84**:96
Pattison, E. M., **84**:332
Patton State Hospital (California), **84**:335, 336
Paul, G. L., **82**:110, 175; et al., **82**:169–70, 175
Paul, N. L., **83**:235
Paul, Steven M., **84**:483, 486, 487, 524; et al., **83**:470; **84**:409, 483n, 485, 487
Pauling, Linus, **82**:142, 145; et al., **82**:143
Pauls, D. L., et al., **84**:408
Paulson, G. W., et al., **83**:115
Paulson, S. M., et al., **84**:357
Pauly, Ira B., **82**:8; **83**:147n
Pausanius, **83**:83
Paykel, E. S., **82**:459, 466; **83**:365, 366; **84**:58, 99, 206, 207, 208, 235, 247; et al., **83**:372, 390, 393, 394, 395, 414; **84**:58, 516
Payne, E. C., et al., **82**:61
PEA (phenylethylamine) hypothesis, *see* Schizophrenia, etiology of
Peake, G. T., **84**:203
Pearce, J., **82**:282, 289
Pearce, T., **84**:273
Pearlin, L. I., **84**:58
Pearson, Jessica, et al., **84**:145, 155
Pecknold, J. C., et al., **82**:205; **84**:518
Pectus excavatum, **84**:275
Pederson, A. M., et al., **83**:415, 417, 419
Pediatrics, **84**:107. *See also* Childhood; Children at risk
Peer relationships, *see* Relationships
Peet, M., et al., **82**:208
Pelligrini, R. V., **84**:264

Pelvic exenteration, *see* Surgery
Pendery, Mary L., **84**:300, 359; et al., **84**:318, 335, 336
Penfield, P. S., **82**:284
Penick, S. B., **84**:229
Penis, **82**:12, 18, 23
    anatomy of, **82**:9–10
    anxiety over size or absence of, **82**:9, 34
    biofeedback regulation of tumescence of, **84**:228
    and clitoral stimulation, **82**:10–11
    nocturnal tumescence (NPT) of, **82**:37–38, 46; **84**:221
    partial amputation of, **84**:275
    stimulation of, in dual-sex therapy, **82**:21–22; **83**:151
    See also Erection
Penis envy, **82**:55; **83**:39
    changing theories regarding, **83**:40–41, 43–48
    Freud's theory of, **83**:40–48 passim
Penman, D., et al., **84**:242
Penn, I., et al., **84**:267
Pennes, H., **82**:458, 462
Pennsylvania Mental Health Procedures Act (1976), **82**:352
Pepitone-Rockwell, F., **84**:259
Peptic ulcer, *see* Gastrointestinal disease
Perception:
    -behavior relationship, **83**:18
    and misperception during trauma, **84**:112, 113, 114, 116
Perceptual-motor dysfunction: and mental retardation, **84**:127
Perel, James M., **83**:356, 492; **84**:416n; et al., **83**:492, 498–504 passim, 508
Perey, B. F. J., et al., **84**:348
Perinatal injury, **84**:101. *See also* Children at risk
Peripheral blood flow: anxiety and, **84**:469
    biofeedback regulation of, **84**:227
Perl, M., **84**:182; et al., **84**:235, 271
Peroutka, S. J., **83**:469
Perret, J. T., **84**:357
Perris, C., **83**:269, 272, 292, 369, 406, 423, 438–41 passim, 447
Perry, C., **84**:446
Perry, E. K., et al., **83**:109, 110
Perry, J. C., **83**:11, 415, 419, 420, 423, 425, 428, 431–36 passim, 456; **84**:299
Persad, E., **83**:303
Persico, M. G., et al., **83**:449
Person, Ethel S., **82**:34; **83**:7, 8, 37, 42, 46, 49
Personality: and alcoholism, **84**:310, 321–22, 325
    alteration of
        in alcoholic, **84**:339
        in cancer patient, **84**:249, 252
        in organ transplant recipient, **84**:269
        in traumatized children, **84**:113
    and cancer risk, **84**:240
    -depression relationship, **83**:364–65, 380, 382, 383, 385–94, 405, 421, 432–33; **84**:59, 66, 216
    evaluation of (in consultation-liaison psychiatry), **84**:180
    interpersonal phenomena and, **83**:170

physical illness correlated with, **84**:216–17, 222, 224
    cancer (and cancer treatment), **84**:239–40
    and surgery, **84**:257–58
    psychotherapy focused on, **84**:66
    of therapist, and type of therapy, **84**:13
    Type A behavior, **84**:216, 220, 230, 265
    Type B behavior, **84**:220
Personality disorders, **82**:14, 429, 470–71; **83**:354
    and alcoholism, **84**:313–14
    in bipolar illness, **83**:281, 282, 286, 288–89, 312
    cancer and, **84**:246
    coexisting, **82**:455
    depression distinguished from, **83**:365, 403
    mental retardation and, **84**:124, 125
    prevalence rate of, **84**:213
    and psychosexual dysfunctions, **82**:15, 17, 18, 19
    and suicide, **83**:429
    See also individual disorders
Personality Factor Questionnaire (16), **83**:387, 392
Persson, E., **82**:207
Peruzza, M., **83**:148
Perversion(s), **82**:32, 33, 34; **83**:190
    as defense against psychosis, **82**:58
    gender dysphoria and, **82**:56
    and transsexualism, **82**:52, 54 (*see also* Transsexualism)
    See also Psychosexual dysfunctions
PET (positron emission tomography), *see* CT (computed tomography) findings
Peterfreund, Emanuel, **84**:104, 108
Peters, J. J., **82**:58, 62; et al., **82**:62
Peters, R. K., et al., **84**:447, 522
Peters, T. J., **84**:324
Peters, W. P., et al., **84**:351
Petersen, F., **84**:486
Peterson, K., **84**:357
Peterson, M. R., **82**:120
Petterson, U., **83**:287, 438
Petti, T. A., **82**:284, 296
Pettinatti, H. M., et al., **84**:313
Pettingale, K. W., et al., **84**:223
Petty, F., **84**:188
Pfeiffer, C. C., **82**:144; et al., **82**:144
Pfeiffer, Eric, **82**:46, 47; **83**:87, 116, 129–30, 141–50 passim; et al., **83**:147, 148
Phallus: symbolism of, **82**:9
Pharmacokinetics: defined, **83**:492
Pharmacotherapy, *see* Drug therapy
Phenylalanine, **84**:127. *See also* Diet
Phenylethylamine (PEA) hypothesis, *see* Schizophrenia, etiology of
Phenylketonuria, **84**:121, 127, 410
Pheochromocytoma: as drug side effect, **83**:128
Philadelphia: Child Guidance Clinic, **82**:264
    studies of anorectic patients in, **84**:225
Philips, Irving, **82**:264, 265, 268, 284, 285; **84**:91, 122–25 passim, 129, 138, 157
Phillips, D., **84**:135
Phillips, L., **82**:108; **84**:133
Phillips, M., **84**:357
Phillips Premorbid Scale, **82**:108

Phobias: psychotherapeutic management of, **84**:23, 299, 439
and school-phobic children, **82**:51; **84**:414–16, 417
sexual, **82**:32–33
Phobic Disorders: DSM-III categories for, **84**:393–400 passim, 410, 419, 518
Simple Phobia, **84**:394, 399–400, 401, 518–19
in children, **84**:410, 411–12
Social Phobia, **84**:394–401 passim, 410, 419
drug therapy for, **84**:510, 518
(*see also* Agoraphobia)
See also Anxiety Disorders
Physical examination, need for, **83**:296
in alcohol withdrawal therapy, **84**:352
of elderly patient, **83**:116–17, 119, 122–23, 125, 143; **84**:234, 235–36, 237
lithium therapy and, **83**:299
sex therapy and, **82**:21, 37
Physical handicap: and childhood depression, **82**:276, 286
Physical harm, *see* Child abuse; Crime; Rape; Violence
Physical illness: and affective disorder, **83**:378; **84**:184, 187, 203, 206, 208, 235
aging and, **83**:109
alcohol and (as exacerbation or complication), **84**:307, 331, 465
and anxiety disorders, **84**:184, 407–08, 467, 482
behavioral approach to, **84**:227, 228–29, 230
consultation-liaison psychiatry and, **84**:183–84
and dementia, **84**:234
and depression, **83**:118–19, 361, 365, 366, 378–80; **84**:49, 184, 206, 208, 217–18, 230, 235, 246–47, 248
childhood depression vs., **82**:306–07
therapy for, **84**:59–50
environmental factors and, **84**:226
and epidemiology of psychiatric illness, *see* Epidemiology
the family and, **83**:169, 193, 195, 213–14
and injury, child's reaction to, **84**:115 (*see also* Children at risk)
mandatory reporting of disease, **82**:332
mania precipitated by, **83**:277, 287
mental retardation secondary to, **84**:126–27
and nervous or mental energy (Janet's concept), **84**:428
personality characteristics and, *see* Personality
the psychiatrist and, **82**:36, 41
psychobiological studies of, **84**:57, 215, 219, 230
developmental psychobiology, **84**:224–25, 230
psychoendocrinology, **84**:221–23
psychoimmunology (behavioral immunology), **84**:223–24, 230
psychophysiology, **84**:219–21
psychological factors in/approach to, **84**:211, 213, 216–17
and psychosexual dysfunctions, **82**:15, 35–38, 41; **83**:150
psychotherapeutic management of, **84**:19, 22, 49

and sexual activity (as "taboo"), **82**:46
stress and, **83**:381; **84**:213, 214, 222, 226
and TCA therapy, **83**:497, 498, 509
See also Cancer; Cardiac disorders; Diet; Drug side effect(s); Endocrine system; Gastrointestinal disorders; Immune system; Infection(s); Mental illness; Pain; Psychosomatic disorders; Sleep disorders; Somatic symptoms; Stroke; Surgery; Vascular disorders; Viruses; *individual diseases*
Physician: as healer, **83**:173, 184
liaison, **84**:180, 181 (*see also* Consultation-liaison psychiatry)
resentment of somatizing patient by, **84**:184
See also Primary care physician; Therapist, the
Physicians' Desk Reference, **83**:484
PI, *see* Paradoxical Intention
Piafsky, K. M., **83**:495, 497; et al., **83**:497
Piaget, Jean, **82**:276, 278; **83**:13, 16
Pick's disease, **83**:109. *See also* Dementia, Primary Degenerative
Pierloot, R. A., **84**:219; et al., **84**:225
Pietruszko, R., **84**:324
Pihl, R. O., et al., **84**:331
Pike, E., **83**:495
Piker, P., **84**:352
Pilcher, J. D., **84**:350
Pills Anonymous, **84**:346
Pilot, M. L., **84**:180
Pincus, N. A., et al., **84**:215
Pinder, R., **84**:516; et al., **83**:486
Pittman, D. J., **84**:362
Pittner, M. S., **84**:220
Pitts, F. N., Jr., **83**:434; **84**:407, 474, 477, 478, 491, 492
Pituitary gland, **83**:99
response of, to stress, 222
P.L. 88-164 (Community Mental Health Centers Act), **82**:371
P.L. 94-142 (Education for all Handicapped Children Act), **84**:123, 126
Plasma factors/levels: age and, **83**:123–24, 128, 498, 499, 509–10
clinical indications of, **83**:508–11
in depressive disorders, **83**:121, 122
in lithium therapy, **83**:299, 316–17
monitoring of, **83**:123, 125, 299, 470–71, 477, 492, 498–500, 503–07
assay methods, **83**:500–503
collection of samples, **83**:501–03
cost of, **83**:508, 509
criteria for studies, **83**:504
preconditions for, **83**:507–08
in schizophrenia etiology and treatment, **82**:118–19, 126–36 passim, 141, 144, 147, 182–83, 190, 200–203
tests of, *see* DST (dexamethasone suppression test); TRH/TSH response test
tricyclics and, **83**:123–24, 125, 477, 480, 486, 491–511
imipramine, **82**:292, 295; **83**:477, 480, 497–500 passim, 504–11 passim
neuroleptics and TCAs combined, **83**:125
Plath, Sylvia, **83**:428–29, 434

Platman, S. B., **83**:300
Platt, J. J., **82**:109; et al., **82**:109
Platt, S., et al., **82**:227
Play, symbolic, **82**:276
  and play therapy, **84**:107, 119–20, 417
  posttraumatic, **84**:113, 114, 119, 120
Ploeger, A., **84**:117
Plotkin, R., **82**:382
Plumb, M. M., **84**:246
Pneumoencephalography, **82**:122
Poetry therapy, **84**:120
Pokorny, A. D., **82**:198
Polatin, P., **82**:444, 462; **83**:326, 328, 331
Polc, P., et al., **84**:489
Police: and civil commitment, **82**:385
  depression and alcoholism among, **82**:385
Polich, J. M., **84**:362; et al., **84**:318, 332
Pollack, M., et al., **83**:479
Pollard, T., et al., **84**:222
Pollin, W., **82**:451; et al., **82**:94, 95, 451
Pollock, H. M., **83**:293
Pollock, V. E., et al., **84**:327
Polvan, O., **82**:291
Polydipsia, **83**:302, 313
Polysomnographic studies, *see* REM (Rapid eye
  movement) sleep
Polyuria, **83**:302, 313, 336
Pomerleau, O. F., et al., **84**:336
POMS (Profile of Mood Stages), **84**:499
Ponce de Leon, Juan, **83**:83
Pontalis, J. B., **82**:488, 489
Pope, H. G., **83**:279, 424; **84**:146; et al., **82**:152
Popkin, M. K., **84**:402
Porjesz, B., **84**:327
Pornography: children and, **84**:116
Porter, R., **83**:133–34
Portnoi, V. A., **84**:233
Positron emission tomography (PET), *see* CT
  (computed tomography) findings
Posner, J. B., **83**:108; **84**:249, 252
Post, F., **83**:108, 118, 131, 132, 136–39 passim,
  285, 287
Post, R. M., **83**:303, 311, 312, 461; et al., **83**:461
Posttraumatic Stress Disorder: drug therapy for,
  84:516
  DSM-III category for, **84**:110, 393, 394, 396,
    401–02, 419, 516
  See also Anxiety Disorders; Trauma, em-
    tional/psychic
Potkin, Steven G., et al., **82**:126, 137, 146
Pottenger, M., et al., **83**:374
Potter, W. Z., **83**:461; et al., **83**:494, 499
Potts, Percival, **84**:239
Pourmand, M., et al., **82**:200
Powell, G. F., et al., **84**:225
Powell, S. F., **84**:237
Powell, W. J., **82**:361, 364n9
Powers, E., **84**:312
Poznanski, Elva, **82**:264, 266, 267, 274, 275, 277,
  284–89 passim, 294, 301; et al., **82**:296–300
  passim, 304, 305
Prange, A. J., **82**:290; **83**:121, 460; **84**:97
Prediction of behavior: adult, by childhood be-
  havior, **84**:95–96

of organ transplant recipient, **84**:266
  See also Children at risk: Psychiatrist, the
Pregnancy: adolescent, and risk, **84**:126
  illegitimate, incestuous relationships and, **82**:58
  lithium treatment during, **83**:314, 321n
  of psychotic mothers, **84**:99, 131, 133, 138, 139,
    143
  stress, and complications of, **84**:229
  See also Birth control
Presbycusis, *see* Hearing loss
Presbyopia, *see* Vision
Present State Examination, *see* PSE
Presidential Commission(s): on Drunk Driving,
  84:367
  on Pornography (1970s), **82**:7
Preskorn, S., **82**:292; **83**:476, 477, 478; **84**:353
Preventative psychiatry, *see* Psychiatry
Price, J., **83**:444
Price, R. A., **84**:252
Price, T. R. P., **83**:107, 109; **84**:236, 357
Prien, Robert F., **82**:188–94 passim; **83**:270, 298,
  300, 311, 312, 316, 482; et al., **82**:188, 210;
  83:298–302 passim, 307–13 passim, 371, 481
Prilipko, L. L., **82**:117
Primary care physician: and donor decision in
  organ transplant case, **84**:267
  and elderly patients, **83**:95
  and emotional dysfunction treatment, **84**:215
  and explanation of treatment (competency),
    82:356
  failure of, to recognize psychiatric disorder,
    84:188, 190, 203, 231
  oncologist as, **84**:243
  referrals by, **84**:180
    of mentally retarded chidlren, **84**:124
    of older patients, **84**:238
    after orthopedic surgery, **84**:275
    for psychiatric disorder, **84**:188
  and sexual adjustments, **82**:47
  and staff burnout, **84**:245
  See also Physician
Primary Degenerative Dementia, *see* Dementia,
  Primary Degenerative
Primary self pathology, **82**:414
  psychoanalytic psychotherapy of, **82**:498–510,
    516
  See also Narcissistic Personality Disorder
Primitive defenses, *see* Defense mechanism(s)
Prince, R. M., Jr., et al., **82**:171
*Principles of Medical Ethics with Annotations Espe-
  cially Applicable to Psychiatry* (American Psy-
  chiatric Association), **82**:329
Prinz, P., et al., **83**:133
Prior, P., **84**:460, 466
Prison(s): bipolar illness in population of, **83**:288
  confinement in, of manic patient, **83**:297
  and effect on child of parent's imprisonment,
    84:135
  and imprisonment of drunk driver, **84**:367
  therapy in, **82**:386, 395–96
  See also Crime
Privacy: elderly right to, **83**:150
  vs. supervision of family therapy, **83**:183
  See also Confidentiality

Privacy Protection Study Commission, **82**:330, 331

PRL, *see* Prolactin

Pro, J. D., **83**:108

Problem of the Aged Patient in the Public Psychiatric Hospital, The (GAP report), **83**:85

Problem-solving skills: schizophrenia and, **82**:108, 109, 112
STAPP and, **84**:31, 33
See also Coping capacities

Procci, W. R., **83**:291

Professional Standards Review Organization, **82**:332

Profile of Mood Stages (POMS), **84**:499

Progesterone: CNS regulation of, **84**:221

Progoff, I., **84**:441

Prohibition, **84**:360–61, 365. *See also* Alcoholism

Projective identification, **82**:474; **83**:22, 190, 218, 235

Projective techniques: in child therapy, **84**:111
in communication, **84**:19 (*see also* Communication)

Prolactin (PRL): CNS regulation of, **84**:221, 222
prolactin response
to drugs, *see* Drugs
to ethanol, **84**:326
See also Hormone(s)

Promiscuity, **82**:58; **83**:190

Propping, P., **84**:326

Prostate problems: drug therapy and, **83**:476
prostatectomy, **82**:39; **84**:275 (*see also* Surgery)

Prostheses, **84**:272, 275. *See also* Surgery

Prostitution: childhood incest or rape and, **82**:58

Protective factors, *see* Children at risk

Protective shield (stimulus barrier), *see* Stimulus-seeking

Protein factors, **82**:117, 119; **83**:110
Duarte protein, **83**:451, 453
tricyclics and, **83**:495, 497

Provence, S., **84**:128

Prudo, R., **83**:400, 401, 404

Prusoff, B. A., **83**:372; et al., **82**:209

Pruyser, P. W., **82**:83

Pryce, I. G., **82**:358

PSE (Present State Examination), **82**:100; **83**:408, 409, 427

Pseudodementia, depressive, *see* Dementia, Primary Degenerative

Psychasthenia: Janet's theory of, **84**:428–29

Psychiatric chemistry: and depressive disorders, **83**:457–71. *See also* Drug therapy

Psychiatric medicine, *see* Medical psychiatry

Psychiatric Status Schedule, **84**:303

Psychiatrist, the: and competency issue, **82**:351–59 passim
as double agent, **82**:393, 396
and gender disturbance cases, **82**:54
and life-threatening illness, **82**:36, 41
-physician cooperation, **82**:36, 61, 356; **83**:478; **84**:177
and postsurgical problems, **82**:38–41 passim
prediction of behavior by, **82**:172, 385, 393, 394, 395, 396; **83**:220, 229; **84**:22, 41, 48, 266

and psychotherapy, **82**:162, 215
in public sector, *see* Psychiatry
responsibility of, toward professionals and public, **82**:287, 388; **84**:186
role of
as consultant, **84**:127–28, 185, 236–38, 243–45, 266
in criminal justice system, **82**:384–96
as specialist best suited to deal with dementia, **83**:117
standard of care for, **82**:329
as teacher, **84**:180, 181, 186
See also Consultation-liaison psychiatry; Therapeutic relationship; Therapist, the

Psychiatry: child, *see* Child psychiatry
consultation, *see* Consultation-liaison psychiatry
effect on, of psychopharmacologic treatment, **83**:269
forensic, **82**:326, 384–96
geriatric, *see* Geriatric psychiatry
German, influence of on nosology, **82**:82
government regulation of, **82**:325–26, 353, 368
history and conceptual background of, **84**:390–91
hostility toward/distrust of, **83**:40, 129
court antipathy to, **82**:322–23, 336, 339
in jails, **82**:386
law and, **82**:321–96
medicine separated from, **84**:177 (*see also* Medical psychiatry)
open-systems theory of, **83**:31
orthomolecular, **82**:142–46
preventative, **82**:281, 287–88; **84**:102 (*see also* Intervention)
and psychiatric classicism, **82**:86
and psychiatric epidemiology, *see* Epidemiology
public health, **82**:281
public-sector, **82**:321, 324, 368, 388, 393
social, **84**:180
in U.S., influences on, **82**:85–86

Psychiatry in Medicine, International Journal of, **84**:182

Psychiatry 1982 (Psychiatry Update: Volume I), **83**:28n, 43n, 131n, 147n, 174n, 242n, 354, 355, 497n; **84**:53n, 95n, 98n, 259n, 325n, 416n

Psychiatry 1983 (Psychiatry Update: Volume II), **84**:35n, 53n, 57n, 58n, 95n, 108n, 178, 225n, 226n, 232, 325n, 358n, 416n, 472n

Psychic numbing: of survivors of disaster, **84**:110, 111

Psychic trauma, *see* Trauma, emotional/psychic

Psychoanalysis, **83**:184, 385; **84**:439
"adultomorphic" approaches in, **84**:104, 105
analyst's task in, **82**:497; **83**:55, 59–60, 65–66
BEP view of, **84**:12
biological assumptions of, **83**:47–48
for bipolar illness, **83**:319–20, 329
and borderline disorders, **82**:436–37, 471, 472, 481, 482
changes in approach to and scope of, **83**:7, 8, 40–44, 48–60, 66, 67

childhood, **83:**55, 192; **84:**105
childhood depression studies influenced by, **82:**266, 272
contraindications for, **82:**56, 481
criticisms of, **83:**39, 40, 46–47; **84:**66, 104, 105
defined, **83:**36, 70
empathic point of view in, **82:**493, 496–97
female psychology and, **83:**38–45, 47–50
group psychology theories and, **83:**7–8, 33
imitation of, in supportive psychotherapy, **82:**485
infancy research implications for, **83:**7, 8–21
interpretation(s) in, **83:**55–56, 59; **84:**29, 417
  bias in, **83:**46
  content of, **83:**62–65, 68
  defined, **83:**61, 67
  Freud's first use of term, **83:**63
  functions of, **83:**61–62, 66–67
  of past and present, **83:**62–65, 66, 68–70
  and selection of what to interpret, **83:**65
  and the therapeutic process, **83:**61–62, 69–70
  of transference, **83:**64–70 passim, 523, 524; **84:**14, 30, 41, 104
Kohut's redefinition of, **82:**495, 496
lack of systematic verification in, **83:**46–47; **84:**391
as "middle (chess) game," **83:**51–59 passim
and narcissism, **82:**487–98, 499, 505–10, 512–20
and Oedipus issue, **82:**489
and the past, **83:**68–70
and psychoanalytic psychotherapy, see Psychotherapy(ies)
and psychological conflict concept, **84:**430
and psychosomatic disorders, **84:**217, 226, 230
psychotherapy distinguished from, **82:**472, 477, 478; **83:**59, 60
role of theory in, **83:**65–66
selection of patient for, **83:**51–52, 60
sexism in, **83:**38–40
and sex therapy, **82:**21, 22, 26, 35
technical essentials for, **82:**476
technical modifications of, **83:**54–58
technical neutrality in, **82:**484
values in relationship to, **83:**8, 36–50
Psychoanalytic Theory of Neurosis, The (Fenichel), **83:**370
Psychodynamic theory, **82:**165; **83:**334–35; **84:**9, 11, 13, 29, 30–31, 66–67, 227
  in alcoholism therapy, **84:**339
  anxiety and, **84:**417, 426–40
    unresolved questions about, **84:**522
  in consultation-liaison therapy, **84:**180, 181
  and depression, **83:**513, 521–24, 525, 526
  and psychic trauma, **84:**118, 119
Psychogenic Pain Disorder: DSM-III category for, **84:**211
  among elderly, **84:**236
  See also Pain; Somatoform Disorders
Psychological, psychobiological, psychosocial studies of illness, *see* Physical illness

Psychological Factors Affecting Physical Condition: DSM-III category for, **84:**211. *See also* Psychosomatic disorders; Somatic symptoms
Psychologie vom empirischen Standpunkte (Brentano), **84:**67
Psychologists: on consultation-liaison team, **84:**182, 215
Psychomotor retardation: depression and, **83:**279, 282, 479, 488; **84:**234, 236
  childhood depression, **82:**303
  of infants at risk, **84:**131
  as predictor of TCA response, **83:**122
Psychopathology, *see* Mental illness
Psychosexual changes: late-life, **83:**147–51
Psychosexual dysfunctions: alcoholism and, **84:**345
  atypical, **82:**16, 20
  classification of, **82:**16 (*see also individual dysfunction*)
  diagnostic complexities of, **82:**14–20
  DSM-III criteria for, **82:**8, 9, 12–21 passim
  depressive disorders and, **82:**16–17; **83:**150, 366, 373
  physiological cause of, **82:**21, 35–41; **83:**149–51
    chemotherapeutic, **84:**255
    postoperative, **84:**260, 265
  of rape victims, **82:**62, 65–66
  separation and divorce and, **82:**44
  treatment of, **82:**20–26; **84:**53
    family therapy, **83:**190, 191
    treatment failures, **82:**25, 26–35
  See also Impotence; Sex therapy; Sexual response
Psychosis(es): atypical, treatment of, **82:**208
  vs. childhood depression, **82:**306
  children at risk for, **84:**131–36 passim (*see also* mental retardation and, *below*)
  CPK activity and, **82:**128–29
  cycloid, **83:**292
  drug-induced, *see* Drug side effect(s)
  fetish or perversion as defense against, **82:**58
  gender dysphoria and, **82:**56
  hormone-induced, **84:**250
  and immunity, **82:**115
  insanity differentiated from, **82:**390
  manic-depressive, *see* Bipolar (manic-depressive) Disorder
  mental retardation and, **84:**124
  paranoid, *see* Paranoid reactions
  psychotherapy and, **84:**17, 23–24
  reactive, **82:**208; **83:**295, 441 (*see also* Grief reaction; Loss)
  schizoaffective, *see* Schizoaffective Disorder
  with systemic lupus erythematosus, **83:**287
  and use of term "psychotic," **83:**370
Psychosocial Collaborative Oncology Group, *see* PSYCOG
Psychosocial factors, **83:**382–85; **84:**53
  and anxiety at hospitalization, **84:**208
  and children at risk, **84:**122, 124, 125, 127, 135–36 (*see also* Children at risk)
  medical disregard of, **84:**177

and psychiatric morbidity rate, **84:**202, 203, 206
   among mentally retarded, **84:**124
social status of parenting, **84:**136, 143
studies of, **84:**97, 215, 216, 225–27
See also Depression; Loss; Role(s); Social class;
   Stress
Psychosomatic disorders: alexithymia and,
   84:437–38
   behavioral approach to, **84:**227, 228–29
   childhood, studies of, **83:**174; **84:**225
   etiology of (studied), **84:**178, 217–18
   family interaction and, **83:**213
   and incidence of psychiatric morbidity, **84:**188,
      198, 202
   panic as symptom, **84:**438
   psychoanalysis and, **84:**217, 226, 230
   studies of (Britain, U.S.), **83:**174; **84:**211, 217
   See also Alexithymia; Physical illness
Psychosomatic medicine: emergence of, **84:**179
   origins of, **84:**227
   research in, **84:**216–18
Psychotherapy(ies), **82:**8
   for alcoholism, **84:**299, 338–46
   alexithymic patients and, **84:**218
   for anxiety/anxiety disorders, **84:**412, 416, 417,
      418–26, 439–40, 521–22
   for bipolar illness, **83:**319–37
   for borderline patients, **82:**425, 467, 470–87
   brief, *see* Psychotherapy(ies), brief
   for cancer patients, **82:**39; **84:**244, 245, 247, 248
   choice of, **83:**526, 527
   conjoint, **82:**26, 35; **83:**170, 190, 191, 193, 215,
      222; **84:**16, 345
   in consultation-liaison psychiatry, **84:**180
   contraindicated, **83:**527; **84:**44
   costs of, **84:**35
   for depression, **83:**252, 319, 511–28
      childhood depression, **82:**302, 307
      negative response to, **83:**369
      short-term, *see* Psychotherapy(ies), brief
   and development of social skills, **82:**302;
      83:517–21 passim, 524
   didactic techniques in, **83:**514, 518, 520
   drug therapy combined with or vs., *see* Drug
      therapy
   efficacy discussed, **82:**157–61, 165–66, 215–28
   existential, **84:**421, 424
   expressive, **82:**471–72, 476–80, 481, 482, 486;
      83:28
      in narcissistic personality disorder, **82:**514,
         520, 522
   family, **84:**225 (*see also* Family therapy)
   genetic counseling within, *see* Genetic factors
   geriatric, **83:**114, 128–30, 138; **84:**238
   goals of, **84:**19, 58, 59–60
   group, *see* Group therapy
   individual
      group vs., **84:**425
      in sex therapy, **82:**21, 24
      for traumatized child, **84:**118, 119–20
   interpersonal, *see* Psychotherapy(ies), brief
   as learning process, **84:**19
   for mentally retarded, **84:**129
   and physical illness, **84:**19, 22, 49

psychoanalysis distinguished from, **82:**472, 477,
   478; **83:**59, 60
psychoanalytic, **82:**22, 26, 35; **83:**65, 193, 519;
   84:11, 30
   of alcoholism, **84:**345
   of borderline disorders, **82:**476–80
   of group/individuals in group, **83:**26–28
   insight-oriented, **84:**226 (*see also* Therapy)
   and interest in symptoms, **83:**62
   interpretation in, **82:**54, 476–81 passim, 507,
      510, 518, 519; **83:**62, 523, 524; **84:**17, 27, 29,
      30, 31, 40, 345
   of primary self pathology, **82:**498–510, 516
psychodynamic approach to/issues in, *see*
   Psychodynamic theory
of schizophrenic disorders, **82:**154–66, 215–28
selection of patient for, **84:**25–27, 44, 440
sexism in, **83:**38–40
shared components of, **84:**422–24
supportive, **82:**471–72, 480–86, 516; **83:**28;
   84:60, 247, 248, 504, 510
   indications and contraindications for, **82:**481–
      82, 520–23
   techniques of, **82:**483–85
and third-party protection, **82:**331 (*see also*
   Confidentiality)
time-limited, *see* Psychotherapy(ies), brief
for transsexualism, **82:**48, 53–54
See also Behavioral approach; Cognitive therapy; Therapy
Psychotherapy(ies), brief, **84:**7–76, 247
   in ancient (Egyptian and Greek) history, **84:**7
   BEP (brief and emergency), **84:**7, 8
      basic concepts of, **84:**12–13
      sequence of sessions in, **84:**14–17
      therapeutic process in, **84:**17–22
   contraindicated, **84:**44
   crisis-oriented, **84:**185
   interpersonal (IPT), **83:**519–21, 524–25, 526;
      84:10
      compared with other psychotherapies,
         84:63–66
      for depression, **84:**56–67
      goals of, **84:**59–60
      phases in, **84:**60–63
      psychodynamic theory and, **84:**66–67 (*see also*
         Psychodynamic theory)
      theoretical and empirical bases for, **84:**57–
         59
   vs. long-term, **84:**13, 64
   multimodal (MMT), **84:**10, 67–76, 318
      bridging and tracking procedures in, **84:**75–
         76
      diagnosis and assessment under, **84:**68–75
      structural profiles in, **84:**73–75
   short-term anxiety-provoking (STAPP), **84:**9,
      24–35
      evaluation process in, **84:**27–29
      follow-up studies of, **84:**32–35
      selection of patient for, **84:**25–27
      technical requirements for, **84:**29–32
   therapeutic relationship/contract in, **84:**15–16,
      29
   time-limited (TLP), **84:**8, 9, 35–44

central issue in, **84:**37–40, 43–44
clinical technique in, **84:**40–43
phases of, **84:**41–42
selection of patients for, **84:**44
See also Cognitive therapy
Psychotherapy by Reciprocal Inhibition (Wolpe), **84:**449
PSYCOG (Psychosocial Collaborative Oncology Group), **84:**242, 246, 247
Public Health Service Grant, **82:**296n, 350n
Public policy: and alcoholism, **84:**359–70
and mental retardation, **84:**122–23
Pugh, T. F., **83:**88, 89, 94, 406; et al., **83:**422
Puig-Antich, Joaquim, **82:**284, 288, 294; **83:**497n; **84:**98, 416n; et al., **82:**264, 269, 284, 289–95 passim, 307; **83:**505, 509
Pulkkinen, E., **82:**115
Pulver, S., **82:**488
Purdy, M. D., **82:**143
Purtell, J. J., et al., **84:**212
Purvis, S. A., **82:**171
Puzantian, V. R., **83:**279, 289, 290
Pynoos, R., **84:**112, 116
Pyridoxine deficiency, **84:**127. *See also* Vitamins

Q

Quality of life, *see* Values
Querido, A., **84:**199
Quilitch, H. R., **83:**114
Quinn, J. T., **84:**351, 354
Quitkin, F., et al., **82:**108, 182, 188, 189, 195, 466; **83:**127, 304, 481

R

Rabin, E. Z., et al., **83:**314
Rabins, P. V., **83:**107, 108; **84:**234
Rabkin, J., **84:**226, 393, 437
Racamier, P. C., **83:**277
Rachlin, S., **82:**384n8
Rachman, S., **84:**449, 453, 456
Racism, **83:**234. *See also* Ethnicity
Rackensperger, W., et al., **82:**207
Racker, H., **82:**474
Radiation therapy, *see* Cancer
Radioimmunoassay, **83:**501
Radloff, L. S., **83:**413; **84:**135
Rado, S., **82:**444, 490, 495; **83:**319, 522
Rae, D., **84:**135
Rafaelson, O., **84:**353; et al., **83:**314
Rage: countertransference, **82:**54
narcissistic, **82:**494, 495, 514–21 passim
See also Anger
Ragheb, M., **82:**214
Rahe, R. H., **83:**394; **84:**94, 213, 226; et al., **83:**394
Rainer, J. D., **83:**277, 438, 444, 446, 447
Rainey, J. M., Jr., **84:**357

Raleigh Hills Hospital (Portland), **84:**334
Raman, A. C., **82:**120
Rama-Rao, V. A., et al., **82:**201, 203
Ramsay, R. A., et al., **82:**181
Ramsey, A. T., **83:**314
Randrup, A., **82:**137
Rand study (of alcoholism), **84:**307, 318, 331
Rangell, L., **84:**108
Rank, O., **83:**55; **84:**7
Rankin, P. P., **84:**145
Rao, A. V., **83:**287
Rape, **82:**56
of child or adolescent, **82:**58, 62, 63; **84:**115, 116
incest as form of, **82:**57 (*see also* Incest)
sexual repercussions of, **82:**61–63
testimonial privilege in cases of, **82:**331
therapeutic considerations for, **82:**63–66
See also Trauma, emotional/psychic
Rapid eye movement, *see* REM sleep
Rappaport, Judith, et al., **84:**512, 513
Rappoport, J. A., **84:**457
Rascovsky, M. and A., **82:**58
Raskin, A. S., **83:**114; et al., **83:**112
Raskin, D., **82:**120
Raskin, M., et al., **84:**401
Raskind, M. A., **83:**106, 506; et al., **83:**139
Rasmussen, A., **82:**58
Raush, H. L., **82:**177
Ravaris, C. L., et al., **83:**479, 482, 483
Ray, W. A., et al., **83:**95
Raynaud's disease, **84:**228, 230, 502. *See also* Physical illness
Rayses, V., **83:**454; **84:**323
Razani, J., **84:**357
Razin, A. M., **84:**229
RDC (Research Diagnostic Criteria): for affective-related disorders, **82:**440; **83:**294, 380, 408, 410, 421, 427, 466; **84:**198, 206
for alcoholism, **84:**303–09 passim
for anxiety neurosis, **84:**494
in borderline disorders, **82:**423, 434
for depression, **82:**289, 296, 305; **83:**294, 411, 465, 466; **84:**49
childhood depression, **82:**270, 290, 293–99 passim
origin of, **84:**303
Reach to Recovery, **84:**271
Reading, A. E., **84:**259
Reality, denial of, *see* Denial
Reality testing: in family therapy, **83:**200–201
loss of, **83:**370
and psychotherapeutic management of feelings of unreality, **84:**23
Rebeta-Burditt, J., **84:**346
Recapitulation (by therapist), **84:**31
Redick, R. W., **83:**130; et al., **83:**94, 95
Redlich, F. C., 93
Redmond, D. E., **84:**471, 472, 512
Reed, D. M., **82:**43
Reed, D. S., **84:**366
Reenactment, **84:**113, 114, 119. *See also* Play, symbolic
Rees, W. D., **84:**217
Referrals, *see* Primary-care physician

Regier, D. A., **83:**94, 95; **84:**92; et al., **84:**189, 396
Regression: "child time" as, **84:**36
  divorce as cause of
    in adult, **84:**148
    in preschool child, **84:**152
  encouragement of, in analysis, **83:**59
  as group reaction, **83:**21, 23, 24, 28, 30, 32, 35
Rehabilitation: of alcoholic, **84:**342–43
  centers for, **84:**184
    halfway houses, **82:**177
  disability benefits as disincentives to, **82:**109–10
  for mentally retarded, **84:**129
  for schizophrenics, **82:**107–10, 176–77
Rehavi, M., et al., **83:**470
Rehfeld, J. F., **84:**223
Rehm, L. P., **83:**516, 517, 524; et al., **83:**524, 527
Reibel, S., **82:**226
Reich, A., **82:**511
Reich, B., **84:**468
Reich, L. H., et al., **83:**286
Reich, Theodore, **82:**290; **83:**269, 443; **84:**320; et al., **83:**447, 448; **84:**406
Reich, Wilhelm, **82:**488; **83:**34
Reichmann, F., **82:**274
Reid, W. H., **84:**96, 135
Reider, N., **82:**475
Reifler, B., **84:**234; et al., **83:**107; **84:**236
Reilly, T. M., **84:**354
Reiman-Sheldon, E., **84:**236
Reinberg, A., **83:**97
Reinforcement: in alcoholism therapy, **84:**330, 345
    contingent, **84:**332, 334, 337
  in avoidance behavior, **84:**449
  and depression, **83:**516–19
Reisberg, B., **83:**112; **84:**234
Reisby, N., et al., **83:**505
Reiser, M. F., **84:**216
Reiser, S. J., et al., **82:**327
Reisine, T. D., et al., **82:**142; **83:**109, 110
Reiss, David J., **82:**173; **83:**171, 174, 181, 242, 245
Relationships: and attachment bonds, **84:**57–58, 59, 100, 127, 128, 420, 423
  cause-effect, **83:**66, 68, 229, 239
  confiding, lack of (and depression), **83:**364, 400, 403, 404, 414, 421–22; **84:**58, 135
  donor-recipient, in organ transplant cases, **84:**266–67, 268–69
  interpersonal, **83:**519
    alcoholism and, **84:**305
    bipolar illness and, **83:**249, 250–51, 279, 286, 302
    depression and, **83:**522, 523; **84:**62, 63
    in family therapy, **83:**181–82
    of geriatric patient, **83:**135–37, 139
    patient-staff, **83:**29–30, 139, 244
    postoperative, **84:**273
    psychotherapy and, **84:**15, 58–59, 62–66 (see also Psychotherapy[ies], brief)
    schizophrenia and, **82:**167–68, 170, 224–25; **83:**130
    and success of therapy, **84:**26
  male-female, within group, **83:**33 (see also Group psychology)

peer, **83:**33, 195; **84:**103, 368
  of child of divorce, **84:**152
  of mentally retarded child, **84:**121–22
psychiatrist-physician, **82:**36, 61, 356; **83:**478 (see also Consultation-liaison psychiatry)
sexual
  conceptualized as dangerous, **82:**473
  of young women from divorced families, **84:**153
See also Communication; Empathy; Expectations; Family, the; Mother-child relationship; Parent(s); Parent-child relationship; Social support networks; Therapeutic relationship; Transference
Relationship therapy, see Therapy
Relaxation therapy, **84:**70, 73, 229
  for anxiety disorders, **84:**258, 439, 440–48, 507, 512
    unresolved questions about, **84:**522–23
  clinical trials of, **84:**447–48
  in consultation-liaison psychiatry, **84:**186
  Eastern religious practices, **84:**441, 443
  for headache, **84:**228
  physiological basis for, **84:**444–45
  secular methods, **84:**443, 446–47
  trophotropic response in, **84:**444–45
  Western mystical practices, **84:**441–43
Religion: and anxiety at hospitalization, **84:**208
  and relaxation response, **84:**441, 442, 447
  and religious prejudice, **83:**234
  sexuality and, **82:**7
REM (rapid eye movement) sleep, **84:**220, 221
  in bipolar and unipolar depressions, **83:**122, 273, 276, 283, 289
  in borderline disorders, **82:**453
  in childhood depression, **82:**290, 294–95
  drug suppression of, **83:**115
  EEG studies of, **83:**122
  late-life, **83:**145
  nocturnal penile tumescence during, **82:**46; **84:**221
  and non-rapid eye movement (NREM) sleep, **84:**220–21
Remove Intoxicated Drivers (RID), **84:**362
Renal disease: delirium caused by, **84:**232
  and depressive symptomatology, **84:**208
  and dialysis, **84:**265–66, 271
  as drug side effect, see Drug side effect(s)
  and kidney transplant, see Surgery
Renard Diagnostic Interview, **83:**408
Rennecker, R., **84:**270
Repetition compulsion, **83:**18
Repetitive phenomena: posttraumatic, **84:**113, 114, 119. See also Trauma, emotional/psychic
Reppucci, N. D., **84:**156
Repression theory, **83:**18
Research, **84:**391, 519
  on children at risk, **84:**87, 90, 91–93, 95–103, 120, 130–31
    methodological issues in, **84:**101–02
    need for (divorce effects), **84:**157–58
  on epidemiology, see Epidemiology
  in medical psychiatry, **84:**186, 215–30

in psychosomatic medicine, **84:**216–18
on separation and divorce, priorities for, **84:**157–58
Research Diagnostic Criteria, *see* RDC
Residual Attention Deficit Disorder, **82:**442. *See also* ADD (Attentional Deficit Disorder)
Resnik, H. L. P., **83:**433
Responsibility: of patient (in therapy), and denial of, **83:**28, 190, 251, 527; **84:**343, 344. *See also* Competency/incompetency; Diminished capacity/responsibility; Psychiatrist, the
Reter, D., **82:**55
Retinopathy: as drug side effect, **82:**169
Reveley, M. A., et al., **83:**467
Review Panel on Coronary-Prone Behavior and Coronary Heart Disease, **84:**216, 217
Rey, J. H., **82:**470
Reynolds, C. M., et al., **84:**358
Reynolds, G. P., **82:**137; et al., **82:**134
Reynynghe de Voxrie, **84:**512
Reznikoff, M., **84:**271
Rheumatic fever: "cure" of, **84:**264
Rheumatic pain modulation disorder (RPMD), **84:**221
Rheumatoid factors: schizophrenia and, **82:**117, 118
Riblet, L. A., **83:**488; et al., **84:**498, 501
Rice, A. K., **83:**22, 30–31, 32, 33, 35
Rice, J. R., et al., **82:**145
Rich, C. L., **83:**434
Richards, M. P. M., **84:**147
Richardson, J. M., **82:**198
Richelson, E., **83:**475
Richmond, J. B., **84:**127
Richmond, Mary E., **83:**169–70
Rickels, K., **84:**484; et al., **84:**499, 516, 517
Riddle, M., et al., **83:**483
Rie, H. E., **82:**272, 274, 278, 289
Rieder, R. O., **82:**448, 450; **83:**450; **84:**99, 100, 101; et al., **82:**448
Rieff, P., **83:**37, 47
Rifkin, A., et al., **82:**459, 463; **83:**142, 288; **84:**474
Right(s): constitutional, *see* Civil commitment of minors, **82:**352
of patient vs. psychiatrist, **82:**334 (*see also* Ethical considerations)
to receive or refuse treatment, *see* Therapy visitation, *see* Separation and divorce
See also Civil rights movement; Informed consent; Law; Law and psychiatry
Rimon, R., **84:**224; et al., **82:**120, 121
Rinieris, P. M., et al., **83:**450
Rinsley, D. B., **82:**470
Rioch, M., **83:**30
Ripley, H. S., **82:**284; **83:**429, 430; **84:**179
Risch, S. C., et al., **83:**463, 469
Risk, **84:**136
concept of, **84:**91, 93–95
and risk factors among medical populations, **84:**214
See also Children at risk; Dangerousness
Ritchie, J., **84:**350
Robbins, D. R., **82:**284; et al., **82:**302

Robbins, G. F., **84:**271
Robbins, M. D., **82:**437
Robert, E., **82:**138
Roberts, B. H., **84:**192, 209, 211, 213
Robertson, A., **83:**174
Robertson, B. M., **82:**286
Robertson, H. A., et al., **84:**485
Robin, A., et al., **82:**103
Robins, Eli, **83:**376, 379, 381, 429, 433; **84:**303, 467; et al., **83:**429, 430, 433
Robins, Lee N., **84:**96, 136, 299, 311, 313, 316; et al., **83:**90, 408; **84:**308, 309
Robinson, D. S., **83:**127, 128; **84:**235; et al., **83:**127, 506
Robinson, J., **84:**259
Robinson, P. A., **83:**34
Rochio, P., **84:**274
Rochlin, G., **82:**266, 272
Rockefeller, John D., Jr., **84:**361
Rockefeller Foundation, **84:**179
Rockwell, D. A., **84:**259
Rodin, J., **84:**219
Rodnick, E. H., **82:**87, 155; **83:**174; **84:**95, 99; et al., **84:**95, 101, 132
Roe v. *Wade*, **82:**328
Roeske, N. A., **84:**274
Roessler, R., **84:**220
Roffman, Mark, **83:**462, 468, 490; et al., **83:**469
Rog, D. J., **82:**177
Rogers, C. R., et al., **82:**158, 216
Rogers, D. E., et al., **83:**106
Rogers, M. P., et al., **84:**223, 275
Rohrbaugh, J. B., **83:**45, 48
Roiphe, H., **82:**55
Roizen, R., et al., **84:**315
Role(s): analyst-patient reversal of, **82:**516 (*see also* Transference)
of consultant, *see* Psychiatrist, the
dual, of psychiatric physician, **83:**173, 183–84
of father, when wife is hospitalized, **84:**133
female
changing concepts of, **83:**38
impairment of (by depression), **84:**58, 62
as parent, **84:**133, 135
gender, *see* Gender identity
and interpersonal role disputes, **84:**58, 62–63
parent-child reversal of, **83:**231–32; **84:**138, 149, 152
and role playing in schizophrenic rehabilitation, **82:**109, 111
and role transition of depressed patient, **83:**521; **84:**63
sick, depression as legitimate, **84:**61
social, and marital disillusionment, **82:**27
of surgeon, in TPN, **84:**272
of therapist, *see* Psychiatrist, the; Therapist, the
Rolf, J. E., **84:**137, 142, 143; et al., **84:**131, 133
Romano, J., **83:**107
Romm, M., **82:**475
Ron, M. A., et al., **83:**107; **84:**235
Room, R., **84:**315, 329, 360
Roose, K., **82:**195
Roose, S., et al., **83:**477
Rorabaugh, W. J., **84:**360

Rorschach test, **82**:433; **84**:19
  of traumatized children, **84**:115
Rorsman, B., **84**:460
Rose, G., **82**:283; **83**:87
Rose, R. M., **84**:222, 488
Rosen, A. M., **83**:325
Rosen, B. M., et al., **84**:195
Rosen, J. N., **82**:217
Rosen, Z. A., **82**:108
Rosenbaum, A. H., et al., **82**:204; **83**:462, 463, 468, 473
Rosenbaum, M., **84**:275
Rosenberger, P., **82**:124
Rosenblatt, M., **82**:213
Rosenfeld, A., **82**:57; **84**:116; et al., **82**:58
Rosenfeld, H., **82**:470, 474, 499n1, 511, 516, 517, 523; **83**:319
Rosenfeld, J. E., **84**:353
Rosenheck, Stephen, **83**:172; **84**:95n
Rosenman, R. H., **84**:216
Rosenthal, D., **82**:445n; **84**:97; et al., **82**:87, 95, 444, 445, 448, 454, 455
Rosenthal, J. B., **84**:218
Rosenthal, N. E., et al., **83**:296, 302
Rosenthal, R. H., **83**:442
Rosenthal, T. L., **84**:453; et al., **83**:275, 276
Rosett, Henry, **84**:303
Rosman, B. L., et al., **84**:225
Ross, H., **83**:108, 114
Ross, H. L., **84**:362, 366, 367
Ross, N., **83**:49
Ross, S. B., et al., **83**:451
Rossor, M. N., et al., **83**:110
Ross-Stanton, J., **82**:129
Roth, E., **84**:115
Roth, Loren H., **82**:324, 326, 330, 331, 351, 354–58 passim; **84**:259n, 260; et al., **82**:351–60 passim
Roth, M., **83**:107, 108, 109, 131, 132, 133, 137, 273, 285
Roth, W. F., **83**:416
Roth, W. T., et al., **84**:468
Rothblum, E. D., et al., **84**:236
Rothschild, M. A., **84**:404
Rothstein, F., **84**:355
Rotrosen, J., et al., **82**:136, 204
Rounsaville, Bruce J., **83**:519; **84**:8, 10; et al., **83**:321
Rovée-Collier, Carolyn K., **83**:16, 18; et al., **83**:16
Rowan, P., et al., **83**:479, 483
Rowe, J. W., **83**:133
Rowland, J., **84**:254, 255; et al., **84**:252
Rowland, M., **83**:492, 493, 500
Roy, A., **83**:402, 403
RPMD (rheumatic pain modulation disorder), **84**:221
Rubin, R. T., **82**:200, 203, 204; **83**:460; et al., **82**:203
Ruddle, F. H., **83**:436
Rüdin, E., **82**:93
Rush, A. John, **82**:161; **83**:512, 527; **84**:8, 9, 45–49 passim, 53; et al., **83**:525; **84**:49, 52
Rush, Benjamin, **84**:177

Rushing, W. A., **82**:100
Russell, G. F. M., **84**:219, 225
Russell, S., **83**:90
Rutenfranz, J., **84**:350
Rutschmann, J., et al., **84**:100
Rutter, M. L., **82**:285, 286; **84**:58, 96, 102, 103, 124, 136, 153, 412; et al., **82**:267, 282, 284; **84**:102, 124, 136
Rybakowski, J., **83**:452
Ryle, A., **83**:525
Rymer, C. A., **84**:179

S

Sacchetti, E., et al., **83**:468
Sachar, E. J., **82**:290; **84**:407, 488; et al., **82**:201, 290, 293
Sadavoy, J., **84**:236
Sadism: characterological, **82**:514–15, 516, 520
  and sadomasochistic sexual exchanges, **82**:30
Sadock, Virginia A., **82**:11
SADS (Schedule for Affective Disorders and Schizophrenia), **82**:432; **83**:408; **84**:61
  Kiddie-SADS, **82**:270
  -RDC, **83**:408, 421, 427
  SADS-L, **84**:198, 206
Sager, C. J., **83**:190, 199, 217, 218, 223; et al., **83**:215; **84**:52
Sainsbury, P., **83**:430, 431
St. Elizabeth's Hospital case (Washington, D.C.), **82**:372–77 passim
St. John, **84**:442
St. Louis studies: alcoholism, **84**:309–10
  anxiety disorders, **84**:404
St. Martin, Alexis, **84**:219
St. Terese of Avila, **84**:442
Salapatek, P., **83**:10
Saldanha, V. F., et al., **82**:204
Salk, D., **83**:110
Salkind, M. R., **84**:204, 206
Salmons, P., **84**:465
Salpêtrière, the, **84**:427, 428
Salt, P., **84**:135
Salzman, C., **82**:209; **84**:235, 237; et al., **84**:237
Salzman, L. F., **84**:132
Salzman, R., **83**:112
Sameroff, A. J., **83**:229, 230; **84**:88, 125; et al., **84**:101, 131, 134, 138
Samorajski, T., **83**:99, 115
Sampliner, R., **84**:355
Sanborn, F. B., **84**:443
Sanchez-Craig, Martha, **84**:337, 338
Sander, L., **83**:14, 18
Sandler, J., **82**:272–73, 503; **84**:108; et al., **83**:61
Sandler, M., **82**:137; **83**:452; et al., **83**:467
Sandoz Pharmaceuticals, **83**:102, 104
Sandt, J. J., **84**:181
Sanger, C. K., **84**:271
Santos, A. D., et al., **84**:481

Santrock, J. W., **84**:153, 156
Sapira, J. D., **84**:353
Saraf, K. R., et al., **84**:415–16
Sargant, W., **84**:507
Sartorius, N., et al., **82**:100
Satir, V., **83**:189
Saunders, G. R., **84**:325
Saunders, J. C., **82**:118
Sawicka, J., et al., **84**:252
Scafa, G. M., **82**:146
Scandinavia: alcoholism studies in, **84**:314, 316–17, 320
  bereavement studies in, **84**:217
  depressive symptom studies in, **83**:407, 413, 423, 426
  postoperative studies in, **84**:264
  risk factors studied in, **84**:96
  schizophrenia studies in, **82**:94, 98, 145
  STAPP studies in, **84**:33
Scapegoating, **83**:210, 233–34, 239, 240
Scarf, M., **84**:61
Scarisbrick, P., **84**:221
Schachter, S., **84**:219
Schaefer, M., **83**:40
Schafer, R., **82**:497; **83**:41, 45, 48, 63
Schaie, K. W., **83**:117
Schanberg, S. M., et al., **83**:460
Schandry, R., **84**:469
Schatzberg, Alan F., **83**:321, 356, 475, 481, 488, 512; **84**:358n; et al., **83**:459, 461, 462, 468, 473, 475, 479, 490
Schechter, M., **84**:115
Schedule(s): for Affective Disorders and Schizophrenia, *see* SADS
  for Interviewing Borderlines (SIB), *see* Borderline Personality Disorder, diagnosis of
  of Recent Experience, **84**:226
  for Schizotypal Personalities (SSP), **82**:432
Scheel-Kruger, J., **84**:486
Scheibel, M. E. and A. G., **83**:100
Schemata: defined, **84**:46–47. *See also* Cognitive therapy
Schenk, G. K., et al., **82**:214
Scherl, D. S., **82**:61
Scherwitz, L., et al., **84**:216
Schiavone, D. J., **82**:128
Schick, J. F. E., **82**:461
Schiebel, D., **84**:219
Schiefelbusch, R. L., **84**:126
Schiele, B. C., **82**:185
Schiff, S. K., **84**:180
Schiffman, S., **83**:104
Schilder, Paul, **84**:311
Schildkraut, Joseph J., **83**:356, 457, 459, 468, 469; et al., **82**:452; **83**:460–67 passim, 473, 474, 512; **84**:472n
Schilsky, R. L., et al., **84**:255
Schizoaffective Disorder, **82**:144, 438, 439; **83**:282, 283, 358; **84**:49, 101
  as bipolar variant, **83**:439, 441–42, 447, 457, 462, 464, 465, 480
  criteria for, **82**:152; **83**:290–92, 302, 376, 441, 462
  genetic studies of, **83**:439–42, 446

medication for, **82**:208, 209; **83**:439
and suicide, **83**:429, 430
Schizophrenia: American concept of, **82**:86; **83**:269
  borderline personality disorder compared to, discriminated from, related to, **82**:416, 436, 439–43 passim, 444–57 passim
  and cancer incidence, **84**:253
  childhood, **82**:108, 263, 306
  children at risk for, **84**:98, 99–101
  communication deviance in, **82**:155; **83**:242, 247, 280; **84**:101, 132
  "core deficit" in, **82**:173, 209
  decompensation in, **82**:88, 100, 103, 106, 163, 177
  definitions (cross-sectional and longitudinal clinical pictures) of, **82**:84, 85–91, 100–101, 108
  depression associated with, **83**:291, 376, 379, 381, 466, 467
  developmental-interactive model of, **82**:161–66
  diagnosis of, **82**:83, 93, 123, 138, 162, 166–68
    in adoptive studies, **82**:445–48
    computerized, **82**:100
    criteria for, **82**:83–91 passim, 98, 101–02, 113, 149, 167, 423, 432, 448; **83**:131, 271, 282; **84**:101, 102, 396
    differential, **83**:131, 278, 282, 285, 289–92, 358–59
    and misdiagnosis, **82**:101–02, 120; **83**:281, 284, 285, 290
    in U.S., **82**:86; **83**:271, 293, 407
  and electrodermal (SCL) response, **84**:131, 470
  epidemiology/prevalence rate of, **82**:93, 95–96, 98, 120–21, 290, 445; **83**:271, 407; **84**:137
    diet (gluten) and, **82**:145–46
    ethnic groups and, **82**:101, 102
    family history and, **83**:132, 283, 439, 441
    outpatient vs. inpatient, **84**:208, 211
    social class and, **82**:98, 100, 101; **83**:426
  (*see also* late-onset, *below*)
  etiology of, *see* Schizophrenia, etiology of, *below*
  genetic studies of (in twins), **82**:94–95; **83**:441
  history of concept of, **82**:82–83
  International Study of (WHO), **82**:100
  late-onset, **83**:91–92, 94–95, 130–32, 138, 140, 144
  and marital status, **83**:427; **84**:132
  and mortality rate, **84**:460
  paranoid, **82**:86
    biochemical factors in, **82**:115, 126, 131, 132, 137–38, 142, 148, 152, 197
    blacks with, **82**:102; **83**:270
    classification of, **82**:86, 149
    late-life, **83**:132, 144
    misdiagnosis of, **83**:281
    paraphrenia differentiated from, **83**:137 (*see also* Paraphrenia)
  of parent (and effect on child), *see* Parent(s)
  prediction of, **82**:172; **83**:175–76; **84**:415
  premorbid functioning and, **82**:89, 90, 98, 100, 108, 109, 122, 149, 150
  prognosis for, **82**:87–89, 115, 167–68

chronicity and, **82:**177; **84:**134
cultural and social factors in, **82:**100, 101, 107, 108
recovery, **82:**88, 89, 90, 101, 115, 154; **83:**282
vocational rehabilitation and, **82:**109–10
(*see also* relapse in, *below*)
pseudoneurotic, **82:**444, 457, 462, 468
relapse in
avoidance of, **82:**163; **83:**171, 244, 245
EE (expressed emotion) and, **82:**103–05, 110, 111, 172, 173–74; **83:**175, 242–47 passim, 249, 256; **84:**95
family factors and, **82:**103–06, 107, 110, 112, 172–74; **83:**171, 175–76, 242–49
medication and, **82:**102, 104, 142–43, 168–72, 190–95
model of, **82:**99
PRL (blood prolactin) as predictor of, **82:**135
rehabilitation efforts (social pressures, social adjustment) and, **82:**107, 108, 110, 176–77
in short-term therapy, **82:**219–20
stress and, **82:**102–03, 106, 112
SPEM impairment in, **82:**453
stress and, **82:**98, 102–03, 106, 107, 112, 156, 163, 165, 173; **83:**381
studies of, **82:**94, 98, 102–09 passim, 128, 145, 173, 205, 215–25, 445–48; **83:**174, 175, 453; **84:**99–102, 303, 405–06
subtypes of, **82:**86, 147, 152; **83:**135, 140
and suicide, **83:**429, 430
symptoms of, **82:**89, 120; **83:**130, 131
brain dopamine increase, **82:**132
delusions and hallucinations, **82:**85, 86, 87, 126, 141, 148, 149, 167, 197, 200, 209; **83:**130, 131, 138
depressive, **83:**291
manic, **83:**376
MAO activity, *see* MAO (monoamine oxidase)
negative and positive, **82:**123, 167–78
Schneiderian and Bleulerian, **83:**279, 289
taraxein and, **82:**118
thought disorder, **82:**199; **83:**279
(*see also* diagnosis of, *above*)
treatment of, *see* Schizophrenia, treatment of, *below*
work and, **82:**109–10
Schizophrenia, etiology of, **82:**84, 85, 91, 215
biochemical and morphological factors in, **82:**112–53
COMT activity and, **82:**128, 131
CPK activity and, **82:**128–29
CT findings in, **82:**120, 122–25
dopamine (DBH) hypothesis of, **82:**123, 126–36 passim, 178–79, 196–97, 200–201
endorphin hypothesis of, **82:**141–42
gluten hypothesis of, **82:**145–46
hallucinogens and, **82:**139–41
hemispheric assymetry and, **82:**124–25
immune system and, **82:**114–22
L-γ-aminobutyric acid (GABA) and, **82:**138–39

MAO activity and, **82:**125–27, 131, 147–52 passim, 452; **83:**467
morphological abnormalities, **82:**148–49
norepinephrine (NE) hypothesis and, **82:**130–32, 152; **83:**132
phenylethylamine (PEA) and, **82:**137–38, 148–52 passim
plasma factors and, **82:**118–19, 126–32 passim, 135–36, 141, 144, 147
prostaglandins (PG) and, **82:**146
serotonin hypothesis of, **82:**129–30
transmethylation hypothesis of, **82:**139–40
ventricular enlargement and, **82:**123–24, 136, 149
cultural factors in, **82:**100–102, 120
environmental factors and, **82:**88–89, 96–97, 99, 106, 155; **83:**138; **84:**100, 134
family role in, **82:**172; **83:**242–43
genetic and biologic factors in, **82:**92–97, 112, 121, 125, 126–27, 155–56, 438, 444–48; **84:**100, 130, 325, 326, 391
and vulnerability, **82:**98–100, 106–08, 161, 165; **84:**87
social factors in, **82:**97–112
treatment linked to, **82:**155 (*see also* Schizophrenia, treatment of, *below*)
Schizophrenia, treatment of, **82:**97, 100, 153–54
behavior therapy, **82:**111
dialysis, **82:**141
dietary, **82:**142, 145–46
drug, *see* Drug therapy
dual mechanism (combined drug and psychotherapy) theory of, **82:**215–28; **83:**243
ECT, **82:**142, 143, 209, 220
family therapy, **82:**106, 110–11, 163, 172–74, 217, 219, 225; **83:**189, 242–49, 252, 253–56 (*see also* Family therapy)
foster care, **82:**225, 227
group therapy, **82:**170–72, 217, 219
hospital/inpatient, **82:**103, 110, 111, 138, 156, 165, 168, 171, 175, 176, 178, 201, 216, 219, 222–23, 225–27, 228; **83:**130; **84:**99
insight-oriented, **82:**111, 217
megavitamin therapy and orthomolecular psychiatry, **82:**142–46
milieu therapy, **82:**110, 172, 174–76
outpatient, **82:**159, 162, 171, 219, 228
patients' understanding of, **82:**357–58
plasma factors in, **82:**182–83, 190, 200–203
psychosocial, **82:**110, 111, 168–69, 170, 176–77, 218
psychotherapy, **82:**154–66, 215–28; **84:**44
response to, GH response and, **82:**136
standard of, **82:**168
termination of, **82:**165
Schizophrenic Disorders, The: Long-Term Patient and Family Studies (Bleuler), **84:**94
Schizophreniform Disorder, **82:**136; **83:**282, 439, 441; **84:**100
in geriatric patients, **83:**131–32, 135, 137, 138
treatment of, **82:**208
Schizotypal (schizoid) Personality Disorder, **82:**429, 434, 439, 441, 452, 455, 456

criteria for, **82**:428, 432, 436, 440, 448–51, 454, 457, 465–66, 471
Schedule for (SSP), **82**:432
and SPEM, **82**:453
Schleidlinger, S., **83**:25, 26, 27
Schleifer, S. J., et al., **84**:187
Schlesinger, H. J., et al., **84**:213
Schlesser, M. A., et al., **83**:273, 280, 291; **84**:314
Schlichter, W., et al., **84**:354
Schmale, A. H., **84**:217, 268; et al., **84**:217
Schmideberg, M., **82**:461
Schmidt, E. H., et al., **83**:433
Schmidt, H. S., **84**:475
Schneck, M. K., et al., **83**:108
Schneider, K., and Schneiderian symptoms, **82**:85, 100; **83**:138, 279, 280, 282, 289, 302, 392
Scholem, G. G., **84**:442
Schomer, J., **83**:190
School, attitude toward or performance in: childhood depression and, **82**:297, 302–03, 306
of children at risk for schizophrenia, **84**:101, 130–31
of children of divorce, **84**:145, 152
of mildly retarded child, **84**:121, 122
and school-phobic children, **82**:51; **84**:414–16, 417
See also Learning disorders
Schooler, N. R., **82**:195; et al., **82**:169, 195
Schopenhauer, Arthur, **83**:47
Schou, M., **83**:304, 313, 314, 315, 326, 327, 368; et al., **83**:298, 314, 328, 331
Schreiner, G. E., **84**:348
Schubert, D. S. P., **84**:182
Schucker, B., **84**:216
Schuckit, Marc A., **83**:116, 454; **84**:300, 312, 320–27 passim, 340; et al., **84**:235, 320, 325, 326, 327
Schulsinger, F., **82**:108, 445n; **84**:130; et al., **83**:432, 445
Schulsinger, H., **82**:108; **84**:99
Schultz, B., **82**:93
Schultz, C. S., et al., **82**:141
Schultz, J. D., et al., **84**:354
Schulz, C., **84**:491
Schwab, J. J., **84**:180; et al., **84**:206, 207, 208, 247
Schwab, K. J. and M. E., **83**:89
Schwaber, E. A., **82**:497; **83**:20
Schwartz, G. E., **84**:227
Schwartz, M., **83**:26, 29
Schwebel, M. and B., **84**:116, 117
Schweitzer, I., **84**:275
Schweitzer, J. W., et al., **82**:137
Schweri, M., et al., **84**:483, 488
Schwimm, C., et al., **82**:204
Schyve, D. M., et al., **82**:202
SCID (Structured Clinical Interview), **84**:61, 402
SCL (skin conductance level), **84**:470. *See also* Electrodermal response
SCL (Symptom Check List), **84**:495, 499
Sclafani, A., **84**:219
Scoggins, B. A., et al., **83**:500
Scoliosis, **84**:275
Scott, A., **84**:361
Scott, A. W., Jr., **82**:342n31

Scott, F. B., et al., **83**:151
Scott, M., et al., **83**:470
Scott, R. A., **83**:173, 184
Scott, R. E., **83**:470
Scott-Strauss, A., **83**:442
Seagal, B., **84**:135
Searles, H. F., **82**:161, 472
Secrets, *see* Confidentiality
Secunda, S. K., et al., **83**:512
Sedvall, G., **82**:201; et al., **83**:452
Seelig, M. S., et al., **84**:355
Seeman, P. P., et al., **83**:134, 196
Segal, H., **82**:474
Segawa, T., et al., **83**:469
Seifter, J., **84**:484
Seixas, Frank, **84**:307
Seldrup, J., **84**:512
Self: bipolar, **82**:491–92, 494, 502–05
and body image, **84**:218–19
changes in, **84**:115, 271
postmastectomy, **84**:270, 271
of traumatized child, **84**:115
concept of, **82**:490–96 passim, 502, 504, 511
defined (Kohut), **82**:500
-ego distinction, Freud and, **82**:488, 489
-idealization, *see* Narcissistic Personality Disorder
narcissistic, **82**:494 (*see also* Narcissism)
-other fusion (in infancy), **83**:14
-representation
in borderline disorders, **82**:473, 474–75, 479
in narcissistic disorder, **82**:493, 511–12, 516, 517, 518
and self pathology, **82**:504–05
sense of (individuation)
adolescent and young adult, **83**:192, 211
infant, **83**:14–15, 19
separation-individuation phase and problems of, **82**:49, 51; **83**:35, 235–36, 247
See also Ego
Self-destructiveness, **82**:345
in alcohol withdrawal, **84**:357
in borderline disorders, **82**:424, 450, 481, 485, 486
in narcissistic personality disorder, **82**:515, 520
See also Suicide and attempted suicide
Self-esteem: of alcoholic patient, **84**:343
in bipolar disorder, **83**:281
in borderline disorders, **82**:462
of children at risk, **84**:103
in depression, **83**:364, 365, 373, 387, 392, 511, 514–15, 517; **84**:19, 63
childhood depression, **82**:272, 276, 277–78, 286, 296, 301, 305
of elderly, **83**:106, 129, 130, 141
invalidism and, **84**:267
narcissism and, **82**:488–94 passim, 504, 515, 522
of rape victim, **82**:66
of schizophrenic patient, **83**:291
sexual, mastectomy and, **84**:270, 271
See also Role(s)

Selfobject, **82:**492, 496, 501–02, 509, 510
    oedipal, **82:**501, 503, 504, 505
    transference, **82:**499–508 passim
Self psychology, **82:**516
    development of, **82:**497–504; **83:**7
    See also Ego psychology
Self-reporting: concept of, **84:**18
    self-rating, **84:**202, 217, 218, 495
        by child, **84:**415
    self-report rating scales, **84:**70, 73–75, 198 (*see also individual scales*)
Self-Reporting Questionnaire, **84:**198
Self-Statement Training (SST), **84:**457–59
Selig, J. W., Jr., **84:**353
Seligman, M. E. P., **82:**267, 286; **83:**364, 383
Seller, R. H., et al., **84:**205, 206
Sellers, E. M., **84:**353; et al., **84:**493
Selman, F. B., et al., **82:**180, 186
Seltzer, B., **83:**109
Selvini-Palazzoli, M., et al., **83:**247
Selye, H., **84:**221
Selzer, M. L., **84:**330
Semantic techniques (cognitive therapy), **83:**515
Senescence, **83:**96. *See also* Aging
Senile dementia, *see* Dementia, Primary Degenerative
Senile macular degeneration, **83:**103. *See also* Vision
Senility, **83:**94, 96. *See also* Aging
Senior, N., et al., **84:**116
Sensate focus exercises, *see* Sex therapy
Sensation-Seeking Scale, **83:**336
Sensitization: in acting-out behavior, **84:**22
    in alcoholism therapy, **84:**356–57
        covert, **84:**328, 333
    and desensitization, **83:**202; **84:**254, 328, 417, 421
        systematic, in treating phobia, **84:**417, 449–50, 451, 470, 504, 507
    and prediction of behavior, **84:**22
Sensorimotor response: of newborn, **83:**11; **84:**131
Sensory deficits: age-related, **83:**102–04, 133–34, 136, 137
    and delirium (in elderly), **84:**232
    and deprivation, psychic trauma and, **84:**109
    and mental retardation, **84:**127
    and paranoia, **83:**133–34, 136, 137, 140
    smell, and taste, sense of, **83:**104
    See also Hearing loss; Vision
Sentencing, psychiatry and, **82:**392–95. *See also* Law and psychiatry
Separation and divorce: bipolar illness and, **83:**250, 286, 426, 456
    and child custody, **84:**149–50, 153, 154–55, 156
        joint, **84:**156–57
    depression and, **83:**366
        and childhood depression, **84:**145, 154
    and depressive symptoms, **83:**380, 399, 413; **84:**58, 148, 206
    effects of, on child, **82:**277
        children at risk, **84:**134, 144–58
    effects of, on partners (males vs. females), **84:**134

family or couples therapy in, **83:**189, 192–93, 226, 227–28
and law, **84:**146–47, 154–57
mediation in, **84:**155–56
of nonpsychotic from psychotic partner, **84:**132, 133
and paranoia, **83:**133
and postmarital sexuality, **82:**41–45
psychiatric disorder and, **84:**155
and psychiatric morbidity rate, **84:**202
psychosexual dysfunction and, **82:**36
research priorities in, **84:**157–58
stages in divorce process, **83:**227–28; **84:**148–49
trial separation, in couples therapy, **83:**226
and use of mental health services, **84:**145
in United States, rate of, **84:**144
and visitation, **84:**149, 150, 154–55, 156
Separation Anxiety Disorder, *see* Anxiety Disorders
Separation fears: adult, **84:**413, 512
    animal research model of, **84:**417
    as childhood anxiety disorder, **84:**411, 412–13, 418
    vs. childhood depression, **82:**306
    of children of divorce, **84:**152
    of prepubertal children, **82:**269
    of "pretranssexual" children, **82:**51
    and sexual dysfunction, **82:**32
    treatment focus on, **84:**16
    treatment termination and, **84:**16, 39, 42, 43 (*see also* Therapy)
    See also Mother-child relationship
Separation-individuation, *see* Self
Seppala, T., et al., **84:**358
Sereny, G., **84:**353
Serotonin: aging and, **83:**96–97, 127
    in Alzheimer's disease, **83:**110
    and depressive disorders, **83:**459, 460, 474, 482, 489
    drug effect on, **82:**196; **83:**474, 482, 483, 489, 490, 508; **84:**497, 511, 515
    hypothesis (of schizophrenia), **82:**129–30
    and serotonin-derived products, **84:**323
    and serotonin metabolite (5-HIAA), **83:**431, 446, 452, 470
Seth, S., et al., **82:**185
Sethy, V. H., **83:**488
Sex: as term, **82:**49
Sex differentiation: in alcoholism, **84:**213
    and anxiety symptoms/disorders, **84:**208, 403–04, 405, 408, 461
    in bipolar illness, **83:**424, 427–28
    in child's reaction to divorce, **84:**153
        and custody, **84:**153
    in child's reaction to mentally ill parent, **84:**133
    in dementia, **83:**107, 115
    in depression, **82:**284; **83:**411–13, 415–20, 422, 427–28; **84:**206, 208
        childhood depression, **82:**284
    in effects (on partners) of separation or divorce, **84:**134

in hypochondriasis, **83**:142
in late-life sexual activity, **83**:148
in lithium side effects/compliance, **83**:333, 334, 335
in mitral valve prolapse, **84**:408
in psychiatric morbidity, **84**:190, 191, 198, 202, 214, 403–04, 461
in schizophrenic illness (among elderly), **83**:132
in sleep patterns, **83**:145
in suicide rate, **83**:433
Sex Information and Education Council of the United States (SIECUS), **82**:7
Sexism: and depression in mothers, **84**:144
in psychotherapies, **83**:38–40
and sex bias in research, **84**:101, 130n
Sex reassignment, **82**:48, 51, 53, 55, 56
therapist's attitude toward, **82**:54
See also Gender identity
Sex therapy, **82**:7, 8, 20–21, 41
in alcoholism cases, **84**:345
analytically oriented, **82**:21, 22, 26, 35
behavioral approach to, **82**:21–26 passim, 35, 40; **84**:53
dual-/couples, **82**:21–22, 25–26, 39, 43; **83**:222n1
effectiveness of, **82**:25
geriatric, **83**:151
group, **82**:21, 24–25, 26
hypnotherapy, **82**:21, 22–23
individual psychotherapy in, **82**:21, 24
in rape cases, **82**:64
sensate focus exercises used in, **82**:36, 37, 40, 41
and treatment failure, **82**:25, 26–35, 64
Sexual abuse, **82**:56–66
and children at risk, **84**:115, 116
and sexual misuse, defined, **82**:57
and therapeutic implications, **82**:59–61
See also Incest; Rape
Sexual conflicts: narcissism and, **82**:514, 519, 522
Sexual deprivation, **82**:30
Sexual dysfunctions, *see* Infertility; Psychosexual dysfunctions
Sexual identity, **82**:49. *See also* Gender identity
Sexuality: aging and, **82**:7, 8, 42, 45–47; **83**:147–51
bisexuality, **82**:55
categorized (as homosexual, heterosexual, or perverse), **82**:33
changing theories of, **83**:41–42, 49, 147
cultural influence on, **83**:49
group intolerance of, **83**:25
postmarital, **82**:41–45
premarital, **82**:43
social attitudes toward, **82**:7; **83**:34, 147, 150
See also Homosexuality; Hypersexuality
Sexual jealousy: divorce and, **84**:148
Sexual phobias, **82**:32–33
Sexual relationships, *see* Relationships
Sexual response: inhibited desire and excitement, **82**:16–18 (*see also* Impotence)
medication and, **82**:8 (*see also* Drug side effect[s])

phases of, **82**:12–14
and sexual assertiveness, **82**:20, 23
See also Ejaculation; Erection; Masturbation; Orgasm
Sexual trauma, *see* Trauma, emotional/psychic
Shadel Sanatorium (Seattle), **84**:328, 333
Shader, R. I., **83**:112, 142; **84**:184, 232, 233, 235, 397, 483, 484, 489; et al., **82**:465; **84**:419
Shakir, S. A., et al., **83**:316, 322, 325
Shammas, E., **84**:495
Shand, D. A., **83**:495
Shapiro, D., **84**:228, 421
Shapiro, Leon N., **83**:8
Shapiro, R. I., **84**:421
Shapiro, Roger W., **83**:33, 189, 235, 276, 512; et al., **83**:449
Shapiro, S., **84**:119–20
Shapiro, T., **83**:67; **84**:108
Sharfstein, S. S., et al., **82**:332
Sharpe, E. F., **82**:475
Shaw, B. F., **83**:524
Shaw, P. M., **84**:450
Sheard, M., et al., **82**:465
Sheehan, David V., **83**:488; **84**:437, 483, 504; et al., **82**:465; **83**:483; **84**:503, 506, 509–11 passim, 518
Sheehy, M., **82**:425; et al., **82**:420, 423–28 passim, 436
Sheiner, L. B., **83**:507
Sheldon, J. H., **83**:91
Shelp, E. E., **84**:182
Shepherd, M., **82**:108; **83**:304; et al., **83**:95; **84**:189, 190, 193, 197, 211
Sherer, D. E. and M. S., **84**:126, 128
Sherman, A. R., **84**:451
Sherman, D. G., **84**:475, 493
Sherman, L., et al., **82**:204
Sherrod, L. R., **83**:10
Sherwin, I., **83**:109
Shetky, D., **84**:116
Shevitz, S. A., et al., **84**:231
Shiefelbusch, R. L., **84**:126
Shields, J., **82**:94, 95, 451
Shigetomi, C. C., **84**:458
Shintoism, **84**:443. *See also* Religion
Shipley Trait Anxiety Scale, **84**:325
Shock: naxolone beneficial in cases of, **84**:351
Shopsin, B., **83**:289; et al., **82**:182, 185, 206, 211; **83**:298, 300, 440, 483
Shore, D., et al., **83**:111
Short Portable Mental Status Questionnaire (SPMSQ), **83**:116
Shulman, K., **83**:285, 287
Shulsinger, O. Z., et al., **84**:356
Shwed, H. J., et al., **82**:331
SIB (Schedule for Interviewing Borderlines), *see* Borderline Personality Disorder, diagnosis of
Sibling(s): depression-HLA studies of, **83**:449–50
reconcilement of struggles between, **83**:212
transference, and marital conflict/sexual dysfunction, **82**:27, 32
See also Family, the

SIECUS (Sex Information and Education Council of the United States), **82:**7
Siegel, H., **84:**12–21 passim
Siegel, J., **82:**109
Siever, Larry J., **82:**413, 425, 438, 446–53 passim; **84:**325n; et al., **82:**453; **83:**469
Sifneos, Peter E., **83:**523; **84:**7–12 passim, 25–34 passim, 218, 227, 437; et al., **84:**34
Signal anxiety, *see* Anxiety
Silber, A., **84:**339
Silberfarb, P., **84:**357; et al., **84:**242, 256, 270
Silverman, C., **83:**406, 420, 426
Silverstein, A. B., **82:**276
Silverstone, B. M., **83:**114
Sime, A. M., **84:**213, 258
Simler, S., et al., **84:**355
Simmel, E., **84:**313
Simmons, O. C., **82:**109
Simmons, R. G., et al., **84:**266
Simon, P., et al., **82:**195
Simonds, J. F., **82:**282, 284
Simons, R., **83:**65
Simpson, G. M., **82:**185; **83:**485, 500; et al., **82:**180, 181, 189, 213; **83:**505
Sims, A., **84:**460, 465, 466
Sinclair, K. G. A., **83:**112
Singer, M. T., **82:**172, 415, 417, 423, 425, 434, 440, 441, 452; et al., **83:**242, 247
Singh, M. M., **82:**145
Single, E., et al., **84:**362
SIP (Special Internal Predisposition) criterion, **84:**34
Siris, S. G., et al., **83:**125, 291
Siskind, M., **84:**217
Sitaram, N., **83:**463
Sitwell, R., **84:**442
Sjoqvist, F., **83:**510
Skeels, H. M., **84:**123
Skin conductance level, *see* SCL
Skin disease, **84:**202, 216
Skinner, B. F., **83:**516
Skirboll, L. R., et al., **82:**134
Skodiak, M., **84:**123
Skodol, A. E., **82:**87
Skolnick, Phil, **84:**483, 486, 487, 524; et al., **84:**487
Skoug, G., **84:**262
Skuterud, B., **83:**495
Skynner, A. C. R., **83:**33, 190, 231, 234; **84:**416
Slade, P. D., **84:**219
Slater, E., **82:**93, 94; **83:**108, 109; **84:**97, 405
Slattery, J. T., et al., **83:**500
Slavson, S. R., **83:**26
Sleep, **83:**355
    EEG studies of, **83:**122, 145, 291; **84:**221
    -induced GH peak, **82:**204
    and memory, **83:**18
    NREM (non-rapid eye movement), **84:**220–21
    physiology of, **84:**219, 220–21
    See also REM (rapid eye movement) sleep
Sleep disorders: age and, **82:**295; **83:**91, 144, 145–47
    in bipolar illness, **83:**277, 279, 281, 282, 297, 423

childhood, **83:**283
in child of divorce, **84:**152
dementia and, **83:**145, 146–47
depression and, **83:**127, 144, 146, 371, 373, 479, 512
    childhood depression, **82:**290, 293–97 passim, 304; **84:**98
as drug side effect, **83:**124, 485
drug therapy for, **84:**495
hypersomnia, **83:**279, 281, 282, 480
and musculoskeletal complaints, **84:**221
sleep apnea, **83:**147; **84:**220–21
See also Insomnia
Sletten, I. W., **84:**353
Sloane, P., **82:**57
Sloane, R. Bruce, **83:**87, 108, 116
Slovenko, R., **82:**330
SMAC (metabolic screening test), **84:**234
Small, J., et al., **82:**209, 211
Small, L., **84:**7, 12, 18
Smart, R., **84:**368
Smell, sense of, *see* Sensory deficits
Smeraldi, E., et al., **83:**273, 438, 446, 449
Smiley, A., **84:**500
Smith, C. B., **83:**474, 489
Smith, C. G., **82:**175
Smith, D., **84:**68
Smith, D. E., **82:**140
Smith, F. W., **84:**357
Smith, G. R., **84:**224
Smith, J. B., **84:**59
Smith, J. M., **82:**147
Smith, J. S., et al., **83:**109
Smith, K., et al., **82:**209
Smith, N. L., et al., **84:**421
Smith, R. C., et al., **82:**135, 183, 196, 202
Smith, R. S., **84:**88, 103, 134
Smith Kline & French Laboratories, **83:**320
Smoking, *see* Tobacco, use of
Smooth pursuit eye movement, *see* SPEM
Smythies, J., **82:**129, 140
Snaith, R. P., et al., **83:**391, 393
Sneznevsky, A. V., **82:**88
Snow, C., **83:**20
Snowden, P. R., et al., **83:**110, 111
Snowdon, J., **83:**107
Snyder, K. K., **82:**98
Snyder, S. H., **82:**196; **83:**101, 469; **84:**485; et al., **82:**196
Soave, R., **84:**233
Sobel, D., **82:**26; **84:**130
Sobel, E., **83:**446
Sobell, Linda C., **84:**299, 300, 318, 332, 335–36
Sobell, Mark B., **84:**299, 300, 318, 331, 332, 335–36
Social class: and alcoholism, **84:**311
    drinking as social custom, **84:**360
    and bipolar illness, **83:**286, 425–28 passim
    and depression, **82:**284–85; **83:**413, 420, 428
    and paranoia, **83:**133
    and psychiatric morbidity rate, **84:**202
        among mentally retarded, **84:**124
    and schizophrenia, **82:**98, 100, 101

selection-drift phenomenon in, **82**:98, 100, 112
See also Psychosocial factors
Social competence, *see* Coping capacities
Social Diagnosis (Richmond), **83**:169–70
Social expectancy, *see* Expectations
Social factors, *see* Environmental factors; Psychosocial factors; Stress
Social isolation: animal model of, **84**:225
  of children at risk, **84**:133, 138
    child of divorce, **84**:151
    retarded child, **84**:121
  geriatric disorders and, **83**:130, 133–40 passim
  See also Withdrawal, social
Social Phobia, *see* Phobic Disorders
Social psychiatry, *see* Psychiatry
Social Readjustment Rating Questionnaire, **84**:226
Social Security, **83**:106
Social skills: and depression, **83**:383, 517, 520, 527
    childhood depression, **82**:302
  family therapy training for, **83**:246–47; **84**:95
  learning techniques for, **83**:517–18, 521, 524
  MAO activity and (introversion, extraversion), **83**:467
  See also Coping capacities
Social support networks: for cancer patients, **84**:246
  for children and family at risk, **84**:102–03, 131, 151
  in consultation-liaison psychiatry, **84**:181, 184–85, 215
  and depression, **83**:364, 414, 521
  in divorce cases, availability or lack of, **84**:151, 154
  and late-life psychiatric disorders, **83**:94
  for patients under stress, **84**:229, 230
  and schizophrenia, **82**:106–07; **83**:244; **84**:95
  See also AA (Alcoholics Anonymous); Education/educational intervention; Family, the; Foster care; Health care system; Relationships
Society for Sex Therapy and Research (SSTAR), **82**:7
Sociopathy, **82**:440; **84**:136
Soft signs: in infants and children, **84**:131, 252
Soininen, H., et al., **83**:109
"Soldier's heart," *see* "Effort syndrome"
Solkoff, N., **84**:110
Solnit, A., **84**:106, 110, 125
Soloff, L. A., **82**:36
Soloff, P. H., **82**:417, 421–29 passim, 443
Solomon, A, **83**:401, 403, 404
Solomon, A. P., **84**:470
Solomon, G. F., **82**:117; et al., **82**:115
Solomon, J., **84**:106
Solomon, L., **83**:195
Solomon, M., **83**:433
Solomon, R. L., **84**:449
Solow, C., **84**:186
Solow, R. A., **84**:156
Solyom, C., et al., **84**:459, 509, 510
Solyom, L., et al., **84**:508, 510
Somatic symptoms: childhood, **82**:304–05; **84**:415

in consultation-liaison psychiatry, **84**:183, 184
drug therapy and, **83**:128; **84**:493–95 (*see also* Drug therapy)
of elderly patient, **83**:119, 127, 140–45 passim
See also Physical illness; Psychosomatic disorders
Somatization Disorder (Briquet's syndrome): among children, **84**:98
DSM-III category for, **84**:211, 460–61
among elderly, **84**:236
and mortality rate, **84**:460, 461, 464
See also Hysteria
Somatoform Disorders: DSM-III category for, **84**:211, 393
epidemiology/prevalence rate of, **84**:208, 211, 212
late-life, **83**:119, 127, 140–45 passim; **84**:231, 236
Sommer, C., **82**:225
Sommer, R., **83**:114
Sonnenberg, S., **84**:110
Sørensen, A., **83**:416
Sorensen, B., et al., **83**:505
Sorensen, S. C., **84**:350
Soskis, D. A., **82**:155, 357
Soteria project, **82**:175; **83**:248
Sourcebook on Aging, **83**:88
South Africa: schizophrenia in, **82**:101
Soviet Union, **83**:34, 84
  immunologic and virus studies in, **82**:119, 120
Sovner, R. D., **83**:289; et al., **82**:357
Spar, J. E., **83**:117; **84**:236; et al., **84**:236
Sparacino, J., **83**:136
Spark, G. M., **83**:199, 219, 223
Spark, R. F., **82**:37
Spaulding, E., **82**:449, 453
Special Internal Predisposition (SIP) criterion, **84**:34
Speech: infant learning of sounds of, **83**:11, 12, 20
  poverty of content (vagueness), **82**:123; **83**:279, 289
  retardation of, childhood depression and, **82**:303
  and verbalizations of small children, **84**:119
  See also Language
Spelke, E. S., **83**:13
SPEM (smooth pursuit eye movement): impaired, **82**:453
Sperling, M., **84**:417
Spicer, C. C., et al., **83**:285, 425
Spiegel, John, **83**:170; **84**:62, 107, 117, 119, 420
Spiegel, K., et al., **84**:249
Spiegelberg, H., **84**:44
Spiker, Duane G., **83**:480; et al., **83**:468, 474, 509
Spina bifida, **84**:275
Spiro, H. R., **82**:288; **83**:286
Spitz, René, **82**:274, 283, 293
Spitzer, R. L., **83**:408; **84**:303, 347, 402, 519, 520; et al., **82**:270, 289, 293, 296, 298, 305, 419–41 passim, 448–53 passim; **83**:273, 278, 407, 408, 512; **84**:49, 303
Spivack, G., et al., **82**:109
Splitting, *see* Defense mechanism(s) (primitive)

SPMSQ (Short Portable Mental Status Questionnaire), 83:116
Spohn, H. E., 82:383n6; et al., 82:199, 383n6
Spradley, J. P., 84:53
Spring, B., 82:98, 103
Spring, G., et al., 83:300
Springarn, N. D., 82:332
Springer, C., 84:152
Springfield, Massachusetts, detoxification center, 84:314
Spruiell, V., 82:489
Spurgeon, C. F. E., 84:443
Squire, L. R., 83:126
Squires, R. F., 84:409, 485
Sri Lanka; schizophrenia in, 82:101
Srole, L., 83:92; et al., 82:283
SSP (Schedule for Schizotypal Personalities), 82:432
SST (Self-Statement Training), 84:457–59
SSTAR (Society for Sex Therapy and Research), 82:7
Stabenau, J. R., 82:451
Stack, J. J., 82:291
Staff, see Health care system; Nursing staff
Staff burnout, 84:245
Stage fright; drug therapy for, 84:496–97, 502. See also Anxiety; Anxiety Disorders
Stahl, M. L., 84:263
Stak, M. H., 84:125
Stallone, F., et al., 83:297, 307, 309
Stam, F. C., 82:208; 83:110
Stampfl, T. G., 84:421, 450
Stancer, H. C., 83:303
Standardized Psychiatric Interview, 84:198, 202, 206
Stanford University, 84:268, 269
Stanley, B., et al., 82:358
Stanton, A. M., 83:29
Stanton, M. D., 83:174
STAPP (short-term anxiety-provoking psychotherapy), see Psychotherapy(ies), brief
Starkman, M. N., 84:182
Steadman, N., 82:387
Stechler, G., 83:10
Stein, B. M., et al., 83:115
Stein, L. I., 82:110, 127, 227; et al., 84:484
Stein, M., 82:495; 84:219; et al., 84:223
Steinberg, E., 84:104
Steinbook, R. M., et al., 82:182, 184; 83:468, 473
Steiner, M., et al., 82:208
Steinglass, P., 83:174, 189
Steinman, S., 84:156
Stekel, Wilhelm, 84:7, 11
Stember, R. H., 83:449
Stengel, E., 83:433
Stenstedt, A., 83:372, 446
"Stéphane, André," 83:35
Stephens, D. A., et al., 82:93
Stephens, J., 82:465
Steptoe, A., 84:219
Sterba, E., 84:110
Stereotype(s): gender, 84:135
    professional trend toward, 83:38, 39

reevaluation of, 82:7; 83:42
of schizophrenic disorders, 82:84, 91
sexual activity, 82:45, 46
See also Role(s)
Stereotyped behavior: amphetamine-induced, 82:137, 144
    mental retardation and, 84:124
Sterility, see Infertility
Stern, Daniel N., 83:7, 10, 14, 16; 84:108; et al., 83:19
Stern, G., 84:110
Stern, M. J., et al., 84:214
Stetzer, S. L., 84:261
Steuer, J., 84:238
Stevens, B., 83:426
Stevens, J., 82:120
Stevens, L. A., et al., 84:271
Stewart, A., 84:135
Stewart, J., 83:445, 446, 450; et al., 82:466; 83:479, 480
Stewart, M. A., 82:282, 284
Stewart, Potter, 82:321
Stewart, W. A., 83:46
Stierlin, H., 82:85
Stiller, R. L., et al., 83:503
Stimulus-seeking: and "stimulus barrier" (in infancy), 83:9–11; 84:108
Stockard, J., 84:327
Stockton, R. A., 84:401
Stoic philosophy, 84:44
Stokes, P. E., et al., 83:298
Stoller, R. J., 82:30, 55, 56; 83:43
Stolorow, R., 82:511
Stone, A., 83:143
Stone, A. A., 82:322nn3, 4, 323n7, 324n11, 326n14, 331, 339n18, 351, 352, 361n2, 366–69 passim, 383, 384
Stone, L., 82:497; 83:50, 61, 65
Stone, Michael H., 82:413, 415, 433–43 passim, 454, 486–87
Stotsky, B., 83:132
Stoyva, J., 84:228
Strachey, J., 82:475
Strahilevitz, M., et al., 82:115
Strain, J. J., 84:182, 183, 188
Straker, G., 83:176–77
Strauss, A., 84:232
Strauss, John S., 82:83–88 passim, 108, 109, 155, 161, 167, 416; 83:130; 84:134; et al., 82:89
Streiner, D. L., et al., 82:102
Streitman, S., 84:99
Stress: and bipolar illness, 83:426
    cancer patients and, see Cancer
    children under, see Children at risk
    as classical cause of psychiatric illness, 83:436
    defined, 83:394; 84:221
    denial of reality under, 84:109, 114
    and depressive disorders, 82:103; 83:126, 361, 362, 364, 371, 381–85 passim, 394–400, 404–05, 412–14, 421–22; 84:58
    endocrine response to, 84:221–23, 225
    family crisis or milestone, 83:188, 197–98, 214–15, 216, 239

genetic vulnerability vs., **83**:436–37
group therapy for, **84**:229
within ICU (intensive care unit), **84**:232, 261–62, 263 (see also Surgery)
and late-life psychiatric disorders, **83**:93–94, 140–41
and life event stress theory, **83**:105, 381, 382, 394–95
caution regarding, **84**:226
and panic or anxiety attacks, **84**:439, 469, 482, 496–97
parents under, see Parent(s)
and physical illness, **83**:381; **84**:213, 214, 222, 226
and psychic trauma, see Trauma, emotional/psychic
and psychosexual dysfunctions, **82**:15, 53
psychotherapeutic management of catastrophe, **84**:24
as risk factor, **84**:94
and schizophrenia, **82**:98, 102–03, 106, 107, 112, 156, 163, 165, 173
social factors and, **83**:400–05
staff burnout, **84**:245
and suicide, **83**:431
See also Adjustment reaction(s); Anxiety; Coping capacities; Environmental factors; Ethnicity; Grief reaction; Loss; Marital problems (disillusionment, mismatch, conflict); Trauma, emotional/psychic
Strickler, D., et al., **84**:332
Strober, M., **83**:284; et al., **82**:291
Stroke, **83**:114, 484; **84**:235. See also Vascular disorders
Stromberg, Clifford D., **82**:323, 326, 339n18
Strömgren, E., **83**:295, 416
Strongin, E., **84**:350
Strong Memorial Hospital (Rochester, N.Y.), **84**:180, 246, 247
Structural Interview, see Borderline Personality Disorder, diagnosis of
Structured Clinical Interview, see SCID
Struening, E. L., **82**:227; **84**:226
Strupp, H. H., **83**:526; et al., **83**:522, 523, 525
Students: and examination "nerves," **84**:496
medical, see Teaching (of medical psychiatry)
rebellion by (French students, 1968), **83**:35
See also Young adults
Study, R. E., **84**:485, 487
Stunkard, A., **84**:219, 229
Stupor, see Catatonic stupor or excitement
Subjective Units of Discomfort (SUDS), **84**:456
Substance abuse: in bipolar illness, **83**:279–86 passim, 290
studies of, **83**:174
See also Alcoholism; Drug abuse/addiction; Tobacco, use of
Substance P, **84**:222
Substance Use Disorders: DSM-III category for, **84**:301, 302. See also Alcoholism; Drug abuse/addiction
Suess, W. M., et al., **84**:220
Sufism, **84**:443. See also Religion

Sugi, Y., **84**:445
Suicide and attempted suicide, **83**:428–34; **84**:217
adolescent or child, **82**:51–52, 278, 285, 300–301, 303, 307; **83**:433
parents' divorce and, **84**:152
alcoholism and, **83**:429, 430, 431, 432; **84**:326, 357, 467
anxiety or panic and, **83**:429; **84**:467
in bipolar illness, **83**:286–87, 320, 329, 330, 334, 429, 430
cancer and, **84**:249
communication of intent, **83**:430–31
depression and, **83**:287, 362–70 passim, 429–34, 527; **84**:326, 460, 467
drug overdose and, **82**:467; **83**:430, 433
drug therapy vs. psychosocial intervention in, **83**:527
as grief reaction, **83**:375, 431
metabolic activity and, **82**:452; **83**:431
nonpsychiatric, defined, **83**:445
parental, effect of, on child, **84**:115
psychotherapeutic management of, **84**:21, 24
risk factors in, **83**:429–33
genetic, **82**:452; **83**:431–33, 443, 445
personality type, **84**:216
suicidal ideation, **82**:463; **83**:280, 281
divorce and, **84**:148
among elderly, **84**:232
See also Self-destructiveness
Sullivan, F. W., **82**:332
Sullivan, Harry Stack, **82**:85, 490; **83**:170, 519; **84**:57, 66, 418
Sullivan, J. L., et al., **83**:467; **84**:325
Sulser, F., **83**:474, 490; et al., **83**:469
Summers, F., **82**:357
Summit, R., **82**:58
Sundby, P., **84**:314
Sunderland, Pearson, **82**:413; **83**:480
Suomi, S. J., et al., **84**:417
Superego, **82**:497, 500, 501, 502; **84**:433
appraisal of (in psychotherapy), **84**:17
in childhood, **82**:272
faulty development of, **83**:35
-ego conflict, **82**:272; **84**:19
formation of, **83**:49
in group psychology, **83**:23, 25, 33, 34, 36
internalization of, **83**:34
narcissism and, **82**:493, 515, 517
Superoxide dismutase, **83**:98
Support groups, see Group therapy; Outpatient treatment; Social support networks
Supreme Court, U.S., **82**:321–24, 337–38, 341, 363–64, 370–79 passim, 383, 386–95 passim
Surgery: amputation, **84**:115, 272–73, 275
and anxiety of patient (pre-, peri-, and post-operative), **84**:222, 229, 254–62, 267
cancer, **82**:39, 40; **84**:273
disfiguring and reconstructive, **84**:276
cardiac, **84**:262–65, 267
and bypass time, **84**:263–64
children undergoing, see Children at risk
cholecystectomy, **84**:262, 274
CJD agent transmitted by, **83**:111

consent to or refusal of, **84:**259–60
hysterectomy, **84:**261, 274
MAOI therapy and, **83:**490
mastectomy, **84:**218
  and choice of treatment, **84:**259, 271
  fears of, **82:**40; **84:**256
  plastic surgery following, **84:**276
  studies of, **84:**269–71
organ transplantation, **84:**265–69
  contraindications for, **84:**266
  donor/donor family reactions to, **84:**266–69
  heart, **84:**265, 268–69
  kidney, **84:**265–68
  and recipient psychopathology, **84:**267–68
  rejection of, **84:**268
orthopedic, **84:**274–75
ostomies, **84:**273
  colostomy, **84:**273
overuse of, **83:**184
pelvic exenteration, **84:**273
perioperative phase of, **84:**260–62, 263
plastic, **84:**275–76
postoperative phase and effects of, **84:**229, 232, 257, 258, 261, 262, 273, 275
  depression, **82:**38–41 passim; **84:**264, 267–68, 269, 272, 274, 275
  in ICU or recovery room, **84:**232, 261–62, 263
  sexual dysfunction, **84:**260, 265
preoperative phase of, **84:**256–60, 263, 264
prognosis for, **84:**218, 264, 268, 274
psychiatric liaison with, **84:**256, 258, 265, 275, 276–77
psychopathology as response to, **84:**184, 208, 262, 262–67 passim
and psychosexual dysfunctions, **82:**38–41, 46; **83:**151
psychotherapeutic management of, **84:**22
as "punishment," **82:**38, 41
sex-reassignment, **82:**7, 48, 53–56
and total parenteral nutrition (TPN), **84:**271–72
urology, **84:**275
"Survivor syndrome," *see* Guilt feelings
Surwit, R. S., **84:**228
Suskind, G. W., **83:**98
Suslak, L., et al., **83:**440
Suspiciousness, *see* Paranoid reactions
Sutherland, A. M., **84:**270; et al., **84:**272
Sutherland, E. W., **84:**350
Sutherland, J. D., **83:**27, 28
Sutherland, S., **82:**61
Suzman, M. M., **84:**493
Suzuki, S., **82:**137
Sveinsson, I. S., **84:**263
Svensson, T. H., **84:**477, 512
Sviland, M. A., **82:**47
Swain, D. B., et al., **84:**87, 88, 89
Swann v. *Charlotte-Mecklenburg Board of Education,* **82:**366
Swanson, D. W., et al., **84:**229
Sweating, *see* Diaphoresis
Sweden, *see* Scandinavia
Sweeney, D. R., et al., **84:**472

Sweeny, G. H., **84:**179
Swift, Jonathan, **83:**83
Swinburne, H., **83:**145
Swinyard, E. A., **84:**354
Switzerland: ADH isoenzyme patterns in, **84:**324
  bipolar illness studies in, **83:**423
Symbiotic phase, *see* Infancy
Symbolic play, *see* Play, symbolic
Symonds, M., **82:**385
Symptom Check List, *see* SCL
Symptom formation: Janet's and Freud's models of, **84:**430–31, 437, 438
  psychosomatic, deficit model of, **84:**438
Symptom substitution: fear of, as consequence of brief psychotherapy, **84:**7
Syndrome approach, **82:**82–83
Syphilis, **84:**234
  congenital, **84:**127
  See also Physical illness
Systems theory: family, *see* Family therapy
  of organizations, **83:**30–32
  and systems level concept of psychopathology, **83:**176, 177
Szasz, T. S., **82:**336, 351
Szulecka, T. K., **82:**108
Szurek, S. A., **84:**129
Szymanski, L. S., **84:**125, 129

T

Tabrizi, M. A., et al., **82:**292
Tachycardia, *see* Heart rate
Taiwan: schizophrenia studies in, **82:**98
Takahashi, R., et al., **83:**299, 300
Takahasi, S., **83:**452, 467; et al., **82:**290
Tall, J., **84:**155
Tallman, J. F., et al., **84:**409, 484, 486
Talvenheimo, J., et al., **83:**470
Tamminga, C. A., et al., **82:**136, 139, 141, 196, 203
Tanguay, P. E., **84:**125
Tanna, V. L., **83:**448; et al., **83:**450; **84:**494
Taoism, **84:**443. *See also* Religion
Taraxein, **82:**118–19
Tardive dyskinesia: and endocrine effects, **82:**136, 203–04
  risk of, **83:**272, 480, 487
  See also Drug side effect(s)
Targum, S. D., **83:**456; et al., **83:**449, 450, 457
Tarnow, J. D., **84:**182
Tartakoff, H., **82:**511
Taste, sense of, *see* Sensory deficits
TAT (Thematic Apperception Test), **82:**216; **84:**19
Taube, C. A., **83:**94, 95
Taube, S. L., et al., **83:**461
Tauchen, G., **84:**363, 364, 365
Tauro, Judge Joseph, **82:**381n3, 383n6
Tavel, M. E., et al., **84:**355
Tavistock Clinic (England), **83:**32; **84:**12, 25

Taylor, B. M., **83**:288
Taylor, D. P., **83**:488
Taylor, J. R., **84**:465
Taylor, L., **82**:332
Taylor, M. A., **82**:152; **83**:273, 279, 440, 443; **84**:208; et al., **83**:279, 438
Taylor Manifest Anxiety Scale, **84**:189, 208
TCA (tricyclic antidepressant) response, **83**:458–59, 472–82, 489, 526
  in anxiety disorders, **84**:248–49, 409, 437, 483, 503–07, 512–19 passim
    childhood, **84**:414–16
    panic disorder, **83**:142; **84**:472, 511, 512
  in bipolar illness, **83**:126, 273–81 passim, 289, 312, 317, 371, 380
  in cancer patients, **84**:248–49
  in combination with other drugs or ECT, **83**:125, 126, 382, 479, 480, 481, 485, 503; **84**:253
  dosage and, **83**:123–26, 317, 476–77, 483, 485, 487, 495, 497, 504, 508, 509
  "first-pass" effect in, **83**:495
  lithium response vs., **83**:308, 311, 481
  in nonbipolar or major depression, **83**:122–25, 289, 359, 369–71 passim, 381, 505, 512, 526
  plasma levels in, **83**:123–24, 125, 474, 477, 480, 486, 491–511
  poor or adverse, **83**:370, 380, 381, 399–400, 479–80, 481, 487, 503, 508; **84**:237 (see also and side effects, below)
  prediction of, **83**:125, 381, 468
  sedative vs. stimulating, **83**:476, 508
  and side effects, **82**:467; **83**:123, 127, 474–77, 480, 485–88 passim, 497, 508; **84**:248, 358
    delirium as, **84**:233
    hypomania as, **83**:273–77 passim, 280, 369, 375, 479
    mania/manic episode as, **83**:126, 311
  stress and, **83**:399–400
  and withdrawal effects, **83**:481
  See also Drugs; Drugs, list of; Drug side effect(s); Drug therapy; Imipramine
Teaching (of medical psychiatry), **84**:180, 181, 186, 238
  and medical student problems, **84**:245
  to surgeons, **84**:277
Teamsters Union, **84**:309
Television, see Videotapes
Tellenbach, H., **83**:374
Temperature: elevation of, in alcohol withdrawal, **84**:352
  skin/finger, biofeedback regulation of, **84**:228
Temple, D., et al., **84**:497, 498
Temple, H., et al., **83**:449
Tenen, S. S., **84**:487
Tennant, C., et al., **83**:404
Teplin, L., **82**:385
Terr, Lenore Cagen, **84**:88, 89, 108–20 passim
Terrorism, see Violence
Terry, R. D., **83**:100, 109, 110
Tessman, L. H., **84**:145, 154
Test, M. A., **82**:110, 227
Testicular removal, **82**:39. See also Surgery

Testimonial privilege, **82**:330–31. See also Confidentiality
Testosterone, **82**:11
  CNS regulation of, **84**:221, 222
Tetrahydroisoquinolines (TIQs), **84**:323–24
Texas custody research project, **84**:153
Thacore, U. R., et al., **83**:416
Tharp, R. G., **84**:329
Thayssen, P., et al., **83**:477, 499, 510
Theander, S., **84**:225
Thematic Apperception Test, see TAT
Therapeutic community, see Health care system; Nursing staff; Therapeutic relationship
Therapeutic relationship: in alcoholism, **84**:343–46
  in bipolar disorder, **83**:302, 323, 326, 329–31, 334
  in borderline disorders, **82**:474, 477–78, 481, 482–86 (see also Transference)
  in cancer management, **84**:242–43
  caregiver-infant dyad as model of, **83**:21
  in child therapy
    of child and therapist, **84**:120
    of parent and therapist, **82**:264; **84**:142–43
  clinical illustration of, **82**:505–10
  in cognitive or behavior therapy, **83**:514–16, 519; **84**:46, 47–48
  and consent to or refusal of treatment, **82**:351; **84**:259–60 (see also Therapy)
  empathy in, see Therapist, the
  ethical principles of, **82**:327–38, 333–34 (see also Confidentiality)
  the family and, **83**:173, 179, 182–84, 194, 198, 205n, 208, 210 (see also Family, the; Family therapy)
  with geriatric patient, **83**:130, 138–39, 144
  in group therapy, **83**:27
  in hypnotherapy, **82**:23
  with hypochondriacal patient, **83**:144
  impact of interpretations on, **83**:61–62
  male-female, **83**:39
  mandatory reporting and, **82**:332
  in "middle game," see Psychoanalysis
  in narcissistic disorder, **82**:516–23
  with psychosomatic patient, **84**:227
  in psychotherapy, **82**:154; **84**:26, 40, 42–43 (see also and therapeutic alliance, below)
  in schizophrenia, **82**:156, 162–65, 358
  sexism in, **83**:38–40
  studies of, **83**:184
  and therapeutic alliance
    with alcoholic, **84**:343–44
    in brief psychotherapy, **84**:15, 16, 29, 38, 40
    concept of, **82**:508
    in depression, **83**:523–24
    development of, **82**:479–80, 482, 485
    in drug therapy, **82**:218, 467; **83**:329
    in family therapy, **83**:194, 198, 205n
  in therapeutic community, **83**:28–30
  and therapeutic contract, **84**:15, 60, 62, 343–44
  third-party payment and, **82**:325
  transference in, see Transference

Therapist, the: active intervention by (in psychotherapy), **84:**29 (*see also* Intervention)
as "anthropologist," **83:**178–79
in childhood disorders, **82:**307; **83:**55
consultation-liaison psychiatrist as, **84:**185
and co-therapist, **82:**21
countertransference problems of, *see* Transference
in depressive disorders, **83:**514–16
empathy of, **82:**477, 508; **83:**55, 59–60; **84:**422, 453
  and ability to listen, **84:**423–24
  in alcoholism, **84:**343
  in bipolar illness, **83:**330
  in brief psychotherapy, **84:**15, 38–39, 47–48
  in data collection, **82:**493, 496
  with family, *see* Family therapy
  and "middle game," *see* Psychoanalysis
  for older patient, **83:**114, 129, 130, 141, 149, 150
experience and ability of, and outcome, **82:**223; **84:**422–23
function of, **82:**482, 484; **84:**422–23
and gender disturbance cases, **82:**54
in group psychotherapy, **83:**27
hostility toward, **82:**156–57, 474; **84:**143 (*see also* Therapeutic relationship)
legal implications concerning, **82:**331 (*see also* Law and psychiatry)
multimodal, **84:**68
note-taking by, **84:**31
-parent relationship (in child therapy), **82:**264; **84:**142–43
and patient-staff relations, **83:**29
personal characteristics of, **82:**161; **84:**13
role of
  in alcoholism psychotherapy, **84:**343, 344, 346
  in group, family or couples therapy, **83:**27, 201, 223–24, 226, 238
in sex therapy, **82:**21, 35, 41
in sexual abuse cases, **82:**60, 64–65
technical neutrality of, **82:**477–78, 480–81, 484
training of, **83:**183; **84:**14, 32, 179–82, 186, 422
violence of patient toward, **83:**196
vulnerability of, to attacks by bipolar patient, **83:**319, 330
See also Analyst, the; Physician; Psychiatrist, the
Therapy: abreactive, **84:**41, 107, 120, 424
aim of, **82:**64
art and poetry, **84:**112, 113, 120
child, **82:**263–65, 289, 305, 307, **84:**120, 142–43

for anxiety disorders, **84:**411–12, 413–18
choice of, vs. restrictions, **82:**378 (*see also* Law and psychiatry)
community care and, **82:**372–78; **83:**94–95; **84:**11–12, 128, 334
consent to or refusal of, **82:**335n3, 347, 348, 350–60, 361, 378, 379–84, 470; **84:**182, 259–60 (*see also* Civil commitment; Informed consent)

in consultation-liaison psychiatry, **84:**185–86
criteria for (family/marital vs. individual), **83:**189–93
exercise as, **83:**142, 146
hospitalization distinguished from, **82:**381 (*see also* Hospitalization)
insight-oriented, **82:**111, 217; **83:**192, 221; **84:**17–18, 26, 119, 226, 424, 440
involuntary, **82:**378, 383, 384
legal doctrine and, **82:**376–78
megavitamin, **82:**142–44
milieu, **82:**110, 172, 174–76
patient's expectations of, *see* Expectations
for person other than patient, **84:**20, 53, 63, 132, 142, 452, 453
play, *see* Play, symbolic
in prison, **82:**386, 395–96
and quality of life, *see* Values
radiation, *see* Cancer
relationship, **82:**42; **83:**114
resistance to or noncompliance with, **83:**528; **84:**13, 239–40 (*see also* Drug therapy)
right to treatment, **82:**322, 323, 347, 361–70, 371–73, 379
  least restrictive alternative, **82:**373, 375–76, 378
  vs. right to refuse, **82:**379–84; **84:**182, 259–60
standards for, **82:**363
termination of, **84:**8, 16, 31–32, 40
  denial of, **84:**42
  schizophrenia, **82:**165
  and separation fears, **84:**16, 39, 42, 43, 254–55
voluntary admission to, **82:**347
See also Behavioral approach; Cognitive therapy; Crisis intervention; Diet; Drug therapy; ECT (electroconvulsive therapy); Exposure treatment (of phobia); Family therapy; Group therapy; Health care system; Hypnosis; Marital therapy; Outpatient treatment; Psychiatry; Psychoanalysis; Psychotherapy(ies); Psychotherapy(ies), brief; Relaxation therapy; Sex therapy; Social support networks; Surgery
Thieden, H., et al., **84:**349
Third-party payment; **82:**325, 331–32; **83:**105–06, 525
  and dementia as insurable illness, **83:**117
Third-party protection, **82:**331. *See also* Confidentiality
Third Spiritual Alphabet, The (Osuna), **84:**441
Thomas, C., et al., **83:**301
Thomas, D. W., **83:**512; **84:**353, 354
Thompson, Clara, **83:**41, 47
Thompson, G. N., **84:**518
Thompson, L. W., et al., **83:**112
Thompson, W. D., et al., **84:**404
Thompson, W. L., **84:**353; et al., **84:**353
Thomsen, K., **83:**313, 314
Thomson, K. C., **83:**395
Thoracic spine films, **83:**126
Thoreau, Henry David, **84:**443

Thoren, P., et al., **84:**512, 513
Thorpe, J. J., **84:**357
Thought disorder: in borderline patients, **82:**417
  and competency, **82:**354
  drug therapy and, **82:**183, 199; **83:**271, 312
  misdiagnosis of (in elderly), **84:**237
  in schizophrenia, **82:**199; **83:**279
Three Mile Island nuclear plant, **83:**403; **84:**116
Thresholds Study, **84:**140
Thromboendarterectomy, **83:**115
Thyroid, *see* Hormone(s)
Thyroxine: CNS regulation of/stress effect on,
  84:222. *See also* Hormone(s)
Ticho, E., **83:**476, 482
Tienari, P., **82:**94, 95, 451; **83:**441
Tiengo, M., **84:**351
Tierney, K., **84:**117
Time: distortions, psychic trauma and, **84:**112,
  114
  meaning and significance of, **84:**35–37
Time-limited psychotherapy (TLP), *see* Psy-
  chotherapy(ies), brief
Tinckler, L. F., **84:**353
TIQs (tetrahydroisoquinolines), **84:**323–24
Tissot, R., **83:**111
Tisza, V., **82:**57
Titchener, J. L., **82:**61; **84:**262
Tizard, J., **84:**124
TLP (time-limited psychotherapy), *see* Psy-
  chotherapy(ies), brief
Tobacco, use of, **84:**313
  and lung cancer, **84:**239
  and mortality rate, **84:**217, 465
Tod, H., **84:**476
Tolwinski, T., **82:**171
Tomlinson, B. E., et al., **83:**109, 110
Tompkins, D., **84:**112
Toohey, M. L., **83:**242
Toolan, J. M., **82:**266, 268
Tooley, K., **84:**145
Toomin, M., **83:**192
Toone, B. K., et al., **84:**470
Torgersen, S., **84:**405
Torrey, E. F., **82:**101, 115, 120; et al., **82:**115, 121
Toru, M., et al., **82:**201
Total parenteral nutrition (TPN), **84:**271–72
Toulmin, S., **82:**351
Tozer, T. N., **83:**492, 507
TPN (total parenteral nutrition), **84:**271–72
Tracey, D., et al., **84:**330
Tracking: defined, **84:**76
Trails Test, **84:**326
Transcendental meditation, **83:**142; **84:**445. *See
  also* Relaxation therapy
Transference: acting out, **82:**475, 476, 478–79, 485
  in alcoholic patients, **84:**345
  in borderline patients, **82:**472–75, 476, 478–81,
    482, 485–86, 489
  and countertransference reactions, **82:**36, 474,
    485, 517
    in bipolar illness, **83:**319, 329–31
    in brief psychotherapy, **84:**15, 31, 42–43
    geriatric patients and, **83:**130

  to mentally retarded, **84:**128
  sexual problems and, **82:**54, 60, 65–66
  toward women, **83:**40
in group therapy, **83:**26, 27, 28
to internist (vs. psychiatrist) in illness, **82:**36
interpretation of, **83:**64–70 passim, 523, 524;
  84:14, 30, 41, 104, 345
narcissistic, **82:**54, 489, 495, 516–22 passim
negative
  in borderline patients, **82:**473, 478, 483, 485
  cognitive therapy and, **84:**48
  in narcissistic patients, **82:**519
  in schizophrenia, **82:**164
  in sex therapy, **82:**35
overintense (transference neurosis or psychosis), **82:**472, 475, 488; **83:**188; **84:**30
parental
  in marital problems, **82:**27, 32
  in psychotherapy (brief), **84:**30–31, 39
positive
  in psychotherapy, **84:**15, 40, 42, 345
  value of, **84:**17
selfobject (mirror and idealizing), **82:**499–508
  passim
and transference relationship, **84:**14
Transference psychosis, **82:**475
Transportation, U.S. Department of, **84:**362
Transsexualism, **82:**49
  "as if" identity represented by, **82:**56
  DSM-III criterion for, **82:**53
  and "pretranssexual"children, **82:**50–51
  stress and, **82:**53
  treatment of, **82:**48, 53–55
  See also Gender identity
Transvestism, **82:**34
Traskman, L., et al., **83:**431
Traub, R. D., et al., **83:**111
Trauma, brain, *see* Brain, the
Trauma, emotional/psychic; anxiety states following, **84:**110–15, 421
  and children at risk, **84:**104–20
  concept of, **84:**107–08
  "contagious," *see* Contagion
  delay in effect of, **84:**117
  and foreshortening of future, **84:**114, 117
  illness and, **82:**35
  sexual
    Freud and, **84:**93, 431
    rape and, **82:**61–63 (*see also* Rape)
  and sexual dysfunction, **82:**15, 28, 31, 32
  surgery and, **82:**38; **84:**272
  treatment of, **84:**118–20
  "vicarious," **84:**107, 116–17
Traumatic neurosis, *see* Posttraumatic Stress
  Disorder
Treatment, *see* Therapy
Treece, J. C., **84:**339
Tremor: during alcohol withdrawal, **84:**351, 352,
  353, 493
  anxiety and, **84:**474, 491, 492, 493, 496, 502
Trevarthan, C., **83:**19
TRH/TSH (thyrotropin-releasing/thyroid-stimu-
  lating) response test, **83:**121–22, 273, 289, 314

Triangulation (in social group), **83**:234
Tricyclics, *see* Drugs; TCA (tricyclic antidepressant) response
Trimingham, J. S., **84**:443
Troen, B. R., **83**:133
Tross, S., **83**:129
Trower, P., et al., **82**:111
Tryptophan, **84**:487, 518
Tsai, L., **83**:117
Tsuang, M. T., **82**:109, 286, 461; **83**:92, 117, 291, 430, 441, 484, 491n; **84**:461; et al., **82**:93; **83**:430, 431, 440; **84**:460, 461
Tuckman, J., **83**:128
Tufo, H. M., **84**:263
Tufts-New England Medical Center conference (1982), **84**:393
Tulchin, S., **84**:115
Tulis, Elaine H., **82**:442, 443, 455
Tuma, A. H., **82**:158, 216, 217
Tumors: and emotional effect of tumor biopsy, **84**:222, 223, 270
  hormone-producing (APUDomas), **84**:250
  lymphomas, **84**:240, 253
    in Alzheimer's disease, **83**:110
  primary brain, and cancer, **84**:249
  See also Cancer; Surgery
Tune, G., **83**:145
Tuomisto, J., et al., **83**:470
Tupin, J., et al., **82**:465
Turgay, A., **84**:272
Turkey: children studied in, **82**:282
Turner, J. A., **82**:332
Turner, P., **84**:494, 495; et al., **84**:492
Turner, W. J., **83**:276, 449
Turn of the Screw, The (James), **84**:104
Turns, D., **83**:406
Turpin, T. J., **84**:274
Turquet, P., **83**:22–23, 24, 30, 32, 33, 35
Twerski, A. J., **84**:339
Twins: affective disorders among, studies of, **83**:435, 441, 443–44, 450, 452; **84**:97
    childhood depression, **82**:286
  in alcoholism studies, **84**:320
  in anxiety disorder studies, **84**:405
  in schizophrenia studies, **82**:93–95, 124, 126, 128, 445, 451–52; **83**:441
  in suicide studies, **83**:432
  See also Genetic factors
Tyrer, P., **83**:467, 479, 483; **84**:494, 496; et al., **84**:469, 507, 508
Tyrer, S. P., **82**:144
Tyrosine hydroxylase: aging and, **83**:96
Tyrrell, D. A. J., **82**:121
Tyson, J. E., **82**:204
Tyson, P., **83**:44
Tzivoni, D., et al., **84**:468

Udry, J. R., **82**:42
UFC (urinary free cortisol) levels, **83**:462–63
Ulcers, *see* Gastrointestinal disorders
Ullman, A. D., **84**:313
Ulrich, D. N., **83**:194
Ulrich, R. F., **82**:417, 421–25 passim, 428, 443; et al., **82**:295
Unadkat, J. D., **83**:500
Unconscious, the, **84**:428
  Freud's concept of, **83**:34; **84**:421, 431
  "history" of, **83**:48
Underhill, E., **84**:443
Unemployment: and depression, **83**:400, 403, 404, 422. *See also* Work
Unfinished Business (Scarf), **84**:61
"Uniform Health Care Consent Act" (proposed), **82**:354
Unipolar/nonbipolar depression, **83**:384, 414
  bipolar compared to (personality, stress effects), **83**:386–92, 395–99, 404
  bipolar distinguished from, **83**:269–70, 272–74, 281, 368–69, 381, 410, 423, 437, 444, 461, 464–66
  bipolar relation to, **83**:271, 438–39, 444, 447, 450
  diagnosis of, **83**:380, 409–10, 414, 437, 462
  epidemiology of, **83**:415–22, 427–28, 437, 447
  etiology of, **83**:252n, 421, 450
  genetic factors in, **83**:272–74, 442–47 passim, 451, 453, 457; **84**:97
  MAO activity in, **83**:467
  and mortality rate, **83**:287; **84**:217
  social factors and, **83**:403
  subtypes or variants of, **83**:92–93, 409–10, 463–64, 468
  and suicide, **83**:430
  treatment of, **83**:252, 274, 319, 321, 368–69, 399, 415; **84**:49 (*see also* Drug therapy)
  unipolar I & II, **83**:274, 292
  urinary MHPG and UFC levels in, **83**:461–65
  See also Bipolar (manic-depressive) Disorder; Depression; Major Depression
United Kingdom, *see* Great Britain
United States: affective disorder studies in, **83**:293, 294, 407, 411, 479; **84**:96, 303
  alcoholism in (and costs of), **84**:300–301, 320, 321, 338, 365
  alcohol policies in, **84**:360–61, 362–65
  arrests (annual) in, **84**:367
  bipolar and unipolar illness in, **83**:271
  depressive disorders overlooked in, **83**:108
  diagnosis systems in, **83**:408, 409
  divorce rate in, **84**:144
  drug-psychotherapy studies in, **83**:321
  elderly population in, **83**:84, 88
  epidemiology studies in, **84**:92, 189–203
  group-relations conferences in, **83**:32
  health care policies of, **82**:160
  interpersonal approach in, **84**:57, 66
  lithium use in, **83**:320
  lung cancer epidemic in, **84**:239
  mental disorder incidence in, **84**:189–98
  psychoanalytic group psychotherapy developed in, **83**:26, 27
  psychosomatic diseases studied in, **84**:211
  schizophrenia in, **82**:86; **83**:132, 407
    misdiagnosis of, **82**:102

studies of, **82:**94, 98, 103–09 passim, 138, 145, 215–25; **83:**407; **84:**303

suicide rate in, **83:**433

See also Census, U.S. Bureau of the; *individual departments*

United States Brewers Association, **84:**362

U.S. Constitution, **82:**365, 381, 383, 386

Univers Contestationnaire, L' ("Stéphane"), **83:**35

University: of California (Los Angeles), **82:**104; **83:**245, 284; **84:**95, 98

Affective Disorders Clinic lithium study, **83:**322, 332–37 passim

of California (San Francisco), Mental Retardation Program, **84:**123, 124

of Cincinnati, **84:**111

of Iowa, **82:**109; **84:**461

of Michigan, **83:**121, 274

of North Carolina, **83:**121

of Oregon Medical School Hospital, **84:**202

of Pennsylvania School of Medicine, **84:**336

of Pittsburgh, **82:**173; **83:**122, 279, 480; **84:**98, 454

of Rochester (NY), **84:**181

Medical Center, **84:**217, 246

of Tennessee, **83:**275, 282, 284

Unraveling Juvenile Delinquency (Glueck and Glueck), **84:**311

Upanishads, the, **84:**443

U'Pritchard, D. C., et al., **83:**470

Urethral surgery: and sexual dysfunction, **82:**38–39. *See also* Surgery

Urinary free cortisol (UFC) levels, **83:**462–63

Urinary MHPG levels, **83:**272–73, 460–66

in anxiety, **84:**472

as predictors of drug response, **83:**468–69, 473–74, 486, 490

Urinary VMA levels, **83:**461, 464–65, 466

Urology, **84:**275. *See also* Surgery

Uterus, removal of, **82:**40–41. *See also* Surgery

V

VA (Veterans Administration), **84:**11

alcoholism studies by, **84:**310

facilities of, **83:**130

-NIMH Collaborative Study of Lithium Therapy, **83:**307, 311, 316–17, 371

schizophrenia studies by, **82:**198, 226, 227

See also War veterans

Vachon, M. L. S., et al., **84:**245

Vagina: aging effects on, **82:**45–46

anatomy of, **82:**10, 12

and vaginal orgasm, **82:**11; **83:**41

Vaginismus: as inhibition, **82:**15, 20, 32

therapy for, **82:**21, 23

Vagueness, *see* Speech

Vaillant, G., **83:**216; **84:**299, 311–19 passim, 329, 339; et al., **84:**299, 315, 318

Valenstein, A. F., **83:**61

Vallee, G. L., **84:**356

Values: conflict of, in couples therapy, **83:**221–22

interpersonal relations and, **84:**66

and quality of life in treatment, **84:**241–42, 255, 264

relationship of, to psychoanalysis, **83:**8, 36–50

traditional, rejection of, **83:**35

See also Ethical considerations; Self-esteem

Valzelli, L., **83:**512

Vandalism, **83:**190. *See also* Crime

Vandenbos, G. R., **82:**158, 217

Vanderstoep, E., **83:**191

Van Der Velde, C. D., **82:**180, 184

Van der Waals, H., **82:**511

Van der Walde, P., et al., **84:**140

Van Dis, H., **84:**477

Van Eerdewegh, M. M., et al., **83:**447

Van Egeren, L. F., **84:**220

van Kammen, D. P., **82:**132

Vannicelli, M., et al., **82:**226

Van Praag, H. M., **82:**195; **83:**273, 452

Van Putten, Theodore, **82:**175; **83:**317, 326, 328, 331, 335

Van Valkenburg, C., et al., **83:**380

Vartanian, M. E., et al., **82:**115, 117

Vascular disorders: cancer and, **84:**250

cardiovascular disorders, **84:**217

alcoholism and, **84:**358, 493

in bipolar illness, **83:**287

among depressives, **83:**361, 366

in drug therapy, **84:**415, 491, 492, 493

drug side effects and, **83:**477–78, 484, 485, 505, 509–10

and metabolism, **83:**509

in panic disorders (and mortality rate), **84:**465–47

personality and, **84:**216, 230

psychophysiological aspects of, **84:**219, 220

and psychosexual dysfunctions, **82:**36–37

and dementia (repeated or multiinfarct), **83:**114–15

DIC (disseminated intravascular coagulation), **84:**250

and vascular amputee, **84:**272, 273

See also Physical illness

Vasectomy, **82:**39. *See also* Birth control

Vasocongestion: as sexual response, **82:**12

Vaughn, C. E., **82:**104, 105, 172; **83:**174, 175; **84:**95; et al., **82:**104; **84:**95

Vaughn, W. T., et al., **82:**115

Vaughter, R. M., **83:**39

Veith, R. C., et al., **83:**478, 503

Venkatesh, A., et al., **84:**408

Verbalization, *see* Speech

Verhoeven, W. M. A., et al., **82:**141, 213

Vermont: children-at-risk programs in, **84:**137, 142

Verrier, R. L., **84:**219

Versiani, M., **82:**185

Verstergaard, P., **83:**314; et al., **83:**313, 314

Verwoerdt, A., **84:**235; et al., **83:**147–48

Veterans, *see* War veterans

Veterans Administration, *see* VA

Vibrator, use of, **82:**21

Vicksburg (Mississippi) tornado, **84**:107
Victor, M., **84**:347, 350, 351, 355
Victoratos, G. C., et al., **83**:109
Videbech, T., **83**:431
Videotapes: as research or teaching tools, **83**:175;
  84:9, 32, 98, 141, 277
Viederman, M., **84**:268
Vierling, L., **82**:352
Vietnam war, **82**:371; **84**:115, 395, 401. *See also*
  War
Vilkin, M. I., **82**:458, 461
Vincent, J. P., et al., **82**:140
Violence: adolescent, **83**:190
    against parent (in divorce), **84**:152
  alcohol-related, **84**:305
  battered wives/husbands, **82**:57; **83**:188, 196
  in bipolar illness, **83**:320
  group potential for, **83**:22, 23, 25
  terrorism and effects of, **84**:109, 118
  toward therapist, **83**:196
  See also Aggression; Child abuse; Dangerous-
    ness; Disaster, studies of; Rape
Virchow, Rudolph, **84**:177
Virginia: preschool children studied in, **84**:152
Viruses: and affective disorders, **83**:379, 453
  and schizophrenia, **82**:119–22
  viral etiology theorized in multiple sclerosis,
    Alzheimer's disease, **82**:121; **83**:111, 453
  See also Physical illness
Vischi, T. R., **84**:213
Visintainer, M. A., **84**:258
Vision: age-related changes in, **83**:102–03, 134
  blindness, psychotherapeutic management of,
    84:49
  cataracts, **83**:103, 134
  color blindness, **83**:436, 448–49
  drug side effects on, **82**:169; **83**:113, 302, 475,
    484; **84**:233
  glaucoma, **83**:103, 113, 475
  paranoia and, **83**:134
  presbyopia, **83**:103
  senile macular degeneration, **83**:103
  See also Sensory deficits
Vital Balance, The (Menninger), **83**:269
Vitamins:
  deficiency of (particularly B vitamins)
    in alcohol withdrawal reactions, **84**:352, 354
    in cancer patients, **84**:250
    and mental retardation, **84**:127
  megavitamin therapy for schizophrenia,
    82:142–44
  ⨍ *See also* Diet
VMA, *see* Urinary VMA levels
Voegtlin, W. L., **84**:328, 333
Vogel, E. F., **83**:233
Vogel, G. W., et al., **82**:290
Vogel, W. H., **82**:126, 144
Vogler, R. E., et al., **84**:336
Vohra, J., et al., **83**:505
Volavka, J., et al., **82**:213
Volicer, L., **84**:350
Volk, W., et al., **82**:206
Volkan, V., **82**:471, 480, 519

Volkmar, F. R., et al., **83**:322, 325
Vollhardt, B. R., et al., **84**:224
Volpe, B. T., **84**:233
Volstead Act, *see* Prohibition
Voluntary admission, **82**:347. *See also* Therapy
von Eschenbach, A. C., **84**:255
von Wartburg, J. P., **84**:320–24 passim, 327
von Zerssen, D., **82**:207
von Zerssen Personality Scale, **83**:387
Vuchinich, R., **84**:331
Vulnerability, **84**:88, 109, 111
  of child of divorce, **84**:151, 153
  of child of mentally ill parent, **84**:133
  defined, **84**:92 (*see also* Risk)
  factors in (social and genetic), **83**:400–403; **84**:97
    (*see also* Genetic factors; Psychosocial fac-
    tors)
  to panic and depression, **84**:511–12
  to psychic trauma, **84**:91–103
  of retarded child, **84**:121, 123
  to schizophrenia, *see* Schizophrenia, etiology
    of
  of therapist, *see* Therapist, the
  See also Children at risk
*Vulnerable but Invincible: A Study of Resilient Chil-
  dren* (Werner and Smith), **84**:103
Vyas, B. K., **82**:186

W

Wachtel, E. F., **83**:216
Wacker, W. E. C., **84**:355, 356
Wadlington, W., **84**:266
Waelder, R., **84**:108
Wahlin, A., **83**:314
Wain, H. J., **84**:186
WAIS (Wechsler Adult Intelligence Scale), **82**:433;
  83:301
Waldmeier, P. C., **83**:469
Walford, R. L., **83**:111
Walinder, J., **82**:211
Walkenstein, S. S., et al., **84**:232
Wallace, J., **84**:339, 343, 344
Wallace, R.K., **84**:445; et al., **84**:445
Wallack, L., **84**:368
Wallerstein, Judith S., **84**:90, 145–54 passim
Wallerstein, R. S., **82**:475, 497, 503
Wallgren, H., **84**:347, 348, 349
Walrath, L. C., **84**:446
Walsh, A. C., **83**:112; et al., **83**:112
Walsh, B. H., **83**:112
Walsh, D., **84**:362
Walsh, F., **83**:222
Walter, C. J. S., **84**:468, 512
Wang, H. S., **83**:102
Wang, Y. C., et al., **83**:470
War: concentration camp experiences (World War
  II), **84**:395

effects on children (World War II), **84:**105–06, 107, 110–11, 115
See also Trauma, emotional/psychic; War veterans
Warburton, C., **84:**360, 364
Ward, A. W. M., **84:**217
Ward, B. E., et al., **83:**110
Ward, N. G., et al., **83:**506
Warheit, G. J., et al., **83:**412, 413, 414
Warren, S. D., **83:**328
Warrenburg, S., et al., **84:**446
Warshak, R. A., **84:**153, 156
War veterans: and alcoholism, **84:**213
   traumatized, **84:**106, 117, 119, 395, 401, 420–21
   Vietnam, treatment of, **84:**395, 401
   See also VA (Veterans Administration)
Washburn, S., **84:**110; et al., **82:**226
Washington University, **83:**282, 293, 376; **84:**303
   Department of Psychiatry, **83:**32, 408, 519; **84:**98
Wasserman, G., et al., **84:**115
Wasserman, M. D., et al., **82:**37
Watcher on the Hills (Johnson), **84:**443
Watson, A., **84:**116, 154
Watson, J. P., **84:**450
Watson, J. S., **83:**14
Watson, R., et al., **83:**461
Watson, S. J., et al., **82:**212
Watt, D. C., **82:**108; **84:**322
Watt, N. F., **82:**89; **84:**101, 130, 132, 134; et al., **84:**94, 99, 131
Watts, C. A. H., **83:**372; et al., **83:**417
Waxler, N. E., **82:**101; **83:**242
Weakland, John, **83:**170
Weaver, J. L., **82:**100
Webb, W., **83:**145
Wechsler, H., **84:**364
Wechsler scales: for adults, *see* WAIS
   for chidlren, **84:**131
Weddington, W. W., et al., **84:**232, 233
Weed, L. L., **84:** 68
Weeke, Anita, **83:**287, 419, 425; et al., **83:**418, 426
Weeks, C., **84:**421
Weeks, G., **83:**223
Weeping: in bipolar disorder, **83:**280
   childhood depression and, **82:**304
Weight gain: depression and, **83:**280
   as drug side effect, *see* Drug side effect(s)
   See also Obesity
Weight loss: depression and, **83:**127, 144, 362, 371, 373, 479; **84:**248
   childhood depression, **82:**297, 304
   as predictor of TCA response, **83:**122
   See also Anorexia nervosa
Weinberg, J., **82:**225; **83:**86–87
Weinberg, W. A., et al., **82:**267, 282, 284, 289–98 passim
Weinberger, Daniel A., **82:**122–24, 148; et al., **82:**123
Weiner, H., **84:**216, 219, 220, 222, 239, 323
Weiner, I., **82:**57
Weiner, R. D., **84:**238

Weingartner, H., et al., **83:**107
Weinmann, B., **82:**177
Weinraub, M., **84:**412
Weinshilboum, R. M., **83:**451; et al., **82:**127
Weinstein, M. R., **83:**314
Weintraub, J. F., **84:**131,132
Weintraub, S., **84:**135
Weisman, A. D., **84:**180, 186, 232, 260, 262, 270
Weiss, J., **84:**104
Weiss, James M. A., **82:**281n
Weiss, R., **82:**452; **83:**467
Weiss, R. S., **84:**149, 152
Weiss, S. M., **84:**227
Weissberg, J. H., **82:**35
Weissman, Myrna M., **82:**161, 281–85 passim; **83:**91, 92, 128, 270, 271, 275, 321, 355, 365, 366, 372, 374, 406–16 passim, 420–27 passim, 438, 519; **84:**8, 10, 58, 99, 100, 133, 135, 206, 214; et al., **82:**281; **83:**128, 391, 393, 398, 400, 409, 416, 420, 424, 437, 438, 512, 525; **84:**99
Weitkamp, L. R., et al., **83:**449
Weitzman, E. D., **84:**221
Weller, E., **82:**292; et al., **82:**307
Weller, H. P., **82:**144
Wellisch, D. K., et al., **84:**270
Wells, C. E., **83:**90, 107, 108, 109, 117; **84:**234, 235
Welner, A., et al., **83:**286, 290
Welner, Z., et al., **82:**289
Wender, P. H., **82:**454; **84:**390; et al., **82:**95, 444, 445, 448, 454, 455, 460, 462–63
Wenger, M. A., **84:**445
Werble, B., **82:**416
Werner, E. E., **84:**88, 103, 134
Werner, Heinz, **83:**14
Werner's syndrome, **83:**110
Wernicke, C., **83:**269
Wertham, F. I., **83:**285
Wertheimer, N. M., **82:**117
Wessels, H., **84:**451
West, D. J., **84:**96
West, D. W., **84:**276
West, E. D., **83:**119, 126; **84:**507
Western beliefs: in continuity of childhood, **84:**130
   and mystical practices (in relaxation response), **84:**441–43
West Virginia Rehabilitation Research and Training Center, **82:**109
Wettstein, Robert M., **84:**177–78
Wetzel, R. D., **83:**433; et al., **83:**390, 392, 393
Wetzel, R. J., **84:**329
Wexler, B., **82:**124
Whaley, K., **82:**117
Whalley, L. J., et al., **83:**111; **84:**351
Wharton, R. N., et al., **83:**480
Wheatley, D., **84:**495, 499, 516
Wheeler, E. O., et al., **84:**404, 464
Whipple, B., **82:**11
Whitaker, Carl, **83:**170, 200, 215
Whitaker, P. M., et al., **82:**130
White, B. J., et al., **83:**110
White, B. V., **84:**468
White, K., **83:**485; et al., **83:**467

White, P., et al., **83**:109
White, P. D., **84**:407, 479
White, R. A., **82**:37
Whiteley, J. S., **83**:25
Whitlock F. A., **84**:217
Whybrow, P. C., **83**:460
Whyte, C. R., **84**:357
Whyte, S. F., et al., **83**:506
Widmer, R. B., **84**:213
Widowhood: and depression, **84**:187, 206
  and mortality rate, **84**:217
  and psychiatric morbidity rate, **84**:202
  and sexuality, **82**:42–43, 44–45
  See also Grief reaction
Wiener, A. D., **84**:276, 277
Wiener, C., **84**:361
Wiens, A. N., et al., **84**:334
Wigmore, J. H., **82**:327
Wilcox, C. B., et al., **83**:111
Wilder, J. F., et al., **82**:225
Wiles, D., et al., **82**:202
Wilkie, F., et al., **83**:133
Wilkinson, G. R., **83**:495
Will, O. A., Jr., **82**:161
Willett, A., et al., **82**:416–17, 418
Williams, A. F., et al., **84**:365
Williams, C. D., **83**:90, 91
Williams, Janet B. W., **84**:397, 402, 519, 520
Williams, J. G. L., **84**:260; et al., **84**:260
Williams, L. T., et al., **83**:470
Williams, M., **83**:115
Williams, N., **84**:123, 124, 125
Williams, R. L., et al., **82**:294, 295; **83**:145
Williams, S. L., **84**:457
Williams, T., **82**:61
Williams, T. A., **82**:287; **84**:188, 204, 206
Williamson, M. J., et al., **84**:485
Willmuth, R. L., **83**:475
Willowbrook (New York), **82**:375
Wilmette, J., **83**:449
Wilson, A., **84**:357
Wilson, E. C., **84**:349
Wilson, G. T., **84**:331, 337; et al., **84**:333
Wilson, J. C., **84**:352
Wilson, J. F., **84**:258
Wilson, R. G., et al., **82**:202
Wilson, W., **83**:144
Wilson's disease, **82**:144
Wiltse, L. L., **84**:274
Wing, J. K., **82**:88, 102, 107, 177; **83**:174, 242; et al., **82**:100; **83**:408–09, 416
Wing, L., **84**:468
Winick, L., **84**:271
Winkelstein, C., et al., **84**:260
Winn, M., **84**:157
Winnicott, D. W., **82**:471, 472, 477, 486, 490, 520; **83**:14, 56
Winokur, A., et al., **83**:442
Winokur, G., **83**:271–78 passim, 282–86 passim, 311, 366, 372, 380, 412, 420–23 passim, 431, 438–48 passim; **84**:97, 357; et al., **82**:438, 443; **83**:118, 269, 279, 283, 287, 293, 304, 368, 380, 446–49 passim; **84**:97, 313, 314

Winokur, M., **84**:68
Winsberg, B. G., et al., **84**:416
Winsor, A., **84**:350
Winter, H., et al., **83**:451, 452
Winter, J., **83**:117; **84**:234
Wirschung, M., et al., **84**:273
Wisconsin: psychiatric morbidity study in, **84**:198
Wise, A., et al., **84**:274
Wise, C. D., **82**:127; et al., **82**:128
Wise, T. N., **84**:182, 218
Wise, T. P., **82**:331
Wisniewski, H. M., **83**:100
Wistedt, B., **82**:191
Withdrawal, alcohol, *see* Alcoholism
Withdrawal, drug: treatment of, **84**:352, 472
  TCA therapy, **83**:481
Withdrawal, social: childhood, and later schizophrenia, **82**:89
  childhood depression and, **82**:297, 302
  in emotionally unstable character disorder, **82**:463
  See also Social isolation
Witmer, H., **84**:312
Wittenborn, J. R., **83**:387, 389, 392
Wittkower, E. D., **84**:226
Wode-Helgodt, B., et al., **82**:183
Wohl, J., **82**:357
Wolberg, L. R., **84**:8
Wold, P. N., **83**:281
Wolf, A., **83**:26
Wolf, E. S., **82**:504, 505, 510, 511
Wolf, G., **82**:293
Wolf, S., **84**:219
Wolfe, H. J., **84**:250
Wolfe, S. M., **84**:347, 351
Wolfensberger, W., **84**:128
Wolfer, J. A., **84**:258
Wolff, H. G., **84**:219
Wolff, P., **83**:9
Wolin, S. J., et al., **83**:176, 177–78
Wolpe, J., **84**:421, 449
Wolpe-Lang Fear Survey, **84**:510
Wolston, E. J., **84**:184, 186
Women, *see* Female(s); Feminist movement
Women for Sobriety, **84**:346
Wood, C. L., et al., **83**:470
Wood, D., et al., **82**:459, 462, 463
Wood, P., **84**:479
Woodman, D., **82**:330
Woodruff, R. A., **83**:372; **84**:212; et al., **83**:426; **84**:465
Woodward, B., **82**:363
Wooley, C. F., **84**:408, 479
Woolson, R. F., **84**:461; et al., **84**:461
Woolverton, W., **84**:501
Worden, J. W., **84**:270
Wordsworth, William, **84**:443
Work: alcoholism and, **84**:305
  continuance of, during depression, **84**:61
  retirement from (age and), **83**:106
  return to, after surgery, **84**:264–65, 272
  and schizophrenia, **82**:109–10
  of women outside home, **84**:135

Worland, J., et al., **84**:132
World Health Organization (WHO), **82**:14, 100–101; **83**:409, 506; **84**:189, 303, 308, 362, 394
World War II, *see* War
Wright, D. J. M., et al., **84**:351
Wright, J. H., et al., **84**:205, 206
Wright, M. R., **84**:276
Wurmser, L., **84**:343
Wyatt, Richard J., **82**:92, 122–24, 125, 130, 143, 147, 148, 452; **83**:131, 132; et al., **82**:118, 119, 126–29 passim, 137, 152
Wyatt right-to-treatment cases, **82**:321, 361–73 passim
Wynne, Lyman C., **82**:172; **83**:170, 190, 191, 193, 235, 242; **84**:130–34 passim, 449; et al., **84**:99

Young adults: affective disorders in, **83**:280, 281, 287, 329, 364, 365, 372, 456
in family therapy, **83**:169, 195, 211–12
See also Adolescent(s); Students
Youngerman, J., **83**:283
Youngs, D. D., **84**:182
Yu, P., et al., **84**:131, 473
Yudofsky, S. C., **84**:263

X

X-chromosome transmission hypothesis, *see* Genetic factors

Y

Yager, J., **84**:203, 204
Yagi, K., **82**:137
Yale University: Department of Psychiatry, **84**:98
depression studies at, **84**:58
disaster studies by, **84**:111
Yale Law Review Journal "Note," **82**:363, 366, 368
Yamada, K., et al., **84**:252
Yanchyshyn, G. W., **82**:284
Yassa, R., **82**:144
Yates, A., **84**:115
Yates, C. M., **83**:111
Yates, P. O., **83**:110
Yeazell, S. C., **82**:324n8
Yelverton, K. C., **83**:446
Yesavage, J. A., et al., **83**:112
Yoga, **84**:443, 445
Yorkston, N. J., et al., **82**:131, 205, 206, 207; **84**:450
Young, D. F., **84**:250, 251, 252
Young, J. E., **83**:513
Young, M., et al., **84**:217
Young, W. S., **84**:486
Young, W. T., **84**:69

Z

Zabarenko, R. N. and L. M., **83**:173
Zackson, H., **82**:62
Zaiden, J., **83**:523
Zajonc, R. B., **83**:16, 17
Zaks, M. S., **84**:262
Zaleznik, A., **83**:33
Zarit, S. N., **83**:132, 133
Zarrabi, M. H., et al., **82**:117, 118
Zeiner, R., **84**:323
Zeisel, S., et al., **83**:113
Zen Buddhism, **84**:443, 445
Zetzel, E. R., **82**:472, 480; **83**:56
Ziegler, V. E., **83**:506; et al., **83**:495, 500, 506
Zigler, E., **82**:108
Zilbach, J. J., **83**:230
Zilbergeld, B., **82**:26; **83**:222n1; **84**:68
Zilboorg, G., **82**:444; **83**:512
Zill, N., **84**:144, 145
Zilm, D., et al., **84**:493
Zimbardo, P. G., **83**:134
Zimberg, Sheldon, **84**:303, 339–45 passim; et al., **84**:343
Zimmer, R., et al., **82**:139
Zimmerman, I., **84**:118
Zinberg, N. E., **84**:186
Zinc concentration, **83**:111
Zinner, J., **83**:218, 235
Zis, A. P., **83**:306
Zitrin, C., et al., **82**:465; **84**:395, 416, 459, 503, 504, 505, 511, 518
Zornetzer, S. F., **83**:110
Zrull, J. P., **82**:266, 267, 274, 277, 284, 285
Zubin, J., **82**:98; **83**:407
Zuk, G. H., **83**:183
Zukin, S. R. and R. S., **82**:140
Zung, W. W. K., **83**:490; et al., **83**:112; **84**:205, 206
Zung scale, **83**:362; **84**:189, 203, 206
Zusman, J., **84**:137
Zyzanski, S. J., et al., **84**:216